AMYOTROPHIC LATERAL SCLEROSIS

Hiroshi Mitsumoto, M.D., D.Sc.

Head, Neuromuscular Diseases/EMG Section
Professor of Neurology
Departments of Neurology and Neurosciences
The Cleveland Clinic Foundation
Cleveland, Ohio

David A. Chad, M.D., F.R.C.P.(C)

Professor of Neurology and Pathology
Department of Neurology
University of Massachusetts Medical Center
Worcester, Massachusetts

Erik P. Pioro, M.D., D.Phil., F.R.C.P.(C)

Departments of Neurology and Neurosciences
The Cleveland Clinic Foundation
Cleveland, Ohio

 F. A. DAVIS COMPANY • Philadelphia

F. A. Davis Company
1915 Arch Street
Philadelphia, PA 19103

Printed in the United States of America

Last digit indicates print number: 10 9 8 7 6 5 4 3 2 1

Senior Medical Editor: Robert W. Reinhardt
Medical Developmental Editor: Bernice M. Wissler
Production Editors: Devorah W. Zuckerman, Nancee A. Morelli
Cover Designer: Louis J. Forgione

As new scientific information becomes available through basic and clinical research, recommended treatments and drug therapies undergo changes. The authors and publisher have done everything possible to make this book accurate, up to date, and in accord with accepted standards at the time of publication. The authors, editors, and publisher are not responsible for errors or omissions or for consequences from application of the book, and make no warranty, expressed or implied, in regard to the contents of the book. Any practice described in this book should be applied by the reader in accordance with professional standards of care used in regard to the unique circumstances that may apply in each situation. The reader is advised always to check product information (package inserts) for changes and new information regarding dose and contraindications before administering any drug. Caution is especially urged when using new or infrequently ordered drugs.

Library of Congress Cataloging-in-Publication Data

Mitsumoto, Hiroshi.
    Amyotrophic lateral sclerosis / Hiroshi Mitsumoto, David A. Chad,
  Erik P. Pioro.
        p.   cm. — (Contemporary neurology series: 49)
    Includes bibliographical references and index.
    ISBN 0-8036-0269-3 (cloth : alk. paper)
    1. Amyotrophic lateral sclerosis.   I. Chad, David A., 1949– .
  II. Pioro, Erik P., 1955– .   III. Title.   IV. Series.
    [DNLM: 1. Amyotrophic Lateral Sclerosis.   W1 CO769N v.49 1998 /
  WE 550 M6845a 1998]
  RC406.A24M58 1998
  616.8'3—dc21
  DNLM/DLC
  for Library of Congress   97-194
                                                                               CIP

CONTEMPORARY NEUROLOGY SERIES AVAILABLE:

AMYOTROPHIC LATERAL SCLEROSIS

The authors dedicate this book to Joseph M. Foley, M.D., Professor Emeritus of Neurology, Case Western Reserve University. A teacher of teachers, Dr. Foley taught us how to dedicate ourselves in caring for the sick and desperately ill and continues to inspire us in our own personal growth and in the joy of practicing neurology.

FOREWORD

In 1967, when Dr. John Walton, now Lord Walton of Detchant, suggested that I start a research program into anterior horn cell and peripheral nerve disease, little did I realize that this would turn into a lifetime commitment to the neuromuscular diseases and, particularly, to what is known in Britain as motor neuron disease and in the United States as amyotrophic lateral sclerosis (ALS). At that time, I was a junior research registrar in the Muscular Dystrophy Group Research Laboratories of the University of Newcastle Upon Tyne in the northeast of England, where the research predominantly dealt with the muscular dystrophies. Very little was known about the causes of most of the peripheral neuropathies or ALS, though theories abounded. It was a very fertile time to launch into a research career.

The research I began in Newcastle has taken me to many parts of the world and into many fields of investigation that I never thought to explore. These have included studies of animal models, including the wobbler mouse, which has proved useful for investigating anterior horn cell degeneration. Investigation of axonal transport mechanisms and the use of neurotoxins proved valuable in those early days. I became involved in research into the etiology of all of the neuromuscular diseases, particularly ALS, and was soon involved not only in the care of ALS patients but also in therapeutic trials.

This work has brought me into contact with many of the most illustrious clinicians and research workers in neurology and has also given me the opportunity to share in the developing careers of many of the best and brightest of the younger generation, including the three authors of this book.

My early period of clinical training with Lord Walton and Dr. David Gardner-Medwin in Newcastle provided me with the skills and empathy needed to care for patients with chronic, progressive, disabling neuromuscular diseases. This has stood me in good stead when caring for what may be one of the most distressing of these diseases, ALS.

Thirty years ago, few knew much about ALS. Patients often confused it with multiple sclerosis or had never even heard of the condition. Now, as more and more prominent people have suffered from this disease, such as David Niven and Senator Jacob Javits, and as the medical knowledge of the population has increased, there are few who have not heard something about the disease. In the United States the disease is particularly known because of the very public development of the symptoms in the "Iron Man of Baseball," Lou Gehrig. The touching film that was made about his life is shown around the time of each World Series.

Like many other neurologists, I find that my heart drops whenever I have to make the diagnosis of ALS. It always seems to be the nice people who are stricken with this disease. It is heartbreaking to give the diagnosis to someone who is quite young. How to face the patient and the family with this diagnosis is one of the most difficult tasks of the neurologist.

Nowadays, with the availability of the Internet and national associations such as the ALS Association and the Muscular Dystrophy Association, patients often know a great deal about their condition even before they come to a specialist. In describing the disease to a patient, one has to relate that the average survival is 3 to 5 years and that there is a progressive physical deterioration that affects all aspects of life, including walking, self-care, speech, swallowing, and breathing. One has to be honest with patients, but one should not take away hope. I always point out that there are patients in whom ALS has remitted; I have seen three, and several others are described in the literature. There is an even greater number of patients in whom the ALS seems to burn itself out; these patients stabilize and remain in whatever state they have reached by this time. A significant proportion of ALS patients have a much slower progression than would be indicated by the average quoted figures for survival; 10% of patients with ALS live 10 years and 5% live 20 years. There are often clinical pointers at the outset that suggest that the patient is going to have a more benign prognosis than the average; these include the presence of *pure* lower motor neuron disease and involvement commencing in the lower limbs.

Neurologists have always been interested in the problem of reaching a diagnosis in patients with ALS, but few have been interested in providing ongoing care. I have heard too many times that a neurologist has told a patient that the disease is called ALS, that it is universally fatal, and that the patient should go home and put his or her affairs in order and prepare to die. These neurologists should remember that doctors are admonished "to cure rarely, to treat often, and to care always." If no cure is available, then the physician must spend even more time with the patient and the family than would generally be needed if there were a cure.

The physician knowledgeable about ALS can provide many things in addition to empathy and information: physical aids so the patient can stay active as long as possible; access to assistance from other health care professionals; mechanisms to improve respiration; help with the problems of insurance and disability. Later, a physician comfortable with the primary goal of caring is needed to guide the patient with ALS in making decisions about parenteral feeding and ventilator support; and at the end of life, the physician can do much to alleviate distress.

From my vantage point, it seems that now is a more exciting period in ALS research than we have seen at any time in the last 30 years. We now are witnessing real advances in our understanding of the disease and its treatment. For the patients and their families, these research advances are the hope to which they inevitably cling. I have always felt it important that the physician make every effort to share research advances with patients. Such foundations as the ALS Association and the Muscular Dystrophy Association provide significant help in this area, both by supporting research and by disseminating information about research. It is particularly helpful when the physician caring for an ALS patient is involved in research; this keeps up the spirits not only of the patient but also of the doctor.

There have been many theories of the cause of ALS, but in the last few years we have begun to feel confident that we are getting closer to a true understanding. This particularly relates to the hypotheses of oxidative damage and glutamate excess. The strongest support for the oxidative hypothesis comes from the discovery of the mutations of the superoxide dismutase-1 gene in familial ALS. The glutamate hypothesis sprang from basic neuroscience research into excitotoxic damage and the finding that in ALS there is a decreased ability to handle the excitatory neurotransmitter, glutamate. In the end, ALS may turn out to be due to many other causes in addition to these two. The disease in some patients may be due to abnormalities of neurofilaments, other specific gene defects, and deficiencies of neurotrophins or neurotrophin receptors. From the patient's point of view, although this plethora of hypotheses may be confusing, any new information raises the spirits.

Even more hope for patients comes from the advances in treatment. Over the last two decades, many of us have undertaken therapeutic trials in ALS that were based mainly on whatever drugs were available that *might* work or whatever treatment was suggested by a new hypothesis. The first small trial of a drug in ALS is often reported to be positive, but until recently, further studies have failed to repeat any positive benefit. With the new development of the science of clinical therapeutic trials, we have come to realize that power calculations are essential to determine whether a study can prove or disprove the efficacy of a drug. In ALS, it appears that between 100 and 300 patients per treatment arm are required for a study to have the power to detect about a 15% slowing in the rate of progression of the disease over a 9-month period of patient follow-up. Hence, at present, therapeutic trials in ALS are very large and extremely costly. What is still needed is a biological marker of the disease process in ALS. Although we have several animal models of ALS, in the final analysis they are no substitute for proof of efficacy of a therapy in humans with the disease.

As we stand here at the end of 1996, we now have the first drug that has been proven to slow the rate of progression of ALS, namely, the antiglutamate agent riluzole. Several other agents are undergoing therapeutic trials, including gabapentin, another antiglutamate agent, as well as various growth factors. The latter include insulin-like growth factor-1, brain-derived neurotrophic factor, and other similar agents that are moving rapidly from the basic research laboratories into the clinical arena. These include small-molecular-weight compounds that can stimulate neurotrophin receptors and pass the blood-brain barrier as well as new growth factors such as glial-derived neurotrophic factor.

An indication of the enormous recent increase in our ability to deal with ALS is provided by the very large audiences that now come to hear about ALS at our neurological meetings and the many national and international meetings currently devoted to research into ALS. Another indication is the appearance of several books on ALS that have been published over the past few years. All are excellent in their own ways, illustrating the multifaceted aspects of ALS and the many approaches to its investigation and management. This book comes at a particularly opportune time, for it presents an excellent and comprehensive review of current information on the clinical features of the disease, its pathology and pathophysiology, and its treatment and management. Now, when we are beginning to see the product of decades of research manifesting as clear insights into the cause of the disease and ways to treat it, the information learned over the decades continues to be crucial in the fight to finally cure and prevent the creeping paralysis, ALS. Even if the cause of ALS were discovered tomorrow and the way to arrest the disease were discovered the day after, the information in this book would still continue to be of importance to all who care for patients with ALS.

Walter G. Bradley, D.M., F.R.C.P.
Miami, Florida
August, 1996

PREFACE

When we began writing this book in the spring of 1994, there were no approved drugs for ALS. A few clinical trials were underway, but their results were still uncertain. In the last 3 years, the neurological community has progressed on a number of fronts, including understanding the basic biology of this disorder; developing novel, effective therapies; and renewing emphasis on patient care. Those of us who look after patients with ALS are now in the midst of some very important developments. Plausible hypotheses of ALS pathogenesis have been proposed, and the process of motor neuron death is now better understood. The first drug for ALS, although modest in its effects, was approved in 1995 by the United States Food and Drug Administration, and several additional medications are now on the horizon. The many aspects of patient care have drawn increasing attention from a diverse array of disciplines, among them physical and occupational therapy, nutritional science, speech-language pathology, psychosocial-spiritual counseling, and hospice care; therefore, in these times of exciting scientific insights, promising therapeutic advances, and multidisciplinary comprehensive patient care, we welcomed the opportunity to write this book. For us, the process of researching, reflecting, and writing has been a richly rewarding educational experience.

Although several excellent books on ALS have already been published, this book is the first written by only a few authors. Taking advantage of the small authorship, we strove to present cohesive and balanced information for every student of ALS. The more we discussed the disease and our approach to writing the book, the more we came to realize the remarkably complex and multifaceted nature of ALS. In an effort to increase our knowledge of the disease and write about it as comprehensively as possible, we carefully considered a host of individual disciplines that we believe are relevant to an understanding of ALS, among them motor system anatomy and physiology, neuropathology, neuroimaging and neurodiagnostic methods, mechanisms of neuronal degeneration and death, epidemiology, biostatistics, and clinical trials. In the final analysis, we wrote the book with the belief that to understand ALS is to understand clinical neurology as well as many of the neurosciences.

Although we brought diverse experience in clinical care, teaching, and research to the task of writing this book, the major emphasis for each of us in our own work is the diagnosis and management of patients with ALS; therefore, we crafted the book mainly for the neurologist who looks after patients with ALS and shares our desire to learn more about its mysterious biology. Although the primary audience for this book is the practicing neurologist, neurology trainees and other health care professionals will also find it useful. The book consists of four major sections: Introduction to ALS, Clinical Features of ALS, Pathology and Pathogenesis, and Treatment and Management. To clarify the material presented, we frequently use summary tables and figures (line drawings and photomicrographs). To help readers recall the main ideas discussed, each chapter has a detailed summary.

We are grateful to many people for their support and assistance during the course of our writing this book. First of all, we are most indebted to Dr. Sid Gilman, Editor-in-Chief of the Contemporary Neurology Series, who encouraged us to start this project, promptly read a series of draft chapters, gave us invaluable suggestions, and set the tone for the entire book. Initial drafts of our chapters were all carefully reviewed by our expert medical editors, Cassandra Talerico, M.A., and Tom Lang, M.A., of the Scientific Publications Department, the Cleveland Clinic Foundation (CCF). We admire their meticulous editing and their helpful comments and suggestions. Ms. Bernice Wissler at the F. A. Davis Company provided additional editorial assistance and encouragement, helping us to craft the final version of the text. We are particularly privileged and honored that our mentor (of H.M. and D.A.C.), Walter G. Bradley, D.M., F.R.C.P., has written the Foreword. He is a consummate clinician, an inspired teacher, and a tireless investigator of ALS, who introduced us to the care of the patient with ALS and to research in the field. We are delighted that Lisa S. Krivickas, M.D., a former neuromuscular and electromyography fellow at CCF, with a special interest in chronic respiratory rehabilitation, contributed Chapter 22, Pulmonary Function and Respiratory Failure.

We are fortunate that many of our colleagues with expertise in the varied aspects of ALS critically reviewed one or more chapters and provided suggestions that we believe strengthened our book. We, however, are solely responsible for the contents and for the accuracy of the material. Those who shared their expertise with us were Neil Aronin, M.D., University of Massachusetts Medical Center (UMMC); Carolyn Benson, M.S., R.N., UMMC; Carolyn Berger, O.T.R./L., CCF; Jesse M. Cedarbaum, M.D., Regeneron Pharmaceuticals; Michelle Secic, M.S., CCF; Vanina DelBello-Haas, M.S., P.T., CCF; Nancy Fontneau, M.D., UMMC; Tom Greene, Ph.D., CCF; Asao Hirano, M.D., Montefiore Medical Center; John Kelemen, M.D., Long Island Neurological Associates; Ann Kloos, P.T., M.S., CCF; David Lacomis, M.D., University of Pittsburgh; Ronald M. Lindsay, Ph.D., Regeneron Pharmaceuticals; Errol Malta, Ph.D., Amgen Inc; Michael T. Modic, M.D., CCF; Dominic Nompleggi, M.D., UMMC; Robert J. O'Hara, M.D., Hines VA Medical Center; Carrie Proch, P.T., CCF; Douglas Seidner, M.D., CCF; Lauren Shockley, R.N., CCF; Teepu Siddique, M.D., Northwestern University; and Asa J. Wilbourn, M.D., CCF.

Other colleagues shared information with us on specific topics or provided figures or photomicrographs to help us illustrate our ideas. For this, we thank Doreen Andrews-Hinders, R.N., CCF; Carmen Blakeley, R.D., CCF; Michael Brooke, M.D., F.R.C.P., University of Edmonton; Benjamin R. Brooks, M.D., University of Wisconsin; Mary Caldwell, R.N., CCF; Amy S. Chappel, M.D., Eli Lilly and Company; Andrew A. Eisen, M.D., University of British Columbia; Mary Jo Hooper, M.A., C.C.C./S.L.P., CCF; Takeo Ishiyama, M.S., CCF; Edward Jones, Pharm. D., CCF; Tony Juneja, M.S., Northwestern University; Jocelyn Kaplan, M.A., Northwestern University; Bogdan Klinkosz, D.V.M., CCF; Kerry H. Levin, M.D., CCF; Michael Maierson, C.O., CCF; Michael J. Meeham, J.D., CCF; Vincent Meininger, M.D., Hôpital de la Pitie-Salpêtrière; Theodore L. Munsat, M.D., New England Medical Center; Richard A. Prayson, M.D., CCF; Carrie Proch, P.T., CCF; Toyakazu Saito, M.D., Kitazato University; Robert W. Shields, Jr., M.D., CCF; Thomas W. Smith, M.D., UMMC; Nancy Stambler, M.S., Regeneron Pharmaceuticals; John S. Stroud, Clarks Summit; Michael Swash, M.D., F.R.C.P., F.R.C.Path., The Royal London Hospital; Mary Wooley, M.A., CCF; and Qiao Yan, Ph.D., Amgen, Inc.

We are fortunate to have had continuous support from the ALS Association, the CCF ALS Center, and the Muscular Dystrophy Association Clinic at the University of Massachusetts Medical Center for our patient care and research efforts. We are grateful to the Steering Committee members of the World Federation of Neurology ALS Treatment Consortia for sharing expertise on broad issues related to the treatment of ALS. The Art and Photography Departments at CCF and UMMC helped us in the design and production of many of our figures and photomicrographs. Ms. Mary Alice Dixon, Ms. Cindy L. Mullins, and Ms. Linda Curnin provided outstanding administrative assistance.

Most of all, we wish to thank the patients with ALS and their families with whom we have had the opportunity to develop a therapeutic partnership. Not only have they taught us volumes about the many clinical aspects of the disease, but they have also shown us that life with ALS can be lived productively, creatively, and with dignity.

Last, we would like to thank our wives, Chizuko, Rita, and Mattie, and our families for their unlimited support and forbearance, which made our work possible.

HM
DAC
EPP

CONTENTS

PART 1

Introduction to ALS

CHAPTER 1

HISTORY, TERMINOLOGY, AND CLASSIFICATION OF ALS

Clinical medicine is made up of anomalies, while nosography is the description of phenomena that occur regularly. What we look for in the clinics is almost always exceptions; what we study in nosography is the rule. It is well to know that, in the practice of medicine, a nosographer is not always a clinician.

Jean Martin Charcot[60]

A BRIEF HISTORY OF ALS
Before Charcot
Charcot's Contribution
Nosologic Controversy
Primary Lateral Sclerosis
Motor System Degeneration, Motor Neuron
   Disease, or ALS?
New Forms of ALS
TERMINOLOGY AND DEFINITIONS
Motor Neuron Disease and ALS
Description of ALS Subsets
WORLD FEDERATION OF NEUROLOGY
   CLASSIFICATION

This chapter briefly reviews the history of amyotrophic lateral sclerosis (ALS). The initial history of ALS is characterized by a series of events that established the nosology. Excellent detailed historic accounts are available in papers by Goldblatt,[27] Norris,[50] and

Tyler and Shefner.[64] Table 1–1 summarizes the early history of ALS in the context of major events in neurology and neuromuscular disease, permitting examination of the historic relationships among disorders. Outstanding books on the history of neurology and neuroscience are also available.[23,30,45,59] This chapter includes a discussion of terminology and definitions of ALS and its subsets, and the World Federation of Neurology classification of motor neuron diseases.[67]

A BRIEF HISTORY OF ALS

Before Charcot

Sir Charles Bell, a British anatomist and surgeon, developed the concept that the anterior nerve roots are involved in movement. In 1830, he described a middle-aged woman with progressive paralysis of the limbs and

3

Table 1–1. TIME LINE OF MAJOR DEVELOPMENTS IN THE HISTORY OF ALS AND OF NEUROLOGY AND NEUROMUSCULAR DISEASES

Decade	Events in ALS	Events in Neurology and Neuromuscular Diseases
1810s		• Parkinson reports shaking palsy (1817)
1820s		• Magendie identifies functional difference between anterior and posterior roots—Bell-Magendie's law (1821)
1830S	• Bell finds anterior spinal cord is involved in movement (1830)	• Remak finds axons to derive from neurons (1838) • Schwann identifies myelin sheath and Schwann cells (1839)
1840s		• Romberg writes the first classic neurology textbook (1840)
1850s	• Aran reports PMA (1850) • Cruveilhier presents neurogenic theory of PMA (1855) • Fromann reports ventral root atrophy, probably in case of ALS (1850) • Duménil agrees with Fromann (1859) • Duchenne reports generalized spinal paralysis and PMA (1859)	• Waller observes axonal degeneration (1851) • Türck identifies corticospinal tracts (1853) • Duchenne publishes full description of acute poliomyelitis (1855)
1860s	• Luys identifies ventral horn cell degeneration in PMA (1860) • Duchenne reports progressive bulbar palsy (1860) • Charcot reports spasmodic tabes dorsalis for primary lateral sclerosis (1865) • Charcot and Joffroy report PMA with anterior spinal cord lesion (1869)	• Broca shows cerebral dominance (1863) • Duchenne establishes pseudohypertrophic muscular paralysis (1868)
1870s	• Charcot concludes progressive bulbar palsy has neurogenic cause (1870) • Leyden reports white matter lesions in the spinal cord both in progressive bulbar palsy and PMA (1870) • Charcot establishes ALS as a distinct condition (1874) • Erb reports a spastic spinal paralytic syndrome (primary lateral sclerosis) (1875)	• Fritsch and Hitzig identify motor cortex (1870) • Golgi invents silver nitrate staining method for neurons and neurites (1873) • Raymond, and Cornil and Lepine report "post-polio" muscular atrophy (1875) • Ranvier identifies interruptions in the medullary sheath in the nerve—the node of Ranvier (1878)
1880s	• Dejerine integrates ALS and progressive bulbar palsy (1883)	• Charcot and Marie describes a special form of PMA, Charcot-Marie-Tooth disease (1886) • Gowers publishes a textbook, *A Manual of Disease of the Nervous System*—"The bible of neurology" (1886)

Decade	ALS	Neuroscience
1890s	• Gowers unifies PMA, progressive bulbar palsy, and ALS as a motor system degeneration (1892)	• Ramon y Cajal publishes *"Axonal Degeneration and Regeneration"* (1890) • Werdnig establishes infantile spinal muscular atrophy as a distinct condition (1891) • Babinski finds extensor plantar response (1896) • Nissl identifies Nissl granules in neurons (1896)
1900s	• ALS-like cases on Guam recorded (1900)	• Brodmann maps cortical localization (1908)
1910s	• Miura reports high incidence of ALS in the Kii peninsula (1911)	• Alzheimer reports senile dementia (1911) • Guillain, Barré, and Strohl describe a syndrome of radicular neuritis (1916) • von Economo reports encephalitis lethargica (1917)
1920s	• First symposium on ALS for the centenary of Charcot's birth in Paris (1925)	• Creutzfeldt and Jakob describe spastic pseudosclerosis (1921) • Sherrington presents concept of motor unit, synapse, and the final common path (1925)
1930s	• Brain advocates the term motor neuron disease for ALS (1933) • Okaya reports a case of Guam parkinsonism (1936) • Lou Gehrig retires from baseball. ALS becomes widely known as Lou Gehrig's disease (1939)	• Denny-Brown and Buchthal both use electromyography in neuromuscular diseases (1938 to 1941) • Ruska and Knoll develop electron microscope (1939)
1940s		
1950s	• Koerner; Arnold, Kurland, Mulder, and Hirano studies on Guamanian ALS and ALS-parkinsonism-dementia complex (1952 to 1954) • Kurland and Mulder report familial ALS (1955) • Symposium on ALS at Mayo Clinic (1957) • Engel et al. report posterior column involvement in familial ALS (1959)	• Levi-Montalcini discovers nerve growth factor (1950) • Watson and Crick determine DNA structure (1953) • Adams, Denny-Brown, and Pearson publish the first textbook on disease of muscle (1953) • Kugelberg and Welander describe juvenile spinal muscular atrophy (1954) • Salk develops formalin-inactivated poliovaccine (1954)
1960s	• Hirano publishes detailed pathology of Guamanian ALS-parkinsonism-dementia complex (1961) • Gajdusek reports ALS in New Guinea (1963) • Hirano et al. describe pathology of familial ALS (1967) • Kurland and Norris organize the first international symposium on ALS (1969) • Lambert establishes electromyographic criteria for ALS (1969)	• Sabin develops oral poliovaccine (1960) • Gajdusek and Gibbs first transmit kuru and Creutzfeldt-Jakob disease to primates (1966)

Abbreviations: ALS = amyotrophic lateral sclerosis; PMA = progressive muscular atrophy.

tongue but with normal sensation.[5] Strengthening his hypothesis were autopsy findings revealing that the anterior portion of the spinal cord had the "consistency of cream," whereas the posterior part was "firm." Bell's idea was further buttressed by his contemporary, the French scientist, François Magendie.[23] These pioneers established the notion that the anterior roots govern motor function, whereas the posterior roots mediate sensory function, a physiologic principle that became known as *Bell-Magendie's law.*[23]

The existence of a progressive muscular weakness accompanied by muscle wasting became clearly recognized by the mid-19th century, but a dispute arose over who was to be credited with first describing this syndrome. François Aran,[1] a well-known French general physician and medical writer, published a description of a new syndrome of progressive muscle weakness in 1848 and correctly suspected a neurogenic cause. In 1850, he published a series on 11 such patients and suggested they had a new syndrome that he termed *progressive muscular atrophy* (PMA).[2] He separated PMA from cerebral palsy, plumbism, and peripheral nerve lesions. After Aran's report on PMA in 1850, Amand Duchenne (de Boulogne) claimed that he had reported this syndrome a year earlier than Aran. However, Duchenne's paper was never published.[50] The 11 patients whom Aran originally described were also seen by Duchenne for galvanic electric therapy. In his 1850 report, Aran acknowledged Duchenne, saying, "I have a thousand obligations to my friend M. le Dr. Duchenne, who had the good will to place at my disposal all the material which he has assembled, and without any officious interference." Duchenne had been privileged to work in close association with Jean Martin Charcot at the Salpêtrière and had already gained prominence in neurology because of his work on muscle disease in 1855.[17] Strongly influenced by Duchenne, Aran reversed his earlier opinion and concluded in his paper of 1850 that PMA was caused by a muscle disease. Thereafter, Aran's interest in and commitment to neurology waned. Duchenne, on the other hand, contributed enormously to the field, and credit for the description of PMA was associated more with Duchenne

than Aran. Charcot,[13] however, later credited both and called PMA the Aran-Duchenne type of progressive muscular weakness.

Duchenne's view that PMA was myogenic held sway for some time. Duchenne even reaffirmed this belief after performing an autopsy on one of the patients reported earlier by Aran. However, Cruveilhier[15] studied the same case in 1853 and suggested a neurogenic cause because of changes in the spinal cord. Other reports of PMA with bulbar dysfunction by Fromann[24] and by Duménil[20] supported this view, but these cases probably represented ALS. In fact, Duchenne did begin to recognize a neural cause of "generalized spinal paralysis," in which the lesion was limited to the spinal cord, but he continued to separate these cases from PMA. In 1860, Bernard Luys,[42] who described the corpus Luysii, reported ventral horn cell degeneration in PMA. In the same year, Duchenne[18] made an unsurpassed description of progressive bulbar palsy (PBP) and distinguished it from PMA by the degree and rapidity of bulbar involvement, but he also reported that one of his patients had both diseases.

Charcot's Contribution

In 1869, Jean Martin Charcot,[14] the first professor of neurology at the Salpêtrière, and Joffroy described two cases of PMA with lesions in the posterolateral spinal cord. They did not name this new syndrome ALS, but they did determine its essential characteristics. In particular, they emphasized that pathologic changes in the posterior portions of the lateral columns and in the anterior horns of the spinal cord occurred together frequently. During a series of lectures in 1874, Charcot clearly established ALS as a distinct syndrome.[12] Goldblatt[27] best expressed Charcot's contribution: "Charcot did not give the first description of ALS, nor did Shakespeare originate the plots of his plays; the elements of the story were known, but it remained for the master to produce a masterpiece." Charcot[12] set forth the clinical and pathologic characteristics of ALS in a form that has since been modified very little. His description of ALS was based on 20 patents

Table 1–2. **CLINICAL FINDINGS OF ALS ACCORDING TO CHARCOT**

Upper Motor Neuron Findings	Weakness of lips
Spasmodic contracture	Drooling
Temporary or permanent rigidity	Nasal voice
Flexibilitas cerea (cataleptic state of limbs)	Thickness to or loss of speech
Exaggerated tendon reflexes	Small, tremulous, wrinkled tongue (or may be of
Spinal epilepsy or trepidation	normal size though weak)
Tremor on movement	Difficulty in swallowing
Involuntary extension or flexion	Respiratory and circulatory disturbances
"Simple" or "pure" paralysis	
	Sensory Findings
Lower Motor Neuron Findings	No loss of sensation
Atrophy of muscles "en masse"	Onset with frequent lively pains, numbness
Fibrillary contractions or "fascicular shaking"	and tingling
(indicating fasciculations)	Muscles tender on pressure and passive movement
Preservation of contractility to faradic stimulation	
	Mental Findings
Bulbar Findings	Intellect undisturbed
Transverse wrinkles on forehead	
Contracture of lower face	*Other Findings*
Widened mouth	No paralysis of bladder or rectum
Crying expression	No bed sores

Source: Adapted from Goldblatt, D: Motor neuron disease: Historical introduction. In Norris, FH and Kurland, LT (eds.): Motor Neuron Diseases. Grune & Stratton, New York, 1969, pp 3–11.

and five autopsy studies; most of the patients were women because Salpêtrière was a women's hospital. Table 1–2 summarizes the clinical manifestations of ALS that Charcot described. The pathologic basis for the clinical findings included white matter lesions of the lateral column (Türck's bundle, the corticospinal tracts), anterior pyramids (in the medulla), pyramidal bundles, and midbrain peduncles. Gray matter changes included atrophy and degeneration of anterior horn cells and neurons of brain-stem motor nuclei. The changes in nerve roots, nerves, and muscles were thought to be secondary to neural degeneration.[13]

In 1870, Charcot studied a patient with PBP and concluded that the primary lesion was atrophy of the medullary motor cells. After Charcot's decisive opinion, Duchenne wrote a paper with Joffroy[19] in 1870 and finally accepted this finding. Thus, a neurogenic cause was also established for PBP.

Charcot separated ALS from PMA on the basis of the slow disease course, the sparing of bulbar function, and the absence of rigid-ity (spasticity) in the latter.[50] He considered PMA as "protopathic" (meaning primary or essential), whereas conditions with both atrophic and spastic features were "deuteropathic" (secondary to another disease), implying a propagation of the lesion from white to gray matter. He also included deuteropathic cases secondary to other conditions such as tumors and syringomyelia. Furthermore, Charcot maintained that PBP was a syndrome distinct from ALS.

Nosologic Controversy

In the mid-19th century, the distinction between bulbar palsy and pseudobulbar palsy was not known. In fact, Charcot considered PBP to be a spastic syndrome because degeneration of motor neurons occurred in the medulla. On the other hand, Leyden,[41] a prominent German neurologist, thought that PBP was an atonic syndrome because of lesions in the corticospinal tracts. In the context of our present knowledge of neuroanatomy, their interpretations were in error and in fact contrary to current thought not only in the interpretation of spasticity but also in the lesions responsible for the clinical symptom, spasticity. Upper motor neuron signs such as the extensor plantar responses described later (in 1896) by Joseph Babinski,[4] a famed student of Charcot, had not yet been appreciated.

Disagreeing with Charcot, in 1870 Leyden[4] insisted that PBP and ALS were not distinct conditions. This opinion was based on his experience with patients with PBP in whom progressive atrophy developed in the small hand muscles. Autopsy examination in these patients disclosed white matter degeneration in areas corresponding to the corticospinal tracts. Joseph Dejerine,[16] who described many new muscle and nerve disorders, integrated PBP and ALS in 1883. He pointed out that autopsy findings in the medullas from patients with these seemingly disparate clinical conditions were indistinguishable. Despite the descriptions suggesting that PBP and ALS were expressions of the same disease process, Charcot continued to maintain that PBP and ALS were distinct syndromes. This controversy among prominent neurologists delayed the development of a unified concept of motor system disease.[27,50]

Primary Lateral Sclerosis

In 1865, Charcot[10] described a woman with "hysterical attacks" who had remitting, and later permanent, "contractures" of the limbs. Autopsy examination showed sclerosis of the lateral columns and atrophic anterior roots but normal cells in the gray matter of the spinal cord. The term *contracture* should be considered as an earlier term meaning "spasticity with hyperreflexia." This case indicated a close association between paralysis and contracture and became one of the defining descriptions of primary lateral sclerosis (PLS). The condition that is now recognized as PLS was described in 1875 by Heinrich Erb,[22] a founder of German neurology. However, the term PLS always included a heterogeneous group of diseases. Until recently, it has been generally agreed that PLS was not a disease separate from ALS.

Motor System Degeneration, Motor Neuron Disease, or ALS?

In 1899, Sir William Gowers,[28] a founder of British neurology, stated in his textbook, *A Manual of Diseases of the Nervous System,* that he never encountered a single case of PMA in which the pyramidal tracts were unaffected. He did not think Charcot's introduction of the term ALS to be very helpful because it implied that the primary lesion was degeneration of the pyramidal tracts and that atrophy of anterior horn cells was secondary or deuteropathic. He felt that Charcot's distinction in effect gave a new name to an old disease.[28,59] He concluded that PMA, PBP, and ALS were "essentially one disease." The clinical manifestations were determined by the timing, extent, and severity of the degeneration in the upper and lower segments of the motor pathway. In 1933 Brain[7] introduced the term "motor neuron disease" so that all these apparently different conditions could be brought together in a single general category; he used the terms motor neuron disease and ALS interchangeably.

A series of studies supported the opinion that PMA, PLS, and PBP were subsets of ALS. In 1943, Swank and Putnam[62] analyzed 197 patients with ALS that was classified according to three types: the Charcot, or completely developed type; the atypical type (monoplegic, hemiplegic, or proximal involvement); and the incomplete type (lateral sclerosis, amyotrophy, or bulbar palsy form). They considered PLS and PMA to be ALS that had yet to develop fully. In 1953, Lawyer and Netsky[40] did a clinicopathologic analysis of 53 patients with ALS and concluded that motor neuron diseases form a group that includes PMA, PLS, ALS, and PBP. In 1963, Mackay[43] reviewed 126 patients with ALS and concluded:

Regardless of the onset, the spastic forms nearly always become atrophic, the atrophic also spastic, while the spinal forms nearly always become bulbar, and the bulbar forms, if the patients live long enough, become also spinal. The entire group is, therefore, best regarded as a single degenerative disease, ALS, which constitutes a spectrum of atrophic process at one end, spastic at the other, and both in the center. With time, cases at each end of the spectrum move towards the center.

In 1970, Brownell and colleagues[9] analyzed the extent of pathologic involvement in motor neuron disease and suggested that "for the time being, we retain the label of 'motor neuron disease'." They thought that "classic" motor neuron disease was not well defined but rather was a prominent band within a wide spectrum of subacute or chronic multiple system degenerations that show a predilection to certain parts of the motor system. In 1971, Metcalf and Hirano[46] reported on two members of a family with PMA and a third member with classic ALS, suggesting that PMA is only a clinical manifestation of ALS.

New Forms of ALS

Guamanian ALS-Parkinsonism-Dementia Complex. Although a nosographic description of ALS and motor neuron disease was in progress in the early part of this century, an ALS-like disease on the Mariana Islands, particularly Guam, was newly recognized. This disease quickly triggered enormous interest among investigators because it provided a unique opportunity to expand the understanding of ALS from a different perspective. In fact, an instance of ALS on the Mariana Islands was recorded in a sanitary report of Guam as early as 1900.[58] In the 1950s, however, a series of reports concerning a high incidence of ALS in Guam started appearing in the medical literature. Among the 38,000 indigenous Chamorro people who lived on Guam, ALS accounted for about 10% of the adult deaths, or about 100 times the ALS death rate reported for any other population.[3,37,38,63] In 1954, Mulder and colleagues[48] were the first to recognize a combination of parkinsonism and ALS, although a case of parkinsonism had been reported previously by Okaya,[52] a Japanese physician, in 1936. The pathologic features of Guamanian ALS were reported by Malamud et al.[44] in 1961. Subsequently the full extent of the clinical and pathologic features of Guamanian ALS-parkinsonism-dementia complex were described by Hirano and colleagues[32,34] in 1961. A strong genetic influence was initially suspected because of the large number of patients within families who developed the disease. However, a genetic and epidemiologic study ruled out such a possibility because offspring of both patients and controls had no increased risk of disease.[53]

ALS in Other Western Pacific Foci. Miura,[47] a Japanese physician and pupil of Charcot, gave the first detailed description of ALS in Japan in 1911. He pointed out the high frequency of ALS in the Kii peninsula on the main island of Honshu. In this form of ALS, however, a combination of parkinsonism and dementia along with ALS is less frequent than in the Mariana Islands.[57] Epidemiologic studies in the Kii peninsula also ruled out a genetic cause of the ALS-parkinsonism-dementia complex in this area.[65] In 1963, another focus of endemic ALS was reported in West New Guinea.[25,26] These endemic forms of ALS in the Western Pacific were most often targeted in the pursuit of an environmental cause for ALS, as pioneered by Yase[68] in 1972. Investigation of environmental causes is discussed in Chapter 16.

Familial ALS. Aran[2] probably first reported familial ALS when he first described PMA. Since then, scattered cases of familial ALS have been reported,[39] and the high incidence of what apparently was familial ALS reported from the Mariana Islands stimulated great interest in possible genetic factors in ALS. In 1959, Engel and colleagues[21] first recognized posterior column involvement in familial ALS. In 1967, Hirano and colleagues[33] further characterized the pathologic features of familial ALS (see Chapter 11). Extensive epidemiologic studies performed by Kurland and Mulder[39] in 1955 established the frequency of familial ALS at 5% to 10%. In 1976, Horton and colleagues[35] recognized the variability among familial ALS cases and attempted to classify reported cases of familial ALS in three categories based on length of the disease and pathologic features.

TERMINOLOGY AND DEFINITIONS

Motor Neuron Disease and ALS

In a 1982 monograph on motor neuron disease, Rowland[56] pointed out the dilemma concerning terminology: "We have a serious problem of terminology, one that affects the title of this volume and the contents of this chapter as well as many of the others. It has to do with the confusion between the singular, 'motor neuron disease,' and the plural, 'motor neuron diseases'."

In 1969, Brain and Walton[8] considered ALS and motor neuron disease to be synonymous, stating that

These two varieties (progressive muscular atrophy and ALS) are now usually regarded as nosologically similar. When the lower motor neuron lesions predominate, or as more rarely happens, occur alone, the term 'progressive muscular atrophy' is still generally applied to the disease, and when the muscles innervated from the medulla are predominantly involved it has been termed 'progressive bulbar palsy'. Some authors then use the term 'amyotrophic lateral sclerosis' for those cases in which signs of corticospinal tract disease predominate in the early stages and in which it may initially be difficult or impossible to find evidence of lower motor neuron involvement. In most cases, however, the symptoms of upper and lower motor neuron lesions are mixed, except in the lower limbs, where the latter are frequently absent until the terminal stages. Greenfield[29] prefers the term ALS to motor neuron disease on the grounds that the pathological changes in the spinal cord are not limited to the motor neurons and many American authors use this term as an inclusive one, embracing all varieties of the disease. Motor neuron disease, however, is a better inclusive term.

The term ALS now is more frequently used than before and is considered to describe the disease more specifically. In this book, we use the following definitions: *Motor neuron diseases* (MNDs) are a heterogeneous group of disorders with diverse signs and symptoms, all in some way affecting the anterior horn cells. *Amyotrophic lateral sclerosis* (ALS) is the most common form of MND of undetermined cause in adults, affecting not only the anterior horn cells but also the corticospinal tracts, resulting in a fairly consistent clinical picture and outcome. Whether ALS is a single disease entity or a syndrome caused by a number of different conditions remains to be determined.

By definition, the features of ALS are signs and symptoms of lower motor neuron dysfunction, including focal and multifocal weakness, atrophy, cramps, and fasciculations associated with the corticospinal tract signs of spasticity and enhanced and pathologic reflexes in the absence of sensory findings (see Chapter 4). The corticobulbar

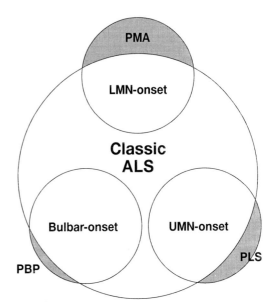

Figure 1–1. ALS manifests generalized upper motor neuron (UMN) and lower motor neuron (LMN) involvement. At onset, however, ALS may present only with UMN, LMN, or bulbar signs. In such situations, ALS can be called UMN-onset, LMN-onset, or bulbar-onset ALS, respectively. In a small number of patients, disease remains exclusively in UMN, LMN, or bulbar involvement over the entire course of the disease. For those patients with exclusively UMN disease, the term "primary lateral sclerosis" (PLS) is designated; for only LMN disease, "progressive muscular atrophy" (PMA); and for disease limited to bulbar muscles, "progressive bulbar palsy" (PBP). PBP is exceedingly rare; usually the limb and paraspinal muscles are affected and thus PBP may not be considered as an independent condition.

tracts may be involved, resulting in dysphagia and dysarthria that aggravates the already established lower motor neuron involvement at the brain-stem level. These features define *classic ALS*, in the sense that it was described by Charcot, and stand in contrast to subsets of ALS.

At onset, ALS presents with lower motor neuron (LMN) involvement (LMN-onset or the PMA form of ALS), upper motor neuron (UMN) involvement (UMN-onset or PLS form), or bulbar involvement (bulbar-onset or PBP form) (Fig. 1–1).

Description of ALS Subsets

Subsets of ALS such as PMA, PLS, and PBP have distinctive clinical pictures, outcomes, and pathologic features, although the definitions and classifications of these subsets remain debatable. In daily clinical practice, precise definitions may not be crucial, but for basic research and clinical trials, strict definitions of ALS and each subset become critical. However, it is important for the clinician to recognize these subsets of ALS because each has a different clinical course and prognosis. In addition, a subset might be included in or excluded from a particular clinical trial.

Progressive muscular atrophy (PMA) is characterized by pure LMN findings only over the entire course of disease. Patients who present with LMN signs and later develop features of classic ALS are considered to have LMN-onset ALS or the PMA form of ALS. It is rare, found by Norris and colleagues[51] in only 2.4% of all ALS patients; Mackay[43] reported that it represented 11% of all cases. Its duration is longer than that of ALS. Based on the World Federation of Neurology El Escorial diagnostic criteria for ALS (see Chapter 6), PMA is not synonymous with ALS and should be considered an independent entity.[66]

Primary lateral sclerosis (PLS) is characterized by pure UMN findings and should be considered an independent condition.[51,54] The diagnosis of PLS should be made by excluding other definable diseases resembling PLS (see Chapter 8); however, it is still difficult to make the diagnosis early in the illness. PLS is found in 2% to 3.7% of all patients with ALS.[43,51] Patients who present with signs of UMN findings and later develop features of classic ALS are considered to have UMN-onset ALS or the PLS form of ALS.

Progressive bulbar palsy (PBP) is characterized by progressive paralysis of bulbar muscles because of involvement of UMNs and LMNs separately or in combination. By definition, the disease must be strictly limited to the bulbar muscles during its entire course. Patients who present with signs of bulbar palsy and later develop features of classic ALS are considered to have bulbar-onset ALS. Even in its early stages, most patients with bulbar-onset ALS have evidence of LMN involvement outside the bulbar musculature.[31] Therefore, PBP is extremely rare and should be considered as one type of presentation of ALS.[51]

Sporadic ALS is nonfamilial; ALS is identified in only one member of the entire family. It constitutes more than 90% of all ALS cases. When the family history is uncertain or the parents of the patient died at an early age, the possibility of familial ALS cannot be excluded (see Chapter 10). Autopsy findings may not be specific enough to distinguish familial from sporadic forms (see Chapter 11), and the clinical features are identical in the two types.

Familial ALS (FALS) constitutes 5% to 10% of all ALS cases. It is typically autosomal-dominant; one additional affected family member needs to be identified in the preceding or successive generation.[49] Generation skipping is rare in FALS[61] (see Chapter 10). When a medical history of the family members, particularly the parents, is not available, FALS cannot be excluded. The key to determining if ALS is familial or sporadic is identifying another family member who is affected by ALS. Until recently, this has been the only method to diagnose FALS.[49] However, the recent discovery of superoxide dismutase mutation (*SOD1*) in approximately 15% of FALS patients may change this situation.[55] If this gene abnormality is identified in a patient with ALS, one can conclude that the patient has FALS, even if the family history is not available (see Chapter 10). However, if such studies are negative, FALS still cannot be excluded. Most FALS patients have no genetic markers; thus, taking a thorough family history is crucial. Autosomal-recessive chronic juvenile ALS has been reported exclusively in Tunisian families.[6]

WORLD FEDERATION OF NEUROLOGY CLASSIFICATION

The World Federation of Neurology Research Group on Neuromuscular Diseases (1994)[67] has published its classification system for neuromuscular diseases. The classification is based on the neuroanatomic locations of the diseases. MNDs are classified under one category, "Spinal Muscular Atrophies and Other Disorders of the Motor Neurons," and then are classified further in nine subcategories based on the mode of inheritance, cause, and expression of other neurologic manifestations (Table 1–3). ALS and related MNDs are subclassified as disorders of

Table 1–3. SPINAL MUSCULAR ATROPHIES AND OTHER DISORDERS OF THE MOTOR NEURONS

Heritable Disorders

Autosomal recessive; biochemical abnormality unknown

- SMA, type 1 (Werdnig-Hoffmann)
- SMA, type 2, late infantile
- SMA, type 3 (Kugelberg-Welander)
- SMA, type 4, proximal, adult form
- Other SMAs, associated with other neurologic features

Autosomal recessive, biochemical abnormality known

- SMA with hexosaminidase deficiency
- SMA with lysosomal enzyme deficiencies
- Other SMAs with known biochemical defects

Autosomal dominant, biochemical abnormality unknown

- Muscular atrophy with other neurological features
- Muscular atrophy, juvenile, proximal type
- Other variations including monomelic form, or segmental distribution
- Muscular atrophy, progressive, malignant, fatal within 1 year, but not clearly different from autosomal dominant ALS
- Muscular atrophy, progressive, not clearly different from ALS
- Amyotrophic dystonic paraplegia
- Familial ALS*
- ALS-parkinsonism-dementia complex of Guam*
- SMAs with or without other neurologic features

X-linked recessive

- Spinal and bulbar muscular atrophy (Kennedy disease)
- Other SMAs with a different distribution, biochemical disorder unknown
- X-linked dominant, lethal in males (infantile SMA in incontinentia pigmenti)

Congenital and Developmental Abnormalities

- Möbius syndrome (agenesis of cranial nerve nuclei)
- Agenesis of muscles
- Other developmental anomalies of the nervous system

Disorders of Motor Neurons Attributed to Physical Causes

- Trauma
- Destruction or compression of the spinal cord
- Ischemia of anterior horns
- Electrical injury
- Amyotrophy after radiation therapy

Disorders of Motor Neurons Attributed to Toxins, Chemicals, or Heavy Metals

- Tetanus
- Strychnine
- Botulinum toxin
- Lead
- Mercury
- Organophosphate
- Saxitoxin
- Dapsone
- Phenytoin

Disorders of Motor Neurons Attributed to Viral Infection

Acute disorders

- Acute paralytic anterior poliomyelitis

Table 1–3—*continued*

Disorders of Motor Neurons Attributed to Viral Infection

Acute disorders

- Amyotrophy in Russian spring-summer encephalitis
- Herpes zoster
- Acute hemorrhagic conjunctivitis
- With asthma, acute transverse myelitis

Subacute or chronic disorders

- Creutzfeldt-Jakob disease
- Amyotrophy or ALS in HIV infection
- HTLV-I infection
- Persistent infection by poliovirus in agammaglobulinemia
- Late post-poliomyelitis muscular atrophy (post-polio syndrome)

Disorders of Motor Neurons with Immunologic Abnormality

- Motor neuron diseases with monoclonal paraproteinemia
- Amyotrophy with Hodgkin's disease
- Carcinomatous motor neuron disease

Disorders of Motor Neurons of Undetermined Etiology

Motor neuron diseases of adults (sporadic)

- ALS, PMA, progressive bulbar palsy*
- Juvenile motor neuron disease
- Amyotrophy in Shy-Drager syndrome
- Amyotrophy in Pick disease
- Chronic neurogenic atrophy of the quadriceps
- Amyotrophy in polyglucosan body disease

Disorders of Motor Neurons in Metabolic Disorders

- Tetany
- Hypoglycemia
- Hyperthyroidism
- Hyperparathyroidism

Disorders of Motor Neurons Manifested by Hyperactivity

- Ordinary muscle cramps
- Benign fasciculation-cramp syndrome (syndrome of Foley and Denny-Brown)
- Occupational cramps and writers' cramp
- Isaacs' syndrome
- Tetanus
- Strychnine intoxication
- Stiff man syndrome
- Satoyoshi syndrome
- Myelopathy with rigidity, spasm, or continuous motor unit activity
- Myokymia
- Black widow spider bite
- Tetany
- Spinal myoclonus, fasciculation myokymia
- Hemifacial spasm
- Painful legs and moving toes
- Restless leg syndrome (Ekbom syndrome)

*ALS and its subsets are marked. This classification is modified for the purpose of the chapter from the original classification.

Source: Adapted from World Federation of Neurology Research Group on Neuromuscular Disease: Classification of neuromuscular disorders. J Neurol Sci 124:109–130, 1994, with permission.

Abbreviations: ALS = amyotrophic lateral sclerosis; HIV = human immunodeficiency virus; HTLV-I = human T-cell lymphoma virus type I; SMA = spinal muscular atrophy.

Table 1–4. **PRACTICAL CLASSIFICATION OF ALS**

Sporadic ALS
- Classic ALS
- Progressive muscular atrophy
- Primary lateral sclerosis
- Progressive bulbar palsy

Familial ALS
- Autosomal dominant
  - Superoxide dismutase (*SOD1*) missense mutation
  - *Non-SOD1* types
- Autosomal recessive
  - Chronic juvenile ALS (Tunisia)

Western Pacific ALS-Parkinsonism-Dementia Complex

Juvenile ALS with Intracytoplasmic Inclusions

ALS-Like Motor Neuron Diseases with Definable Causes
- Polyradiculopathy and myelopathy
- Post-polio syndrome
- Motor neuropathy with multifocal conduction block, anti-GM1 antibody, or both
- Motor neuron disease with gammopathy or paraproteinemia
- Heavy metal intoxication
- Hexosaminidase-A deficiency
- Paraneoplastic motor neuronopathy syndrome
- Syringomyelia and syringobulbia

Source: Adapted from Hudson, AJ: Amyotrophic lateral sclerosis: Clinical evidence for differences in pathogenesis and etiology. In Hudson, A (ed): Amyotrophic Lateral Sclerosis. University of Toronto Press, Toronto, 1990, pp 108–143.

motor neurons of undetermined cause. In the daily practice of neurology, a classification originally suggested by Hudson[36] is perhaps more practical and simple because it includes only ALS and its differential diagnoses (Table 1–4).

SUMMARY

The history of the description of ALS is closely associated with the founders of neurology, including Bell, Aran, Charcot, Duchenne, Erb, Gowers, and Brain. These investigators contributed to establishing ALS as an independent disease, although they disagreed on the definition of the disorder and site of pathology. Subsequent progress has been achieved by extensive clinical and pathologic investigation in ALS, endemic

ALS–Parkinson's disease–dementia complex, and familial ALS, particularly in the past several decades.

ALS is the most common motor neuron disease of undetermined cause in adults. Diagnosis requires evidence of widespread upper motor neuron (UMN) and lower motor neuron (LMN) involvement. At onset, however, ALS may present exclusively with LMN signs, in which case it may be called LMN-onset ALS or the progressive muscular atrophy (PMA) form of ALS. If UMN signs develop during the disease course, the disease, by definition, becomes ALS. Similarly, when ALS presents solely with UMN signs, it may be called UMN-onset ALS or the primary lateral sclerosis (PLS) form. Again, if LMN signs develop subsequently, the designation of ALS is indicated. In a small number of patients in whom the disease has an LMN onset, UMN signs never develop; then the condition is referred to as PMA. Similarly, in a small percentage of patients with UMN-onset disease, LMN signs do not develop, and the disease is termed PLS. Although PMA and PLS may be the opposite ends of the spectrum of ALS (the subsets of ALS), we believe they should be viewed as independent conditions. When symptoms begin in bulbar muscles, the disease should be called bulbar-onset ALS because in most cases the extremity and paraspinal muscles are eventually affected. The term *progressive bulbar palsy* (PBP) should be reserved for conditions in which motor neurons in the lower brain stem are exclusively affected over the entire course of the disease. PBP is exceedingly rare; some investigators do not consider it to be an independent condition, unlike PMA or PLS. However, the definitions of these ALS subsets are still debatable.

Most ALS cases (approximately 90%) are sporadic, in that no other family member had or develops ALS. Familial ALS is defined as ALS affecting at least two members of one family in the preceding or successive generation or ALS in which a genetic abnormality (e.g., *SOD1* mutation) is identified in a patient even when the family history is not available. This chapter also briefly reviewed the classification of MNDs (a part of an extensive classification of neuromuscular diseases) recommended by the World Federation of Neurology and a classification of ALS that is useful for practicing neurologists.

REFERENCES

1. Aran, FA: Revue clinique des hôpitaux et hospices. Un Med 2:553–554, 557–558, 1848.
2. Aran, FA: Recherches sur une maladie non encore décrite du système musculaire (atrophie musculaire progressive). Arch Gen Med 24:15–35, 1850.
3. Arnold, A, Edgren, DC, and Palladino, VS: Amyotrophic lateral sclerosis: Fifty cases observed on Guam. J Nerve Ment Dis 117:135–139, 1953.
4. Babinski, JEF: Sur le réflexe cutané plantaire dans certains affections organiques due système nerveux central. CR Soc Biol (Paris) 3:207–208, 1896.
5. Bell, C: The nervous system of the human body. Longman, London, 1830, pp 132–136, pp 160–161.
6. Ben Hamida, M, Hentati, F, and Ben Hamida, C: Hereditary motor system diseases. (Chronic juvenile amyotrophic lateral sclerosis). Conditions combining a bilateral pyramidal syndrome with limb and bulbar amyotrophy. Brain 113:347–363, 1990.
7. Brain, WR: Diseases of the Nervous System. Oxford University Press, London, 1933.
8. Brain, WR and Walton, JN: Brain's Disease of the Nervous System. Oxford University Press, London, 1969, pp 595–606.
9. Brownell, B, Oppenheimer, DR, and Hughes, JT: The central nervous system in motor neurone disease. J Neurol Neurosurg Psychiatry 33:338–357, 1970.
10. Charcot, JM: Sclerose des cordons lateraux de la moelle epiniere chez une femme hysterique atteinte de contracture permanente des quatres membres. L'Union Med 25:451–467, 461–472, 1865.
11. Charcot, JM: Note sur un cas de paralysie glosso-laryngée suivi d'autopsie. Arch Physiol 3:247–260, 1870.
12. Charcot, JM: De la sclérose latérale amyotrophique. Prog Med 23:235–237, 24:341–342, 1874; 29:453–455, 1874.
13. Charcot, JM: Lectures on the Diseases of the Nervous System. Sigerson, S (ed, trans). Hafner, New York, 1962.
14. Charcot, JM and Joffroy, A: Deux cas d'atrophie musculaire progressive. Arch Physiol 2:354–367, 1869.
15. Cruveilhier, J: Sur la paralysie musculaire progressive atrophique. Arch Gen Med 91:561–603, 1853.
16. Dejerine, J: Etude anatomique et clinique sur la paralysie labio-glosso-laryngée. Arch Physiol Norm Pathol 2:180–227, 1883.
17. Duchenne, G: De l'Electrisation Localisée. Paris: Baillière, 1855.
18. Duchenne, G: Paralysie musculaire progressive de la langue, du voile du palais et des lèvres. Arch Gen Med 16:283–296, 431–445, 1860.
19. Duchenne, G and Joffroy, A: De l'atrophie aigue et chronique des cellules nerveuses de la moelle et du bulbe rachidien. Propos d'une observation de paralysie labio-glosso-laryngée. Arch Physiol 3:499, 1870.
20. Duménil, DR: Atrophie des nerfs hypoglosses, faciaux et spinaux. Gax Hebd Med Chir 6:390–392, 1859.
21. Engel, WK, Kurland, LT, and Klatzo, I: An inherited disease similar to amyotrophic lateral sclerosis with a pattern of posterior column involvement. An intermediate form? Brain 82:203–222, 1959.
22. Erb, WH: Über einen wenig bekannten spinalen symptomen-complex. Berl Klin Wochenschr 12:357–359, 1875.
23. Finger, S: Origin of neuroscience. A history of explorations into brain function. Oxford University Press, New York, 1994.
24. Fromann, M: Atrophie musculaire progressive (autopsie). Med Chir Mschr 1 (1858) summary in Arch Gen Med 13:96, 1859.
25. Gajdusek, DC: Motor-neuron disease in native of New Guinea. N Engl J Med 268:474–476, 1963.
26. Gajdusek, DC and Salazar, AM: Amyotrophic lateral sclerosis and parkinsonian syndromes in high incidence among the Auyu and Jakai people of West New Guinea. Neurology 32:107–126, 1982.
27. Goldblatt, D: Motor neuron disease: Historical introduction. In Norris, FH and Kurland, LT (eds): Motor Neuron Diseases. Grune & Stratton, New York, 1969, pp 3–11.

28. Gowers, WR: A Manual of Diseases of the Nervous System, vol 1, ed 3. Plakiston, Philadelphia, 1899, pp 531–558.

29. Greenfield, JG: Amyotrophic lateral sclerosis. In Greenfield, JG, Blackwood, W, McMenemey, WH, et al (eds): Neuropathology. Arnold, London, 1958, pp 545–548.

30. Haymaker, W and Schiller, F: The Founders of Neurology, ed 2. Charles C Thomas, Springfield, IL, 1970.

31. Heitzman, D, Wilbourn, A, and Mitsumoto, H: A retrospective study examining the clinical and electrodiagnostic features of patients with bulbar-onset amyotrophic lateral sclerosis. Neurology 45(suppl 4):A447, 1995.

32. Hirano, A, Kurland, LT, Krooth, RS, et al: Parkinsonism-dementia complex, an endemic disease on the island of Guam. I. Clinical features. Brain 84:642–661, 1961.

33. Hirano, A, Kurland, LT, and Sayre, GP: Familial amyotrophic lateral sclerosis. A subgroup characterized by posterior and spinocerebellar tract involvement and hyaline inclusions in the anterior horn cells, Arch Neurol 16:232–243, 1967.

34. Hirano, A, Malamud, N, and Kurland, L: Parkinsonism-dementia complex, an endemic disease on the Island of Guam. II Pathological features. Brain 84:662–679, 1961.

35. Horton, WA, Eldridge, R, and Brody, JA: Familial motor neuron disease. Neurology 26:460–465, 1976.

36. Hudson, AJ: Amyotrophic lateral sclerosis: Clinical evidence for differences in pathogenesis and etiology. In Hudson, A (ed): Amyotrophic Lateral Sclerosis. University of Toronto Press, Toronto, 1990, pp 108–143.

37. Koerner, DR: Amyotrophic lateral sclerosis on Guam: A clinical study and review of the literature. Ann Intern Med 37:1204–1220, 1952.

38. Kurland, LT and Muldeer, DW: Epidemiologic investigations of amyotrophic lateral sclerosis. Preliminary report on geographic distribution, with special reference to the Mariana Islands, including clinical and pathological observations. Neurology 4:355–378 (part 1), 438–448 (part 2), 1954.

39. Kurland, LT and Mulder, DW: Epidemiologic investigations of amyotrophic lateral sclerosis. Familial aggregation indicative of dominant inheritance. Neurology 5:182–196, 1955.

40. Lawyer, JR, Netsky, T, and Netsky, MG: Amyotrophic lateral sclerosis. Arch Neurol Psychiatry 69:171–192, 1953.

41. Leyden, EV: Über progressive Bulbarparalysie. Arch Psychiatr i:648; ii:657; iii:338, 1870.

42. Luys, J: Atrophie musculaire progressive. Gaz Med Fr 3 & 4: 505, 1860.

43. Mackay, RP: Course and prognosis in amyotrophic lateral sclerosis. Arch Neurol 8:17–27, 1963.

44. Malamud, N, Hirano, A, and Kurland, LT: Pathoanatomic changes in amyotrophic lateral sclerosis on Guam: Special reference to the occurrence of neurofibrillary changes. Arch Neurol 5:401–415, 1961.

45. McHenry, LC: Garrison's History of Neurology. Charles C Thomas, Springfield, IL, 1969.

46. Metcalf, CW and Hirano, A: Amyotrophic lateral sclerosis. Arch Neurol 24:518–523, 1971.

47. Miura, K: Amyotrophische Lateralsklerose unter dem Bilde von sog. Bulbärparalyse. Neurol Jpn 10:366–369, 1911.

48. Mulder, DW, Kurland, LT, and Iriarte LLG: Neurologic diseases on the island of Guam. US Armed Forces Med J 5:1724–1739, 1954.

49. Mulder, DW, Kurland, LT, Offord, KP, et al: Familial adult motor neuron disease: Amyotrophic lateral sclerosis. Neurology 36:511–517, 1986.

50. Norris, FH: Adult spinal motor neuron disease. In Vinken, PJ, Bruyn, GW, DeJong, JMBV (eds). System Disorders and Atrophes, vol 22. Amsterdam: North-Holland, 1975, pp 1–56.

51. Norris, F, Shepherd, R, Denys, E, et al: Onset, natural history and outcome in idiopathic adult motor neuron disease. J Neurol Sci 118:48–55, 1993.

52. Okaya, N: Gamu shimajima min chamoro-zoku (mikuronesyajin) ni okeru shinsen mahi no shorei (A case of paralysis agitans in a Chamorro, Micronesia, from Guam, US Territory). Tokyo Med J 2997:2517–2518, 1936.

53. Plato, CC, Cruz, MT, and Kurland, LT: Amyotrophic lateral sclerosis/parkinsonism-dementia complex of Guam: Further genetic investigations. Am J Hum Genet 21:133–141, 1969.

54. Pringle, CE, Hudson, AJ, Munoz, DG, et al: Primary lateral sclerosis. Clinical features, neuropathology and diagnostic criteria. Brain 115:495–520, 1992.

55. Rosen, DR, Siddique, T, Patterson, D, et al: Mutations in Cu/Zn superoxide dismutase gene are associated with familial amyotrophic lateral sclerosis. Nature 362:59–62, 1993.

56. Rowland, LP (ed): Human Motor Neuron Diseases. Advances in Neurology, Vol 36. Raven Press, New York, 1982.

57. Shiraki, H and Yase, Y: Amyotrophic lateral sclerosis and parkinsonism-dementia in the Kii Peninsula: Comparison with the same disorders in Guam and Alzheimer's disease. In Vinken, PJ, Bruyn, GW, and Klawans, HL (eds): Disease of the Motor System. Handbook of Neurology 15. Elsevier, Amsterdam, 1991, pp 273–300.

58. Spencer, PS: Guam ALS/Parkinsonism-Dementia: A long-latency neurotoxic disorder caused by "slow toxin(s)" in food? Can J Neurol Sci 14:347–357, 1987.

59. Spillane, JD: The History of Neurology. Oxford University Press, London, 1981.

60. Strauss, MB: Familiar Medical Quotations. Little, Brown, Boston, 1968.

61. Strong, MJ, Hudson, AJ, and Alvord, WG: Familial amyotrophic lateral sclerosis, 1850–1989: A statistical analysis of the world literature. Can J Neurol Sci 18:45–58, 1991.

62. Swank, RL and Putnam, TJ: Amyotrophic lateral sclerosis and related conditions. Arch Neurol Psychiatry 49:151–177, 1943.

63. Tillema, S and Wijnberg, CJ: "Epidemic" amyotrophic lateral sclerosis on Guam: Epidemiologic data. Doc Med Geog Trop 5:366–370, 1953.

64. Tyler, HR and Shefner, J: Amyotrophic lateral sclerosis. In Vinken, PJ, Bruyn, GW, and Klawans, HL,

(eds): Diseases of the Motor System, vol 59. Elsevier, New York, 1975, pp 169–216.

65. Uebayashi, Y: Epidemiological investigation of motor neuron disease in the Kii Peninsula, Japan and on Guam: The significance of long survival cases. Wakayama Med Rep 23:13–27, 1980.

66. World Federation of Neurology Research Group on Neuromuscular Diseases Subcommittee on Motor Neuron Disease: El Escorial World Federation of Neurology criteria for the diagnosis of amyotrophic lateral sclerosis. J Neurol Sci 124 (suppl):96–107, 1994.

67. World Federation of Neurology Research Group on Neuromuscular Diseases: Classification of neuromuscular disorders. J Neurol Sci 124:109–130, 1994.

68. Yase, Y: The pathogenesis of amyotrophic lateral sclerosis. Lancet 2:292–296, 1972.

CHAPTER 2

EPIDEMIOLOGY

The epidemiology of ALS has been of interest for a number of decades. Not only have epidemiologic studies provided information on the frequency (incidence, prevalence, and mortality rates) of ALS, but they have also contributed to our understanding of its clinical expression (see Chapter 4) and natural history (see Chapter 9). Numerous population-based epidemiologic studies have revealed the pattern of ALS occurrence in relation to age, sex, race, and geographic area. The association of ALS with specific factors, such as genetics, occupation, and exposure to toxins, has been investigated using case control and cohort studies. Although ALS is considered to be relatively rare, its personal and socioeconomic impact is greater

than its annual incidence of about 1 per 100,000 population. For example, assuming that an extended nuclear family consists of three generations, that each individual has two siblings, and that the generation time is about 20 years, it can be calculated that approximately 1 in 200 individuals have a nuclear family member afflicted by ALS.[9]

When discussing ALS epidemiology, it is useful to distinguish three distinct forms of disease: classic sporadic ALS, familial ALS, and Western Pacific ALS. Although usually similar clinically,[125] these forms of ALS differ in epidemiology, pathology (see Chapter 11), and possibly in pathogenesis (see Chapter 12). One must be aware that some epidemiologic studies, particularly those from Europe, refer to ALS in the generic sense as "motor neuron disease" or include other forms of motor neuron degeneration (e.g., progressive bulbar palsy, progressive spinal muscular atrophy) in reporting the epidemiology of motor neuron disease. Here, we will use the term ALS to encompass all these types of motor neuron degeneration because most cases eventually progress to become classic ALS. This pattern is particularly evident in epidemiologic studies in which patients have been repeatedly examined and disease progression monitored.[84,110,131] True progressive bulbar palsy is rare and progressive spinal muscular atrophy is uncommon (see Chapter 1). Therefore, any risk factor identified for ALS will likely apply for motor neuron disease and vice versa.[106] The terminology and definition of ALS are discussed in detail in Chapter 1. Further discussion of the epidemiology of ALS can be found in several comprehensive reviews.[12,20,92,105–107,155]

DEFINITIONS AND CASE IDENTIFICATION IN ALS EPIDEMIOLOGY

Definitions

The frequency of ALS in the population can be represented by its incidence (the number of newly identified patients per year) or by its prevalence (the number of surviving patients at any given time). Both measures are usually expressed per 100,000 population and are determined from observational morbidity studies. ALS mortality rates, also expressed per 100,000 population, are calculated from existing national vital statistics and have been used to estimate the frequency of ALS, although not without error. Such population-based morbidity studies and mortality rate analyses constitute the majority of epidemiologic studies of ALS from North America, Mexico, Europe, Australia, the Middle East, and the Western Pacific.

Potential risk factors in ALS have been examined using case control and cohort studies. Such analytic studies are appropriate after an unusually high occurrence of ALS has been identified either in a geographic area (e.g., the Western Pacific or other clusters) or in specific patient groups (e.g., occupational). In case control studies, a retrospective analysis of possible risk factor exposure is performed in individuals who already have the disease. These studies are suited for studying rare conditions such as ALS but are subject to inaccuracies because of several types of bias, including recall, sampling, and ascertainment bias. Furthermore, because many comparisons must be performed in case control studies, chance occurrences may appear to be statistically significant if no statistical procedure is used to control for the problem of multiple comparisons.[3] Cohort studies, on the other hand, introduce less bias because initially healthy individuals who have or have not been exposed to risk factors are observed prospectively to determine which group develops the disease. Although they provide more valid data, cohort studies are labor-intensive and take long to complete, especially for rare diseases.[44]

Case Identification

Accurate epidemiologic studies begin with accurate case ascertainment, which in turn depends on correctly diagnosing ALS in the individual. Diagnosis can either be done clinically, as in population (morbidity) studies, or pathologically after death, as in mortality studies. Postmortem neuropathologic examinations of patients suspected of having ALS obviously provide the most definitive means of diagnosis.

Because of the variability in clinical presentation and the absence of any single diagnostic test for ALS, an algorithm has been established by the World Federation of Neurology to provide internationally accepted diagnostic criteria, the El Escorial criteria.[13] Similar criteria have been used in genetic studies of patients with familial ALS.[157] According to the El Escorial criteria, clinical findings in a patient being evaluated for ALS can be supplemented with laboratory, electrodiagnostic, radiologic, and even pathologic tests to increase the level of diagnostic certainty (see Chapter 6). The increasing international use of these criteria, which have been field-tested in several North American and European clinical trials,[12] will improve the consistency of ALS diagnosis and make case ascertainment more reliable for epidemiologic studies.[114]

Mortality rates in ALS may provide accurate estimates of disease incidence because ALS is correctly diagnosed in most advanced cases, survival is relatively short, and death certificates are generally reliable.[84,95,121] Studies have shown that 70% to 90% of patients diagnosed as having ALS had this condition recorded on their death certificate.[14,73,95,133] However, errors in mortality rates can occur because of diagnostic inaccuracy and incomplete recording of all conditions affecting a patient at death.[73,110]

SPORADIC ALS

Frequency

Except for specific endemic areas in the Western Pacific where a unique form of ALS has been characterized, the worldwide frequency of ALS is notably uniform despite cli-

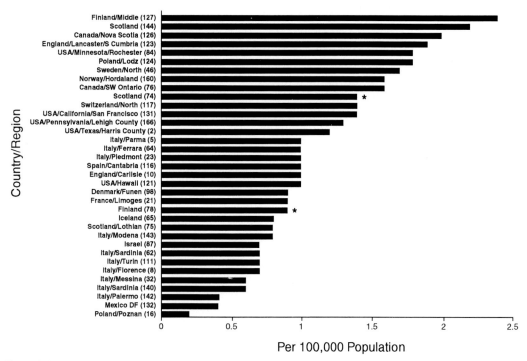

Figure 2–1. Annual incidence rates of ALS reported from 1966 until 1994 in various countries (except in the Western Pacific) are diagrammed according to decreasing frequency. Reference numbers of the respective studies are indicated in parentheses. *Represents mortality rates.

matic, geographic, racial, and socioeconomic differences. Reports from the United States (including Hawaii), Canada, Mexico, Europe, and the Middle East indicate annual incidence rates from 0.2 to 2.4 per 100,000 population (1.1 ± 0.5, mean ± standard deviation) (Fig. 2–1) and prevalence rates from 0.8 to 7.3 per 100,000 (3.6 ± 1.8) (Fig. 2–2).

The observed variability may be related, at least in part, to the extent of bias in case ascertainment because incidence and prevalence rates of ALS seem to be proportional to the level of health care provided and the type of data sources analyzed.[84,165] In other words, individuals with ALS are more likely to be identified when neurologic evaluation by well-trained medical personnel is available. In addition, complete case ascertainment is more likely when cases are identified from a combination of sources, including patient registries, physician-patient databases, hospital discharge data, and death certificates. The lower rates reported in some European[140,142,161] and Mexican[132] studies may

be the result of incomplete case ascertainment, which can occur when using predominantly hospital-based surveys.[7,19] On the other hand, these findings have been suggested to represent a northwest-to-southeast gradient of decreasing incidence.[12] ALS frequency as determined from death certificate data also shows a gradient in the United States: mortality is lower east of but higher west of the Mississippi River. This pattern is not associated with any specific factor, such as socioeconomic status, rural location, physician-patient ratio, or environmental toxins.[6]

AGE-RELATED ONSET

Most studies indicate that the age-specific incidence and mortality rates in classic sporadic ALS increase until the eighth decade, with a peak occurring between 55 and 75 years of age (Fig. 2–3).* These rates marked-

---

*References 19,20,37,46,66,70,87,106,110,131,140.

Prevalence of ALS

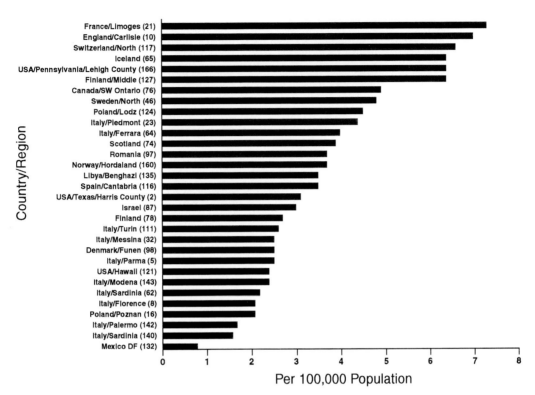

Figure 2–2. Prevalence rates of ALS reported from 1964 until 1994 in various countries (except in the Western Pacific) are diagrammed according to decreasing frequency. Reference numbers of the respective studies are indicated in parentheses.

Figure 2–3. Age-specific incidence of sporadic ALS for males and females is seen to increase until the eighth decade, with a dramatic decline after a peak between 55 and 75 years of age. Sex-related incidence is higher in males, although this is less pronounced over 65 years of age. General population data based on United States census (US Department of Commerce, 1982). (Reprinted from J Neurol Sci 118 (1), Norris, F, Shepherd, R, Denys, E, et al: Onset, natural history and outcome in idiopathic adult motor neuron disease, pp 51, 1993, with kind permission of Elsevier Science - NL, Sara Burgerhartstraat 25, 1055 KV Amsterdam, The Netherlands.)

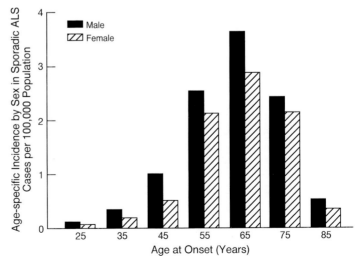

ly drop in individuals over 75 years of age. Although a 1980 population-based study found that the incidence continued to rise with age,[84] an updated survey from the same institution in 1986 revealed a maximal occurrence in the eighth decade.[165] Kurtzke[106,107] has suggested that a peak onset of ALS that occurs between 65 and 75 years of age is more consistent with an acquired or environmental pathogenic factor than if ALS occurred more frequently at progressively older ages. A peak incidence in the sixth decade was noted in 23 ALS patients from Libya.[135]

The decreasing frequency of ALS in the eighth and ninth decades has been proposed to be a result of false-negative diagnosis.[14,129] It is difficult to estimate the amount of false-negative diagnosis in ALS,[95] but it may be high in the elderly,[9,14,19] particularly if signs and symptoms are minimal; up to 90% of deaths from ALS are probably unrecorded at age 85 years.[129] Alternatively, a diagnosis of ALS may be missed in the elderly if the findings are attributed to the debility of old age or other more frequent pathologies, such as cerebrovascular disease or radiculomyelopathy.[19]

Age is the most significant risk factor for ALS,[92,107,139] although genetic predisposition is also important (see Chapter 10). In addition, the duration of ALS appears to be age-related, with survival being approximately three times longer in patients with onset age less than 41 years compared to those with onset age over 60 years[38] (see Chapter 9). The progressive "exhaustion" of motor neurons in the aging nervous system of at-risk individuals may contribute to the high incidence and poor prognosis of ALS in the elderly population.[94,131]

SEX PREDOMINANCE

Most patient series indicate that ALS occurs predominantly in males, with male-to-female ratios adjusted for age-related incidence of 1.4 to 2.5.* With increasing age, the proportions of male and female ALS patients over 65 years of age become more equal (see Fig. 2–3).[19,86,131] However, bulbar-onset ALS has been reported to be more frequent in women than in men in some,[25,113] but not all,[131] studies. This apparent female predominance is unexplained, but it may be related to the effects of sex hormones on bulbar motor neurons, which possess androgen receptors[26,120] (see Chapter 16).

Men have more false-positive diagnoses than women,[95] but this alone cannot account for the consistently greater proportion of men with sporadic ALS. Furthermore, studies in which ALS was identified clinically and confirmed pathologically indicate that the overall occurrence of false-positive diagnosis is low.[14,84] Thorough clinical evaluation should exclude conditions that can resemble ALS, such as spondylotic cervical myeloradiculopathy (see Chapter 6).

RACIAL PREDISPOSITION

There is evidence that the frequency of non–Western Pacific ALS is higher in whites than in nonwhites, at least in the United States.[106] Age-adjusted ALS death rates in various regions of the country are 20% to 60% lower for nonwhites than for whites, although both groups share the age-related onset and male predominance. In some cases, the lower frequency in nonwhites may be a result of under-reporting because earlier surveys in the continental United States did not include blacks.[106] The higher incidence of ALS reported among Filipino men in Hawaii[121] has been disputed,[106] and no difference was found in ALS incidence rates in Israel when rates were examined according to the patient's ethnic origin.[87]

Although it has been proposed that the lower incidence and prevalence of ALS in Mexico[132] and certain European countries like Poland[16,161] and Italy[140,142] represent incomplete case ascertainment,[7,19,84,165] this may truly reflect a lower susceptibility in these populations.

DURATION OF ILLNESS

Based on the mean and median durations from several worldwide studies,* the average survival after onset of ALS symptoms is approximately 3 years. The mean duration

---

*References 16,37,47,62,65,84,87,94,111,135,140

*References 8,16,84,87,98,121,132,140

of disease has generally been reported to be 31 to 43 months, except in two relatively small surveys from Carlisle, England,[10] and Iceland,[65] where the mean duration was 84 and 96 months, respectively. Norris and colleagues[131] observed that approximately 5% of all patients have a long survival and suggested that these patients have a more benign form of ALS. Onset of ALS in patients less than 50 years of age is generally associated with a longer survival. A detailed discussion of the duration of ALS can be found in Chapter 9.

Observed Increases in Sporadic ALS Frequency

Several studies from various countries found that the frequency of sporadic ALS has been increasing over the past several decades. Most of these data have come from mortality rates, which are believed to be representative of incidence rates. Kurtzke[107] has suggested that this increased frequency is the result of unidentified exogenous or environmental factors. These factors may either be new to the environment in the past few decades or may simply be exerting greater detrimental effects on the central nervous system.

Because ALS has been coded in the death statistics since 1949 according to the International Classification of Diseases, mortality rates are available from many countries for the past five decades. Early reviews of ALS mortality rates in various countries, including the United States, revealed a modest increase (20% to 40%) from 1949 to 1976.[63,93,106] Increasing mortality has also been noted in more recent studies from Scotland,[74] England and Wales,[14,40,119] the Republic of Ireland,[40] Australia and New Zealand,[30] Finland,[80] Sweden,[66] France,[37] and the United States.[115,152] In addition, population-based incidence rates have been reported to be increasing in the United States,[165] in Canada (Nova Scotia),[126] Scotland,[74] and Israel.[86] The increased rates were found almost exclusively in patients over 65 years of age.

Whether this increase in mortality is a true increase because of undefined pathogenic factors or is merely an apparent increase for reasons unrelated to the disease process per se is debatable. For example, an apparent increase in the number of individuals dying from ALS could result from more accurate disease identification on death certificates. Riggs[139] has argued that another reason for an apparent increase in deaths from ALS is the increased life expectancy of the general population, which allows more of the "susceptible population subset" to live long enough to develop the disease. Statistical modeling methods that adjust for increased mortality as a result of aging (the Gompertz method) have shown that increased ALS mortality rates in England, Wales, France, and the United States are almost entirely associated with increased life expectancy in the examined populations.[128–130,139] However, this determination does not exclude the existence of a subgroup of the population that is susceptible to ALS.

In our practices, we have informally observed an increase in the frequency of young adults (younger than 45 years) with sporadic ALS. This increase may simply reflect a referral bias, but this trend has been more prevalent in the past few years, when referral practices should not have altered significantly. Some of these patients have abnormal hyperintensities of the descending (corticospinal) motor tracts on magnetic resonance imaging of the brain. As discussed in detail in Chapter 8, this relatively uncommon finding occurs more frequently in younger ALS patients and may identify individuals with a different form of ALS.

FAMILIAL ALS

Although familial ALS (FALS) superficially resembles classic sporadic ALS, careful analysis of its natural history (see Chapter 9), pathology (see Chapter 11), and genetics (see Chapter 10) suggests that it may be a distinct disease. This concept is supported by the biochemical and molecular biologic characterization of a proportion of FALS patients who have mutations in the copper, zinc-superoxide dismutase (*SOD1*) gene (see Chapter 10).

Familial ALS has been reported worldwide and comprises approximately 5% to 10% of all ALS cases, with the reported range being

0.8% to 12%.[18,41,103,125,131,155] Inheritance is predominantly autosomal dominant, although recessive forms of ALS have been identified. The mean age at onset of autosomal-dominant ALS is approximately 47 years[41,103,155] and may be influenced by a parental sex effect.[109] Earlier onset of FALS is more likely when the abnormal gene is inherited from male ancestors than from female ancestors with the disease.[112] In contrast to sporadic ALS, men are no more likely to develop FALS than women.[14,22,125] Symptoms more often begin in the legs,[125] although not always.[41] After symptom onset, patients with FALS survive an average of 1 to 2 years, although almost 25% of individuals survive 5 years; a small number of patients have a much more aggressive course and die within 1 year of disease onset.[155] The molecular mechanisms underlying phenotypic variability in FALS are under investigation, as discussed in Chapter 10.

Superoxide Dismutase 1 Gene Mutations

Genetic studies by Siddique and collaborators[146] of patients with autosomal-dominant FALS identified a linkage to chromosome 22q22.1–22.2. The *SOD1* gene, located in this chromosomal region, was subsequently discovered to be mutated in an estimated 10% to 20% of FALS patients.[33,141] An increasing number of point mutations are being identified in the *SOD1* gene, and relationships have been found between certain mutations and the clinical course.[85] It is not known what proportion of patients with apparently sporadic ALS actually have new mutations in the *SOD1* gene or incomplete penetrance of known familial *SOD1* mutations, but such cases are increasingly being recognized.[83,156] Further epidemiologic studies of autosomal-dominant and autosomal-recessive FALS will undoubtedly provide information on genetic causes of ALS in addition to the *SOD1* mutations.

ALS IN TWINS

Rarely, ALS is reported in twins with no family history of neuromuscular disease.[28,34,42,81] Except for ALS occurring in both dizygotic twins of consanguineous parents,[34] the other cases of ALS in twins suggest that an environmental factor may be the cause. For example, the onset of ALS in dizygotic twins within 2 years of each other during the sixth decade of life suggests the delayed effects of a prenatal insult (perhaps infectious or toxic) to the anterior horn cells or an environmental factor to which both were exposed during childhood.[42] One report of monozygotic twins discordant for ALS raises the possibility that external factors (such as snakebite or more frequent infections in the affected twin) may have had a pathogenic role.[81]

In an extensive study of 17 risk factors in 24 twin pairs (11 monozygotic and 13 dizygotic) discordant for ALS, Currier and Conwill[28] found that histories of either an acute influenza-like illness (usually less than 3 years before the onset of ALS) or more vigorous physical activity were more frequent among affected twins than among their unaffected siblings. Although neither of these risk factors was statistically significant when analyzed alone, the occurrence of both together was significantly ($p < .04$) more frequent in the twins with ALS. Comparing various job-related or non–job-related activities revealed that the ALS-affected twins were significantly ($p < .02$) more active than their unaffected siblings.

HIGH-RISK FOCI OF ALS IN THE WESTERN PACIFIC

The incidence of ALS in the Western Pacific has been 50-fold to 150-fold higher than in most other world regions. Three major foci have been identified: the Chamorro people on the islands of Guam, Rota, and Tinian in the Marianas chain of Micronesia[101,102]; Japanese villagers in the Hobara and Kozagawa districts on the Kii Peninsula of Honshu Island in Japan[57,106]; and the Auyu and Jakai people living inland on the coastal plain of southern West New Guinea (Irian Jaya), Indonesia[51,52,55] (Fig. 2–4). The clinical and pathologic features of this Western Pacific ALS have been most extensively studied on Guam and the Kii Peninsula, where the incidence rates until the mid-1960s ranged from

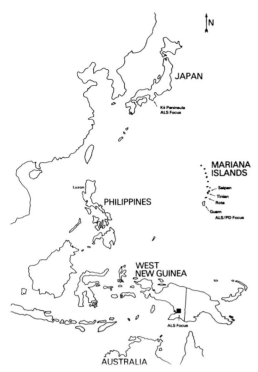

Figure 2–4. Geographic locations of the three high-incidence foci of Western Pacific ALS: the Kii Peninsula in Japan, Mariana Islands (Guam, Rota, and Tinian), and southern West New Guinea, where the frequency of ALS has been 50 to 100 times greater than in other world regions. (Reprinted from Neurology V35, page 194, 1985, by permission of Little, Brown and Company [Inc.].)

14 to 55 per 100,000.[60] Afflicted individuals often have both ALS and parkinsonism-dementia. An essentially identical form of ALS occurs in West New Guinea, but the incidence rate of 147 per 100,000 is up to 10 times higher than in the two other regions.[51,52,55] Although Western Pacific ALS resembles sporadic ALS clinically, it is a distinct disease because the parkinsonism-dementia complex is often associated with it[71] and, pathologically, Alzheimer's disease–like changes (neurofibrillary tangles) are seen (see Chapter 11).

Over the past 40 years, the high incidence of Western Pacific ALS has decreased five-fold to ten-fold, to rates only slightly higher than those in North America.[58,60,68] For example, the incidence on the Kii Peninsula in Hobara has decreased from 55 per 100,000 to 14 per 100,000, with no new cases recorded in the Kozagawa district since 1982.[60] On Guam, the greatest decrease in ALS has occurred in men born after 1920, so that the male-to-female ratio is approaching unity.[58] A similar decrease in the frequency of parkinsonism-dementia has been reported[58] but is controversial.[137] ALS and parkinsonism-dementia have also decreased in villages of West New Guinea where there has been increasing exposure to western lifestyles and foods.[53] Numerous analytic studies of possible risk factors have been performed to identify a common underlying cause of ALS in these high-risk foci (for reviews, see References 52, 57, 145), but these diseases may disappear before the cause or causes are discovered.[154]

Genetic Factors

It is unlikely that Western Pacific ALS has a significant genetic component.[60] Even though affected individuals have a migration pattern and genotype in common, the disease occurs in a restricted region of the Mariana Islands.[101,102,162] Also, Western Pacific ALS is not transmitted by mendelian inheritance,[138] although an additive genetic component, probably enriched in the gene pool through intermarriage, may influence pathogenic environmental factors.[4] No mutations in the *SOD1* gene have been identified in patients from Guam.[43]

Environmental Factors

In contrast to genetic causes, one or more environmental factors are probably implicated in the development of Western Pacific ALS.[100] Long-term exposure seems to be required because the disease did not develop in Americans living on Guam for a short period.[11] However, a United States naval veteran developed pathologically confirmed ALS parkinsonism approximately 2 years after having cruised throughout the Pacific for 13 years, a period that included a 3-week visit to Guam.[45] In studies of Chamorran natives in whom ALS developed after they migrated from Guam to the United States, the age of onset indicated that the putative environmental insult would have to have occurred in childhood or adolescence.[39,56,159] Therefore, if the disease is caused by environmental factors on Guam, most reports suggest its latency period to be at least three decades. Adoption of a more western lifestyle on Guam since the end of World War II, including a change in diet, has coincided with the diminishing frequency of Western Pacific ALS but not of parkinsonism-dementia.[137] Comprehensive studies have excluded a conventional viral cause of this disease.[58]

An exogenous factor proposed in the pathogenesis of Western Pacific ALS is an excitatory neurotoxin, β-N-methylamino-L-alanine (BMAA), found in the seed of the false sago palm (*Cycas circinalis* and *Cycas revoluta*).[99,149] Ground cycad seeds have been used extensively on Guam and in other high-risk Western Pacific regions for flour or as a topical medicine (poultice) for wounds.[57,149–151] It is estimated that more than 80% of the Chamorro population was exposed to cycad.[136] However, the regular practice on Guam and Rota of washing the cycad seeds before grinding removes almost all the BMAA,[36] making the doses available for human ingestion several orders of magnitude lower than those producing neurotoxicity in primate studies.[149] Other countries in the Asia-Pacific basin, such as Malaysia, south India, Sri Lanka, and the Philippines, where cycad is eaten and used medicinally, do not have an unusually high incidence of ALS.[54] Further, Chammoran Guamanians who apparently never ingested cycad seeds have developed ALS.[92] For these and other reasons discussed in Chapter 12, cycad-derived BMAA as a cause of Western Pacific ALS has been seriously questioned.[35,59]

Another environmental factor implicated in ALS and parkinsonism-dementia in high-incidence Western Pacific foci is the mineral composition of the soil and drinking water, which is unusually low in calcium and magnesium and unusually high in aluminum, lead, and silicon.[57,164] Secondary hyperparathyroidism and abnormalities of vitamin D metabolism, as documented in about one-third of Guamanian patients with ALS,[163] have been proposed to increase the intestinal absorption and tissue deposition of aluminum and silicon[57] (see Chapter 16). However, epidemiologic evidence against mineral imbalance as the common environmental cause of Western Pacific ALS includes the relative persistence of parkinsonism-dementia despite the marked decrease in the incidence of Guamanian ALS[137] and the development of ALS and parkinsonism-dementia in Filipino migrants to Guam who lived in low-risk areas where the soil calcium level was high.[136] Furthermore, the dietary intake of calcium is probably high because Guamanians regularly consume fish along with the bones.[69]

In summary, no genetic or exogenous factors have yet been definitely identified in the pathogenesis of Western Pacific ALS, but environmental causes are more likely to have a role.

RISK FACTORS FOR SPORADIC ALS

Investigators have searched for potential risk factors in ALS in the hope of identifying clues to its pathogenesis that may lead to disease prevention. To establish risk factors as such, a statistical association must be demonstrated between a specific event and the subsequent occurrence of disease[158] (for review, see Reference 91). With this criterion in mind, only age and sex have been conclusively established as risk factors for sporadic ALS. Risk factors identified in FALS and the lack of such factors in Western Pacific ALS have been discussed previously.

Although no exogenous factors have been identified as significantly influencing the development or course of sporadic ALS, a few have shown positive correlations (not always of statistical significance) in most risk studies. This finding is particularly true for trauma, especially mechanical trauma and fractures,[1,31,49,61,64,96,108] more often involving the shoulder and upper arm[110] or head, neck, and spine.[96] Except for a prospective study by Kurtzke and Beebe,[108] these studies have been retrospective and so are more subject to error, including recall bias. For example, at least one study found that ALS patients were more likely to recall prior trauma than were controls.[31] In addition, a recent critical review of previous studies has shown no relationship between ALS and antecedent trauma.[104]

Other potential risk factors implicated in some studies but not others include electri-

Table 2–1. **RISK FACTORS EXAMINED IN RELATION TO THE DEVELOPMENT OF ALS**

Possible Association	Unlikely or No Association
Farming	Alcohol
Heavy labor	Allergies
Toxins or chemicals (solvents, plastics)	Anesthesia (spinal anesthesia)
Trauma (mechanical, electrical)	Animal or pet exposure
	Athletics
	Blood product transfusions
	Childhood diseases
	Dental procedures (prostheses)
	Dietary (milk ingestion)
	Electromagnetic field exposure
	Gastric resection
	Glucose intolerance
	Heavy metals (lead, mercury)
	Immunizations
	Infections (influenza)
	Leather processing (carcasses or hides)
	Malignant tumors
	Marital status
	Parental age (at patient's birth)
	Poliomyelitis
	Rural residence
	Smoking
	Sun exposure
	Surgery

Source: Based on data from References 1, 24, 29, 31, 49, 61, 64, 88, 96, 107, 108, 110, 148, 153.

cal injury, particularly when it results in unconsciousness[31,50,61,148]; physical exertion, particularly heavy labor[28,64,67,108]; and exposure to chemicals used in plastics manufacture.[31] Kurtzke[107] has presented a detailed analysis of these putative risk factors. Table 2–1 ranks the likelihood that these and other putative risk factors are associated with ALS development. Except for sex and age, as discussed above, no other risk factors have been consistently found for sporadic ALS.

ALS CLUSTERS

There have been a few reports of geographic clustering of sporadic ALS patients. Such clustering occurs when a higher-than-expected number of affected individuals is observed in a geographic area. The occurrence of ALS in clusters is potentially significant if it can be shown to result from an underlying epidemiologic factor rather than from chance alone. For example, the early observation by Koerner of an ALS cluster on Guam[90] led to the extensive studies of potential risk factors in Western Pacific ALS, including excitotoxin exposure and mineral imbalance in the soil and water supplies.

Most non–Western Pacific ALS clusters have consisted of three or four individuals living[72,122] or working[77] in close proximity, although other clusters have involved individuals playing on the same sports team[48] or who have been war evacuees.[82] No significant risk factors were identified in these ALS patients. A case control study of a cluster in Wisconsin implicated trauma and the frequent consumption of freshwater fish, but no specific toxin was identified.[147] ALS developed in four unrelated male farmer-ranchers living within a 15-km radius of each other in a region where chronic selenium intoxication had been endemic in farm animals for the preceding 40 years.[89]

Conjugal ALS

ALS occurring in both spouses of a nonconsanguineous marriage (conjugal ALS) can be considered a rare form of ALS clustering. The spouses, who have been from the United States,[17,27] France,[15] Sardinia,[134] and Libya,[118] lived together between 10 and 40 years before developing classic ALS within a median of 2 years (range, 8 months to 13 years) of each other. Unfortunately, no exogenous factors common to both spouses have been identified as a cause. The few reported cases may be coincidental; statistical calculations indicate that four American couples each year could develop ALS by chance alone.[27] As with other ALS clusters, conjugal ALS is of interest as an unusual occurrence, but it has not revealed further clues to the pathogenesis of ALS.

SUMMARY

Numerous studies of the worldwide epidemiology of the three major categories of ALS—sporadic classic ALS, FALS, and Western Pacific ALS—have identified the incidence, prevalence, mortality rates, natural history, potential risk factors, and geographic distribution (including clustering) that are unique to each category. Accurate clinical and pathologic diagnosis using standardized criteria is important in maximizing case ascertainment to ensure the most representative and accurate epidemiologic studies possible. The El Escorial criteria for the diagnosis of ALS is an international effort to achieve this goal.

Sporadic ALS, the most extensively studied form of ALS, has relatively constant incidence and prevalence rates worldwide, except for isolated regions in the Western Pacific. Onset is most likely in the seventh and eighth decades of life, is slightly more frequent in males than in females, and usu-ally results in death an average of 3 years after symptoms begin. The frequency of sporadic ALS, as reflected by worldwide mortality rate and incidence rate analyses, appears to have been increasing moderately over the past 50 years. Although this rise may indicate the increasing effect of some unidentified exogenous factor, it may simply reflect the greater life expectancy of the general population, which allows longer survival of a subpopulation susceptible to ALS.

Familial ALS, which is primarily inherited as a dominant trait, comprises approximately 5% to 10% of all ALS cases. Because of epidemiologic, clinical, and molecular differences, it may be a disease distinct from sporadic ALS. Onset of FALS peaks at a younger age, and FALS affects both sexes about equally. Approximately 25% of patients with FALS have a mutation in the *SOD1* gene on chromosome 21. The rare occurrence of ALS in monozygotic and dizygotic twins generally supports an environmental cause of ALS.

An exceptionally high incidence of ALS had been identified in the Western Pacific, on the Mariana Islands, the Kii Peninsula of Japan, and in West New Guinea, although its occurrence, at least on Guam, has decreased markedly over the past 40 years. This Western Pacific ALS is distinct from sporadic ALS because it is frequently associated with a parkinsonism-dementia complex and neurofibrillary tangles. Major genetic factors have been excluded, but environmental causes, such as an excitotoxin from the cycad seed and mineral imbalances in the soil and water, are the subjects of continued research and debate.

Numerous risk factors have been excluded as possible causes of ALS. Only age and sex are considered to be definite risk factors, although farming, heavy labor, certain toxins or chemicals, and some types of trauma may be associated with the development of ALS. The occurrence of ALS in clusters or in both spouses has not provided any clues to ALS pathogenesis.

REFERENCES

1. Angelini, C, Armani, M, and Bresolin, N: Incidence and risk factors of motor neuron disease in the Venice and Padua districts of Italy, 1972–1979. Neuroepidemiology 2:236–242, 1983.

2. Annegers, JF, Appel, S, Lee JR-J, et al: Incidence and prevalence of amyotrophic lateral sclerosis in Harris County, Texas, 1985–1988. Arch Neurol 48:589–593, 1991.
3. Armon, C, Daube, JR, O'Brien, PC, et al: When is an apparent excess of neurologic cases epidemiologically significant? Neurology 41:1713–1718, 1991.
4. Bailey-Wilson, JE, Plato, CC, Elston, RC, et al: Potential role of an additive genetic component in the cause of amyotrophic lateral sclerosis and parkinsonism-dementia in the Western Pacific. Am J Med Genet 45:68–76, 1993.
5. Bettoni, L, Bazzani, M, Bortone, E, et al: Steadiness of amyotrophic lateral sclerosis in the province of Parma, Italy, 1960–1990. Acta Neurol Scand 90:276–280, 1994.
6. Bharucha, NE, Schoenberg, BS, Raven, RH, et al: Geographic distribution of motor neuron disease and correlation with possible etiologic factors. Neurology 33:911–915, 1983.
7. Bobowick, AR and Brody, JA: Epidemiology of motor-neuron diseases. N Engl J Med 288:1047–1055, 1973.
8. Bracco, L, Antuono, P, and Amaducci, L: Study of epidemiological and etiological factors of amyotrophic lateral sclerosis in the province of Florence, Italy. Acta Neurol Scand 60:112–124, 1979.
9. Bradley, WG: Recent views on amyotrophic lateral sclerosis with emphasis on electrophysiological studies. Muscle Nerve. 10:490–502, 1987.
10. Brewis, M, Poskanzer, DC, Rolland, C, et al: Neurological disease in an English city. Acta Neurol Scand 42(suppl 24):1–89, 1966.
11. Brody, JA, Edgar, AH, and Gillespie, MM: Amyotrophic lateral sclerosis. No increase among US construction workers in Guam. JAMA 240:551–560, 1978.
12. Brooks, BR: Clinical epidemiology of ALS. In Riggs, JE (ed): Neurologic Clinics Vol 14. WB Saunders, Philadelphia, 1996, pp 399–420.
13. Brooks, BR: El Escorial World Federation of Neurology criteria for the diagnosis of amyotrophic lateral sclerosis. J Neurol Sci 124(suppl):96–107, 1994.
14. Buckley, J, Warlow, C, Smith, P, et al: Motor neuron disease in England and Wales, 1959–1979. J Neurol Neurosurg Psychiatry 46:197–205, 1983.
15. Camu, W, Cadilhac, J, and Billiard, M: Conjugal amyotrophic lateral sclerosis: A report on two couples from southern France. Neurology 44:547–548, 1994.
16. Cendrowski, W, Wender, W, and Owsianowski, M: Analyse épidémiologique de la sclérose latérale amyotrophique sur le territoire de la Grand-Pologne. Acta Neurol Scand 46:609–617, 1970.
17. Chad, D, Mitsumoto, H, and Adelman, LS: Conjugal motor neuron disease. Neurology 32:306–307, 1982.
18. Chancellor, AM, Fraser, H, Swingler, RJ, et al: Clinical heterogeneity of familial motor neuron disease: Report of 11 pedigrees from a population-based study in Scotland. The Scottish Motor Neuron Disease Research Group. J Neurol Sci 124(suppl):75–76, 1994.
19. Chancellor, AM, Hendry, A, Caird, FI, et al: Motor neuron disease: A disease of old age. Scot Med J 38:178–182, 1993.
20. Chancellor, AM and Warlow, CP: Adult onset motor neuron disease: Worldwide mortality, incidence, and distribution since 1950. J Neurol Neurosurg Psychiatry 55:1106–1115, 1992.
21. Chazot, F, Vallat, JM, Hugon, J, et al: Amyotrophic lateral sclerosis in Limousin (Limoges area, France). Neuroepidemiology 5:39–46, 1986.
22. Chiò, A, Brignolio, F, Meineri, P, et al: Familial ALS. Clinical, genetic and morphological features. Acta Neurol Scand 75:277–282, 1987.
23. Chiò, A, Brignolio, F, Meineri, P, et al: Epidemiology of motor neuron disease in two Italian provinces: Analysis of secular trend and geographic distribution. Neuroepidemiology 8:79–86, 1989.
24. Chiò, A, Meineri, P, Tribolo, A, et al: Risk factors in motor neuron disease: A case-control study. Neuroepidemiology 10:174–184, 1991.
25. Christensen, PB, Hojer-Pedersen, E, and Jensen, NB: Survival of patients with amyotrophic lateral sclerosis in two Danish counties. Neurology 40:600–604, 1990.
26. Clancy, AN, Bonsall, RW, and Michael RP: Immunohistochemical labeling of androgen receptors in the brain of rat and monkey. Life Sci 50:409–417, 1992.
27. Cornblath, DR, Kurland, LT, Boylan, KB, et al: Conjugal amyotrophic lateral sclerosis: Report of a young married couple. Neurology 43:2378–2380, 1993.
28. Currier, RD and Conwill, DE: Influenza and physical activity as possible risk factors for amyotrophic lateral sclerosis: A study of twins. In Rose, FC and Norris, FH (eds): ALS. New Advances in Toxicology and Epidemiology. Smith Gordon, London, 1990, pp 23–28.
29. Davanipour, Z, Sobel, E, Vu, H, et al: Electromagnetic field exposure and amyotrophic lateral sclerosis [letter]. Neuroepidemiology 10:308, 1991.
30. Dean, G and Elian, M: Motor neuron disease and multiple sclerosis mortality in Australia, New Zealand and South Africa compared with England and Wales. J Neurol Neuosurg Psychiatry 56:633–637, 1993.
31. Deapen, DM and Henderson, BE: A case-control study of amyotrophic lateral sclerosis. Am J Epidemiol 123:790–799, 1986.
32. De Domenico, P, Malara, CE, Marabello, L, et al: Amyotrophic lateral sclerosis: An epidemiological study in the province of Messina, Italy, 1976–1985. Neuroepidemiology 7:152–158, 1988.
33. Deng, H-X, Hentati, A, Tainer, JA, et al: Amyotrophic lateral sclerosis and structural defects in Cu, Zn superoxide dismutase. Science 261:1047–1051, 1993.
34. Dumon, J, Macken, J, and De Barsy, T: Concordance for amyotrophic lateral sclerosis in a pair of dizygous twins of consanguineous parents. J Med Genet 8:113–116, 1971.
35. Duncan, MW, Kopin IJ, Garruto, RM, et al: 2-Amino-3-(methylamino)-propionic acid cycad-derived foods is an unlikely cause of amyotrophic lateral sclerosis/parkinsonism [letter]. Lancet 2:631, 1988.
36. Duncan, MW, Steele, JC, Kopin, IJ, et al: 2-Amino-3-(methylamino)-propanoic acid (BMAA) in cycad flour: An unlikely cause of amyotrophic lateral sclerosis and parkinsonism-dementia of Guam. Neurology 40:767–772, 1990.

37. Durrleman, S and Alperovitch, A: Increasing trend of ALS in France and elsewhere: Are the changes real? Neurology 39:768–773, 1989.

38. Eisen, A, Schulzer, M, MacNeil, M, et al: Duration of amyotrophic lateral sclerosis is age dependent. Muscle Nerve 16:27–32, 1993.

39. Eldridge, R, Ryan, E, Rosario, J, et al: Amyotrophic lateral sclerosis and parkinsonism dementia in a migrant population from Guam. Neurology 19:1029–1037, 1969.

40. Elian, M and Dean, G: The changing mortality from motor neuron disease and multiple sclerosis in England and Wales and the Republic of Ireland. Neuroepidemiology 11:236–243, 1992.

41. Emery, AEH and Holloway, S: Familial motor neuron diseases. In Rowland, LP (ed): Human Motor Neuron Diseases. Raven Press, New York, 1982, pp 139–147.

42. Estrin, WJ: Amyotrophic lateral sclerosis in dizygotic twins. Neurology 27:692–694, 1977.

43. Figlewicz, DA, Garruto, RM, Yanagihara, R, et al: The Cu/Zn superoxide dismutase gene in ALS and parkinsonism dementia of Guam. Neuroreport 5:557–560, 1994.

44. Fletcher, RH, Fletcher, SW, and Wagner, EH: Clinical Epidemiology. The Essentials, ed 2. Williams & Wilkins, Baltimore, 1988.

45. Forno, LS and O'Flanagan, TJ: Amyotrophic lateral sclerosis of the Guam type in a US veteran. Neurology 23:876–880, 1973.

46. Forsgren, L, Almay, BGL, Holgren, G, et al: Epidemiology of motor neuron disease in northern Sweden. Acta Neurol Scand 68:20–29, 1983.

47. Friedman, AP and Freedman, D: Amyotrophic lateral sclerosis. J Nerv Ment Dis 111:1–18, 1950.

48. Gallagher, JP: ALS [letter]. South Med J 81:417, 1988.

49. Gallagher, JP and Sanders, M: Trauma and amyotrophic lateral sclerosis: A report of 78 patients. Acta Neurol Scand 75:145–150, 1987.

50. Gallagher, JP and Talbert, OR: Motor neuron syndrome after electric shock. Acta Neurol Scand 83:79–82, 1991.

51. Gajdusek, DC: Motor-neuron disease in natives of New Guinea. N Engl J Med 268:474–476, 1963.

52. Gajdusek, DC: Foci of motor neuron disease in high incidence in isolated populations of East Asia and the Western Pacific. In Rowland, LP (ed): Human Motor Neuron Diseases. New York: Raven Press, 1982, pp 363–393.

53. Gajdusek, DC: Environmental factors provoking physiological changes which induce motor neuron disease and early neuronal aging in high incidence foci in the Western Pacific. In Rose, FC (ed): Research Progress in Motor Neurone Disease. Pitman Press, London, 1984, pp 44–69.

54. Gajdusek, DC: Cycad toxicity not the cause of high incidence of amyotrophic lateral sclerosis/parkinsonism-dementia on Guam, Kii Peninsula of Japan, or in West New Guinea. In Hudson, AJ (ed): Amyotrophic Lateral Sclerosis: Concepts in Pathogenesis and Etiology. University of Toronto, Toronto, 1990, pp 317–325.

55. Gajdusek, DC and Salazar, AM: Amyotrophic lateral sclerosis and parkinsonian syndromes in high incidence among the Auyu and Jakai people of West New Guinea. Neurology 32:107–126, 1982.

56. Garruto, RM, Gajdusek, DC, and Chen K-M: Amyotrophic lateral sclerosis among Chamorro migrants from Guam. Ann Neurol 8:612–619, 1980.

57. Garruto, RM and Yanagihara, R: Amyotrophic lateral sclerosis in the Mariana islands. In Vinken, PJ, et al (eds): Handbook of Clinical Neurology, vol 59: Diseases of the Motor System. Elsevier, Amsterdam, 1991, pp 253–271.

58. Garruto, RM, Yanagihara, R, and Gajdusek, DC: Disappearance of high-incidence amyotrophic lateral sclerosis and parkinsonism-dementia on Guam. Neurology 35:193–198, 1985.

59. Garruto, RM, Yanagihara, R, and Gajdusek, DC: Cycads and amyotrophic lateral sclerosis/parkinsonism dementia [letter]. Lancet 2:1079, 1988.

60. Garruto, RM and Yase, Y: Neurodegenerative disorders of the western Pacific: The search for mechanisms of pathogenesis. Trends Neurosci 9:268–374, 1986.

61. Gawel, M, Zaiwalla, Z, and Rose, FC: Antecedent events in motor neuron disease. J Neurol Neurosurg Psychiatry 46:1041–1043, 1983.

62. Giagheddu, M, Mascia, V, Cannas, A, et al: Amyotrophic lateral sclerosis in Sardinia, Italy: An epidemiologic study. Acta Neurol Scand 87:446–454, 1993.

63. Goldberg, ID and Kurland, LT: Mortality in 33 countries from diseases of the nervous system. World Neurol 3:444–465, 1962.

64. Granieri, E, Carreras, M, Tola, R, et al: Motor neuron disease in the province of Ferrara, Italy, in 1964–1982. Neurology 38:1604–1608, 1988.

65. Gudmundsson, KR: The prevalence of some neurological diseases in Iceland. Acta Neurol Scand 44:57–69, 1968.

66. Gunnarsson, L-G, Lindberg, G, Söderfelt, B, et al: The mortality of motor neuron disease in Sweden. Arch Neurol 47:42–46, 1990.

67. Gunnarsson, L-G and Palm, R: Motor neuron disease and heavy manual labor: An epidemiologic survey of Värmland County, Sweden. Neuroepidemiology 3:195–206, 1984.

68. Haddock, RL and Santos, JV: Are the endemic motor neuron diseases of Guam really disappearing? Southeast Asian J Trop Med Publ Health 23:278–281, 1992.

69. Hankin, J, Reed, D, Labarthe, D, et al: Diet and disease patterns among Micronesians. Am J Clin Nutr 23:346–357, 1970.

70. Haverkamp, LJ, Appel, V, and Appel, SH: Natural history of amyotrophic lateral sclerosis in a database population. Validation of a scoring system and a model for survival prediction. Brain 118:707–719, 1995.

71. Hirano, A, Kurland, LT, Krooth, RS, et al: Parkinsonism-dementia complex, endemic disease on the island of Guam: I. Clinical features. Brain 84:642–661, 1961.

72. Hochberg, FH, Bryan II, JA, and Whelan, MA: Clustering of amyotrophic lateral sclerosis [letter]. Lancet 1:34, 1974.

73. Hoffman, PM and Brody, JA: The reliability of death certificate reporting for amyotrophic lateral sclerosis. J Chronic Dis 24:5–8, 1971.

74. Holloway, SM and Emery, AEH: The epidemiology of motor neuron disease in Scotland. Muscle Nerve 5:131–133, 1982.

75. Holloway, SM and Mitchell, JD: Motor neuron disease in the Lothian Region of Scotland 1961–81. J Epidemiol Comm Health 40:344–350, 1986.

76. Hudson, AJ, Davenport, A, and Hader, WJ: The incidence of amyotrophic lateral sclerosis in southwestern Ontario, Canada. Neurology 36:1524–1528, 1986.

77. Hyser, CL, Kissel, JT, and Mendell, JR: Three cases of amyotrophic lateral sclerosis in a common occupational environment. J Neurol 234:443–444, 1987.

78. Jokelainen, M: The epidemiology of amyotrophic lateral sclerosis in Finland. J Neurol Sci 29:55–63, 1976.

79. Jokelainen, M: Amyotrophic lateral sclerosis in Finland. I. An epidemiological study. Acta Neurol Scand 56:185–193, 1977.

80. Jokelainen, M: Amyotrophic lateral sclerosis in Finland. Adv Exp Med Biol 209:341–344, 1987.

81. Jokelainen, M, Palo, J, and Lokki, J: Monozygous twins discordant for amyotrophic lateral sclerosis. Eur Neurol 17:296–299, 1978.

82. Jokelainen, M, Wikstrom, J, and Palo, J: Effect of birthplace on the development of amyotrophic lateral sclerosis and multiple sclerosis. A study among Finnish war evacuees. Acta Neurol Scand 60:283–288, 1979.

83. Jones, CT, Swingler, RJ, and Brock DJH: Identification of a novel *SOD1* mutation in an apparently sporadic amyotrophic lateral sclerosis patient and detection of *Ile1 13Thr* in three others. Hum Molec Genet 3:649–650, 1994.

84. Juergens, SM, Kurland, LT, Okazaki, H, et al: ALS in Rochester, Minnesota, 1925–1977. Neurology 30:463–470, 1980.

85. Juneja, T, Pericak-Vance, MA, Laing, NG, et al: Prognosis in familial amyotrophic lateral sclerosis: Progression and survival in patients with glu100gly and ala4val mutations in Cu, Zn superoxide dismutase. Neurology 48: 55–57, 1997.

86. Kahana, E and Zilber, N: Changes in the incidence of amyotrophic lateral sclerosis in Israel. Arch Neurol 41:157–160, 1984.

87. Kahana, E, Alter, M, and Feldman, S: Amyotrophic lateral sclerosis, a population study. J Neurol 212:205–213, 1976.

88. Kalfakis, N, Vassilopoulos, D, Voumvourakis, C, et al: Amyotrophic lateral sclerosis in southern Greece: An epidemiological study. Neuroepidemiology 10:170–173, 1991.

89. Kilness, AW and Hochberg, FH: Amyotrophic lateral sclerosis in a high selenium environment. JAMA 237:2843–2844, 1977.

90. Koerner, DR: Amyotrophic lateral sclerosis on Guam: A clinical study and review of the literature. Ann Intern Med 37:1204–1220, 1952.

91. Kondo, K: Environmental factors in motor neuron disease. In Gourie-Devi, M (ed): Motor Neuron Disease. Oxford University Press, New Delhi, 1987, pp 54–60.

92. Kondo, K: Epidemiology of motor neuron disease. In Leigh, PN and Swash, M (eds): Motor Neuron Disease: Biology and Management. Springer-Verlag, New York, 1995, pp 19–33.

93. Kondo, K: Motor neuron disease: Changing population patterns and clues for etiology. In Schoenberg, BS (ed): Neurological Epidemiology. Raven Press, New York, 1978, pp 509–542.

94. Kondo, K and Hemmi, I: Clinical statistics in 515 fatal cases of motor neuron disease. Neuroepidemiology 3:129–148, 1984.

95. Kondo, K and Tsubaki, T: Changing mortality patterns of motor neuron disease in Japan. J Neurol Sci, 32:411–424, 1977.

96. Kondo, K and Tsubaki, T: Case-control studies of motor neuron disease: Association with mechanical injuries. Arch Neurol 38:220–226, 1981.

97. Kreindler, A, Ionasecu, V, and Drinca-Ionescu, M: Repartita bolilor neurologice eredo-familiale in Romînia: Nota preliminara. Stud Cercet Neurol 9:401–410, 1964.

98. Kristensen, O and Melgaard, B: Motor neuron disease: Prognosis and epidemiology. Acta Neurol Scand 56:299–308, 1977.

99. Kurland, LT: An appraisal of the neurotoxicity of cycad and the etiology of amyotrophic lateral sclerosis on Guam. Fed Proc 31:1540–1542, 1972.

100. Kurland, LT and Molgaard, CA: Guamanian ALS: Hereditary or acquired? In Rowland, LP (ed): Human Motor Neuron Diseases. Raven Press, New York, 1982, pp 165–171.

101. Kurland, LT and Mulder, DW: Epidemiologic investigations of amyotrophic lateral sclerosis: I. Preliminary report on geographic distribution with special reference to the Mariana islands, including clinical and pathologic observations. Neurology 4:355–378, 1954.

102. Kurland, LT and Mulder, DW: Epidemiological investigations of high-incidence amyotrophic lateral sclerosis and parkinsonism-dementia on Guam. Neurology 5:182–196, 1955.

103. Kurland, LT, and Mulder, DW: Epidemiological investigations of amyotrophic lateral sclerosis. Familial aggregations indicative of dominant inheritance. Part II. Neurology 5:249–268, 1955.

104. Kurland, LT, Radhakrishnan, K, Smith, GE, et al: Mechanical trauma as a risk factor in classic amyotrophic lateral sclerosis: Lack of epidemiologic evidence. J Neurol Sci 113:133–143, 1992.

105. Kurland, LT, Radhakrishnan, K, Williams, DB, et al: Amyotrophic lateral sclerosis-parkinsonism-dementia complex on Guam: Epidemiologic and etiological perspectives. In Williams, AC (ed): Motor Neuron Disease. Chapman and Hall Medical, London, 1994, pp 109–130.

106. Kurtzke, JF: Epidemiology of amyotrophic lateral sclerosis. In Rowland, LP (ed): Human Motor Neuron Diseases. Raven Press, New York, 1982, pp 281–302.

107. Kurtzke, JF: Risk factors in amyotrophic lateral sclerosis. In Rowland, LP (ed): Amyotrophic Lateral Sclerosis and Other Motor Neuron Diseases. Raven Press, New York, 1991, 245–270.

108. Kurtzke, JF and Beebe, GW: Epidemiology of amyotrophic lateral sclerosis: 1. A case-control comparison based on ALS deaths. Neurology 30:453–462, 1980.

109. Leone, M: Parental sex effect in familial amyotrophic lateral sclerosis. Neurology 41:1291–1294, 1991.

110. Leone, M, Chandra, V, and Schoenberg, BS: Motor neuron disease in the United States, 1971 and 1973–1978: Patterns of mortality and associated conditions at the time of death. Neurology 37:1339–1343, 1987.

111. Leone, M, Chiò, A, Mortara, P, et al: Motor neuron disease in the Province of Turin, Italy, 1971–1980. Acta Neurol Scand 68:316–327, 1983.

112. Leone, M, De Angelis, MS, Giordano, M, et al: Influence of ancestral gender on transmission of familial amyotrophic lateral sclerosis [letter]. Lancet 34:1639, 1994.

113. Li, T-M, Alberman, E, and Swash, M: Clinical features and associations of 560 cases of motor neuron disease. J Neurol Neurosurg Psychiatry 53:1043–1045, 1990.

114. Li, T-M, Swash, M, Alberman, E, and Day, SJ: Diagnosis of motor neuron disease by neurologists: A study in three countries. J Neurol Neurosurg Psychiatry 54:980–983, 1991.

115. Lilienfeld, DE, Chan, E, Ehland, J, et al: Rising mortality from motoneuron disease in the USA, 1962–84. Lancet 1:710–713, 1989.

116. Lopez-Vega, JM, Calleja, J, Combarros, O, et al: Motor neuron disease in Cantabria. Acta Neurol Scand 77:1–5, 1988.

117. Lorez, A: Ein Beitrag zu Klinik und Vorkommen der amyotrophischen Lateralsklerose (isolierte und familiäre Fälle). Schweiz Med Wochenschr 99:51–57, 1969.

118. Maloo, JC, Radhakrishnan, K, Poddar, SK, et al: Conjugal motor neuron disease. J Assoc Physicians India 35:303–304, 1987.

119. Martyn, CN, Barker, DJP, and Osmond, C: Motor neuron disease and past poliomyelitis in England and Wales. Lancet 1:1319–1322, 1988.

120. Matsuura, T, Ogata, A, Demura, T, et al: Identification of androgen receptors in the rat spinal motor neurons. Immunohistochemical and immunoblotting analyses with monoclonal antibody. Neurosci Lett 158:5–8, 1993.

121. Matsumoto, N, Worth, RM, Kurland, LT, et al: Epidemiologic study of amyotrophic lateral sclerosis in Hawaii: Identification of high incidence among Filipino men. Neurology 22:934–940, 1972.

122. Melmed, C and Krieger, C: A cluster of amyotrophic lateral sclerosis. Arch Neurol 39:595–596, 1982.

123. Mitchell, JD, Gibson, HN, and Gatrell, A: Amyotrophic lateral sclerosis in Lancashire and South Cumbria, England, 1976–1986. A geographical study. Arch Neurol 47:875–880, 1990.

124. Mochecka-Thoelke, A: Clinical pattern and epidemiological analysis of amyotrophic lateral sclerosis in the Lódz Region in 1980–1986. Neurol Neurochir Pol 28:189–194, 1994.

125. Mulder, DW, Kurland, LT, Offord, KP, et al: Familial adult motor neuron disease: amyotrophic lateral sclerosis. Neurology 36:511–517, 1986.

126. Murray, TJ, Cameron, J, Heffernan, LP, et al: Amyotrophic lateral sclerosis in Nova Scotia. Adv Exp Med Biol 209:345–349, 1987.

127. Murros, K and Fogelholm, R: Amyotrophic lateral sclerosis in Middle-Finland: An epidemiological study. Acta Neurol Scand 67:41–47, 1983.

128. Neilson, S, Robinson, I, and Alperovitch, A: Rising amyotrophic lateral sclerosis mortality in France 1968–1990: Increased life expectancy and interdisease competition as an explanation. J Neurol 241:448–455, 1994.

129. Neilson, S, Robinson, I, Clifford Rose, F, et al: Rising mortality from motor neurone disease: An explanation. Acta Neurol Scand 87:184–191, 1993.

130. Neilson, S, Robinson, I, and Hunter, M: Longitudinal Gompertzian analysis of ALS mortality in England and Wales, 1963–1989: Estimates of susceptibility in the general population. Mech Ageing Dev 64:201–216, 1992.

131. Norris, F, Shepherd, R, Denys, E, et al: Onset, natural history and outcome in idiopathic adult motor neuron disease. J Neurol Sci 118:48–55, 1993.

132. Olivares, L, Esteban, ES, and Alter, M: Mexican "resistance" to amyotrophic lateral sclerosis. Arch Neurol 27:397–402, 1972.

133. O'Malley, F, Dean, G, and Elian, M: Multiple sclerosis and motor neuron disease: Survival and how certified after death. J Epidemiol Community Health 41:14–17, 1987.

134. Paolino, E, Granieri, E, Tola, MR, et al: Conjugal amyotrophic lateral sclerosis. Ann Neurol 14:699, 1983.

135. Radhakrishnan, K, Ashok, PP, Sridharan, R, et al: Descriptive epidemiology of motor neuron disease in Benghazi, Libya. Neuroepidemiology 5:47–54, 1986.

136. Reed, DM and Brody, JA: Amyotrophic lateral sclerosis and parkinsonism-dementia on Guam, 1945–1972. I. Descriptive epidemiology. Am J Epidemiol 101:287–301, 1975.

137. Reed, D, LaBarthe, D, Chen, KM, et al: A cohort study of amyotrophic lateral sclerosis and parkinsonism-dementia on Guam and Rota. Am J Epidemiol 125:92–100, 1987.

138. Reed, DM, Torres, JM, and Brody, JA: Amyotrophic lateral sclerosis and parkinsonism-dementia on Guam, 1945–1972. II. Familial and genetic studies. Am J Epidemiol 101:302–310, 1975.

139. Riggs, JE: Longitudinal Gompertzian analysis of amyotrophic lateral sclerosis mortality in the U.S., 1977–1986: Evidence for an inherently susceptible population. Mech Ageing Dev 55:207–220, 1990.

140. Rosati, G, Pinna, L, Granieri, E, et al: Studies on epidemiological, clinical and etiological aspects of ALS disease in Sardinia, Southern Italy. Acta Neurol Scand 55:231–244, 1977.

141. Rosen, DR, Siddique, T, Patterson, D, et al: Mutations in Cu/Zn superoxide dismutase are associated with familial amyotrophic lateral sclerosis. Nature 362:59–62, 1993.

142. Salemi, G, Fierro, B, Arcara, A, et al: Amyotrophic lateral sclerosis in Palermo, Italy: An epidemiologic study. Ital J Neurol Sci 10:505–509, 1989.

143. Scarpa, M, Colombo, A, Pancetti, P, et al: Epidemiology of amyotrophic lateral sclerosis in the province of Modena, Italy. Influence of environmental exposure to lead. Acta Neurol Scand 77:456–460, 1988.

144. Scottish Motor Neuron Disease Research Group: The Scottish motor neuron disease register: A prospective study of adult onset motor neuron disease in Scotland. Methodology, demography and clinical features of incident cases in 1989. J Neurol Neurosurg Psychiatry 55:536–541, 1992.

145. Shiraki, H and Yase, Y: Amyotrophic lateral sclerosis and parkinsonism-dementia in the Kii Peninsula: Comparison with the same disorders in Guam

and with Alzheimer's disease. In Vinken, PJ, et al (ed): Handbook of Clinical Neurology: Diseases of the Motor System, Vol 59. Elsevier, Amsterdam, 1991, pp 273–300.

146. Siddique, T, Figlewicz, DA, Petricek-Vance, MA, et al: Linkage of a gene causing amyotrophic lateral sclerosis to chromosome 21 and evidence of genetic-locus heterogeneity. N Engl J Med 324:1381–1384, 1991.

147. Sienko, DG, Davis, JP, Taylor JA, et al: Amyotrophic lateral sclerosis. A case-control study following detection of a cluster in a small Wisconsin community. Arch Neurol 47:38–41, 1990.

148. Sirdofsky, MD, Hawley, RJ, and Manz, H: Progressive motor neuron disease associated with electrical injury. Muscle Nerve 14:977–980, 1991.

149. Spencer, PS, Nun, PB, Hugon, J, et al: Guam amyotrophic lateral sclerosis-parkinsonism-dementia linked to a plant excitant neurotoxin. Science 237:517–522, 1987.

150. Spencer, PS, Ohta, M, and Palmer, VS: Cycad use and motor neuron disease in the Kii Peninsula of Japan. Lancet 2:1462–1463, 1987.

151. Spencer, PS, Palmer, VS, Herman, A, et al: Cycad use and motor neuron disease in Irian Jaya. Lancet 2:1273–1274, 1987.

152. Stallones, L, Kasarkis, EJ, Stipanowich, C, et al: Secular trends in mortality rates from motor neuron disease in Kentucky 1964–1984. Neuroepidemiology 8:68–78, 1989.

153. Steiner, I, Birmanns, B, and Panet, A: Sun exposure and amyotrophic lateral sclerosis [letter]. Ann Intern Med 120:893, 1994.

154. Stone, R: Guam: Deadly disease dying out. Science 261:424–426, 1993.

155. Strong, MJ, Hudson, AJ, and Alvord, WG: Familial amyotrophic lateral sclerosis, 1850–1989: A statistical analysis of the world literature. Can J Neurol Sci 18:45–58, 1991.

156. Suthers, F, Laing, N, Wilton, S, et al: "Sporadic" motor neuron disease due to familial *SOD1* mutation with low penetrance [letter]. Lancet 344:1773–1994.

157. Swash, M and Leigh, N: Criteria for diagnosis of familial amyotrophic lateral sclerosis. European FALS Collaborative Group. Neuromusc Disord 2:7–9, 1992.

158. Tandan, R and Bradley, WG: Amyotrophic lateral sclerosis: Part 2, etiopathogenesis. Ann Neurol 18:419–431, 1985.

159. Torres, J, Iriarte, D, Chen, K-M, et al: A cohort study of amyotrophic lateral sclerosis among Guamanians in California. Calif Med 86:385–388, 1986.

160. Tysnes, OB, Vollset, SE, and Aarli, JA: Epidemiology of amyotrophic lateral sclerosis in Hordaland county, western Norway. Acta Neurol Scand 83:280–285, 1991.

161. Wender, M, Pruchnik, D, Kowal, P, et al: Comparative analysis of the epidemiology of amyotrophic lateral sclerosis in the province of Poznan. (English abstract). Neurol Neurochir Pol 24:297–302, 1990.

162. Yanagihara, RT, Garruto, RM, and Gajdusek, DC: Epidemiological surveillance of amyotrophic lateral sclerosis and parkinsonism-dementia in the Commonwealth of the Northern Mariana islands. Ann Neurol 13:79–86, 1983.

163. Yanagihara, RT, Garruto, RM, Gajdusek, DC, et al: Calcium and vitamin D metabolism in Guamanian Chamorros with amyotrophic lateral sclerosis and parkinsonism-dementia. Ann Neurol 15:42–48, 1984.

164. Yase, Y: The pathogenesis of amyotrophic lateral sclerosis. Lancet 2:292–296, 1972.

165. Yoshida, S, Mulder, DW, Kurland, KT, et al: Follow-up study on amyotrophic lateral sclerosis in Rochester, Minn., 1925 through 1984. Neuroepidemiology 5:61–70, 1986.

166. Zack, MM, Levitt, LP, and Schoenberg, B: Motor neuron disease in Lehigh County, Pennsylvania: An epidemiologic study. J Chronic Dis 30:813–818, 1977.

CHAPTER 3

FUNCTIONAL NEUROANATOMY OF THE MOTOR SYSTEM

UPPER MOTOR NEURONS
CORTICOSPINAL AND CORTICOBULBAR
    TRACTS
BRAIN-STEM SOMATIC MOTOR CONTROL
LIMBIC MOTOR CONTROL
INTERNEURONS
LOWER MOTOR NEURONS

Comprehension of the neuroanatomy of the motor system is a prerequisite to grasping the signs and symptoms of ALS.[3,5,6,10] Contracting skeletal muscles are required for movements of our bodies, whether as reflex actions, maintenance of balance and posture, or complex motion of the limbs, eyes, face, or tongue. The motor system transforms neural information into physical energy by sending commands that are transmitted via the brain stem and spinal cord to skeletal muscles. The motor control system has three distinct features. First, motor neurons and their tracts are somatotopically organized. Second, the motor system has proprioceptive inputs for both feedback control (for adjusting slow movement and posture) and feed-forward control (essential for preparing for rapid movements). Third, the motor system is organized hierarchically and in parallel with cortical motor neurons, the brain stem, and the limbic system to control the interneuron system and alpha motor neurons in the brain stem and spinal cord[3,10,18] (Fig. 3–1).

The cerebellum and basal ganglia regulate motor functions but have no direct input to lower motor neurons. The cerebellum improves the accuracy of movement by signaling to the brain stem and cortical motor areas via the thalamus, after analyzing output from the motor cortex itself and sensory feedback from the spinal cord via the spinocerebellar tracts. The basal ganglia also monitor inputs from all cortical areas and project fibers to the frontal cortex through the thalamus to assist in motor planning and execution (see Fig 3–1). These two systems are crucial to control body movement but are not affected in ALS; hence, this chapter will focus on the neuroanatomy of the motor system directly or indirectly influencing lower motor neurons.

UPPER MOTOR NEURONS

Upper motor neurons (a somewhat ill-defined term) are located in the motor cortex and brain stem; thus, they are rostral to the lower motor neurons and exert direct or indirect supranuclear control over them.[18] The highest level of motor control occurs in the motor areas of the cerebral cortex, in-

34

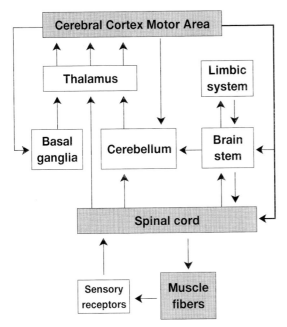

Figure 3–1. A schematic representation of the motor control system. Arrows indicate afferent or efferent direction of the neural control. The cerebellum and basal ganglia have no direct input to the lower motor neurons. The brain stem and spinal cord lower motor neurons receive supranuclear control from the cerebral cortex through the corticospinal tracts (heavy line) and brain-stem descending tracts. The principal areas where lesions occur in ALS are shaded.

muscles and control the force of contraction by varying the signal intensity. They also make direct synaptic contacts on several distinct motor nuclei at the same spinal segment and even at different spinal segments, although such divergence is less apparent in neurons innervating distal muscles.[5,10]

Voluntary movements differ from reflex movements because they are under conscious control, improve in effectiveness with experience and learning, and do not require external stimuli to be initiated. Whereas only 120 to 150 ms may elapse before a reflex action occurs in response to external stimuli, several hundred milliseconds are required to initiate any voluntary movement. The more complex the voluntary action, the longer the processing time for its initiation. Such motor planning is a major function of the premotor areas. Although the size of the primary motor cortex is similar between nonhuman primate and human brains, the premotor areas in humans are six times as large. The supplementary motor cortex is involved in the programming of complex sequences of movements rather than their execution. The premotor cortex, the most poorly understood of the premotor areas, probably controls proximal and axial muscles during the initial phases of orienting the body and arm to a target. In nonhuman primate studies, lesions of the primary cortex greatly diminish muscle actions, whereas those in the premotor areas result in the inability to develop an appropriate strategy for movement, resembling apraxia in the human.[5,24]

cluding the *primary motor cortex* (Brodmann's area 4) and the *premotor areas* (Brodmann's area 6), which are subdivided into the *supplementary motor area* (sometimes called the *secondary motor cortex*) and the *premotor cortex*.[5,19] All these motor areas are somatotopically organized. The topographic specificity of the corticospinal projection appears to be far more complex and broader than has been previously mapped onto muscles.[12,20,21] The upper motor neuron cortical cytoarchitecture differs from that of neurons in the sensory cortex because the internal granular layer (layer 4) is absent in motor cortex. Instead, the primary motor cortex has a distinct group of neurons in layer 5 known as the giant pyramidal neurons, or *Betz cells*. However, these neurons represent only a small portion of all primary motor neurons. Most are in layer 5, adjacent to the Betz cells. Individual motor neurons in the primary motor cortex trigger the contraction of small groups of skeletal

CORTICOSPINAL AND CORTICOBULBAR TRACTS

Axons from motor areas form the largest descending tracts of the brain, called the corticospinal and corticobulbar tracts (Fig. 3–2). Axons arising from neurons in the primary motor cortex, however, constitute only one-third of all the corticospinal and corticobulbar tracts. In fact, Betz cell axons make up only 3% to 5% of the approximately 1 million fibers in the tract, the rest arising from neurons in layer 5 of the primary motor cortex. Another one-third of the axons are derived from Brodmann's area 6, including the supplementary motor and lateral premotor cor-

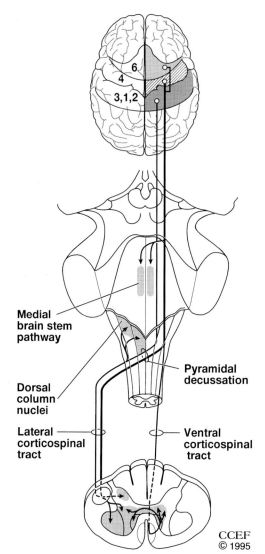

Medial
brain stem
pathway

Pyramidal
decussation

Dorsal
column
nuclei

Lateral
corticospinal
tract

Ventral
corticospinal
tract

CCEF
© 1995

Figure 3–2. The corticospinal and corticobulbar tracts originate in the broad areas of the cerebral cortices, including the primary motor cortex (area 4), premotor areas (area 6), primary sensory cortex (areas 1, 2, 3), and temporal cortex. The lateral corticospinal tract controls the interneurons and alpha motor neurons that are located in the lateral portion of the anterior horn and regulate extremity muscles. The nondecussating ventral corticospinal tract arises mainly from neck and trunk areas of the primary motor cortex and the premotor cortex, to signal the ipsilateral and contralateral motor neurons and control axial and truncal muscles. This tract also projects collateral to the medial brain-stem pathways. The corticospinal tract arising from the sensory cortex gives collateral to dorsal column nuclei and projects to the medial dorsal horn. The corticobulbar tract is not shown. (Adapted from Ghez, C: The control of movement. Posture. Voluntary movement. In Kandel, ER, Schwartz, JH, and Jessell, TM (eds): Principles of Neural Science, ed 3. Elsevier, New York, 1991, p 544.) (Copyright © the Cleveland Clinic Educational Foundation.)

tex. The remaining third is derived from the somatic sensory cortex (areas 1, 2, and 3) and the adjacent temporal lobe region.

The corticospinal and corticobulbar tracts converge in the internal capsule, specifically in its posterior limb, then pass through the ventral portion of the midbrain (the cerebral peduncle) and separate into small bundles in the basis pontis. The corticobulbar tract departs from the other main tracts at the level of the pons and medulla and projects bilaterally to the motor neurons of cranial nerves V, VII, IX, X , and XII. However, motor neurons innervating the lower face receive a predominantly contralateral input from the corticobulbar tract. Small bundles of the corticospinal tract at the pontine level regroup in the medulla to form a prominent medullary pyramid. Most corticospinal fibers (75% to 90%) decussate in the lower medulla (pyramidal decussation) and form the lateral corticospinal tract. The remaining fibers descend in the ipsilateral ventral corticospinal tract (see Fig. 3–2). The lateral corticospinal tract projects to ipsilateral motor neurons that innervate extremity muscles and their associated interneurons in the lateral anterior horn, whereas the anterior corticospinal tract ends bilaterally on ventromedial motor neurons and interneurons, which control axial and postural muscles. These corticospinal axons provide direct and strong glutamatergic excitatory input to alpha motor neurons[25] (Table 3–1). At the same time, they excite gamma motor neurons through polysynaptic pathways so that when extrafusal muscle-fiber shortening occurs, the muscle spindle length is adjusted and its afferent sensitivity is maintained. Axons originating from the somatic sensory cortex terminate primarily on Ia-inhibitory interneurons in the dorsal horn to regulate afferent input to motor neurons. The corticospinal tracts also give collateral inputs to the brain-stem nuclei that provide the brain-stem somatic motor control (see Fig 3–2).

BRAIN-STEM SOMATIC MOTOR CONTROL

Motor neurons of the spinal cord are influenced by the brain-stem nuclei through several control systems[4] (Fig. 3–3). There-

Table 3–1. **NEUROTRANSMITTERS IN THE MOTOR SYSTEM**

Neuronal System	Neurotransmitter
EXCITATORY	
Corticocortical association pathways	Glutamate
Corticospinal tract	Glutamate
Excitatory interneuron	Glutamate, aspartate
Primary sensory or afferent, excitatory	Glutamate
Nociceptive small-fiber afferent	Substance P
Lower motor neuron to muscle	Acetylcholine
Lower motor neurons to Renshaw cells	Acetylcholine
INHIBITORY	
Renshaw cells	Glycine, taurine
Primary sensory inhibitory	Glycine, taurine
Inhibitory interneurons	GABA
BRAIN-STEM DESCENDING PATHWAY	
Raphe nuclei	TRH, serotonin, substance P
Locus coeruleus	Norepinephrine

Abbreviations: GABA = gamma-aminobutyric acid; TRH = thyrotropin-releasing hormone.

fore, the neurons belonging to these brain-stem nuclei are upper motor neurons in a broad sense. The projections from the brain stem to motor neurons are highly complex. Somatic upper motor neuron control is organized mediolaterally.[10,14] The fibers originating in the medial and inferior vestibular nuclei in the medulla descend in the medial vestibulospinal tract, which terminates on medial cervical and thoracic motor neurons and medial interneurons. These fibers excite the corresponding ipsilateral cervical motor neurons and inhibit the contralateral neurons. The lateral vestibulospinal tracts originate in the lateral vestibular nucleus (Deiter's nucleus) and provide polysynaptic facilitation to the extensor motor neurons and inhibition to the flexor motor neurons in both upper and lower extremities.

The brain-stem reticular formation also strongly influences spinal motor neurons (see Fig. 3–3). The pontine reticular formation, located in the ventral pontine tegmentum, gives rise to the medial reticulospinal tract, which descends along the ventral column of the spinal cord; this tract facilitates the firing of axial muscle and limb extensor muscle motor neurons. In contrast, the medullary reticular formation, which origi-

nates from the gigantocellular nucleus, projects to the lateral reticulospinal tracts in the lateral column of the spinal cord and causes monosynaptic inhibition of cervical and thoracic motor neurons. This tract also exerts widespread polysynaptic inhibitory inputs on extensor motor neurons and exerts excitatory inputs on flexor motor neurons. The reticulospinal tracts modulate various reflex actions during ongoing movements. The brain-stem reticular formation receives supranuclear control from the motor cortex, via the corticoreticulospinal pathway, to act as a major inhibitor of spinal reflexes and activity (see Fig 3–2). Therefore, a lesion of the corticoreticular pathway can disinhibit reticulospinal control of lower motor neurons.

The tectospinal tract originates in the superior colliculus and controls eye and head movement. Although in other mammals the rubrospinal tract begins in the red nucleus and projects to distal limb muscle motor neurons, in humans it is vestigial.

LIMBIC MOTOR CONTROL

The limbic system is closely involved in emotional experience and expression and is

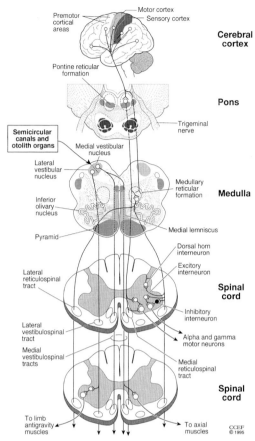

Figure 3–3. Brain-stem somatic motor control. The reticulospinal tract and vestibulospinal tract are the two key brain-stem tracts. Both tracts are organized mediolaterally. The medial tracts regulate the interneuron system located in the medial portion of the anterior horn, controlling axial muscles, whereas the lateral tracts regulate the interneurons located in the lateral anterior horn, to control the extremity muscles. (Copyright © the Cleveland Clinic Educational Foundation.)

associated with a wide variety of autonomic, visceral, and endocrine functions.[10,16] Recent studies clearly indicate that the limbic system strongly influences somatic motor neurons; this organization is termed the *limbic motor control system*.[9,10] According to Holstege,[10] this system is independent of other major descending somatic brain-stem tracts and corticospinal and corticobulbar tracts, which form another major motor control system. These two motor control systems overlap very little, the exception being the monoaminergic projections originating in the raphe system and locus coeruleus complex.

The limbic motor control system can be generally organized into the lateral and medial components.[10] The medial component originates in the medial hypothalamus and mesencephalon and terminates in the area of the locus coeruleus and subcoeruleus, in the ventral caudal pontine, and in the medullary medial tegmental field. This component sends monoaminergic projections into the somatosensory and motor neurons and thus globally affects their activity by changing their membrane potential. The emotional status and experience of an individual determines the overall spinal cord activity. The lateral component, in contrast to the medial component, originates in the lateral limbic system—the lateral hypothalamus, central nucleus of the amygdala, and bed nucleus of the stria terminalis. The prefrontal cortex is also involved, but the extent of the involvement is unclear. These structures project onto the lateral tegmental fields of the caudal pons and medulla. The lateral component of the limbic motor system influences respiration, vomiting, swallowing, chewing, and licking.

In addition to the mediolateral components, the periaqueductal gray (PAG) of the mesencephalon is important in limbic motor control. The limbic system has strong reciprocal connections with mesencephalic structures, particularly the PAG, that are considered as part of the limbic system itself.[10] Crying and laughing are expressive behaviors, which are called vocalization in animal behavior.[8,9] Stimulating the caudal PAG in many species, including primates, produces similar vocalization. Holstege[8] found that a specific group of neurons in the lateral area (and, to a limited extent, the dorsal area) of the caudal PAG sends fibers to the nucleus retroambiguus in the caudal medulla. The nucleus retroambiguus in turn projects to the somatic motor neurons that innervate the pharynx; soft palate; intercostal, diaphragmatic, and abdominal muscles; and probably the larynx (Fig. 3–4). The generation of pseudobulbar signs is closely related to abnormality in this system (see Chapter 4).

A large number of neurotransmitters or neuromodulators are involved in the limbic motor control system. Glutamate and aspartate, but not acetylcholine, are found throughout the system. Descending tracts of

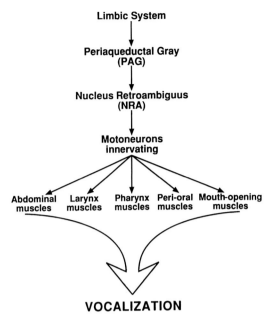

VOCALIZATION

Figure 3–4. Electrical stimulation of the periaqueductal gray (PAG) in many animal species induces automatic vocalization. The PAG has strong reciprocal control from the limbic system. The PAG fibers end at the nucleus retroambiguus (NRA), which functions as the coordinating center for vocalization, stimulating muscle groups involved in vocalization. (From Holstege, G: Somatic motor neurons and descending motor pathways. Limbic and non-limbic components. In Leigh, PN and Swash, M (eds): Motor Neuron Disease. Biology and Management. Springer-Verlag, London, 1995, p 305, with permission.)

the limbic motor control system, however, consist mainly of serotonergic fibers. Serotonin exerts an excitatory influence on motor neurons. Other peptides are also involved with the descending tracts. They include substance P, thyrotropin-releasing hormone, somatostatin, and enkephalin, and to a limited degree, vasoactive intestinal peptide and cholecystokinin. In these descending fibers, sometimes more than one peptide appears to coexist in the same neuron.[7,10]

INTERNEURONS

The interneurons are of paramount importance in determining the final output of the motor neurons. Interneurons residing in the anterior horn of the spinal cord and brain stem constitute the major motor control system, along with the other two motor control systems, the motor control system involving descending somatic brain-stem tracts and corticospinal and corticobulbar tracts, and the limbic motor control system.[10] The interneuron system receives hierarchical and parallel motor control by the brain-stem descending tracts and corticospinal tracts and by the limbic motor control.[10] These interneurons also receive direct or indirect afferent information from the afferent peripheral nerves. Interneurons form intricate neuronal circuits involving the automatic and stereotyped spinal reflexes. These reflexes can function even when the spinal cord is separated from the brain. The interneuron circuit coordinates the integrated activation of synergist muscles and inhibition of antagonist muscles (Fig. 3–5) and controls the timing of these integrated actions. These interneurons are not always located close to the projecting motor neurons; for example, some interneurons controlling back muscles send axons over a great distance.

Depending on the pattern of motor action, the interneurons can also control contralateral motor pools. Renshaw cells, which are unique interneurons, provide a negative feedback loop to motor neurons by regulating their excitability and stabilizing their firing rates.[3] Renshaw cells use glycine and perhaps taurine for inhibitory neurotransmission[7] (see Table 3–1). The interneuron circuit receives excitatory and inhibitory descending inputs and afferent muscle signals to control the overall excitability of motor neurons.[17,23] It also controls protective and postural reflexes triggered by noxious cutaneous stimuli. The same network of interneurons that mediates such stereotyped reflex behavior now is known also to provide the basic functional units involved in highly skillful voluntary movements. In 1947, Sherrington[22] showed that virtually all reflexes involve an integrated activation and inhibition of different muscle groups, largely coordinated by the spinal interneurons. Ultimately, all interneuronal paths converge on the motor neurons that innervate the skeletal muscles. He called this terminal path the *final common path* and said "the motor nerve to a muscle is a collection of such final common paths."

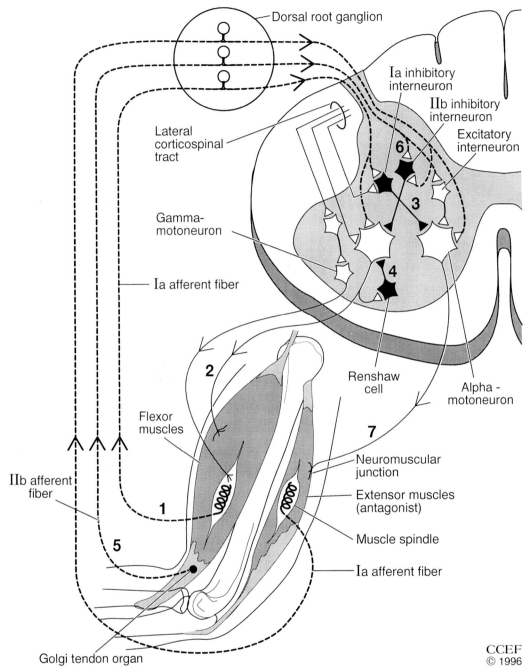

Figure 3–5. A simplified diagrammatic presentation of the interneurons and alpha motor neurons. The Ia afferent and corticospinal tract fibers transmit monosynaptic excitatory signals to alpha motor neurons, resulting in direct muscle contractions. All muscle contractions are coordinated by the interneuron system. When a flexor muscle is stretched, as shown, the stretch stimulates intrafusal spindle fibers, sending excitatory impulses through Ia afferent fibers (1), which stimulates the contraction of the same muscle (2). The Ia afferent fibers simultaneously stimulate Ia inhibitory interneurons, which inhibit the alpha motor neurons of antagonist extensor muscles (3), so that flexor muscle contraction can be carried out without resistance. The excitation of alpha motor neurons sends collateral signals to Renshaw cells that regulate their own excitation (4). At the same time, the mechanical contraction of the flexor muscle stretches the Golgi tendon organ, which then sends IIb inhibitory signals (5). This signal stimulates the IIb inhibitory interneurons (6), which exert polysynaptic inhibitory inputs on the original alpha motor neurons and polysynaptic excitatory inputs on alpha motor neurons controlling antagonist extensor muscles (6); the antagonist con-

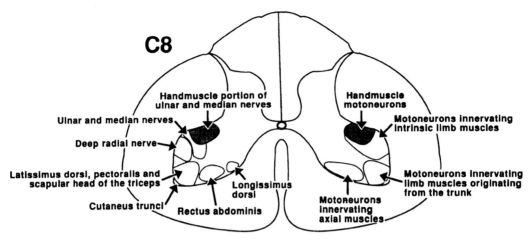

Figure 3–6. Lower motor neurons in the anterior horn are clustered in the motor nucleus and somatotopically organized. Anatomical tracing techniques identified motor nuclei in the cervical spinal cord as shown in this diagram. (From Holstege, G: Somatic motor neurons and descending motor pathways. Limbic and nonlimbic components. In Leigh, PN and Swash, M (eds): Motor Neuron Disease. Biology and Management. Springer-Verlag, London, 1995, p 262, with permission.)

LOWER MOTOR NEURONS

The lower motor neurons are located in the brain stem and spinal cord and send out motor axons directly to innervate skeletal muscle fibers. These motor neurons are lowest in the hierarchy of motor control. Those in the spinal cord are clustered in nuclei or motor neuron pools, forming longitudinal columns extending from one to four spinal segments (Fig. 3–6). Because lower motor neurons are located in the anterior gray matter, or anterior horn, they are also known as *anterior horn cells.* Anterior horn cells vary in size.[11] Large motor neurons are the most common and often are called *alpha motor neurons;* they are the principal motor neurons innervating muscle fibers. Medium-sized motor neurons, conventionally called the *beta motor neurons,* innervate both muscle fibers and intrafusal (muscle spindle) fibers.[6] Intermediate and small motor neurons innervating the spindle fibers constitute approximately one-third of the lower motor neurons. They are called *gamma motor neurons* or *fusimotor neurons.* The rest of the small anterior horn cells are *interneurons.* The alpha motor neuron is among the largest neurons of the nervous system. It has a single axon extending to its innervated muscles and a number of large dendrites that sometimes reach more than 1 mm in width and extend well into the white matter of the spinal cord to provide an extensive receptive field[1] (Fig. 3–7). A great number of synaptic boutons (estimated at up to 10,000) contact the dendritic surface. Synapses that relay excitatory inputs to motor neurons are located at the proximal portion of the dendrites or at the soma itself, whereas inhibitory synapses are concentrated along the initial segment of the axon.[1] In alpha motor neurons, acetylcholine is the excitatory neurotransmitter at the neuromuscular junction and Renshaw cells (see Table 3–1).

In general, motor neurons innervating the distal muscles of the extremities are located in the dorsal anterior horn, whereas those

---

traction (7) inhibits further flexor contraction and restores the flexor muscle to the original position. In another mechanism, flexor muscle contraction shortens intrafusal spindle muscle fibers, which stimulates another feedback system, signaling gamma motor neurons to contract the intrafusal spindle fibers so that the sensitivity of the spindle fibers to stretch is restored. The corticospinal tract fibers also stimulate polysynaptic excitatory interneurons to stimulate gamma motor neurons so that the sensitivity to stretch is increased, causing hyperreflexia. (Copyright © the Cleveland Clinic Educational Foundation.)

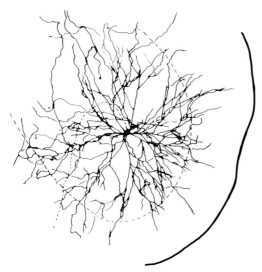

Figure 3–7. A typical alpha motor neuron in a transverse section. Note the extensive dendritic system, some of which extends into the white matter. The thick dotted line indicates an axon arising from the perikaryon. A gray and white matter junction is shown by the thin line of dashes. (From Brown, AG: Organization in the Spinal Cord. Springer-Verlag, Berlin, 1981, p 199, with permission.)

innervating proximal muscles of the extremities reside in the more ventral anterior horn. Motor neurons innervating axial and truncal muscles are the most medially located. The cervical enlargement of the spinal cord is the result of a markedly enlarged lateral anterior horn, which contains motor neurons for the arm and hand muscles (see Fig. 3–6).

One alpha motor neuron innervates one group of muscle fibers.[3,13] This group constitutes the smallest unit of the motor system. The combination of the motor axon and all the muscle fibers it innervates was termed the *motor unit* by Liddell and Sherrington.[15] The size of a motor unit depends on the type of muscle and is measured by the innervation ratio, which is the number of muscle fibers innervated by a single motor neuron. In the exquisitely sensitive small extraocular muscles, this ratio is approximately 1:10; in the intrinsic hand muscles, it rises to about 1:100; in moderately large muscles (e.g., biceps muscle), it increases to about 1:500; and in the largest muscles (e.g., gastrocnemius muscle), it may exceed 1:2000. The muscle fibers belonging to one motor unit are not grouped together but rather are dispersed over a limited area in the skeletal muscle. This area is known as the *motor unit territory* and reaches an area approximately 20 mm^2 in the biceps brachii.[2] Thus, many motor units overlap their territories within the muscle. Such an arrangement allows the muscle to contract smoothly and evenly.

The motor neuron determines the characteristic physiology of muscle contraction in its motor unit. Functionally, there are three types of muscle fibers: slow nonfatigable, fast fatigable, and intermediate, fast nonfatigable.[3] The differences between the two distinct functional types are shown in Table 3–2. Proximal and axial muscles that sustain body posture contain predominantly slow nonfatigable motor units, whereas extremity muscles involved in fast phasic or ballistic contractions that quickly generate large force possess largely fast fatigable motor units.

Table 3–2. PHYSIOLOGIC AND METABOLIC PROPERTIES OF MOTOR UNIT TYPES

Characteristic	Slow Nonfatigable	Fast Fatigable
Histochemical type	Type I	Type II
Contraction time	Long	Fast
Tetanic contraction	Easy	Difficult
Fatigue	Hard	Fast
Motor axon size	Small	Large
Force generation	Small	Large
Muscle metabolism	Oxidative	Glycolytic
Muscle type	Axial, postural	Distal, phasic

SUMMARY

Muscle contraction is the final event of the highly elaborate and hierarchical motor control system, and to understand the signs, symptoms, and disease process of ALS, the clinician must understand this system. The motor areas of the cerebral cortex exert the highest level of control, are somatopically organized, and initiate voluntary movements. The premotor area is involved with motor planning, and the supplementary motor cortex programs complex sequences of muscle movements.

The corticospinal tract arises from not only the motor areas but also the neighboring areas of cerebral cortex, and exerts direct and indirect control over interneurons and lower motor neurons. It divides into two tracts: the lateral, which controls extremity muscle contractions, and the anterior, which controls axial and postural muscle contractions.

The brain-stem descending tracts originate in the vestibular nuclei and brain-stem reticular formation and are organized mediolaterally in the spinal cord. The medial tracts control involuntary reflex motions of the head, neck, and trunk, and influence axial muscles. The lateral tracts control spinal reflexes and extensor and flexor muscles of both extremities.

The limbic system provides independent motor control; is closely involved in emotional expression; and is associated with autonomic, visceral, and endocrine functions. The mesencephalic PAG, which has strong reciprocal input from the limbic system, exerts unique control over pharyngeal, laryngeal, respiratory, and abdominal muscles through the nucleus retroambiguus located in the caudal medulla. This system is closely associated with the generation of forced crying and laughter.

The interneuron system is key in determining the final output of the lower motor neurons. This system coordinates agonist-antagonist and ipsilateral-contralateral muscle contractions. It also controls automatic and stereotyped spinal reflexes to produce highly skilled movements. The motor control system ultimately converges on motor neurons that innervate muscle, forming the *final common path*.

Lower motor neurons vary in size. Alpha motor neurons are among the largest and have a broad dendritic receptive field. One alpha motor neuron innervates one group of muscle fibers to form the motor unit. The alpha motor neuron determines the physiologic properties of its motor unit. Gamma motor neurons innervate intrafusal muscle fibers, controlling the sensitivity of the muscle spindle.

REFERENCES

1. Brown, AG: Organization in the Spinal Cord. Springer-Verlag, Berlin, 1981.
2. Buchthal, F, Guld, C, and Rosenfalck, P: Multielectrode study of the territory of a motor unit. Acta Physiol Scand 39:83–104, 1957.
3. Ghez, C: The control of movement. Posture. Voluntary movement. In Kandel, ER, Schwartz, JH, and Jessell, TM (eds): Principles of Neural Science. Elsevier, New York, 1991, pp 533–547.
4. Ghez, C: Posture. In Kandel, ER, Schwartz, JH, and Jessell, TM (eds): Principles of Neural Science. Elsevier, New York, 1991, pp 598–607.
5. Ghez, C: Voluntary movement. In Kandel, ER, Schwartz, JH, and Jessell, TM (eds): Principles of Neural Science. Elsevier, New York, 1991, pp 609–625.
6. Gilman, S and Newman, SW: Manter and Gatz's Essentials of Clinical Neuroanatomy and Neurophysiology, ed 9. FA Davis, Philadelphia, 1992.
7. Guiloff, RJ: Clinical pharmacology of motor neurons. In Leigh, PN and Swash, M (eds): Motor Neuron Disease. Biology and Management. Springer-Verlag, London, 1995, pp 245–373.
8. Holstege, G: An anatomical study of the final common pathways for vocalization in the cat. J Camp Neurol 284:242–252, 1989.
9. Holstege, G: Descending motor pathways and the spinal motor system. Limbic and non-limbic components. In Holstege, G (ed): Role of the Forebrain in Sensation and Behavior. Elsevier, Amsterdam, 1991, pp 307–421.
10. Holstege, G: Somatic motoneurons and descending motor pathways. Limbic and non-limbic components. In Leigh, PN and Swash, M (eds): Motor Neuron Disease. Biology and Management. Springer-Verlag, London, 1995, pp 259–330.
11. Kawamura, Y, O'Brien, P, Okazaki, H, et al: Lumbar motor neurons of man. II. The number and diameter distribution of large- and intermediate-diameter cytons in "motoneuron columns" of spinal cord of man. J Neuropathol Exp Neurol 36:861–870, 1977.
12. Kew, JJM, Leigh, PN, Playford, ED, et al: Cortical function in amyotrophic lateral sclerosis. Brain 116:655–680, 1993.
13. Krnjevic, K: Transmitters in motor systems. In Burke, RE (ed): Handbook of Physiology. Sec I, The Nervous System, Vol 2. Motor System. Ameri-

can Physiological Society, Washington, 1981, pp 107–154.

14. Kuypers, HGJM: Anatomy of the descending pathways. In Burke, RE (ed): Handbook of Physiology. Sec I, The Nervous System. Vol 2, Motor System. American Physiological Society, Washington, 1981, pp 597–666.

15. Liddell, EGT and Sherrington, C: Reflexes in response to stretch (myotatic reflexes). Proc R Soc Lond [Biol] 96:212–242, 1924.

16. MacLean, PD: Some psychiatric implications of physiological studies on frontotemporal portion of limbic system. EEG Clin Neurophysiol 4:407–418, 1952.

17. O'Brien, RJ and Fischbach, GD: Modulation of embryonic chick motor neuron glutamate sensitivity by interneurones and agonists. J Neurosci 6:3290–3296, 1986.

18. Phillips, CG and Landau, WM: Upper and lower motor neurons: The little old synecdoche that works. Neurology 40:884–886, 1990.

19. Porter, P: Brain mechanisms of voluntary motor commands—A review. Electroenceph Clin Neurophysiol 76:282–293, 1990.

20. Remy, P, Silbovicius, M, Leroy-Willig, A, et al: Movement- and task-related activations of motor cortical areas: A positron emission tomographic study. Ann Neurol 36:19–26, 1994.

21. Schieber, MH and Hibbard, LS: How somatotopic is the motor cortex hand area? Science 261:489–492, 1993.

22. Sherrington, C: The integrative action of the nervous system, ed 2. Yale University Press, New Haven, 1947.

23. Storm-Mathison, J and Otterson, OP: Localization of excitatory amino acid transmitters. In Lodge, D (ed): Excitatory Amino Acids in Health and Disease. John Wiley & Sons, Chichester, 1988, pp 107–143.

24. Weis, SP and Strick PL: Anatomical and physiological organization of the non-primary motor cortex. Trends Neurosci 7:442–446, 1984.

25. Young, AB, Penney, JB, Dauth, GW, et al: Glutamate or aspartate as a possible neurotransmitter of the cerebral cortico-fugal fibers in the monkey. Neurology 33:1513–1516, 1983.

PART 2

Clinical Features of ALS

CHAPTER 4

CLINICAL FEATURES: SIGNS AND SYMPTOMS

A grasp of the clinical features of ALS is more important than any technology for the clinician who is involved in the diagnostic evaluation of patients who may have this disease. This chapter thus reviews the clinical features of ALS in detail. Sporadic and familial ALS manifest no features to distinguish one from another clinically,[63] and therefore the discussion in this chapter is applicable to both types of ALS.

UPPER MOTOR NEURON SYNDROME

When upper motor neuron control is lost suddenly, as in the case of acute spinal cord trauma, muscle movements completely cease, a condition called *spinal shock*. This condition results from an abrupt loss of normal function (performance) of the upper motor neurons at the spinal cord level. In ALS, however, upper motor neuron dysfunction develops slowly, resulting in an imbalance between inhibitory effects on stretch reflexes mediated

Table 4–1. **SIGNS OF UPPER AND LOWER MOTOR NEURON SYNDROME**

Upper Motor Neuron Syndrome	Lower Motor Neuron Syndrome
Loss of dexterity	Loss of muscle strength
Loss of muscle strength	Muscle atrophy
Spasticity	Hyporeflexia
Hyperreflexia	Muscle hypotonia
Pathologic reflex	Fasciculations
Pseudobulbar sign	Muscle cramps
Flexor spasms	

by the dorsal reticulospinal tract and facilitatory effects on extensor spasticity that are mediated by the medial reticulospinal tract, and to some extent, by the vestibulospinal tract.[5] Slowly progressive loss of upper motor neuron control is clinically manifested as the signs and symptoms listed in Table 4–1.

Loss of Dexterity

Voluntary skillful movements result from the integrated activation of many interneuron circuits in the spinal cord, but the corticospinal tract ultimately controls such actions. Thus, a prominent upper motor neuron dysfunction is loss of dexterity. When dexterity is impaired, voluntary and even reflex motions become awkward. This loss may be expressed as stiffness, slowness, and clumsiness in any skillful motor actions. The loss of dexterity is demonstrated by testing the patient's ability to perform rapid repetitive motions with fingers, feet, or even lip or tongue. For example, when the patient is asked to flex and extend both thumb and index finger repetitively as fast as possible, slow and clumsy motion can be detected easily. Similar impairment can be detected by repetitive pronation and supination of the forearm or by tapping the floor with the foot.

Loss of Muscle Strength (Weakness)

Another manifestation of the upper motor neuron syndrome is loss of muscle strength. The degree of muscle weakness resulting from upper motor neuron dysfunction is generally mild and not as severe as that seen in lower motor neuron involvement because the motor units are preserved (Table 4–2). A patient's subjective complaint of "muscle weakness" may not indicate a true loss of muscle strength (Table 4–3). A careful neurologic history and examination are essential to exclude other neurologic causes for subjectively felt weakness. In the upper motor neuron syndrome, extensor muscles of the upper extremities and flexor muscles of lower extremities may become weaker than their antagonist muscles because the upper motor neuron lesion disinhibits brain-stem control of the vestibulospinal and reticulospinal tracts, thus increasing muscle spasticity in the flexor muscles of the upper extremities and the extensor muscles of the lower extremities. In patients with severe upper motor neuron syndrome, accurately assessing muscle strength becomes difficult because spasticity and loss of dexterity prevent effective activation of the motor units.

Table 4–2. **MUSCLE WEAKNESS IN UPPER OR LOWER MOTOR NEURON DYSFUNCTION**

Characteristic	Upper Motor Neuron	Lower Motor Neuron
Mechanism	Spasticity Disinhibition Loss of voluntary control	Loss of motor units
Degree of weakness	Modest	Severe
Muscle atrophy	Mild	Severe
Stretch reflexes	Exaggerated	Diminished

Table 4–3. **CAUSES OF "MUSCLE WEAKNESS" DESCRIBED BY PATIENTS**

Loss of muscle strength
Variation of muscle strength
Fatigability
Diminished range of movement
Slowed rate of movement
Loss of coordination
Clumsiness
Lack of ability to carry out skilled acts

Table 4–4. **ASHWORTH SPASTICITY SCALE**

Value	Observation
0	Passive movement of joint impossible
1	Increased tone sufficient to require effort on part of examiner to overcome resistance
2	Definite resistance to passive movement
3	Slight catch: passive movement of limb otherwise unimpeded
4	Normal

Spasticity

Spasticity is the central feature of the upper motor neuron syndrome. The pathophysiology of spasticity is complex and controversial.[5,50] A lesion of the upper motor neurons or their descending fibers can result in disinhibition of the facilitatory vestibulospinal and medial reticulospinal tracts, leading to spasticity usually involving flexors of the upper extremities and extensors of the lower extremities.[5,49] The loss of corticospinal tract integrity between the upper and lower motor neurons blocks the major excitatory input over both alpha and gamma motor neurons. This block may result in remodelling of interneuron circuits and denervation hypersensitivity that may enhance overall excitability of lower motor neurons. Furthermore, the upper motor neuron lesion disinhibits a polysynaptic Ia-inhibitory input normally exerted by the corticospinal tract, again resulting in spasticity. Experimentally, abnormal muscle resistance to passive manipulation in the form of rigidity and spasticity can be abolished by dorsal root transection (rhizotomy), indicating that Ia afferents are essential to maintain spasticity—the defining feature of the upper motor neuron syndrome.[82]

Spasticity is a state of sustained increase in muscle tension when the muscle is lengthened. Electrophysiologic studies in patients with upper motor neuron lesions show that passive movement elicits a tonic reflex that predominates during muscle stretch and muscle shortening. In these patients, movement is primarily impaired not because of an abnormal stretch reflex in antagonist muscles, but rather because of prolonged recruitment and delayed relaxation of agonist contraction.[74] Clinically, muscles lose normal smoothness during passive movement and suddenly increase their resistance and resist further passive movement. This resistance is referred to as a "catch." However, when a sustained passive stretch is applied to spastic muscles, they quickly release the tension and relax, an event often described as the "clasp-knife phenomenon." In muscles with severe spasticity, passive movement becomes more difficult and even impossible. Rigidity, a key manifestation of extrapyramidal disease, is another important type of increased resistance to passive manipulation, but in contrast to spasticity, it is plastic to passive movement and often is described as having a "lead-pipe" quality. The Ashworth spasticity scale,[1] graded from 0 to 4, is helpful in classifying spasticity severity (Table 4–4). In a spastic gait, the lower extremities lose their natural flexion movement at the hips and knees; instead, the legs stiffen and, with each step, circumduct at the hip.

Pathologic Hyperreflexia (Increased Muscle Stretch Reflexes)

Pathologic hyperreflexia is another crucial manifestation of the upper motor neuron syndrome (see Table 4–1). When the muscle tendon is tapped, muscle spindles are stretched and an afferent impulse is generated from the primary ending of the spindle fiber. In healthy people, this impulse produces a typical monosynaptic stretch reflex through excitation of the alpha motor neuron. When upper motor neuron control is interrupted, stretch reflexes are exaggerated because polysynaptic Ia-inhibitory input is reduced. In pathologic hyperreflexia, only a slight or distant stimulus is needed to elicit a reflex response. For example, an ordinary tendon tap elicits reflexes in neighboring muscles (spreading), and manual stretching of the muscle induces repeated, rhythmic muscle contraction (muscle clonus). Such responses are considered pathologic, indicating that upper motor neurons are affected. In ALS, one finds a unique situation: severely wasted, nearly paralyzed muscles, from which one would expect no or minimal stretch reflex activity, instead have markedly brisk stretch reflexes, a feature indicating that both upper and lower motor neurons are involved.[87] A variety of cutaneous reflexes, such as superficial abdominal and cremasteric reflexes, are usually intact in ALS.

Pathologic Reflexes

So-called pathologic reflexes, which actually are primitive reflexes normally present during early development, are released only when the upper motor neuron control over these reflexes is disinhibited. The Babinski sign (extensor plantar response) is the most important sign in clinical neurology and is characterized by extension of the great toe, often accompanied by fanning of the other toes, in response to stroking the outer edge of the ipsilateral sole upward from the heel with a blunt object.[2,13] In healthy adults, great-toe flexion is the expected response. Toe extension in the Babinski response therefore results from the mechanical overpowering of the toe flexor muscle. This sign is sometimes associated with foot dorsiflexion and contraction of the tensor fascia latae and other extensor muscles (the triphasic response). The Babinski sign, if present, is a definitive sign of upper motor neuron disease. Its importance in identifying upper motor neuron involvement in ALS recently has been re-emphasized by Rowland,[73] who found that most cases demonstrating a Babinski sign had corticospinal involvement at autopsy. Several eponymic reflexes, such as Oppenheim's,

Chaddock's, and Gordon's reflexes, are modifications of the Babinski sign and indicate upper motor neuron involvement.[13]

"No toe movement" is often considered as a positive upper motor neuron sign, but only when the contralateral side shows normal toe flexion. It is not unusual to find patients with ALS who have all the classic upper motor neuron signs except the Babinski sign. Landau[51] electrophysiologically studied this issue in depth and found that lower motor neuron involvement weakens the toe extensor muscles, which results in factitious toe flexion when the plantar surface is stimulated. In this situation, plantar stimulation triggers a vigorous motor unit firing pattern in both toe flexor and extensor muscles, identical to that found in patients with a typical extensor plantar response in ALS. Therefore, a flexor plantar response accompanied by other signs of upper motor neuron dysfunction does not imply that the crucial upper motor neuron sign is missing. In the upper motor neuron syndrome, the same plantar stimulation may trigger the reflex contraction of the ipsilateral tensor fascia latae, which is a particularly helpful test when toe extensor muscles are paralyzed. This response involves a few repetitive contractions of the tensor fascia latae muscle in the lateral aspect of the thigh. This reflex has the same clinical significance as the Babinski sign.

In the upper extremities, Hoffmann's sign may be considered to be a pathologic reflex. This reflex is triggered by a quick release after the forceful flexion of the most distal phalangeal joint of the middle finger. A reflex flexion and adduction of the ipsilateral thumb is a positive reflex. Tapping the belly of the tip of the middle finger can also elicit a similar thumb flexion (Trömner's sign). When these reflexes appear ipsilaterally, they are always abnormal. However, bilateral positive reflexes may not be abnormal because they are not unusual in healthy, young, anxious individuals. When upper motor neuron signs also exist, these reflexes should be considered pathologic.[13]

Spastic Bulbar Palsy

When upper motor neurons and the corticobulbar fibers controlling speech, mastication, and deglutition are affected, a unique upper motor neuron syndrome, spastic bulbar palsy, appears. The term *pseudobulbar palsy* is often used to distinguish it from bulbar palsy, which is a result of lower motor neuron involvement in the brain stem (see p 53).

Tonic Flexor Spasms

When the corticospinal tract is partially damaged at the spinal cord level, sometimes tonic flexor spasms are released. They are characterized by sudden spasmodic flexion of the legs at the hips, knees, and ankles: a typical mass avoidance reflex.[13] They may occur spontaneously but often are triggered by various painful stimuli to the lower extremities. These flexor spasms are not present in patients with ALS.

LOWER MOTOR NEURON SYNDROME

In ALS, the upper and lower motor neuron syndromes always manifest themselves in combination and in varying degrees, resulting in a complex clinical syndrome. The diagnostic process for ALS is discussed separately in Chapter 6.

Loss of Muscle Strength (Weakness)

The loss of a motor neuron means the loss of its motor unit, whereas impaired motor neuron function leads to abnormal or impaired activation of the motor unit. In either case, a progressive decrease in the number of functional motor units reduces the muscle twitch tension (muscle strength). Weakness caused by the lower motor neuron involvement differs from that seen in the upper motor neuron syndrome (see Table 4–2). Studies in patients with acute poliomyelitis indicate that more than 50% of lower motor neurons must be lost before muscle weakness is clinically detected.[81] In healthy individuals, more than enough motor units are available to generate the necessary muscle twitch tension and offset an unexpected loss of motor neurons. In a disease causing chronic motor unit depletion, denervated muscle fibers

Table 4–5. **MEDICAL RESEARCH COUNCIL SCALE FOR MUSCLE STRENGTH TESTING**

Value	Observation
0	No movement
1	Flicker of motion
2	Movement with gravity eliminated
3	Strength against gravity only but no resistance to passive force
4	Strength with resistance to passive force but can be overcome
5	Normal

belonging to a diseased motor unit are reinnervated by neighboring healthy motor neurons so that existing motor units are continually modified[4] (see Chapter 5).

Muscle weakness is the cardinal sign and symptom of ALS (see Table 4–1). It is almost always focal in onset and is followed by progressive weakness of contiguous muscles.[3,84] Weakness in ALS is not associated with pain, but patients may complain of muscle cramps and ill-defined pain. As mentioned before, "muscle weakness" may be an expression of many different conditions underlying motor abnormalities (see Table 4–2).

The degree of muscle weakness is assessed at the bedside by manual muscle strength testing. For this purpose, most neurologists use the Medical Research Council (MRC) scale[56] (Table 4–5) or modifications of it. Because of the subjectivity of manual muscle strength testing and the large difference between MRC scale values 4 and 5, the maximum voluntary isometric contraction measurement is used to obtain more accurate quantitative measurement (see Chapter 20).

Truncal Muscle Weakness

Whereas weakness in cervical flexor muscles is seen in many neuromuscular diseases, such as muscular dystrophy and polymyositis, cervical extensor weakness is rare and seen almost exclusively in ALS and myasthenia gravis. Weakness of the neck extensors causes heaviness of the head and often allows the head to fall forward (head droop): patients frequently support their heads with one

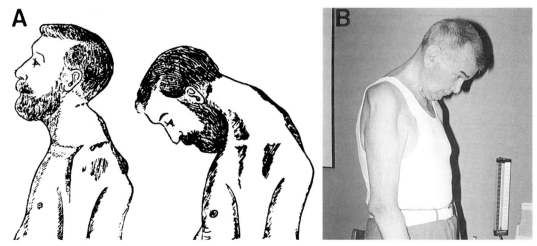

Figure 4–1. (*A*) A typical posture shown in an 1888 textbook by William Gowers is the most revealing of this difficult problem. The head tends to fall forward because the neck extensor and thoracic paraspinal muscles are weak. (From Kuncl, RW, et al.: Assessment of thoracic paraspinal muscles in the diagnosis of ALS. Muscle Nerve 11:485, 1988. © 1988. Reprinted by permission of Wiley-Liss, Inc., a subsidiary of John Wiley & Sons, Inc.) (*B*) Marked head droop in a 65-year-old man with ALS who first developed progressive weakness in both upper extremities. Head droop causes neck pain and marked functional impairment.

hand. In advanced stages, the neck becomes completely flexed with the head dropped forward, which limits the patient's ability to look more than a few feet away. Consequently, walking, eating, and even breathing are seriously impaired. Muscle pain in the overstretched neck extensors is common. A compensatory lordosis may occur as patients attempt to maintain their posture while walking. This unusual head position was originally described by Gowers[23] and its importance was recently re-emphasized by Kuncl and colleagues[47] (Fig. 4–1).

Muscle Atrophy

When muscle fibers are denervated, they atrophy. Loss of a motor neuron leads to atrophy of the entire motor unit; partial damage to a motor unit causes limited atrophy of the corresponding muscle fibers. In ALS, progressive loss of motor neurons results in a reduction of muscle volume and size that is clinically observed as wasting of affected skeletal muscles. Atrophy of the intrinsic hand muscles is easily recognized by patients and physicians, even in early stages of the disease (Fig. 4–2). Proximal and lower-extremity muscles also atrophy.

Hyporeflexia

If the disease involves the lower motor neurons only, muscle stretch reflexes are reduced or absent. This is a result of the loss of active motor units and insufficient muscle contraction, even when the excitatory afferent arc is intact. When muscles become totally paralyzed or atrophied, the hyperreflexia noted earlier in the course of the disease may disappear.

Muscle Hypotonicity or Flaccidity

Hypotonicity or flaccidity refers to the decrease or complete loss of normal muscle resistance to passive manipulation. In contrast to spasticity, the muscle lies inert and flaccid.

Fasciculations

Fasciculations are observed clinically as fine, rapid, flickering, and sometimes vermicular twitching movements of a muscle portion that occur irregularly in time and location. Fasciculations are the result of spontaneous contractions of a group of muscle fibers belonging to a single motor unit. The

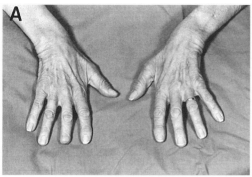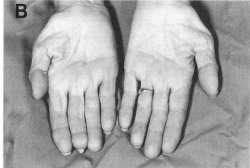

Figure 4–2. (*A*) Marked intrinsic hand muscle atrophy is seen, particularly in the interosseous muscles. (*B*) The palm of the hand shows that the thenar eminence is markedly atrophied because of atrophy of the abductor pollicis brevis.

impulse for the fasciculation appears to arise from hyperexcitable distal motor axons and is perhaps multifocal in origin.[12,72,85] The underlying mechanism of fasciculations is not fully understood, but we discuss them further in Chapter 5.

In general, the larger the muscle, the greater the size of the fasciculations. In tongue muscles, for example, fasciculations produce small vermicular movements on its surface. Fasciculations are found in nearly all ALS patients, but rarely are they a presenting symptom. If fasciculations are not found in a patient who is suspected to have ALS, one must be cautious in the diagnostic process. Fasciculations can be easily induced after forceful muscle contraction or focal tapping over the muscles. When their presence cannot be confirmed by clinical examination, needle electromyographic examination is important. However, fasciculations are common and occur in healthy persons. In the absence of neurologic findings, such as weakness or atrophy, they are termed *benign fasciculations* and usually have no serious clinical implications.

Muscle Cramps

Muscle cramps are another positive sign of the lower motor neuron syndrome. Their pathogenesis is poorly understood, although cramps and fasciculations are likely to share a similar mechanism, that is, hyperexcitability of distal motor axons (see Chapter 5). In a true muscle cramp, the abrupt, involuntary, and painful shortening of the muscle is accompanied by visible or palpable knotting, often with abnormal posture of the affected joint; it can be relieved by stretching or massaging. Adopting a practical definition is useful when discussing this with patients: a muscle cramp, otherwise known as a "charley horse," is a sudden, involuntary, sustained muscle contraction with severe pain that interrupts activity or sleep. Sudden muscle pains often described as "muscle spasms" are not associated with severe muscle contraction, and so are not true muscle cramps.

As with fasciculations, muscle cramps (especially in the calves) are an ordinary and common phenomenon in healthy people. In ALS, the same muscle cramps occur not only in usual sites, such as the calf, but also in the thighs, arms, hands, abdomen, neck, jaw, or even tongue. Muscle cramps are one of the most frequently encountered symptoms in ALS, and if patients report no cramps, one must be cautious in making a diagnosis of ALS.

BULBAR SIGNS AND SYMPTOMS

Muscles controlling articulation, mastication, and deglutition are innervated by the VII (facial), IX (glossopharyngeal), X (vagus), and XII (hypoglossal) cranial nerves, whose nuclei are located mostly in the medulla. Because the medulla is also known as the "bulb," neurologic signs and symptoms

Table 4–6. SIGNS OF BULBAR PALSY

Dysarthria

Dysphagia

Sialorrhea (drooling)

Aspiration

Pseudobulbar signs

resulting from the loss of medullary neurons and their axons are referred to as *bulbar palsy* (Table 4–6). Although its nucleus is not in the medulla, cranial nerve V (trigeminal) is also usually implicated because it controls jaw movement. When the medullary lower motor neurons are primarily affected, the condition is called *flaccid* or *paretic bulbar palsy*. In contrast, when upper motor neurons and their descending tracts (the corticobulbar tracts) are affected, *spastic bulbar palsy* develops (Table 4–7). In ALS, a mixed bulbar palsy is usually seen, which consists of a varying mixture of flaccid and spastic components.

The Examination of Bulbar Muscles

In pure flaccid bulbar palsy (see Table 4–7), facial muscles are flaccid and weak. This weakness is easily found by determining the orbicularis oculi muscle strength. Using the fingers, an examiner cannot open tightly closed eyes in a healthy person, whereas facial muscle weakness allows the examiner to open the eyes easily. When facial muscles are markedly weak, even voluntary eye closure becomes impossible; that is, the eyes are left partially open. Muscle strength of the lower facial muscles may be tested by assessing the orbicularis oris. Patients with lower facial muscle weakness cannot whistle or pucker their lips, and resistance to passive opening of tightly closed lips is negligible. When the examiner presses the patient's puffed cheeks from both sides, air held in the mouth easily leaks out between the lips or escapes into the nose through the velopharyngeal port. Those who have advanced bulbar palsy cannot retain any air in their mouths. On rare occasions, fasciculations are found in facial muscles.

Examination of the tongue begins with a careful inspection. The normal tongue has a smooth surface, whereas the atrophied tongue has an irregular, wavy surface with smooth furrows (Fig. 4–3). When the normal tongue is at rest inside the mouth, its surface is smooth, and it does not move. With tongue fasciculations, the tongue surface may quiver or undergo wavy motions. In typical fasciculations, the muscle twitches are irregular, multifocal in distribution, and extend only a short distance, from a few to several millimeters. In restless or nervous individuals, or those with extrapyramidal tremor, movements can occur that resemble fasciculations. Generally one should be skeptical about the presence of tongue fasciculations unless there is definite tongue atrophy. Tongue atrophy does not develop in spastic bulbar palsy. Examination of volitional tongue movement is also important, and the ability to move the tongue side to side or in and out should be determined. The speed of

Table 4–7. CHARACTERISTIC DIFFERENCES BETWEEN FLACCID AND SPASTIC BULBAR PALSY

Clinical Symptoms	Flaccid	Spastic
Lesion location	Lower motor neuron	Upper motor neuron
Weakness	Severe	Mild
Gag reflex	Absent	Brisk
Tongue	Atrophied	No atrophy
Fasciculations	Present	Absent
Jaw reflex	Absent	Brisk
Forced crying	Absent	Present

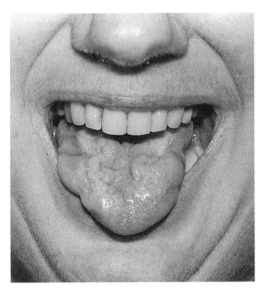

Figure 4–3. Advanced tongue atrophy is evident in this patient.

tongue movement is decreased by the presence of weakness, spasticity, or both. The strength of the tongue is tested by having the patient press it against the inside of the cheek against the examiner's finger. In advanced stages of bulbar palsy, the tongue is markedly atrophic and lies on the floor of the mouth with frequent fasciculations.

Recently, a reliable quantitative measurement was developed to analyze bulbar muscle strength.[14] Gag and jaw reflexes are usually absent in flaccid bulbar palsy but markedly exaggerated in the spastic form, even to the point of causing jaw clonus in jaw reflex. The muscles innervated by the trigeminal nerve can be tested by examining the competence of jaw opening and closure.

Dysarthria

Impaired articulation, or dysarthria, can be flaccid or spastic. Initial complaints include the inability to shout or sing, a weakened voice, and difficulty with enunciation. When the vocal cords become paretic, the voice takes on either a hoarse or whispering quality. Incompetence of the velopharyngeal port allows air in the mouth to leak into the nose during enunciation, which results in a

nasal tone. In spastic dysarthria, the voice sounds forced because much effort is needed to force air through the upper airway. Repetitive movements of the lips, tongue, and pharynx become particularly slow because of reduced dexterity. In either case, enunciation becomes progressively more difficult and in advanced stages, speech becomes unintelligible and finally nonexistent (anarthria) (see Chapter 23).

Dysphagia

Impaired mastication and deglutition, or dysphagia, usually accompanies dysarthria in ALS patients. Manipulating food inside the mouth becomes difficult, and food may pool between the gum and cheek. Patients may be unable to move food into the throat and experience weak or uncoordinated movements when swallowing. Small pieces of dry, crumbly food are more difficult to handle and are far more problematic than food with a soft, smooth consistency. Patients with neurogenic dysphagia generally have more difficulty swallowing liquids than solids. Liquids regurgitate into the nose if the velopharyngeal port is incompetent. Eventually, swallowing may trigger reflex coughing, a warning that dysphagia is serious and has led to aspiration. At this stage, patients require increasingly more time than before to finish a meal, and eating becomes a great chore. Eating while talking, a bulbar function requiring skillful coordination, eventually becomes impossible. When the cough reflex is weakened by flaccid paralysis of pharyngolaryngeal and respiratory muscles, the risk of aspirating food and saliva into the airway becomes significant. Speech pathologists should be consulted to evaluate swallowing dysfunction in detail; a modified barium swallowing test is useful to analyze dysphagia and aspiration objectively (see Chapter 23).

Sialorrhea (Drooling)

Patients with ALS frequently complain of drooling that is both disabling and embarrassing.[83] It results from the absence of spontaneous, automatic swallowing to clear excessive saliva and is aggravated by the drooping head posture caused by cervical extensor muscle weakness.

Aspiration and Laryngospasm

The epiglottis closes automatically upon swallowing. Incomplete or uncoordinated closure may allow liquid, saliva, or food to pass into the larynx. This aspiration usually triggers the cough reflex or an overt choking episode. Although aspiration can be a life-threatening event and may result in aspiration pneumonia, when the amount aspirated is small, it may be asymptomatic. To investigate a possible aspiration, a modified barium swallowing test, which should be attended by an experienced speech pathologist, is required.

Cough attacks, an exaggerated gag reflex, or aspiration to the larynx may trigger laryngospasm, which is clinically characterized by loud inspiratory stridor. Although laryngospasm in ALS has been generally considered as a non–life-threatening event, recently sudden death has been reported after episodes of laryngospasm in several ALS patients. The physician should give serious attention to laryngospasm, not only because it may cause death but also because patients with laryngospasm greatly fear respiratory distress.

Spastic Bulbar Palsy (Pseudobulbar Palsy)

As discussed previously, bulbar symptoms in ALS most often consist of a combination of upper and lower motor involvement. However, a pure upper motor neuron involvement causing bulbar dysfunction or spastic bulbar palsy is associated with a unique symptomatology. The symptoms include difficulties with articulation, mastication, and deglutition that are similar to those in flaccid bulbar palsy. However, the impairment in spastic bulbar palsy is generally milder and qualitatively different (see Table 4–7). The term *pseudobulbar palsy*, which is commonly used and widely accepted, is used to describe a complex of symptoms resembling bulbar palsy; however, the underlying mechanism differs from that in bulbar palsy because the anatomic location causing the symptoms in spastic bulbar palsy is not in the bulb itself.

The spastic bulbar palsy syndrome is caused by bilateral lesions that interrupt corticobulbar pathways between the upper motor neurons and the bulbar nuclei. The lack of highly coordinated bulbar muscle movements results in stiffness in enunciation, mastication, and deglutition.

Patients with spastic bulbar palsy appear to have poor emotional control, as characterized by spontaneous or unmotivated crying and laughter. In daily life, discussions or questions about subjects with emotional content often trigger a highly stereotyped crying or laughter that is embarrassing to patients. The underlying mechanism may be a clonic laryngorespiratory (vocalization) muscle contraction, resembling crying or laughter.[35,36] This phenomenon is caused by the disinhibition of the limbic motor control, which controls primitive vocalization muscles[29,36] (see Chapter 3). The term *emotional incontinence* has been used to describe the above specific symptom in spastic bulbar palsy, but it is probably a misnomer because the term "incontinence" is conventionally used to denote an inability to restrain from the urge to defecate or urinate, or yielding to normal impulse, as sexual desire.

RESPIRATORY SYMPTOMS

Loss of respiratory muscle strength is the cause of respiratory symptoms in ALS. Exertional dyspnea is common and frequent sighs at rest may represent respiratory symptoms at an early stage in the disease. Signs and symptoms of respiratory muscle weakness are shown in Table 4–8. Measurements of forced

Table 4–8. **RESPIRATORY SIGNS AND SYMPTOMS OF ALS**

Frequent sighs
Exertional dyspnea
Dyspnea at rest
Use of accessory respiratory muscles
Inability to sleep supine (diaphragmatic paralysis)
Orthopnea
Sleep apnea
Morning headaches
Hypoxemia
CO_2 narcosis

vital capacity are useful to identify early respiratory problems and are highly useful to follow a patient's respiratory status clinically.[16,77] Sometimes measuring the patient's phonation time ("ah") with a single deep breath can be performed as a simple but informative bedside test.[32] The diaphragm may be particularly vulnerable in ALS patients who have reported dyspnea when supine. In the early stages, patients prefer lying in a lateral decubitus position or may use a few extra pillows to make their upper body partially upright. Subsequently they may develop frank orthopnea. A careful examination may detect paradoxical respiration in those with more advanced diaphragmatic weakness. Paradoxical respiration is a reverse movement of the abdomen during inspiration; when the patient is supine, the abdomen normally elevates during inspiration because the abdominal contents are displaced downward during diaphragmatic contraction. In paradoxical respiration, diaphragmatic weakness allows the abdomen to draw inward, displacing the abdominal contents upward because of increasing intrathoracic negative pressure. Forced vital capacity measurements in both sitting and supine positions are useful in detecting early diaphragmatic weakness in ALS patients (see Chapter 22). Severe hypopnea may develop during sleep, primarily because of nocturnal diaphragmatic weakness.[9] In patients with moderately advanced respiratory distress, accessory respiratory muscle contraction is visible in the anterior neck, along with shoulder movements during respiration.

Rarely, patients present with impending respiratory failure as the first manifestation of ALS.[19,31,66] This presentation is associated with a poor prognosis. These patients often need immediate respiratory support in the intensive care unit, and it is not unusual for them to become completely ventilator dependent. In such cases, the cause of respiratory failure is unknown, and the correct diagnosis of ALS can often be significantly delayed.[46]

CONSTITUTIONAL SIGNS AND SYMPTOMS

Ongoing reduction of muscle mass and diminished caloric intake secondary either to dysphagia or loss of appetite can cause progressive weight loss in ALS patients. Occasionally, however, the weight loss is far more pronounced than would be expected in those with little or only mild muscle wasting. This unusual weight loss, called ALS cachexia, primarily involves subcutaneous and peritoneal fat and was first described by Gowers[23] and then Norris and coworkers.[67] Weight loss exceeding 20% of body weight within 6 months from the onset of weakness is not unusual in this form of cachexia. The body weight in all ALS patients should be checked at every office visit because the rate of weight loss provides a useful indicator of general prognosis and nutritional management.

Fatigue is a common complaint in neuromuscular diseases. In ALS, however, a fatigue identical to that occurring in myasthenia gravis may occur early on. The similarity exists between ALS and myasthenia gravis because the neuromuscular junctions in muscles undergoing denervation and reinnervation are likely to be unreliable in impulse transmission. Furthermore, newly sprouted motor axons reinnervating denervated muscle fibers are also electrophysiologically unstable. Such a pathophysiologic situation results in typical fatigue upon repetitive muscle contractions.[64] However, recent studies of fatigue in patients with ALS showed that the source of fatigue is not at the neuromuscular junction or within the muscle membrane. It appears to result from activation impairment, caused in part by alterations distal to the muscle membrane.[79]

MUSCULOSKELETAL SIGNS

Foot and hand deformities are common in ALS. Patients with a relatively slow course of the upper motor neuron syndrome develop extensor stiffness of the lower extremities. Such stiffness shortens posterior compartment muscles more than anterior compartment muscles and results in Achilles tendon shortening. Claw hand deformity is a fairly common hand deformity seen in ALS patients. It occurs because of weakness of lumbricus and interosseous muslces (Fig. 4–4). Metacarpophalangeal joints are hyperextended, whereas distal joints are flexed because of the tenodesis mechanism. Almost invariably, secondary joint contracture develops and further complicates the hand deformity.

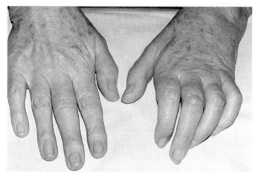

Figure 4–4. The left hand shows an early claw-hand deformity with the metacarpophalangeal joints hyperextended and the fingers (third through fifth) flexed. Atrophy of the first dorsal interosseous muscle is evident.

Contracture develops relatively quickly in joints immobile as a result of muscle paralysis. Joint contracture and pericapsulitis can cause severe pain and discomfort on attempted voluntary action or passive movement. Painful pericapsulitis often involves the shoulder joints. The pain prevents voluntary joint movements and further aggravates joint contracture.

RARE MANIFESTATIONS OF ALS

Clinically, ALS is a pure motor neuron syndrome; that is, the sensory system, higher cortical function, and the extrapyramidal system are not affected. Furthermore, certain motor neurons, such as those innervating external ocular muscles and the bladder and anal sphincter muscles, are typically spared. Interestingly, decubitus ulcers are rare, even in totally paralyzed ALS patients (Table 4–9). Charcot[10] pointed out the absence of these

Table 4–9. **SIGNS AND SYMPTOMS RARE IN ALS***

Sensory impairment
Dementia
Ocular palsy
Bladder and bowel dysfunction
Decubiti

*If seen, they argue against ALS in general.

complications when he first described ALS more than 120 years ago. All these signs and symptoms are "negative manifestations" of ALS; that is, they must be absent. However, in some patients with otherwise typical ALS, these signs and symptoms do occur. If the diagnosis of ALS is still to be accepted in such instances, it should be considered atypical. At present, the significance of these rare or negative manifestations remains unknown because the pathogenesis and the clinical limits of ALS are not yet defined.[61] In the following section, we discuss these atypical signs and symptoms that may occur in patients with otherwise typical ALS.

Sensory Impairment

A small proportion of patients with ALS complain of numbness or ill-defined pain in the distal part of their extremities. Patients' use of the word "numbness" does not necessarily imply sensory impairment; patients may even be describing muscle weakness. Sensory impairment has not been found in ALS patients,[17,62] but sensory complaints are not unusual. In our retrospective studies, nearly 20% of motor neuron disease patients (180 with ALS and 36 with progressive muscular atrophy) had ill-defined sensory symptoms of paresthesia or focal pain. None of these patients, however, had abnormal findings on a sensory examination, except for a decreased vibratory sense in the toes, which is not unusual in healthy elderly people.

Although a routine neurologic examination reveals no sensory abnormalities in most patients with ALS, more sophisticated quantitative sensory testing reveals clear abnormalities in some patients. With such testing, Mulder and colleagues[62] reported that 14 of 80 patients with ALS did indeed have abnormally elevated sensory thresholds, particularly to vibratory stimuli. On the other hand, cutaneous touch-pressure and thermal-cooling thresholds were normal.[62] Electrophysiologic tests also suggest that subtle sensory impairment can occur in ALS patients.[24,80] Furthermore, somatosensory evoked potentials are abnormal in some patients with typical disease, indicating that the ascending afferent sensory system is also involved. Pathologic studies reveal that peripheral sensory nerves have a decreased number of myelinated fibers (see Chapter 10). All these findings support the opinion that ALS is not a pure motor neuron syndrome but rather a generalized neuronal disease primarily involving the motor neurons.

We have seen several patients with otherwise typical ALS who complained of modest distal paresthesia and mild sensory impairment on neurologic examination but had marked abnormalities in sensory nerve conduction studies. These patients may represent one end of the range of sensory involvement in ALS. However, we emphasize that these cases should not be considered as being typical ALS.

Dementia

Although rare, dementia can also occur in patients who have otherwise typical ALS. Epidemiologic data on concomitant dementia are scarce, but its frequency is reportedly less than 5%.[43,44] In our experience, at most 1% or 2% of ALS patients have dementia. However, as Hudson[39] pointed out, mild dementia may elude detection, particularly in patients with bulbar palsy whose impaired ability to communicate verbally makes assessment of mentation particularly difficult. In addition, because the dementia in ALS seems to be more common in those with bulbar palsy than in those with predominantly extremity involvement, dementia may not have been detected in some of these patients.

When dementia develops, confusion, forgetfulness, and poor memory retention are usual early symptoms. Behavioral changes and psychotic manifestations occur rarely. The Mini-Mental Status Examination should be given to all patients who are being evaluated for ALS. Care must be taken to exclude depression as a cause of the symptoms because it is one of the most common psychologic processes in these patients. When psychomotor retardation is present, psychiatric and neuropsychologic evaluations are required. Several investigations have analyzed cognitive function in ALS patients. Although the number of patients tested was relatively small, all studies except one[71] showed impairment in memory, calculation, and overall cognitive function in those tested.[20,40,41]

Verbal and nonverbal fluency was also impaired.[55] Iwasaki and colleagues[40,41] found that cognitive dysfunction was positively correlated with the presence of upper motor neuron involvement. Positron emission tomography scan studies by Ludolph et al.[55] revealed a decreased glucose consumption in cortex regions serving higher cognitive functions as well as in the motor cortex. These investigations suggest that ALS is not restricted to motor neurons.

Table 4–10 lists a variety of dementias that may be associated with ALS. Dementia is a part of the parkinsonism-dementia complex in the Western Pacific.[11,33] Clinically about 5% of patients with parkinsonism-dementia develop ALS, whereas 38% of patients with ALS in this region develop parkinsonism-dementia. However, after detailed postmortem study of the brain in these patients, Hirano and Kurland[34] concluded that Guamanian ALS and the parkinsonism-dementia complex in the Western Pacific are the same disease process because both showed the same histopathologic changes (see Chapter 10). Although the ALS-parkinsonism-dementia complex most commonly occurs in the Western Pacific in an endemic form, both familial and sporadic cases of a clinically identical syndrome have been reported outside this region.[21,78] Hudson[39] reviewed this topic extensively and concluded that ALS dementia and ALS-parkinsonism-dementia are the same disease process, both characterized by striking cortical and subcortical neuronal degeneration.

To add further complexity, the dementia

Table 4–10. **FORMS OF DEMENTIA ASSOCIATED WITH ALS**

Guam ALS-parkinsonism-dementia complex

ALS associated with dementia and parkinsonism

Alzheimer's disease

Presenile dementia with motor neuron disease of non-Alzheimer type

Aphasic dementia in motor neuron disease

Thalamic dementia

Creutzfeldt-Jakob's disease*

Gerstmann-Straussler-Scheinker syndrome*

*A combination of amyotrophy, upper motor neuron signs, and dementia may be seen in these conditions.

in ALS and in Alzheimer's disease can be identical.[18,65] However, non-Alzheimer's dementia, histopathologically characterized by neuronal degeneration in the frontal and temporal lobes, which was originally described by Mitsuyama,[6,59,86] is perhaps the most common form of dementia in ALS. A unique form of dementia presenting with aphasia in patients with predominantly bulbar ALS has recently been reported.[9] Even in this situation, the histopathology may resemble that of non-Alzheimer's dementia in ALS. Essentially, dementia in ALS can be associated with many different pathologic conditions, and autopsy study appears to be the only way of identifying the underlying cause at present[15,38,45,75] (see Chapter 10).

Extrapyramidal (Parkinsonian) Signs

Parkinsonism is another key feature of the parkinsonism-dementia complex in the Western Pacific.[11,33] Although parkinsonian signs are not usually seen in patients with classic ALS outside the Mariana Islands, such cases have been reported in the western world[7,21,39,78]; we also have seen such patients who have features of parkinsonism in addition to typical ALS. Parkinsonian features include bradykinesia, cogwheel rigidity, increased glabella reflex (poor suppression of blink response to glabella tapping with an examiner's finger), diminished facial expression, and postural instability. These features, however, are often masked by marked spasticity and soon dominated or replaced by progressive lower motor neuron signs.

Ocular Palsy

Ocular muscles are typically spared in ALS. When ocular motility is tested in depth, however, the velocity of saccadic or smooth pursuit movement is decreased in about 50% of patients with typical ALS.[42,53] Such ocular abnormalities are thought to be caused by extrapyramidal or supranuclear dysfunction. Although Gizzi and colleagues[22] found ocular motor function to be normal in most ALS patients tested, those with additional par-

kinsonian features had abnormal saccadic and pursuit ocular movements, suggesting that these ocular abnormalities are probably secondary to extrapyramidal involvement. Hayashi and colleagues[30] found a high frequency of ocular abnormalities, such as an absence of voluntary eye closure and complete ocular palsy (ophthalmoplegia), in those who were on a ventilator for long periods. Ocular motor control is affected in the later stages of ALS, primarily as the result of supranuclear involvement. In other patients with ALS associated with nystagmus, no specific pathology was identified.[48]

In our clinical practice, we occasionally find patients who have ocular apraxia, or the inability to look voluntarily at a target from side to side without turning the head, which involves the oculovestibular reflex (voluntary turning of the head followed by reflex ocular movement). Occasionally, patients cannot voluntarily perform or maintain eye closure (apraxia of eye closure). These patients invariably have predominantly spastic bulbar-onset ALS. Their ocular abnormalities, such as the inability to close the eyes, suggest supranuclear involvement.[52]

Several autopsy studies of patients who had ALS and ophthalmoplegia showed, in addition to ALS-related changes, widespread neuronal loss in the deep subcortical nuclei, substantia nigra, olivary nuclei, Clarke's columns, and spinocerebellar tracts, suggesting a multisystem neurodegeneration[26,60,68] (see Chapter 11).

Bladder and Bowel Dysfunction

A group of motor neurons in the Onufrowicz nucleus is located in the medial sacral spinal cord and controls vesicourethral and anal sphincter muscles, and muscles of the pelvic floor.[37] These motor neurons are generally spared in ALS. Although Charcot stated that no bladder dysfunction exists in ALS, micturition symptoms are not unusual. Swank and Putnum[83a] reported micturition symptoms in 27 (17%) of 160 patients, and recently Hattori et al.[28] noted urinary symptoms in nearly half of 38 patients with ALS. These symptoms included urgency, obstructive micturition, or both; only one patient had urge incontinence. The fact that micturition symptoms are generally subtle and incontinence is rare may explain why bladder function has often been thought to be normal in these patients. However, detailed analyses of bladder function showed abnormal urodynamics in nearly one-third of 38 patients with ALS.[27,28] All these data indicate that supranuclear control over sympathetic, parasympathetic, and somatic neurons may be abnormal in ALS. Although bowel function in ALS has not been systematically studied, in our experience, bowel dysfunction is very rare.

Decubiti

Intact sensory perception and normal cutaneous autonomic function may prevent decubiti in ALS patients. Recent studies suggest that cutaneous collagen fibrils and the biochemical properties of collagen in ALS patients differ from those in healthy people.[69] However, decubiti do occasionally occur, particularly in patients with ALS who are kept alive on a ventilator for a long period.[60,76]

PRESENTING SYMPTOMS

Many studies have analyzed the frequency of initial symptoms of ALS. Table 4–11 summarizes several recent studies providing such data. The most frequent presenting symptom is weakness, which occurs in approximately 60% of patients with ALS. Typically, clinical presentation is a focal weakness beginning in the arm, leg, or bulbar muscles. A generalized onset with simultaneous involvement of the arms, legs, and bulbar muscle occurs in only 1% to 9% of all patients (Table 4–12).

Weakness involving only one side of the body in the initial stages is uncommon; called *Mills' variant* (hemiparetic form),[57] it may cause diagnostic difficulty[70] (see Table 4–11). When the distribution of involved muscles at onset resembles a major nerve palsy, such as radial (with wrist drop), ulnar (with a claw hand), or peroneal nerve (with footdrop), it may be called a *pseudoneuritic form*. A detailed electrodiagnostic analysis of such cases reveals that the true involvement is far more widespread than the clinical presentation of a nerve palsy, perhaps justifying the term *pseudoneuritic*. However, such cases often cause a diagnostic dilemma because widespread motor neuron involvement occurs slowly.[70] Although ALS patients develop weakness of cervical extensor muscles during the course of the disease, initial manifestation in the neck and truncal muscles is rare.

According to Gubbay et al.,[25] 9% of patients present with pain or muscle cramps. In our experience, pain and cramps are relatively rare as initial symptoms, but muscle cramps are one of the most common symptoms as the disease progresses and occur in more than 80% or 90% of patients. Fasciculations and weight loss are the first symptoms in a small percentage of patients. Respiratory distress as the first symptom is rare. Norris and colleagues[67] found only one patient who presented with respiratory failure out of 613 patients with ALS.

We have seen several patients who had upper and lower motor neuron dysfunction limited to one extremity, usually one of the upper extremities, for a year or more before typical widespread muscle involvement en-

Table 4–11. **LOCATION OF INITIAL SYMPTOM**

Location (%)	Jokelainen[43] (n = 255)	Gubbay et al.[25] (n = 318)	Li et al.[54] (n = 560)	Norris et al.[67] (n = 613)
Arms	29	20	44	34
Legs	37	32	37	41
Neck and trunk	2	—	—	—
Generalized	4	9	—	1
Bulbar	28	23	19	24
Others or unknown	—	16	—	—

Table 4–12. Unusual Initial Signs and Symptoms

Hemiparetic form (Mills' variant)
Pseudoneuritic form
Head drop (cervical extensor muscle weakness)
Fasciculations
Weight loss
Respiratory failure
Monomelic presentation

sued. This unusual presentation could be termed a *monomelic form* of ALS.

SUMMARY

This chapter covered both typical and atypical signs and symptoms of ALS. The upper and lower motor neuron syndromes manifest in combination and in varying degrees. Muscle cramps and focal or multifocal muscle weakness and atrophy accompanied by fasciculations, pathologic hyperreflexia, and spasticity are crucial clues in diagnosis. Progressive bulbar palsy and respiratory failure may complicate the clinical presentation. Patients may have constitutional signs and musculoskeletal changes. Although by definition ALS solely affects motor neurons, one should be aware that other neuronal systems can be affected. Thus, a careful evaluation based on knowledge of ALS symptomatology is the key to correct diagnosis.

REFERENCES

1. Ashworth, B: Trial of crisoprodol in multiple sclerosis. Practitioner 192:540–542, 1964.
2. Babinski, JEF: Sur le réflexe cutané plantaire dans certains affections organiques due système nerveux central. CR Soc Biol (Paris) 3:207–208, 1896.
3. Brooks, BR: The role of axonal transport in neurodegenerative disease spread: A meta-analysis of experimental and clinical poliomyelitis compares with amyotrophic lateral sclerosis. Can J Neurol Sci 18:435–438, 1991.
4. Brown, MC, Holland, RL, and Hopkins, WG: Motor nerver sprouting. Ann Rev Neurosci 4:17–42, 1981.
5. Brown, P: Pathophysiology of spasticity. J Neurol Neurosurg Psychiatry 57:773–777, 1994.
6. Brun, A: Frontal lobe degeneration of non-Alzheimer type revisited. Dementia 4:126–131, 1993.
7. Burrow, JNC and Blumbergs, PC: Substantia nigra degeneration in motor neurone disease: A quantitative study. Aust NZ J Med 22:469–472, 1992.
8. Carre, PC, Didier, AP, Tiberge, YV, et al: Amyotrophic lateral sclerosis presenting with sleep hypopnea syndrome. Chest 93:1309–1312, 1988.
9. Caselli, RJ, Windebank, AJ, Petersen, C, et al: Rapidly progressive aphasic dementia and motor neuron disease. Ann Neurol 33:200–207, 1993.
10. Charcot, J-M: De la sclérose latérale amyotrophique. Prog Med 23:235–237, 24:341–342, 1874; 29:453–455, 1874.
11. Chen, KM: Amyotrophic lateral sclerosis and parkinsonism-dementia and its relationship to Guam amyotrophic lateral sclerosis. In Tsubaki, T and Tokyokura, Y (eds): Amyotrophic Lateral Sclerosis. University of Tokyo Press, Tokyo, 1984, pp 319–344.
12. Conradi, S, Grimgy, L, and Lundemo, G: Pathophysiology of fasciculations in ALS as studied by electromyography of single motor units. Muscle Nerve 5:202–208, 1982.
13. DeJong, RN: The neurologic examination. Hoeber Medical, New York, 1970.
14. DePaul, R, Abbs, JH, Caligiuri, M, et al: Hypoglossal, trigeminal, and facial motor neuron involvement in amyotrophic lateral sclerosis. Neurology 38:281–283, 1988.
15. Deymeer, F, Smith, TW, DeGirolami, U, et al: Thalamic dementia and motor neuron disease. Neurology 39:58–61, 1989.
16. Fallat, RJ, Jewitt, B, Bass, M, et al: Spirometry in amyotrophic lateral sclerosis. Arch Neurol 36:74–80, 1979.
17. Fincham, RW and Van Allen, MW: Sensory nerve conduction in amyotrophic lateral sclerosis. Neurology 14:31–33, 1964.
18. Frecker, MF, Fraser, FC, Anderman, E, et al: Association between Alzheimer disease and amyotrophic lateral sclerosis? Can J Neurol Sci 17:12–14, 1990.
19. Fromm, GB, Wisdom, PJ, and Block AJ: Amyotrophic lateral sclerosis presenting with respiratory failure. Chest 71:612–614, 1977.
20. Gallassi, R, Montagna, P, Ciardulli, C, et al: Cognitive impairment in motor neuron disease. Acta Neurol Scand 71:480–484, 1985.
21. Gilbert, JJ, Kish, SJ, Chang, LJ, et al: Dementia, parkinsonism, and motor neuron disease: Neurochemical and neuropathological correlates. Ann Neurol 24:688–691, 1988.
22. Gizzi, M, DiRocco, A, Sivak, M, et al: Ocular motor function in motor neuron disease. Neurology 42:1037–1046, 1992.
23. Gowers, WR: A Manual of Diseases of the Nervous System, Vol 1, ed 3. Plakiston, Philadelphia, 1899.
24. Gregory, R, Mills, K, and Donaghy, M: Progressive sensory nerve dysfunction in amyotrophic lateral sclerosis: A prospective clinical and neurophysiological study. J Neurol 240:309–314, 1992.
25. Gubbay, SS, Kahana, E, Zilber, N, et al: Amyotrophic lateral sclerosis. A study of its presentation and prognosis. J Neurol 232:295–300, 1985.
26. Harvey, DG, Torack, RM, and Rosenbaum, HE: Amyotrophic lateral sclerosis with ophthalmoplegia. Arch Neurol 36:615–617, 1979.

27. Hattori, T: Negative symptoms and signs of amyotrophic lateral sclerosis. Clin Neurol 24:1254–1256, 1984.

28. Hattori, T, Hirayama, K, Yasuda, K, et al: Disturbance of micturition in amyotrophic lateral sclerosis. Clin Neurol 23:224–227, 1983.

29. Hayashi, H: Long-term in-hospital ventilatory care for patients with amyotrophic lateral sclerosis. In Mitsumoto, H and Norris, FH, Jr (eds): Amyotrophic Lateral Sclerosis. A Comprehensive Guide to Management. Demos, New York, 1994, pp 127–138.

30. Hayashi, H, Kato, S, Kawada, T, et al: Amyotrophic lateral sclerosis: Oculomotor function in patients in respirators. Neurology 37:1431–1432, 1987.

31. Hill, R, Martin, J, and Hakim, A: Acute respiratory failure in motor neuron disease. Arch Neurol 40:30–32, 1983.

32. Hillel, AD, Yorkston, K, and Miller, RM: Using phonation time to estimate vital capacity in amyotrophic lateral sclerosis. Arch Phys Med Rehabil 70:618–620, 1989.

33. Hirano, A, Kurland, LT, Krooth, RS, et al: Parkinsonism-dementia complex, an endemic disease on the island of Guam. I. Clinical features. Brain 84:642–661, 1961.

34. Hirano, MN and Kurland, LT: Pathoanatomic changes in amyotrophic lateral sclerosis on Guam. Arch Neurol 15:401–415, 1961.

35. Holstege, G: An anatomical study on the final common pathways for vocalization in the cat. J Camp Neurol 284:242–252, 1989.

36. Holstege, G: Somatic motoneurons and descending motor pathways. Limbic and non-limbic components. In Leigh, PN and Swash, M (eds): Motor Neuron Disease. Biology and Management. Springer-Verlag, London, 1995, pp 259–330.

37. Holstege, G and Tan, J: Supraspinal control on motoneuron innervating the striated muscles of pelvic floor including urethral and anal sphincters in the cat. Brain 110:1323–1344, 1987.

38. Horoupian, DS, Thal, L, Katzman, R, et al: Dementia and motor neuron disease: Morphometric, biochemical and Golgi studies. Ann Neurol 16:305–313, 1984.

39. Hudson, AJ: Amyotrophic lateral sclerosis and its association with dementia, parkinsonism and other neurological disorders. Brain 104:217–247, 1981.

40. Iwasaki, Y, Kinoshita, M, Ikeda, K, et al: Cognitive impairment in amyotrophic lateral sclerosis and its relation to motor disabilities. Acta Neurol Scand 81:141–143, 1990.

41. Iwasaki, Y, Kinoshita, M, Ikeda, K, et al: Neuropsychological dysfunctions in amyotrophic lateral sclerosis: Relation to motor disabilities. Intern J Neurosci 54:191–195, 1990.

42. Jacobs, L, Bozian, D, Heffner, RR, et al: An eye movement disorder in amyotrophic lateral sclerosis. Neurology 31:1282–1287, 1981.

43. Jokelainen, M: Amyotrophic lateral sclerosis in Finland. 2. Clinical characteristics. Acta Neurol Scand 56:194–204, 1977.

44. Kondo, K, and Hemmi, I: Clinical statistics in 515 fatal cases of motor neuron disease. Neuroepidemiology 3:129–148, 1984.

45. Kretzschmar, HA, Kufer, P, Reithmüller, G, et al: Prion protein mutation at codon 102 in an Italian family with Gerstmann-Sträussler-Scheinker syndrome. Neurology 42:809–810, 1992.

46. Kuisma, MJ, Saarinen, KV, and Teirmaa, HT: Undiagnosed amyotrophic lateral sclerosis and respiratory failure. Acta Anaesthesiol Scand 37:628–630, 1993.

47. Kuncl, RW, Cornblat, DR, and Griffin, JW: Assessment of thoracic paraspinal muscles in the diagnosis of ALS. Muscle Nerve 11:484–492, 1988.

48. Kushner, MJ, Parrish, M, Burke, A, et al: Nystagmus in motor neuron disease: Clinicopathological study of two cases. Ann Neurol 16:71–77, 1984.

49. Lance, JW: Pathophysiology of spasticity and clinical experience with Baclofen. In Feldman, RG, Young, RR, and Klella, WP (eds): Spasticity: Disorder of Motor Control, 1980, pp 185–203.

50. Landau, WM: Spasticity: The fable of a neurological demon and the emperor's new therapy. Arch Neurol 31:217–219, 1974.

51. Landau, WM and Clare, MH: The plantar reflex in man, with special reference to some conditions where the extensor response is unexpectedly absent. Brain 82:321–355, 1959.

52. Lessell, S: Supranuclear paralysis of voluntary lid closure. Arch Ophthalmol 88:241–244, 1972.

53. Leveille, A, Kiernan, J, Goodwin, A, et al: Eye movements in amyotrophic lateral sclerosis. Arch Neurol 39:684–686, 1982.

54. Li, TM, Alberman, E, and Swash, M: Clinical features and associations of 560 cases of motor neuron disease. J Neurol Neurosurg Psychiatry 53:1043–1045, 1990.

55. Ludolph, AC, Lange, KJ, Regard, M, et al: Frontal lobe function in amyotrophic lateral sclerosis: A neuropsychologic and positron emission tomography study. Acta Neurol Scan 85:81–89, 1992.

56. Medical Research Council. Aid to the investigation of peripheral nerve injuries. War Memorandum, ed 2 (revised). London, His Majesty's Stationary Office, 1943, pp 11–46.

57. Mills, CK: Unilateral ascending paralysis and unilateral descending paralysis. JAMA 47:1638–1645, 1906.

58. Mitsuyama, Y: Presenile dementia with motor neuron disease. Dementia 4:137–142, 1993.

59. Mitsuyama, Y: Presenile dementia with motor neuron disease in Japan: Clinico-pathological review of 26 cases. J Neurol Neurosurg Psychiatry 47:953–959, 1984.

60. Mizutani, T, Aki, M, Shiozawa, R, et al: Development of ophthalmoplegia in amyotrophic lateral sclerosis during long-term use of respirators. J Neurol Sci 99:311–319, 1990.

61. Mulder, DW: Clinical limits of amyotrophic lateral sclerosis. In Rowland, LP (ed): Human Motor Neuron Diseases. Raven Press, New York, 1982, pp 15–27.

62. Mulder, DW, Bushek, W, Spring, E, et al: Motor neuron disease (ALS): Evaluation of detection thresholds of cutaneous sensation. Neurology 33:1625–1627, 1983.

63. Mulder, DW, Kurland, LT, Offord, KP, et al: Familial adult motor neuron disease: Amyotrophic lateral sclerosis. Neurology 36:511–517, 1986.

64. Mulder, DW, Lambert, EH, and Eaton, LM: Myas-

thenic syndrome in patients with amyotrophic lateral sclerosis. Neurology 9:627–631, 1959.

65. Müller, M, Vieregge, P, Reusche, E, et al: Amyotrophic lateral sclerosis and frontal lobe dementia in Alzheimer's disease. Eur Neurol 33:320–324, 1993.

66. Nightingale, S, Bateman, DE, Ellis, DA, et al: Enigmatic dyspnoea: An unusual presentation of motor-neurone disease. Lancet 1:933–935, 1982.

67. Norris, FH, Shepherd, R, Denys, E, et al: Onset, natural history and outcome in idiopathic adult motor neuron disease. J Neurol Sci 118:48–55, 1993.

68. Okuda, B, Yamamoto, T, Yamasaki, M, et al: Motor neuron disease with slow eye movements and vertical gaze palsy. Acta Neurol Scand 85:71–76, 1992.

69. Ono, S, Toyokura, Y, Mannen, T, et al: Amyotrophic lateral sclerosis: Histologic, histochemical and ultrastructural abnormalities of skin. Neurology 36:948–956, 1986.

70. O'Reilly, DF, Brazis, PW, and Rubino, FA: The misdiagnosis of unilateral presentation of amyotrophic lateral sclerosis. Muscle Nerve 5:724–726, 1982.

71. Poloni, M, Capitani, E, Mazzini, L, et al: Neuropsychological measures in amyotrophic lateral sclerosis and their relationship with CT scan-assessed cerebral atrophy. Acta Neurol Scand 74:257–260, 1986.

72. Roth, G: The origin of fasciculations. Ann Neurol 12:542–547, 1982.

73. Rowland, LP: Babinski and the diagnosis of amyotrophic lateral sclerosis. Ann Neurol 33:108–109, 1993.

74. Sahrmann, SA and Norton, BJ: The relationship of voluntary movement to spasticity in the upper motor neuron syndrome. Ann Neurol 2:460–465, 1977.

75. Salazar, AM, Masters, CL, Gajdusek, C, et al: Syndromes of amyotrophic lateral sclerosis in dementia: Relation to transmissable Creutzfeldt-Jacob disease. Ann Neurol 14:17–26, 1983.

76. Sasaki, S, Tsutsumi, Y, Tamane, K, et al: Sporadic amyotrophic lateral sclerosis with extensive neurological involvement. Acta Neuropathol 84:211–215, 1992.

77. Schiffman, PL and Belsh, JM: Pulmonary function at diagnosis of amyotrophic lateral sclerosis. Chest 103:508–513, 1993.

78. Schmitt, HP, Emser, W, and Heimes, C: Familial occurrence of amyotrophic lateral sclerosis, parkinsonism, and dementia. Ann Neurol 16:642–648, 1984.

79. Sharma, KR, Kent-Braun, JA, Maumdar, S, et al: Physiology of fatigue in amyotrophic lateral sclerosis. Neurology 45:733–740, 1995.

80. Shefner, JM, Tyler, R, and Krarup, C: Abnormalities in the sensory action potential in patients with amyotrophic lateral sclerosis. Muscle Nerve 14:1242–1246, 1991.

81. Sharrard, WJW: The distribution of the permanent paralysis in the lower limb in poliomyelitis; a clinical and pathological study. J Bone Joint Surg 37b:540–548, 1955.

82. Sherrington, C: The Integrative Action of the Nervous System, ed 2. New Haven: Yale University Press, 1947.

83. Smith, RA and Goode, RL: Sialorrhea. N Engl J Med 283:917–918, 1970.

83a. Swank, RL and Putman, TJ: Amyotrophic lateral sclerosis and related conditions. Archives of Neurology and Psychiatry 49:151–177, 1943.

84. Swash, M, Leader, M, Brown, A, et al: Focal loss of anterior horn cells in the cervical cord in motor neuron disease. Brain 104:939–952, 1986.

85. Wettstein, A: The origin of fasciculations on motor neuron disease. Ann Neurol 5:295–300, 1979.

86. Wilkström, J, Paetau, A, Palo, J, et al: Classic amyotrophic lateral sclerosis with dementia. Arch Neurol 39:681–683, 1982.

87. Younger, DS, Rowland, LP, Latov, N, et al: Motor neuron disease and amyotrophic lateral sclerosis: Relation of high CSF protein content to paraproteinemia and clinical syndromes. Neurology 40:595–599, 1990.

CHAPTER 5

ELECTRO-DIAGNOSIS

Although the diagnosis of ALS is based primarily on clinical assessment, electrodiagnostic techniques such as nerve conduction studies and needle electrode examination are important in supporting the diagnosis and excluding other conditions that resemble ALS. These studies also help monitor clinical progression and provide prognostic information. The conventionally used electromyographic techniques of nerve conduction studies and concentric needle electrode examination assess essentially only lower motor neuron involvement in ALS. These techniques will be discussed in detail because they are used regularly in virtually all electromyography (EMG) laboratories. Other specialized, although more time-consuming,

techniques can provide additional information about lower motor neuron function (e.g., motor unit number estimation, repetitive stimulation, single-fiber EMG, macro EMG) and upper motor neuron function (e.g., transcranial magnetic stimulation). In ALS, these studies are used primarily for research.

This chapter will first deal with the commonly used techniques, stressing their strengths and limitations, and then outline special procedures that can provide important neurophysiologic information in ALS (Table 5–1). Electrodiagnostic abnormalities generally parallel the activity, progression, and stage of the disease. If the disease is mild and progresses slowly or if lower motor neuron involvement is slight, changes may be limited. Rapidly evolving or advanced stages of ALS produce dramatic changes on EMG. Furthermore, the needle electrode examination is essential to reveal lower motor neuron abnormalities in muscles that are not yet affected clinically. It is important to reach an accurate diagnosis when assessing a patient with suspected ALS and to identify other causes of progressive weakness. The electrodiagnostic evaluation is essential to that process.

MOTOR NERVE COMMUNICATION STUDIES

Conventional Studies

The results of routine motor nerve conduction studies, including compound motor

Table 5–1. ELECTRODIAGNOSTIC TECHNIQUES USED IN ALS

Nerve Conduction Studies	Needle Electrode Examination	Techniques for Central Nervous System Evaluation
Motor Studies	Concentric	Evoked potentials
Conventional (including F-waves)	Single-fiber EMG	Somatosensory
Motor unit estimation	Macro EMG	Brain-stem auditory
Repetitive stimulation	Scanning EMG	Visual
Collision techniques		Transcranial magnetic stimulation
Sensory studies		
Conventional (including H-reflexes)		
Near-nerve recording		
Quantitative sensory testing		

Abbreviation: EMG = electromyography.

action potential amplitudes, distal latencies, and conduction velocities, reflect the functional capacity of large myelinated motor axons. Early in the course of ALS, these studies are normal. In advancing disease, compound motor action potential amplitudes begin to drop because of progressive motor neuron loss, axon loss, muscle denervation, and atrophy.[52,53] The motor nerves we routinely study in three limbs (arm and leg on the side most affected, contralateral arm or leg) of individuals with suspected ALS are listed in Table 5–2. F-wave responses, resulting from antidromic (retrograde) firing of lower motor neuron neurons, are also included in the motor evaluation. If accessible, other nerves supplying clinically weak muscles are also studied to improve the diagnostic yield. For example, the peroneal nerve study in a patient presenting with footdrop should include evaluation of the tibialis anterior muscle in addition to the extensor digitorum brevis.

COMPOUND MOTOR ACTION POTENTIAL AMPLITUDES

The result of progressive motor neuron loss in ALS is muscle atrophy and concomitant decrease in compound motor action potential amplitude (Fig. 5–1). Patients with advanced disease and low-amplitude compound motor action potentials have a poor prognosis.[67] Patients with progressive ALS may show decreased motor nerve responses and normal sensory nerve amplitudes, the so-called generalized low motor-normal sensory pattern.[110] Although uncommon, this pattern is noteworthy because it is almost invariably associated with a poor outcome. Most patients with this pattern have progressive ALS, but some have a potentially treatable disorder (Table 5–3). For example, multifocal motor neuropathy with conduction block, which can be clinically mistaken for a lower motor neuron form of ALS (see Chapter 6), often has multifocal conduction

Table 5–2. SUGGESTED ROUTINE MOTOR NERVE CONDUCTION STUDIES IN ALS

Nerve	Recording Site	Characteristic Studied
Median	Abductor pollicis brevis	Amp, DL, CV, F-wave
Ulnar	Abductor digiti minimi	Amp, DL, CV, F-wave
Peroneal	Extensor digitorum brevis	Amp, DL, CV
Posterior tibial	Abductor hallucis	Amp, DL, CV, F-wave
Posterior tibial	Soleus	Amp, DL: M-component of H-response

Abbreviations: Amp = amplitude, CV = conduction velocity, DL = distal latency.

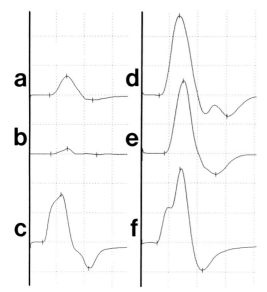

Figure 5–1. Motor nerve compound motor action potential amplitudes recorded from intrinsic hand muscles (stimulating at the wrist), including the abductor pollicis brevis (a, d), first dorsal interosseus (b, e), and abductor digiti minimi (c, f), are decreased in a patient with advanced ALS (a, b, c) and normal in a healthy age-matched individual (d, e, f). Note that the amplitudes from the abductor pollicis brevis (a) and first dorsal interosseus (b) muscles are disproportionately lower than the amplitude from the abductor digiti minimi muscle (c); this difference reflects the split-hand pattern of greater denervation of muscles in the lateral half of the hand, which is occasionally seen in ALS. Each division represents gain = 5 mV, sweep speed = 5 ms.

blocks on motor nerve conduction studies and normal sensory responses.[54,76,100]

Another pattern of motor nerve conduction involvement specific to ALS is characterized by decreased compound motor action potential amplitudes in the lateral half of the hand (thenar, median innervation and the first dorsal interosseous, ulnar innervation) and relatively normal values in the medial half (hypothenar, ulnar innervation) (see Fig. 5–1). This results from dissociated wasting of the medial and lateral hand muscles with evidence of denervation in the latter group of muscles.[112] Why the first dorsal interosseous and abductor digiti minimi (hypothenar eminence) are so unequally involved is unclear, given that the ulnar nerve innervates them both. It may be that anterior horn motor neurons supplying the first dorsal interosseous are anatomically closer to those supplying the median-innervated thenar muscles than to those supplying the ulnar-innervated hypothenar muscles.[112] Presumably, motor neurons innervating the lateral hand muscles are affected earlier and more severely in ALS than neurons innervating the medial hand muscles.

NERVE CONDUCTION VELOCITIES AND DISTAL LATENCIES

Conduction velocities slow only when compound motor action potential amplitudes are markedly decreased (less than 20% of the

Table 5–3. DIFFERENTIAL DIAGNOSIS OF CONDITIONS CAUSING GENERALIZED LOW MOTOR-NORMAL SENSORY AMPLITUDES ON NERVE CONDUCTION STUDIES

Motor neuron disease
    ALS
    Werdnig-Hoffman disease
    Poliomyelitis/post-polio syndrome
Diffuse myelopathy
Polyradiculopathies
    Cervical and lumbar canal stenoses
    Meningeal metastases
"Pure" motor polyneuropathy (e.g., multifocal motor neuropathy with conduction block)
Guillain-Barré syndrome
Lambert-Eaton (myasthenic) syndrome
Myopathy (especially polymyositis, dermatomyositis, inclusion-body myositis)

lower limit of normal),[53] reflecting loss of the fastest-conducting motor fibers. The slowing therefore may represent conduction along the remaining smaller fibers. Impulse collision techniques have been used in ALS to determine whether the conduction velocity is also diminished in these normally slower-conducting fibers (see below). In conventional nerve conduction studies, slowed conduction and prolonged distal latency are proportional to the reduction in compound motor action potential amplitudes, and throughout the course of ALS, fast- and slow-conducting fibers degenerate randomly.[52] ALS alone does not produce conduction velocities less than 70% of the lower limit of normal, and an alternative explanation, such as polyneuropathy, should be sought. In one study, distal latency prolongation, multifocal motor conduction slowing, and conduction blocks occurred in up to 20% (6 of 31) of patients with clinically classic ALS who had no other features of multifocal motor neuropathy with conduction block.[113]

Distal latencies may be prolonged out of proportion to the degree of conduction velocity slowing for various reasons, including cool extremities (which occurs frequently when muscle atrophy is pronounced), distal compressive nerve lesions (e.g., carpal tunnel syndrome in which sensory nerve action potential amplitudes are decreased), or nerve terminal sprouting.[82] In the last scenario, incompletely myelinated new collateral sprouts conduct nerve impulses inefficiently, increasing distal latencies.[11,97] Dying back of distal nerve terminal axons, which has been suggested to occur in ALS,[12,20] could also prolong distal latency.

F-WAVE RESPONSES

F-wave responses can be useful in evaluating the proximal ventral root or neuronal pool generating them. In ALS, both the frequency and latency of F-wave responses can be abnormal, particularly in advanced cases.[37,69,75] The progressive loss of spinal cord motor neurons probably accounts for the overall decrease in response frequency and amplitude;[36,75] however, F-wave amplitudes increase when motor neuron excitability is enhanced (e.g., spasticity), as occurs in ALS.[31] With progressive motor axon loss and

the resultant decrease in compound motor action potential (CMAP) amplitudes, F-wave responses become undetectable.

As with conventional motor conduction velocities, F-wave latencies remain within normal limits until axon loss severely reduces CMAP amplitudes. A detailed prospective analysis of F waves and CMAP amplitudes in the peroneal, ulnar, and median nerves of 95 ALS patients revealed that F-wave latencies recorded from 202 nerves were only rarely (1%, $n = 2$) greater than 125% of the upper limit of normal over a range of decreased CMAP amplitudes.[23]

Specialized Studies

MOTOR UNIT NUMBER ESTIMATION

Conventional motor nerve conduction studies usually do not detect motor unit dysfunction until clinical weakness exists.[17,60,89] Methods have been developed, however, to estimate the number of motor units and, by inference, the number of functional spinal cord motor neurons innervating a given muscle. In this context, motor unit number estimation has been applied primarily to identifying and monitoring motor neuron degeneration in ALS.[13,15,62,99] The original manual technique of McComas and colleagues[60,61] has certain limitations. The technique is based on submaximal electrical stimulation of motor axons, which produces incremental increases that represent individual motor units. The manual technique is best applied to distal muscles but is limited because motor fiber thresholds overlap extensively. This makes it difficult to separate individual motor units from one another,[16] and the results are sometimes nonspecific.[60]

Daube[25] described a variation of the manual technique using a computer-based statistical (Poisson) analysis of motor units recorded from distal upper and lower extremity muscles of ALS and post-poliomyelitis patients. This analysis revealed a high correlation with clinical dysfunction and earlier methods of motor unit number estimation. Decreased motor unit numbers could be detected even in the absence of weakness or reduced CMAP amplitudes. This method was used to monitor progression of motor neuron degeneration in patients enrolled in neurotrophic factor treatment trials.[87]

The manual techniques use surface recording, making it difficult to apply them to proximal muscles because the nerves are not easily accessible, and graded motor nerve stimulation may activate multiple rather than individual motor units. Therefore, the spike-triggered averaging technique was developed.[17,89] An intramuscular needle electrode is used to identify individual motor units after isometric contraction, thus allowing surface-recorded motor unit potentials that correspond to a chosen spike (hence "spike-triggered") to be averaged. The motor unit estimate is then calculated by dividing the mean of several (e.g., 10) surface-recorded motor unit potentials into the CMAP amplitude obtained by supramaximal nerve stimulation (Fig. 5–2). Motor unit numbers in proximal (biceps-brachialis) muscles of ALS patients are usually substantially reduced when compared to those of age-matched controls.[13,99]

REPETITIVE STIMULATION

Motor nerve stimulation at slow rates (2 to 3 Hz) causes decrement of CMAP amplitude (usually less than 10%) in up to half of patients with ALS.[53] Although this decrease is generally less than that occurring in patients with myasthenia gravis, it shares similar characteristics: it is greatest after three to five stimuli, improves after brief exercise or anticholinesterase drug administration, and worsens after prolonged exercise or curare administration.[53] The decrement probably results from unstable neuromuscular transmission through immature nerve terminal sprouts or neuromuscular junctions[65,71] but could also be caused by abnormal neuronal function.[7] Its presence suggests active disease, and the decrease is found almost exclusively in patients with rapidly progressive symptoms.[7,71]

COLLISION TECHNIQUES

Routine measurements of motor conduction velocities evaluate the fastest-conducting large myelinated nerve fibers, but slower-conducting axons also contribute to the CMAP amplitude and form. A specialized technique based on impulse collision was introduced to determine the velocity of small, slow-conducting (thinly myelinated or unmyelinated) motor nerve fibers that are also affected in ALS.[104] By stimulating the same nerve fiber at two points, the faster-conducting, larger (thickly myelinated) fibers can be blocked selectively by a preceding submaximal stimulus given distally. This makes it possible to examine the conduction velocity of the slower fibers (i.e., the minimum conduction velocity) in isolation.[104] Modifications of this collision method have been introduced.[2]

The minimum conduction velocity usually is significantly reduced in ALS as compared to age-matched controls,[73] particularly in younger patients.[46] This suggests either preferential involvement of smaller motor nerve fibers or an increase in suboptimally conducting regenerating, remyelinating axons and terminal sprouts.[114] The latter explana-

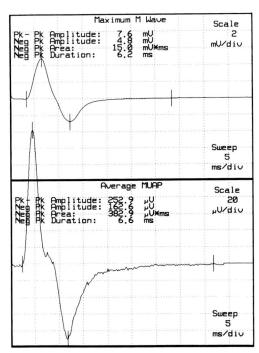

Figure 5–2. Motor unit number estimate in the adductor digiti minimi of a patient with ALS is calculated from the ratio of the compound motor action potential (7.6 mV) (*Top*) and average motor unit action potential (252.9 μV) (*Bottom*). The abnormally low ratio (30, as measured by peak-to-peak amplitude) reveals motor unit loss in this muscle.

tion is more likely because axonal regeneration is more robust in younger individuals after either nerve crush[11] or transection,[18] as well as in the early stages of ALS.[101]

Results of collision experiments have been inconsistent, probably because of the relative positions of fibers in nerve trunks rather than their sizes.[60] Fibers closer to the stimulating electrode are likely to undergo depolarization earlier than those farther away, regardless of fiber diameter. Therefore, the clinical utility of the collision technique for studying conduction velocities is limited in ALS. It has, however, been useful in identifying both distal and proximal sites of origin of fasciculations in ALS.[80,109]

SENSORY NERVE CONDUCTION STUDIES

General Studies

Although some patients with ALS experience sensory symptoms, most have normal sensory nerve action potential amplitudes and conduction velocities on routine studies.[52] Indeed, significantly abnormal sensory nerve function indicates the existence of other conditions and raises doubts about the diagnosis of ALS. For example, another motor neuron disease, X-linked bulbospinal neuronopathy (Kennedy's disease) is associated with characteristic and often widespread sensory nerve action potential amplitude reductions on routine sensory nerve testing.[43] Nerve conduction studies are useful in differentiating Kennedy's disease from other forms of motor neuron disease because of the characteristic sensory abnormalities, even in the absence of sensory symptoms (see Chapter 6). We have observed a subset of patients with a form of focal motor neuron disease (not Kennedy's disease) who have decreased sensory nerve action potential amplitudes only along sensory nerves at the spinal level in which muscle weakness is present.[66] The explanation for this finding is unknown.

Whether stimulating sensory nerves orthodromically (in the natural direction of transmission) or antidromically, conventional studies use surface electrodes and evaluate the fastest-conducting, large myelinated sensory nerve axons. With these methods, a small proportion of patients with clinically definite ALS and no underlying illnesses predisposing them to peripheral neuropathy (e.g., diabetes mellitus) have electrophysiologic evidence of sensory abnormalities.[40,68] The more sensitive technique of near-nerve recording with needle electrodes revealed abnormally decreased minimum conduction velocities in 9 of 18 ALS patients studied.[83,84] Another technique, quantitative sensory testing, is a psychophysical method for evaluating modality-specific (vibratory, warming and cooling) detection thresholds.[41] In one study of ALS patients ($n = 80$), almost one-fifth ($n = 14$) had significantly impaired vibratory detection but normal detection thresholds for touch pressure and thermal cooling.[70] The finding of degeneration in some peripheral sensory nerve fibers provides a pathologic basis for the sensory nerve dysfunction seen electrodiagnostically (see Chapter 11).[12,29] Furthermore, a prospective clinical and electrophysiologic study of 12 patients with sporadic ALS revealed that such sensory nerve dysfunction progresses in parallel with motor decline.[40] Thus, electrophysiologic evidence of sensory involvement, albeit limited, has been adduced in some cases of typical sporadic ALS.

H-Reflex

The H-reflex, which is a monosynaptic response, assesses the integrity of proximal sensory nerve fibers and motor neuronal excitability at the S1 spinal level.[55] Stimulating a mixed peripheral nerve (posterior tibial) at low intensity mostly depolarizes afferent sensory fibers. These then activate the corresponding spinal alpha motor neuron pool via a monosynaptic reflex loop that produces the low-amplitude H-reflex recorded over the soleus muscle. Progressively more intense stimulation results in the direct muscle or M-response, which eventually overcomes and blocks the H-reflex.

Early in ALS, the H-reflex amplitude relative to the M-response is normal. The H-reflex amplitude may be greater than would be expected for age or the M-response amplitude, probably because disturbance of upper motor neuron function disinhibits the

Table 5–4. **SUGGESTED SENSORY NERVE CONDUCTION STUDIES IN ALS**

Nerve	Recording Site	Characteristic Studied
Median	Index finger	Amp, DL, CV
Ulnar	Fifth finger	Amp, DL, CV
Radial	Thumb	Amp, DL, CV
Sural	Lateral malleolus	Amp, DL, CV
Posterior tibial	Soleus	Amp, DL: H-response

Abbreviations: Amp = amplitude, CV = conduction velocity, DL = distal latency.

spinal motor neuron.[1] We have observed H-reflex loss in patients with advanced disease, particularly those with the generalized low motor–normal sensory pattern on nerve conduction study; this loss does not seem age-related because many of these patients were less than 65 years old. Increased latency fluctuation and variability (jitter) of repetitive H-reflex responses are found in patients with ALS, implying an abnormality either of synaptic input summation onto motor neurons or an intrinsic defect of motor neuron electrical properties.[88] A modified H-reflex technique, in which paired stimuli of low and high intensity cause impulse collision and repeated activation of the same alpha motor neuron pool, was used to measure inhibitory Renshaw cell function in patients with clinically definite ALS.[78] This technique, called a "conditioned" H-reflex because a submaximal conditioning stimulus precedes the maximal one, revealed markedly reduced recurrent inhibition in ALS patients compared to control subjects, suggesting that their spasticity may result from decreased Renshaw cell activity at the spinal cord level.

The sensory nerves we routinely record antidromically in three limbs of patients undergoing evaluation for ALS are listed in Table 5–4. We also regularly evaluate the H-response along the posterior tibial nerve.

NEEDLE ELECTRODE EXAMINATION

Assessing motor unit integrity by needle electrode examination is vital to the electrophysiologic diagnosis of ALS. The recorded abnormalities, however, are not specific for ALS, but also occur in disorders affecting spinal cord motor neurons (e.g., spinal muscular atrophy, poliomyelitis, syringomyelia), motor nerve roots (e.g., polyradiculopathies), and even peripheral nerves (e.g., axonloss neuropathies). These conditions are discussed in Chapter 6 as part of the differential diagnosis of ALS. The progressive nature of the anterior horn cell degeneration in ALS at multiple levels of the neuraxis results in widely distributed abnormal findings on needle electrode examination. These abnormalities can be observed when the muscle is at rest (abnormal spontaneous activity) and in varying degrees of contraction (abnormalities of motor unit firing rate, size, and form). The abnormalities are not confined to a single nerve root or peripheral nerve territory. In ALS, a constellation of findings indicating motor denervation (fibrillation potentials, decreased numbers of motor units) and reinnervation (increased duration, amplitude, and complexity of motor unit potentials) characteristically are observed. Common but not diagnostic changes include fasciculation potentials and insertional positive waves (Fig. 5–3).

Conventional studies using concentric (or less commonly, monopolar) needles provide important information for routine electrodiagnosis of ALS and are used most frequently. However, the concentric needle's 2.5-mm semicircular uptake area[74] detects only part of a normal motor unit's territory, which extends 2 to 10 mm[95] because only fibers within 0.5 mm of the electrode tip generate the "spiky" part of the motor unit potential.[74] More specialized techniques (single-fiber

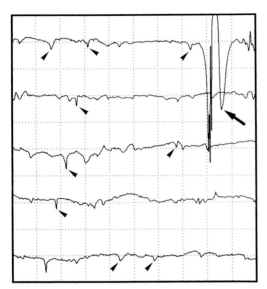

Figure 5–3. Abnormal spontaneous activity in the denervating pronator teres muscle of a patient with moderately advanced ALS with frequent fibrillation potentials (arrowheads) and a fasciculation (arrow). Note that the fibrillation potentials are 50 to 100 μV in amplitude. Each division represents gain = 200 μV, sweep speed = 10 ms.

EMG, macro EMG, scanning EMG) can reveal features of the disease process not appreciated otherwise. The techniques of single-fiber EMG, macro EMG, and scanning EMG have been particularly helpful in research settings to study motor unit pathophysiology and provide quantitative information of disease progression.[13,91,94,95]

Needle Electrode Studies of Relaxed Muscle

GENERAL

Normally, electrical activity is not detectable in resting muscle after termination of the brief (200 to 300 ms) insertional activity, which results from distortion or trauma of muscle fiber membranes by the needle electrode. The exceptions include miniature end-plate potentials and end-plate spikes caused by nearby nerve terminals and occasional fasciculations, particularly after muscle exertion. In addition, an irregular "sputtering" of a few individual or grouped motor unit potentials occasionally occurs (especially in the medial gastrocnemius muscle of

men) immediately after insertional activity has subsided. These benign discharges have been termed "snap, crackle, pop" because of their characteristic sound[111] and should not be confused with pathologic insertional activity such as fibrillation potentials. We have evaluated several patients referred with a diagnosis of ALS (based primarily on EMG findings) who only had the benign snap, crackle, pop discharges.

In ALS of long duration, and particularly in chronic neurogenic atrophies (e.g., spinal muscular atrophy), complex repetitive discharges, previously called "bizarre" repetitive discharges, and myotonic potentials can be seen. Complex repetitive discharges are regularly fired multispike discharges that have a variety of morphologies and characteristically distort the baseline of the waveform. Although their site of origin is uncertain, these discharges likely arise from the lateral or ephaptic spread of spontaneous activity in adjacent muscle fibers that act as pacemakers.[98] They are relatively nonspecific and can occur normally in some muscles such as the iliacus and paraspinalis, particularly in older individuals. Myotonic potentials, with their characteristic waxing and waning amplitudes and firing frequencies, occur infrequently in ALS, but can be seen when fibrillation potentials and insertional positive waves are prominent.[24] Grouped repetitive discharges and similar phenomena rarely occur in ALS and have no specific significance.[24] Myokymic discharges, a subset of the grouped repetitive discharge, are usually comprised of intermittent, brief, single, double, or triple discharges of single motor units. They probably do not occur in ALS but have been observed in Kennedy's disease and other conditions such as post-irradiation plexopathy.[86] Table 5–5 lists types of intramuscular electrical activity observed at rest and the likelihood that each type is pathologic.

FIBRILLATION POTENTIALS

Fibrillation potentials were originally defined by Denny-Brown and Pennybacker as the "periodic rhythmical twitch excitation of each muscle fiber sensitized by neural atrophy."[28] Fibrillation potentials are shorter in duration (0.5 to 2.0 ms) and lower in amplitude (50 to 150 μV) than motor unit poten-

Table 5–5. **INTRAMUSCULAR ELECTRICAL ACTIVITY AT REST**

Always Pathologic	Sometimes Pathologic	Benign
Fibrillation potentials*	Complex repetitive discharges[†]	End-plate spikes
Insertional positive waves*	Cramps*	Miniature end-plate potentials
Myokymia	Fasciculations*	Snap, crackle, pop discharges
Myotonic potentials[†]	Grouped repetitive discharges	

*Occurs frequently in ALS.
[†]Occurs occasionally in ALS.

tials (see Fig. 5–3). The presence of fibrillation potentials is essential for an electrodiagnosis of ALS. They are found in almost all muscles with less than half normal strength but also in about 25% of clinically unaffected muscles.[52] They represent spontaneous discharges of individual muscle fibers that have been denervated by anterior horn cell degeneration. Fibrillation potentials are believed to arise at former neuromuscular junction sites[6] from electrophysiologic and biochemical changes, including decreased resting membrane potential and increased synthesis of extrajunctional acetylcholine receptors, respectively.[39,103] Denervated muscle fiber membranes can thus be spontaneously depolarized by acetylcholine, generating fibrillation potentials.

Insertional positive waves are probably the earliest indicators of denervation, arising when the needle electrode injures a partially denervated muscle. First described by Jasper and Ballem,[48] they last longer than fibrillation potentials (2 to 15 ms). Early in ALS, when denervation is still incomplete, insertional positive waves are particularly prominent, intermixed with varying proportions of fibrillation potentials. In clinically obvious disease, fibrillations and insertional positive waves can be numerous, particularly if the course is rapidly progressive. In advanced ALS or if the course is protracted, however, fibrillation potentials may be sparse because ongoing denervation is reduced. If even partial reinnervation accompanies the denervation, further denervation and generation of fibrillation potentials occur.

FASCICULATIONS

Fasciculations are often benign, but they also are seen in pathologic conditions and frequently accompany other neurophysiologic findings in ALS.[27,28,80,109] They are spontaneous, irregularly discharging motor unit potentials that are often manifest clinically as a focal twitching or superficial contraction of a muscle belly. Even when not evident symptomatically or clinically, however, fasciculation potentials can be detected electrically (see Fig. 5–3). They can be so abundant and frequent that other spontaneous activity is obscured. They occur "so regularly in ALS that one rarely accepts the diagnosis unless fasciculation is demonstrated."[52] We have seen the occasional patient, however, who has few if any fasciculations (but significant fibrillation potentials) and subsequently develops clinically definite ALS with or without enhancement of the fasciculation potentials.

Denny-Brown and Pennybacker[27,28] were among the first to discuss the physiologic causes of fasciculations and their differentiation from fibrillation potentials and other forms of spontaneous activity. Although their site of origin has been debated (for review, see Reference 86), fasciculations in ALS can probably arise from the anterior horn cell, nerve trunk,[14] and distal nerve terminal.[22,27,38,109] Special studies, such as impulse collision techniques[80] and macro EMG,[42] have revealed an axonal origin that is generally distal to nerve branching points, although more proximal sites also have been documented.[109]

Benign fasciculation potentials cannot be differentiated from those found in ALS. Large polyphasic fasciculation potentials can occur in advanced ALS,[52] although they can also occur in relatively benign disorders.[106] However, specialized electrodiagnostic techniques such as single-fiber EMG have revealed increased jitter and fiber density in fasciculations of ALS patients.[47,98] Of course, benign fasciculations would not be associated with any electromyographic indicators of denervation such as fibrillation potentials.

CRAMPS

Cramps, which frequently occur in patients with ALS and are related pathophysiologically to fasciculations, are often seen on EMG as high-frequency (200 to 300 Hz) repetitive motor unit potentials. They usually occur with voluntary muscle contraction but can begin spontaneously as single motor unit potentials, then doublets, and finally a full cramp potential involving larger areas of a muscle.[86] Their clinical characteristics and presentation are discussed in Chapter 4.

Needle Electrode Studies with Voluntary Muscle Contraction

Normally, a mild-to-moderate degree of voluntary effort results in the synchronous firing of all muscle fibers in an activated motor unit. Action potentials of individual muscle fibers sum to produce motor unit potentials whose biphasic or triphasic waveform appearance (including duration and amplitude) is essentially constant with successive firing. As voluntary effort and therefore the motor unit potential firing rate increases, progressively more and more motor units are recruited, producing screen-fill and the so-called full interference pattern. The ratio of the firing rate of individual motor unit potentials to the number of firing motor unit potentials (recruitment ratio) in most normal muscles is 5 or less.[24] For example, if the overall firing frequency is 50 Hz, at least 10 motor unit potentials should be firing. Alternatively, if individual motor units are firing at 15 Hz each, at least three should appear. When maximal voluntary effort activates all available motor units, individual motor unit potentials may become indistinguishable because of the full interference pattern.

FIRING PATTERN

In patients with ALS, degeneration of anterior horn cells and loss of motor units results in proportionately fewer motor unit potentials firing for any given degree of effort than in healthy individuals. This reduction increases the firing rate of the remaining motor unit potentials and results in impaired recruitment, a so-called neurogenic firing pattern. Although typical of any denervating condition, this pattern may be one of the earliest changes detected by needle electrode examination in ALS. With disease progression, fewer and fewer motor units remain, so that in advanced cases, it is not uncommon to find only one or two motor unit potentials firing at a frequency of 30 Hz or higher. The neurogenic firing pattern is particularly striking during maximal effort[24,52] (Fig. 5–4).

Patients with upper motor neuron pathology may be unable to produce a full interference pattern because of difficulty activating the motor units. The resulting firing rate of motor unit potentials is slower than normal. Although suggestive of upper motor neuron dysfunction, poor activation of motor units can also result from pain or poor patient performance for other reasons.[24,52]

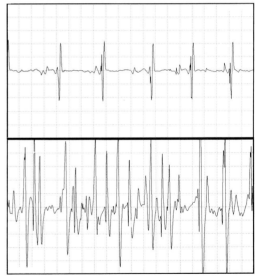

Figure 5–4. Firing patterns of motor unit potentials at maximal effort of contraction in the abductor pollicis brevis muscles of a 50-year-old patient with rapidly progressive ALS. Recruitment is markedly impaired in the severely denervated left abductor pollicis brevis (*Top*) whereas the interference pattern is full in the relatively normal muscle on the right (*Bottom*). Note that the increased firing rate of the remaining single motor unit potential (neurogenic firing pattern) in the denervated muscle (*Top*) is approximately 30 Hz. Each division represents gain = 500 μV, sweep speed = 10 ms.

NEUROGENIC MOTOR UNIT POTENTIALS

After degeneration of some anterior horn cells in ALS, the remaining cells have the potential to sprout collaterals at their nerve terminals and reinnervate nearby recently denervated muscle fibers.[114] This incorporation of muscle fibers into an established motor unit, a process termed remodeling, is reflected by increased duration and amplitude of the reformed or neurogenic motor unit potential. Motor unit potential duration[85] and amplitude[49] indicate the extent of motor unit denervation and reinnervation. Because the newly formed sprouts and neuromuscular junctions conduct more slowly and less efficiently than normally innervated junctions, particularly in the early stages of reinnervation (probably less than 3 months), several characteristic changes occur in motor unit potential configuration. They become complex and polyphasic (greater than four phases) because of asynchrony in muscle fiber potentials. Their amplitude and shape vary on consecutive discharges because impulse transmission is intermittently blocked. This moment-to-moment variation generally indicates early regeneration of nerve terminals. If the motor unit potentials remain unstable, even after sufficient time has elapsed (at least 3 months) for improvements in myelination and neuromuscular transmission, the disease is likely to be evolving rapidly and therefore has a poor prognosis. Stable motor unit potentials suggest a slower progression. Late components (satellite or linked potentials), time-locked after the main motor unit potential, can be seen because reinnervated portions of the motor unit conduct more slowly than areas that retain their innervation.[24,52]

Low-amplitude, polyphasic motor unit potentials of reinnervated motor units in some cases of ALS may be confused with those seen in myopathic conditions.[52] This differentiation is even more difficult in the case of necrotizing myopathies, in which fibrillation potentials also occur. For example, needle electrode examination of inclusion body myositis, a condition that occasionally resembles ALS (see Chapter 6), reveals fibrillation potentials and a mixed population of motor unit potentials with myopathic (low amplitude and polyphasic) and neurogenic features.

The muscles we routinely study with needle electrode examination in three limbs (arm and leg on side most affected and a contralateral arm or leg) and sometimes in the bulbar and thoracic regions are listed in Table 5–6. Although the total number of muscles studied varies between EMG laboratories, we have found this selection of muscles to be useful because of the variety of nerve root levels and peripheral nerve territories that can be identified. Other muscles may be added as directed by findings on the conventional needle electrode examination. As indicated for nerve conduction studies, when possible it is important to study clinically involved muscles and thereby enhance the diagnostic yield.

The nerve conduction study and needle electrode examination can vary depending on the stage of ALS (Table 5–7). Specific cri-

Table 5–6. **MUSCLES SUGGESTED FOR NEEDLE ELECTRODE EXAMINATION IN THE DIAGNOSIS OF ALS**

Upper Extremity	Lower Extremity	Other (Optional)
First dorsal interosseous	Extensor digitorum brevis	Frontalis
Abductor pollicis brevis	Abductor hallucis	Masseter
Extensor indicis	Flexor digitorum longus	Orbicularis oris
Flexor pollicis longus	Tibialis anterior	Tongue
Pronator teres	Gastrocnemius medialis	Mid-thoracic paraspinals
Biceps brachii	Vastus lateralis	
Triceps	Gluteus medius	
Low cervical paraspinal	High sacral paraspinal	

Table 5–7. **ELECTRODIAGNOSTIC CHANGES AT DIFFERENT STAGES OF ALS**

Study	STAGE		
	Early	Clinically Obvious	Advanced
Motor NCS			
CMAP amplitude	N or ↓	↓ or ↓↓	↓↓ or ↓↓↓
Conduction velocity	N	N	N or
Distal latency	N	N or ↑	N or ↑
Sensory NCS			
SNAP amplitude	N	N	N or ↓
Conduction velocity	N	N	N or ↓
H-reflex	N	N or ↓	N to ↓↓
NEE			
Fasciculations	N or +	N to ++	N to ++
Insertional positive sharp waves	+ or ++	+ to +++	+ to +++
Fibrillations	N or +	+ to +++	+ to +++
Motor unit potentials			
Recruitment	N or ↓	↓ or ↓↓	↓↓ or ↓↓↓
Duration	N or ↑	↑ or ↑↑	↑↑ or ↑↑↑
Amplitude	N	↑ or ↑↑	↑↑ or ↑↑↑
Complexity	N	+ or ++	+ or ++

Abbreviations: CMAP = compound motor action potential; N = normal/none; ↓/↑ = decreased/increased: 1 arrow = mild, 2 arrows = moderate, 3 arrows = marked; + = mild; ++ = moderate; +++ = marked; NCS = nerve conduction study; NEE = needle electrode examination; SNAP = sensory nerve action potential.

teria[35,52] have been established to assist in the diagnosis of ALS based on the distribution of such abnormalities, as described below.

Specialized Needle Electrode Techniques

SINGLE-FIBER EMG

Individual muscle fiber potentials in a single motor unit can be recorded using a single-fiber electrode with a side-port whose uptake area is restricted. The single-fiber EMG technique allows study of motor unit microphysiology, including the fiber density, jitter, and blocking of neuromuscular transmission.[34] Fiber density represents the number of muscle fibers belonging to a single motor unit or the number innervated by one anterior horn cell within a 300-μm radius. Jitter is an abnormally increased interval between action potentials of two repeatedly firing muscle fibers that belong to the same motor unit. Blocking occurs when the action potential is not propagated and neuromuscular transmission intermittently fails. Single-fiber EMG does not give information about the total size of the motor unit.

Single-fiber EMG is not useful for clinical diagnosis in ALS because other conditions cause abnormalities of increased fiber density (for instance, any cause of denervation and reinnervation) and increased jitter or blocking (Fig. 5–5). Single-fiber EMG has been used to study the distribution and extent of denervation and reinnervation in ALS. It can complement the conventional needle electrode examination in differentiating rapidly from slowly evolving ALS (Table 5–8).

Fiber Density

Fiber density increases to two to four times normal in approximately 75% of muscles

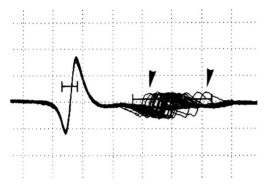

Figure 5–5. Single-fiber EMG recording of the brachioradialis muscle in a 59-year-old patient with rapidly progressing ALS revealing increased jitter between two muscle fibers innervated by the same motor unit. Firing of the muscle fiber used as the trigger is stable (*Left*) but that of the nearby muscle fiber (*Right*) is markedly variable (between arrowheads), indicating inefficient conduction through newly sprouted nerve terminals and related neuromuscular junctions. Also, approximately 10% of the motor units are blocked and do not fire (seen as the flat line through the region of increased jitter). Each division represents gain = 500 μV.

Jitter and Blocking

Jitter and blocking of neuromuscular transmission occur in 90% of ALS patients because the newly sprouted nerve terminals and immature neuromuscular junctions conduct inefficiently.[57,94] Patients with rapidly progressive disease show the most significant jitter and blocking on single-fiber EMG (see Fig. 5–5). These findings are essentially identical to those seen in myasthenia gravis, although the cause is different.

MACRO EMG

In macro EMG, a modified single-fiber electrode is used to record nonselectively from all muscle fibers in a motor unit.[90,92] The number, size, and density of the studied fibers can be determined from the area of the macro motor unit potential (calculated from its duration and amplitude). Macro EMG studies can be useful in ALS in estimating the extent of motor unit loss and, therefore, the extent of (or the degree of) motor neuron abnormality. A twofold to fourfold increase in motor unit potential amplitude probably corresponds to a 50% to 70% loss of anterior horn cells[95] (Fig. 5–6).

Patients with slowly progressing ALS may have increased macro motor unit potential amplitudes (e.g., 10 or more times normal) because of fiber grouping.[91,92] The increase represents the ongoing process of denervation and reinnervation. Studies comparing macro motor unit potential values with fiber density measured by single-fiber EMG can also reveal how well reinnervation is compensating for the ongoing denervation.[102] For example, patients with relatively stable

(tibialis anterior and biceps brachii) in ALS patients.[94,95] This increase occurs as collateral sprouts reinnervate nearby recently denervated muscle fibers to create fiber grouping.[101] Single-fiber studies can detect these changes even in clinically normal muscles or before motor unit potentials appear neurogenic by conventional needle electrode examination. Fiber densities tend to be higher in slowly progressing cases of ALS because the reinnervating anterior horn cell has time to produce a dense motor unit before its own death.[96]

Table 5–8. **INDICATORS OF DENERVATION AND REINNERVATION ON SINGLE-FIBER EMG**

Finding	Rapidly Progressive ALS	Slowly Progressive ALS
Fibrillations	Numerous	Few
Motor unit potentials		
Instability	Marked	Mild to moderate
Duration/amplitudes	Slightly increased	Significantly increased
Fiber density	Slightly increased	Significantly increased
Jitter or block	Marked	Mild to moderate

Abbreviation: EMG = electromyography.

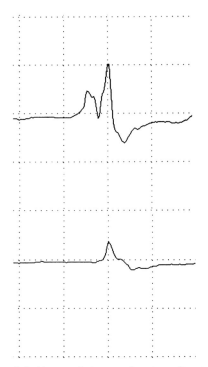

Figure 5–6. Abnormally increased motor unit potential amplitude recorded with macro EMG from the tibialis anterior muscle of a 44-year-old ALS patient (*Top*) compared with a normal recording from the same muscle in a healthy age-matched individual (*Bottom*). Compared with the normal peak-to-peak macro amplitude (80 to 575 μV) for an individual of this age, the patient's motor unit potential amplitude is markedly increased (800 μV), consistent with denervation and reinnervation secondary to motor neuron degeneration. Each division represents gain = 500 μV, sweep speed = 10 ms.

strength but parallel increases in macro motor unit potentials and fiber densities have ongoing denervation with compensatory reinnervation. Minimal weakness in the first dorsal interossei muscles of patients with early ALS, as revealed by relatively high twitch forces, was accompanied by enlarged macro motor unit potentials.[26] In contrast, little increase in macro motor unit potentials despite increasing fiber density indicates failing reinnervation. Such failure frequently occurs in patients with rapidly progressing disease when fiber grouping is limited.

In advanced disease, motor unit potentials measured by macro EMG can decrease, particularly when muscle strength diminishes significantly. This decrease is believed to result when an entire muscle fascicle supplied by a single motor unit because of repeated reinnervation (resulting in dense fiber grouping) is totally denervated after the motor neuron degenerates.[95] Motor units do not seem able to extend beyond the original fascicle during reinnervation attempts, as shown in rat muscle.[50] This finding is supported by scanning EMG studies,[91] which revealed that motor units are seldom reinnervated outside their original territory.

SCANNING EMG

Scanning EMG[91,93] provides information about the spatial distribution of muscle fibers in the entire motor unit territory and can reveal electrical evidence of fiber grouping. The process of repeated muscle denervation and reinnervation of a motor unit results in fiber grouping. While the muscle is mildly contracted, a single-fiber electrode is used as a trigger to identify the motor unit limits and a recording concentric needle electrode—the scanning electrode—samples motor unit potentials from many sites, each spaced 50 mm apart. Subsequent computer analysis of these motor unit potentials and three-dimensional plotting of their distribution provides an electrophysiologic profile of the motor unit.

In ALS, as in other chronic anterior horn cell disorders, scanning EMG has revealed that reinnervation occurs distally in the denervated motor unit but is limited to the territory originally innervated.[91] Scanning and macro EMG, therefore, are not useful to differentiate the denervation in ALS from that found in other diseases. Their utility is in monitoring the progression of ALS and potentially determining if experimental drug treatments can retard it.[13]

TECHNIQUES FOR CENTRAL NERVOUS SYSTEM EVALUATION

Sensory Evoked Potentials

Lesions of central sensory pathways can occur in ALS, as shown by abnormal somatosensory[10,58,77] or brainstem auditory[58,77] evoked potentials in patients with clinically definite ALS who had normal peripheral sensory nerve conduction studies and no other identifiable pathology. Abnormal lower extremity somatosensory evoked potentials suggest lesions in the posterior columns, whereas abnormal long-latency cortical potentials suggest lesions in the thalamocortical projections. Each of these projection pathways is affected pathologically, particularly in patients with familial ALS (see Chapter 11). Most patients undergoing these evoked potential studies had sporadic ALS and usually no sensory findings on clinical examination. Visual evoked potentials were rarely abnormal, and then only mildly so.[58] Clearly, these findings are not universal because earlier evoked potential studies of ALS patients revealed no abnormalities.[21,59,107]

Transcranial Magnetic Stimulation

Transcranial magnetic stimulation of the motor cortex for analysis of central motor pathway conduction was first devised by Barker and colleagues[4] in 1985, although high-voltage electrical stimulation had been previously reported.[63,64] This latter technique is painful. Both procedures allow noninvasive evaluation of upper motor neuron pathways in awake individuals, but magnetic stimulation is virtually pain-free. Recording motor evoked potentials over extremity muscles after cortical stimulation of patients with ALS can reveal amplitude abnormalities (absolute or relative to the compound motor action potential), prolonged latency, and central conduction delay of the excitatory postsynaptic potential.[30,33] Based on response latency in healthy individuals, conduction is believed to occur along the largest-diameter, fast-conducting monosynaptic component of the corticospinal tract.[56] It is essential to exclude the presence of any peripheral nerve dysfunction with conventional nerve conduction tests because such dysfunction would influence the motor evoked potential results.

Compared to age-matched controls, patients with ALS frequently have low motor evoked potential amplitudes, sometimes less than 10% CMAP amplitude.[33] (Normal motor evoked potential amplitude is generally greater than 50% of CMAP amplitude, depending on muscle, age, and measurement technique). Latency of the potential and central conduction delay can be prolonged. Prolonged central conduction time is significantly correlated with pyramidal signs, as revealed by extensor plantar responses.[108] Greater threshold intensities are usually needed to elicit the motor evoked potential in most, but not in all, ALS patients.[19,32] Characteristically, the ratio of the motor evoked potential to the CMAP amplitude decreases. In patients with prominent pseudobulbar features, responses may not be elicitable in limb muscles, even when muscle bulk and strength are preserved.[81] Low-amplitude motor evoked potentials probably result from loss or dysfunction of cortical motor neurons.[33,81] Approximately 15% of ALS patients, however, have motor evoked potentials that are normal or even higher in amplitude than expected for age, obtained with normal or reduced stimulation thresholds.[19,32]

Magnetic stimulation of motor cortex during the voluntary discharge of a single motor unit alters its firing probability, and this can be revealed by peristimulus time histograms.[8,9,30] Normally, motor neuron firing is increased in the early poststimulus period, about 20 ms after the cortical stimulus, representing compound excitatory postsynaptic potentials generated by cortical motor neurons that project onto the anterior horn cell being studied.[3] Peristimulus time histogram analyses have further delineated abnormalities of the descending cortical motor neuron system in ALS.[30] In addition to identifying patients with decreased or absent poststimulus firing probability, consistent with loss or dysfunction of cortical motor neurons, Eisen et al.[30] have found a subset of ALS patients with a *higher* than expected number of excitatory postsynaptic potentials, suggesting hyperexcitability of the cortical motor neuron, anterior horn cell, or both (Fig. 5–7).

Pathology affecting the upper motor neuron pathway at almost any level between the cortical motor and spinal motor neurons can cause low or absent motor evoked potentials. In addition, abnormalities in motor evoked potentials are not specific for ALS. Rarely, patients with early manifestations of ALS may have amplitudes higher than normal, possibly because of spinal motor neuron disinhibition if cortical motor neurons still function.[33] Those with a predominantly lower motor neuron form of ALS usually retain motor evoked potentials, although they are

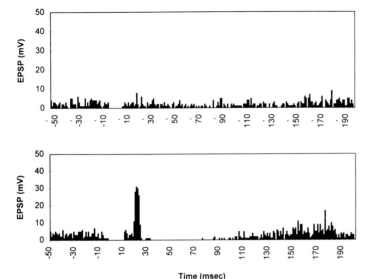

Figure 5–7. Peristimulus time histograms obtained during transcranial magnetic stimulation of two patients with ALS while recording a voluntarily activated single motor unit in the contralateral extensor digitorum communis muscle. Absence of increased excitatory postsynaptic potential firing in one patient (*Top*) suggests cortical motor neuron loss or dysfunction; higher than normal excitatory postsynaptic potential firing in the other patient (*Bottom*) is consistent with hyperexcitability of the corticospinal pathway. (Courtesy of Dr. Andrew Eisen, University of British Columbia).

often reduced and dispersed. In some of these patients, central motor studies can reveal unsuspected upper motor neuron involvement.[81] The inhibition of tonic muscle activity recorded by surface EMG that occurs in the immediate poststimulation period,[45] termed the "silent period,"[79] is prolonged in ALS[105] and in other upper motor neuron lesions.[44]

Although the diagnostic role of transcranial magnetic stimulation is limited in ALS because the technique is not widely available and frequently produces nonspecific results, it provides a relatively noninvasive means of studying the function of the upper motor neuron.[72] Further studies will be important to explore fully the potential of this technique in the electrodiagnosis of ALS.

ELECTROMYOGRAPHIC DIAGNOSTIC CRITERIA

As indicated above, the major role of electrodiagnosis in ALS, particularly of nerve conduction studies and needle electrode examinations, is to confirm the clinical diagnosis and exclude conditions that can be mistaken for ALS. These studies may provide prognostic information and even reveal evidence (on needle electrode examination) of active denervation in muscles not suspected to be clinically involved. Because EMG eval-

uates only the lower motor neuron component of ALS, objectively assessing the coexistent upper motor neuron pathology is not possible. Other techniques, such as transcranial magnetic stimulation, may prove useful in this regard.

Because the EMG changes commonly observed in ALS are not specific for this disease, electrical criteria to establish the diagnosis have been proposed. The original criteria, proposed initially by Lambert in 1957[53] and expanded in 1969[52] (Table 5–9), have been

Table 5–9. **LAMBERT CRITERIA FOR EMG DIAGNOSIS OF ALS***

- Fibrillation and fasciculation in muscles of the lower and the upper extremities, or in the extremities and the head
- Reduction in number and increase in amplitude and duration of motor unit action potentials
- Normal electrical excitability of the remaining fibers of motor nerves, and motor fiber conduction velocity within the normal range in nerves of relatively unaffected muscles and not less than 70% of the average normal value according to age in nerves of more severely affected muscles
- Normal excitability and conduction velocity of sensory nerve fibers even in severely affected extremities

*From Refs. 5, 52.
Abbreviation: EMG = electromyography.

the most widely used and have remained essentially unaltered until recently. Although the strict nature of these criteria ensures a very high degree of specificity (few false positives), sensitivity is relatively low (few true positives) because only the more clinically aggressive or advanced ALS cases fulfill all criteria. For example, in one study more than one-third of patients with a clinical diagnosis of ALS did not fulfill the Lambert criteria on EMG testing.[5] This discrepancy resulted most frequently (40/133, 30%) because "patients failed to have widespread denervation," particularly early in the course of disease. Those patients generally had fibrillation potentials in one or occasionally two limbs at the same level or in bulbar muscles but not elsewhere.[5] We have also seen this pattern because active denervation may be limited to one or both extremities at two levels (upper and lower) but not three (thoracic or bulbar).[67] In these circumstances, finding fibrillation potentials in thoracic paraspinal muscles can be especially useful because an additional level of involvement is identified.[51]

We have frequently observed active fasciculation potentials in muscles that initially showed few or no fibrillation potentials but had active denervation on subsequent studies. Repeating the EMG approximately 6 to 12 months later is usually useful, particularly to document disease progression. After the first nerve conduction study and needle electrode examination on 29 patients with clinically definite or probable ALS, we were not able to make an EMG diagnosis (using Lambert criteria) on any of these patients.[67] A repeat EMG an average of 12 months (range, 3 to 36 months) later, when all patients had clinically definite ALS, was diagnostic in 25 (87%) patients. The remaining 4 (13%) patients still had insufficient electrodiagnostic evidence of motor neuron degeneration. This follow-up EMG evaluation suggests the strictness of Lambert's criteria for electrophysiologic diagnosis of ALS.

Making a correct diagnosis of ALS in individuals in whom the disease is advanced and the clinical findings therefore obvious is usually not difficult for an experienced neurologist, even in the absence of an EMG. Early in the course of the disease, however, before widespread denervation and reinnervation

have occurred, or in slowly evolving cases, the ability of EMG to provide definite confirmation of the diagnosis provides an advantage. The ability to diagnose ALS early is a particularly important issue with the advent of research-treatment protocols; timely enrollment of patients may improve the chances of detecting a drug's benefit. In an effort to address this issue and have universally accepted guidelines for EMG diagnosis, the El Escorial diagnostic criteria for the electrophysiologic features of ALS have been established.[35]

The El Escorial criteria were agreed upon at the World Federation of Neurology Subcommittee on Motor Neuron Disease (ALS) meeting in El Escorial, Spain, in 1990. Electrophysiologic studies are recommended for patients with clinically suspected, possible, probable, or definite ALS (see Chapter 6). To confirm the diagnosis, electrophysiologic evidence of lower motor neuron degeneration (active and chronic) should be present in "at least two muscles of different root or spinal nerve and different cranial or peripheral nerve innervation in two or more of the four (bulbar, cervical, thoracic, lumbosacral) regions."[35] Evidence of denervation (fibrillation potentials, neurogenic motor unit potentials) in only one muscle in each of two nerve root territories in any two regions of bulbar, cervical, thoracic, or lumbosacral myotomes would satisfy the El Escorial EMG diagnostic criteria. Table 5–10 summarizes combinations of needle electrode examination findings of denervation-reinnervation required by El Escorial criteria to identify definite, probable, or possible primary lower motor neuron degeneration.

Although reduced recruitment (neurogenic firing pattern) is considered important enough alone to support the identification of probable lower motor neuron degeneration, it may be seen in motor conduction block. Motor conduction block is usually identifiable on motor nerve conduction studies, but if the lesion is very proximal (i.e., at the nerve root level), it may be missed, even with F-wave studies. To avoid such misdiagnosis, the El Escorial criteria include electrophysiologic features, summarized in Table 5–11, whose presence would be inconsistent with the diagnosis of ALS or would suggest other concomitant disease processes (see Chapter 6).

Table 5–10. **EL ESCORIAL WORLD FEDERATION OF NEUROLOGY CRITERIA FOR THE ELECTRODIAGNOSIS OF ALS: FEATURES FOUND ON CONVENTIONAL NEEDLE ELECTRODE EXAMINATION**

Diagnosis	Needle Electrode Exam Requirements
Definite ALS	Decreased recruitment, large (large amplitude, long duration) MUPS, fibrillation potentials *and* unstable MUPs
Probable ALS	Decreased recruitment *or* large MUPs, fibrillation potentials and unstable MUPs
Possible ALS	Decreased recruitment *or* large MUPs *or* fibrillation potentials *or* unstable MUPs

Abbreviation: MUPs = motor unit potentials.
Source: From El Escorial World Federation of Neurology: Criteria for the diagnosis of amyotrophic lateral sclerosis. J Neurol Sci 124 (suppl): 96–107, 1994, with permission.

The El Escorial EMG criteria are particularly useful because they (1) allow for varying degrees of diagnostic certainty that can be upgraded (e.g., two regions with probable or one region with probable and one region with possible EMG evidence of lower motor neuron degeneration are equivalent to one region with definite EMG evidence) and (2) incorporate findings of more specialized electrodiagnostic techniques (e.g., reduced motor unit estimates, increased macro EMG motor unit potentials, increased central motor conduction velocity, increased sensory evoked potential latencies). In addition, they can be used to supplement the clinical findings for a more definite diagnosis (e.g., one region with probable or two regions with possible EMG evidence of lower motor neuron degeneration can upgrade the certainty of clinical diagnosis from possible to probable). As stated in the El Escorial World Federation of Neurology criteria, "Definite LMN [lower motor neuron] degeneration by EMG has the same significance as clinical LMN degeneration and can upgrade the certainty of the clinical diagnosis of ALS in the same fashion as if the clinical signs of LMN degeneration were present in that region."[35]

SUMMARY

Electromyography (EMG), including nerve conduction studies and needle electrode ex-

Table 5–11. **ELECROPHYSIOLOGIC FEATURES *INCONSISTENT* WITH THE DIAGNOSIS OF ALS ACCORDING TO EL ESCORIAL CRITERIA**

- Focal decrease in CMAP $\leq$ 10% in a 4-cm segment of nerve
- Motor CVs, F-wave latencies or H-response amplitudes >30% of established normal values
- >20% decrease on repetitive stimulation at 2 Hz
- SNAP latencies >20% above or SNAP amplitudes >20% below established normal values
- Unstable MUPs with no other electromyographic changes
- Small MUPs with no other electromyographic changes
- >30% increase of central motor CV
- >10% decrease in sensory evoked potential latency or >10% decrease in sensory evoked potential amplitude
- Moderate or greater abnormalities in autonomic function or electronystagmography.

Abbreviations: CMAP = compound motor action potential, CV = conduction velocity, MUP = motor unit potential, SNAP = sensory nerve action potential.
Source: From El Escorial World Federation of Neurology: Criteria for the diagnosis of amyotrophic lateral sclerosis. J Neurol Sci 124 (suppl): 96–107, 1994, with permission.

amination, has a major role in confirming the clinical diagnosis of ALS, excluding similar-appearing conditions, and monitoring progression. It may provide prognostic information by identifying abnormalities in clinically uninvolved regions.

The mainstays of electrodiagnosis for the clinician assessing a patient for ALS are conventional motor studies, including F-waves; sensory nerve conduction studies, including H-responses; and concentric needle electrode examination. EMG essentially evaluates only the lower motor neuron degeneration in ALS. Predominant findings include normal sensory nerve conduction studies and varying degrees of abnormality on motor nerve conduction studies (e.g., low compound motor action potentials) and needle electrode examination (e.g., fibrillation potentials and neurogenic motor unit potentials) that reflect the degree of muscle denervation. Other abnormalities on needle electrode examination frequently seen in ALS, although not specific for it, include insertional positive waves and fasciculations. In evaluating patients with suspected ALS, our laboratories routinely examine specific nerves and muscles in at least three limbs to document the characteristic multifocal lower motor neuron degeneration of this disease.

Specialized but time-consuming techniques predominantly used in ALS research include motor unit estimation, repetitive stimulation, collision techniques, near nerve recording, quantitative sensory testing, single-fiber EMG, macro EMG, scanning EMG, sensory evoked potentials, and transcranial magnetic stimulation. The central nervous system diagnostic techniques of sensory evoked potentials and transcranial magnetic stimulation provide the only direct means of electrically assessing the upper neuron component of neuronal degeneration in ALS.

Because no single EMG abnormality is diagnostic for ALS, it is the combination and widespread distribution of electrodiagnostic abnormalities that distinguish this disease from other conditions affecting the lower motor neuron. To assist clinicians in making a correct diagnosis of ALS, particularly when the disease is not advanced, certain criteria have been proposed. The earliest and still most often used Lambert criteria allow for a high degree of specificity but low sensitivity.

Strict adherence to these criteria results in very little overdiagnosis but probably some underdiagnosis of early cases of ALS. This problem is particularly germane as early enrollment of patients into therapeutic drug trials becomes common. The recently proposed World Federation of Neurology (El Escorial) EMG criteria expand on the Lambert criteria and are less restrictive in regard to the distribution of certain typical changes. Moreover, they specify which findings are incompatible with an electrical diagnosis of ALS. The El Escorial criteria also provide levels of diagnostic certainty that can be modified as other clinical and laboratory information is obtained. Because no single test definitively identifies the presence of ALS, EMG is one of the most important means the clinician has to arrive at an accurate and timely diagnosis.

REFERENCES

1. Angel, RW and Hofmann, W: The H reflex in normal, spastic, and rigid subjects. Arch Neurol 8: 591–596, 1963.
2. Arasaki, K and Iwamoto, H: Motor nerve conduction studies using a new collision method: Principles and application to motor neuron disease. In Rose, FC (ed): ALS—from Charcot to the Present and into the Future. Smith-Gordon, London, 1994, pp 59–71.
3. Ashby, P and Zilm, D: Characteristics of postsynaptic potentials produced in single human motoneurons by homonymous group I volleys. Exp Brain Res 47:41–48, 1982.
4. Barker, AT, Jalinous, R, Freeston, IL, et al: Noninvasive magnetic stimulation of the human motor cortex. Lancet 1:1106–1107, 1985.
5. Behnia, M and Kelly, JJ: Role of electromyography in amyotrophic lateral sclerosis. Muscle Nerve 14:1236–1241, 1991.
6. Belmar, J and Eyzaguirre, C: Pacemaker site of fibrillation potentials in denervated mammalian muscle. J Neurophysiol 29:425–441, 1966.
7. Bernstein, LP and Antel, JP: Motor neuron disease: Decremental responses to repetitive nerve stimulation. Neurology 31:202–204, 1981.
8. Boniface, SJ, Schubert, M, and Mills, KR: Responses of single motoneurons to magnetic brain stimulation in healthy subjects and patients with multiple sclerosis. Brain 114:643–662, 1991.
9. Boniface, SJ, Schubert, M, and Mills, KR: Suppression and long latency excitation of single spinal motoneurons by transcranial magnetic stimulation in health, multiple sclerosis and stroke. Muscle Nerve 17:642–646, 1994.
10. Bosch, EP, Yamada, T, and Kimura, J: Somatosensory evoked potentials in motor neuron disease. Muscle Nerve 8:556–562, 1985.

11. Bowe, CM, Hildebrand, C, Kocsis, JD, et al: Morphological and physiological properties of neurons after long-term axonal regeneration: Observations on chronic and delayed sequelae of peripheral nerve injury. J Neurol Sci 91:259–292, 1989.

12. Bradley, WG, Good, P, Rasool, CG, et al: Morphometric and biochemical studies of peripheral nerves in amyotrophic lateral sclerosis. Ann Neurol 14:267–277, 1983.

13. Bromberg, MB, Forshew, DA, Nau, KS, et al: Motor unit number estimation, isometric strength, and electromyographic measures in amyotrophic lateral sclerosis. Muscle Nerve 16:1213–1219, 1993.

14. Brown, RJ and Johns, RJ: Abnormal motor nerve excitability. Johns Hopkins Med J 127:55–63, 1970.

15. Brown, WF and Jaatoul, N: Amyotrophic lateral sclerosis. Arch Neurol 30:242–248, 1974.

16. Brown, WF and Milner-Brown, HS: Some electrical properties of motor units and their effects on the methods of estimating motor unit numbers. J Neurol Neurosurg Psychiatry 39:249–257, 1976.

17. Brown, WF, Strong, MJ, and Snow, R: Methods for estimating numbers of motor units in biceps-brachialis muscles and losses of motor units with aging. Muscle Nerve 11:423–432, 1988.

18. Buchthal, F and Kühl, V: Nerve conduction, tactile sensibility, and the electromyogram after suture or compression of peripheral nerve: A longitudinal study in man. J Neurol Neurosurg Psychiatry 42:436–451, 1979.

19. Caramia, MD, Cicinelli, P, Paradiso, C, et al: "Excitability" changes of muscular responses to magnetic brain stimulation in patients with central motor disorders. Electroencephalogr Clin Neurophysiol 81:243–250, 1991.

20. Cavanagh, JB: Morphological problems posed by "motor neurone disease." In Rose, FC (ed): Motor Neuron Disease. Pitman Medical, London, 1977, pp 73–78.

21. Chiappa, K: Evoked Potentials in Clinical Medicine. Raven Press, New York, 1982, pp 84, 174, and 296.

22. Conradi, S, Grimby, L, and Lundemo, G: Pathophysiology of fasciculations in ALS as studied by electromyography of single motor units. Muscle Nerve 5:202–208, 1982.

23. Cornblath, DR, Kuncl, RW, Mellits, D, et al: Nerve conduction studies in amyotrophic lateral sclerosis. Muscle Nerve 15:1111–1115, 1992.

24. Daube, JR: Electrophysiologic studies in the diagnosis and prognosis of motor neuron disease. Neurol Clin 3:473–493, 1985.

25. Daube, J: Statistical estimates of number of motor units in thenar and foot muscles in patients with amyotrophic lateral sclerosis or the residual of poliomyelitis [abstract]. Muscle Nerve 11:957–958, 1988.

26. Dengler, R, Konstanzer, A, Küther, G, et al: Amyotrophic lateral sclerosis: Macro-EMG and twitch forces of single motor units. Muscle Nerve 13:545–550, 1990.

27. Denny-Brown, D: Clinical problems in neuromuscular physiology. Am J Med 15:368–390, 1953.

28. Denny-Brown, D and Pennybacker, JB: Fibrillation and fasciculation in voluntary muscle. Brain 61: 311–332, 1938.

29. Dyck, PJ, Stevens, JC, Mulder, DW, et al: Frequency of nerve fiber degeneration of peripheral motor and sensory neurons in amyotrophic lateral sclerosis. Neurology 25:781–785, 1975.

30. Eisen, A, Entezari-Taher, M, and Stewart, H: Cortical projections to spinal motoneurons: Changes with aging and amyotrophic lateral sclerosis. Neurology 46:1396–1404, 1996.

31. Eisen, A and Odusate, K: Amplitude of the F-wave—A potential means of documenting spasticity. Neurology 29:1306–1309, 1979.

32. Eisen, A, Pant, B, and Stewart, H: Cortical excitability in amyotrophic lateral sclerosis: A clue to pathogenesis. Can J Neurol Sci 20:11–16, 1993.

33. Eisen, AA and Shtybel, W: AAEM Minimonograph 35: Clinical experience with transcranial magnetic stimulation. Muscle Nerve 13:995–1011, 1990.

34. Ekstedt, J and Stålberg, E: Single-fibre electromyography for the study of the microphysiology of the human muscle. In Desmedt, JE (ed): New Developments in Electromyography and Clinical Neurophysiology, Vol 1. Karger, Basel, 1973, pp 89–112.

35. El Escorial World Federation of Neurology: Criteria for the diagnosis of amyotrophic lateral sclerosis. J Neurol Sci 124(suppl):96–107, 1994.

36. Feasby, TE and Brown, WF: Variation of motor unit size in the human extensor digitorum brevis and thenar muscles. J Neurol Neurosurg Psychiatry 37:916–926, 1979.

37. Fisher, MA: F response latencies and durations in upper motor neuron syndromes. Electromyogr Clin Neurophysiol 26:327–332, 1986.

38. Forster, FM and Alpers, BJ: Site of origin of fasciculations in voluntary muscle. Arch Neurol Psychiatry 51:264–267, 1944.

39. Froehner, SC: Molecular studies of acetylcholine receptors from denervated muscle. In Culp WJ and Ochoa, J (eds): Abnormal Nerves and Muscles as Impulse Generators. Oxford University Press, Oxford, 1982, pp 663–667.

40. Gregory, R, Mills, K, and Donaghy, M: Progressive sensory nerve dysfunction in amyotrophic lateral sclerosis: A prospective clinical and neurophysiological study. J Neurol 240:309–314, 1993.

41. Gruener, G and Dyck, PJ: Quantitative sensory testing: Methodology, applications, and future directions. J Clin Neurophysiol 11:568–583, 1994.

42. Guiloff, RJ and Modarres-Sadeghi, H: Voluntary activation and fiber density of fasciculations in motor neuron disease. Ann Neurol 31:416–424, 1992.

43. Harding, AE, Thomas, PK, Baraitser, M, et al: X-linked recessive bulbospinal neuronpathy: A report of ten cases. J Neurol Neurosurg Psychiatry 45:1012–1019, 1982.

44. Haug, BA and Kukowski, B: Latency and duration of the muscle silent period following transcranial magnetic stimulation in multiple sclerosis, cerebral ischemia, and other upper motor neuron lesions. Neurology 44:936–940, 1994.

45. Holmgren, H, Larsson, LE, and Pedersen, S: Later muscular responses to transcranial cortical stimulation in man. Electroencephalogr Clin Neurophysiol 75:161–172, 1990.

46. Iijima, M, Arasaki, K, Iwamoto, H, et al: Maximal and minimal motor nerve conduction velocities in patients with motor neuron disease: Correlation

with age of onset and duration of illness. Muscle Nerve 14:1110–1115, 1991.

47. Janko, M, Trontelj, JV, and Gersak, K: Fasciculations in motor neuron disease: Discharge rate reflects extent and recency of collateral sprouting. J Neurol Neurosurg Psychiatry 52:1375–1381, 1989.

48. Jasper, H and Ballem, G: Unipolar electromyograms of normal and denervated human muscle. J Neurophysiol 12:231–244, 1949.

49. Kopec, J and Hausmanowa-Petrusewicz, I: 1. Computer-analyse des EMG and klinische Ergerbnisse. Elektroenzeph Elektromyogr 14:28–35, 1983.

50. Kugelberg, E, Edstrom, L, and Abruzzese, M: Mapping of motor units in experimentally reinnervated rat muscle. J Neurol Neurosurg Psychiatry 33:319–329, 1970.

51. Kuncl, RW, Cornblath, DR, and Griffin, JW: Assessment of thoracic paraspinal muscles in the diagnosis of ALS. Muscle Nerve 11:484–492, 1988.

52. Lambert, EH: Electromyography in amyotrophic lateral sclerosis. In Norris, FH Jr and Kurland, LT (eds): Motor Neuron Disease. Grune and Stratton, New York, 1969, pp 135–153.

53. Lambert, EH and Mulder, DW: Electromyographic studies in amyotrophic lateral sclerosis. Staff Meet Mayo Clin 32:441–446, 1957.

54. Lewis, RA, Sumner, AJ, Brown, MF, et al: Multifocal demyelinating neuropathy with persistent conduction block. Neurology 32:958–964, 1982.

55. Magladery, JW, Teasdall, RD, Park, AM, et al: Electrophysiological studies of the H-reflex activity in patients with lesions of the nervous system. I. A comparison of spinal motor neurone excitability following afferent nerve volleys in normal persons and patients with upper motor neurone lesions. Bull Johns Hopkins Hosp 91:219–244, 1952.

56. Marsden, CD, Merton, PA, and Morton, HB: Direct electrical stimulation of corticospinal pathways through the intact scalp in human subjects. Adv Neurol 339:387–391, 1982.

57. Massey, JM, Sanders, DB, and Nadedkar, SD: Sensitivity of various EMG techniques in motor neuron disease. Electroencephalogr Clin Neurophysiol 61: S74–S75, 1985.

58. Matheson, JK, Harrington, HJ, and Hallett, M: Abnormalities of multimodality evoked potentials in amyotrophic lateral sclerosis. Arch Neurol 43:338–340, 1986.

59. Matthews, WB: The cervical somatosensory evoked potential in clinical diagnosis. In Aminoff, MW (ed): Electrodiagnosis in Clinical Neurology. Churchill-Livingstone, New York, 1980, pp 451–467.

60. McComas, AJ, Fawcett, PR, Campbell, MJ, et al: Electrophysiological estimation of the number of motor units within a human muscle. J Neurol Neurosurg Psychiatry 34:121–131, 1971.

61. McComas, AJ, Scia, REP, and Currie, S: An electrophysiological study of Duchenne dystrophy. J Neurol Neurosurg Psychiatry 34:461–468, 1971.

62. McComas, AJ, Upton, ARM, and Sica REP: Motor neurone disease and aging. Lancet 2:1447–1480, 1973.

63. Merton, PA, Hill, DK, Morton, HB, et al: Scope of technique for electrical stimulation of human brain, spinal cord, and muscle. Lancet 2:597–600, 1982.

64. Merton, PA and Morton, HB: Stimulation of cerebral cortex in the intact human subject. Nature 285:227, 1980.

65. Milner-Brown, H, Stein, R, and Lee, R: Pattern of recruiting human motor units in neuropathies and motor neurone disease. J Neurol Neurosurg Psychiatry 37:665–669, 1974.

66. Mitsumoto, H, Wilbourn, AJ, Hanson, MR, et al: Spectrum of sensory abnormalities in adult motor neuron disease (MNDs) [abstract]. Neurology 39(suppl 1):111, 1989.

67. Mitsumoto, H, Schwartzman, MJ, Levin, K, et al: Electromyographic (EMG) changes and disease progression in ALS [abstract]. Neurology 40 (suppl 1):318, 1990.

68. Mondelli, M, Rossi, A, Passero, S, et al: Involvement of peripheral sensory fibers in amyotrophic lateral sclerosis: electrophysiological study of 64 cases. Muscle Nerve 16:166–172, 1993.

69. Morimoto, K: Clinical application of the F-wave. II. Frequency of the F-wave. Kawasaki Med J 6:49–64, 1980.

70. Mulder, DW, Bushek, W, Spring E, et al: Motor neuron disease (ALS): Evaluation of detection thresholds of cutaneous sensation. Neurology 33:1625–1627, 1983.

71. Mulder, DW, Lambert, EH, and Eaton, LM: Myasthenic syndrome in patients with amyotrophic lateral sclerosis. Neurology 9:627–631, 1959.

72. Murray, NMF: The clinical usefulness of magnetic cortical stimulation. Electroencephalogr Clin Neurophysiol 85:81–85, 1992.

73. Nakanishi, T, Tamaki, M, and Arasaki, K: Maximal and minimal motor nerve conduction velocities in amyotrophic lateral sclerosis. Neurology 39:580–583, 1989.

74. Nandedkar, S, Sanders, and D, Stålberg, E: Selectivity of electromyographic recording techniques: A simulation study. Med Biol Eng Comput 23:536–540, 1985.

75. Peioglou-Harmoussi, S, Fawcett, PRW, Howel, D, et al: F-response frequency in motor neuron disease and cervical spondylosis. J Neurol Neurosurg Psychiatry 50:593–599, 1987.

76. Pestronk, A, Cornblath, DR, Ilyas, AA, et al: A treatable multifocal motor neuropathy with antibodies to GM1 ganglioside. Ann Neurol 24:73–78, 1988.

77. Radtke, RA, Erwin, A, and Erwin, CW: Abnormal sensory evoked potentials in amyotrophic lateral sclerosis. Neurology 36:796–801, 1986.

78. Raynor, EM and Shefner, JM: Recurrent inhibition is decreased in patients with amyotrophic lateral sclerosis. Neurology 44:2148–2153, 1994.

79. Rossini, PM: Methodological and physiological aspects of motor evoked potentials. In Rossini, PM and Mauguiere, F (eds): New Trends and Advanced Techniques in Clinical Neurophysiology. Elsevier, Amsterdam, 1990, pp 124–133.

80. Roth, G: The origin of fasciculations. Ann Neuro 12:542–547, 1982.

81. Schriefer, TN, Hess, CW, Mills, KR, et al: Central motor conduction studies in motor neuron disease using magnetic brain stimulation. Electroencephalogr Clin Neurophysiol 74:431–437, 1989.

82. Shahani, BT, Young, RR, Potts, F, et al: Terminal latency index (TLI) and late response studies in

motor neuron disease (MND), peripheral neuro-pathies, and entrapment syndromes [abstract]. Acta Neurol Scand 60(suppl 73):118, 1979.

83. Shefner, JM, Buchthal, F, and Krarup, C: Slowly conducting myelinated fibers in peripheral neuropathy. Muscle Nerve 14:534–542, 1991.

84. Shefner, JM, Tyler, HR, and Krarup, C: Abnormalities in the sensory action potential in patients with amyotrophic lateral sclerosis. Muscle Nerve 14:1242–1246, 1991.

85. Sica, REP, McComas, AJ, and Ferreira, JCD: Evaluation of automated method for analysing the electromyogram. Can J Neurol Sci 5:275–281, 1978.

86. Sivak, M, Ochoa, J, and Fernandez, JM: Positive manifestations of nerve fiber dysfunction: clinical, electrophysiologic, and pathologic correlates. In Brown, WF and Bolton, CF (eds): Clinical Electromyography. Butterworth-Heinemann, Boston, 1993, pp 117–147.

87. Smith, BE, Stevens, JC, Litchy, WJ, et al: Longitudinal electrodiagnostic studies in amyotrophic lateral sclerosis patients treated with recombinant ciliary neurotrophic factor [abstract]. Neurology 45:A448, 1995.

88. Soliven, B and Maselli, RA: Single motor unit H-reflex in motor neuron disorders. Muscle Nerve 15:656–660, 1992.

89. Stålberg, E: Electrogenesis in human dystrophic muscle. In Roland, LP (ed): Pathogenesis of Human Muscular Dystrophies. Excerpta Medica, Amsterdam-Oxford, 1976, pp 570–587.

90. Stålberg, E: Macro EMG, a new recording technique. J Neurol Neurosurg Psychiatry 43:469–474, 1980.

91. Stålberg, E: Electrophysiological studies of reinnervation in ALS. In Roland, LP (ed): Human Motor Neuron Diseases. Raven Press, New York, 1982, pp 47–59.

92. Stålberg, E: Macro EMG. Muscle Nerve 6:619–630, 1983.

93. Stålberg, E: Single fiber EMG, macro EMG, and scanning EMG. New ways of looking at the motor unit. CRC Crit Rev Clin Neurobiol 2:125–167, 1986.

94. Stålberg, E and Sanders, DB: The motor unit in ALS studies with different neurophysiological techniques. In Rose, FC (ed): Research progress in Motor Neurone Disease. Pitman, London, 1984, pp 105–122.

95. Stålberg, E and Sanders, DB: Neurophysiological studies in amyotrophic lateral sclerosis. In Smith, RA (ed): Handbook of Amyotrophic Lateral Sclerosis. Marcel Dekker, New York, 1992, pp 209–235.

96. Stålberg, E, Schwartz, MS, and Trontelj, JV: Single fibre electromyography in various processes affecting the anterior horn cell. J Neurol Sci 24:402–415, 1975.

97. Stålberg, E and Thiele, B: Transmission block in terminal nerve twigs: Single fibre electromyographic finding in man. J Neurol Neurosurg Psychiatry 35:52–59, 1972.

98. Stålberg, E and Trontelj, JV: Abnormal discharges generated within the motor unit as observed with single-fiber electromyography. In Culp, WJ and Ochoa, J (eds): Abnormal Nerves and Muscles as Impulse Generators. Oxford University Press, Oxford, 1982, pp 443–474.

99. Strong, MJ, Brown, WF, Hudson, AJ, et al: Motor unit estimates in the biceps-brachialis in amyotrophic lateral sclerosis. Muscle Nerve 11:415–422, 1988.

100. Sumner, AJ: Separating motor neuron diseases from pure motor neuropathies. Multifocal motor neuropathy with persistent conduction block. Adv Neurol 56:399–403, 1991.

101. Swash, M and Schwartz, MS: A longitudinal study of changes in motor units in motor neuron disease. J Neurol Sci 56:185–197, 1982.

102. Tackman, W and Vogel, P: Fibre density, amplitudes of macro-EMG motor unit potentials and conventional EMG recordings from the anterior tibial muscle in patients with amyotrophic lateral sclerosis. J Neurol 235:149–154, 1988.

103. Thesleff, S: Fibrillation in denervated mammalian skeletal muscle. In Culp, WJ and Ochoa, J (eds): Abnormal Nerves and Muscles as Impulse Generators. Oxford University Press, Oxford, 1982, pp 678–694.

104. Thomas, PK, Sears, TA, and Gilliatt, RW: The range of conduction velocity in normal motor nerve fibres to the small muscles of the hand and foot. J Neurol Neurosurg Psychiatry 22:175–181, 1959.

105. Triggs, WJ, Macdonell, RA, Cros, D, et al: Motor inhibition and excitation are independent of magnetic cortical stimulation. Ann Neurol 32:345–351, 1992.

106. Trojaborg, W and Buchthal, F: Malignant and benign fasciculations. Acta Neurol Scand 41(suppl 13):251–254, 1965.

107. Tsuji, S, Muracka, S, Kuroina, Y, et al: Auditory brainstem evoked response of Parkinson-dementia complex and amyotrophic lateral sclerosis in Guam and Japan. Clin Neurol (Tokyo) 21:37–41, 1981.

108. Ugawa, Y, Shimpo, T, and Mannen, T: Central motor conduction in cerebrovascular disease and motor neuron disease. Acta Neurol Scand 78:297–30, 1988.

109. Wettstein, A: The origin of fasciculations in motor neuron disease. Ann Neurol 5:295–300, 1979.

110. Wilbourn, AJ: Generalized low motor-normal sensory conduction responses: The etiology in 55 patients [abstract]. Muscle Nerve 7:564, 1984.

111. Wilbourn, AJ: An unreported, distinctive type of increased insertional activity. Muscle Nerve 5:S101–S105, 1982.

112. Wilbourn, AJ and Sweeney, PJ: Dissociated wasting of the medial and lateral hand muscles with motor neuron disease [abstract]. Can J Neurol Sci 21(suppl 2):S9, 1994.

113. Wirguin, I, Breener, T, Argov, Z, et al: Multifocal motor nerve condition abnormalities in amyotrophic lateral sclerosis. J Neurol Sci 112:199–203, 1992.

114. Wohlfart, G: Collateral regeneration from residual motor nerve fibers in amyotrophic lateral sclerosis. Neurology 7:124–134, 1957.

CHAPTER 6

THE DIFFERENTIAL DIAGNOSIS OF ALS

DIAGNOSIS
DISEASES CONSIDERED IN THE
   DIFFERENTIAL DIAGNOSIS OF ALS
Disorders of Muscle Tissue
Disorders of the Neuromuscular Junction
Disorders of Nerve Roots, Plexuses, and the
   Peripheral Nerves
Disorders of Anterior Horn Cells
Spinal Cord Disorders
Other Disorders of the Central Nervous
   System
Systemic Disorders
THE DIFFERENTIAL DIAGNOSIS OF
   SYMPTOMS AND SIGNS IN ALS

A variety of neurologic disorders present with features similar to ALS. Because no specific test is available to prove whether an individual has ALS, it remains a diagnosis of exclusion. The process of differential diagnosis is, therefore, particularly important because ALS may present with different patterns of weakness that include a focal onset restricted to bulbar muscles or to a single limb (mononeuritic form), a bibrachial paresis, hemiparesis (Mills variant), or paraparesis. Moreover, the weakness seen in ALS may be exclusively lower motor neuron in type at the outset, simulating a disorder of the nerve roots or plexuses, or it may be upper motor neuron in type, suggesting a myelopathy. In addition, certain characteristic findings such as fasciculations may be scattered or difficult to detect, leading the physician to consider an alternative diagnosis. Indeed, although ALS is generally viewed as a diagnosis made with a high degree of accuracy (approaching 95%) in major neurologic centers,[116] among a varied group of physicians (generalists, neurologists, and other specialists), the percentage of patients with ALS diagnosed correctly on initial evaluation is closer to 60%,[9] especially when the presentation is unilateral or predominantly asymmetric.[99]

DIAGNOSIS

The El Escorial World Federation of Neurology (WFN) criteria[17] (Table 6–1) were established because of the need for precise diagnostic criteria to apply in order for clinical research and therapeutic trials to proceed. The WFN sought to develop workable, internationally acceptable diagnostic criteria that would enhance clinical and research studies in the field of ALS.[17]

To make the diagnosis of ALS, a combination of lower and upper motor neuron signs with evidence of spread within a region or to other regions of the body is required. The four cardinal regions are defined in Table

Table 6–1. **EL ESCORIAL WORLD FEDERATION OF NEUROLOGY CRITERIA FOR THE DIAGNOSIS OF ALS**

Features Present	Features Absent
• Signs of lower motor neuron degeneration by clinical, EMG, or neuropathologic examination • Signs of upper motor neuron degeneration by clinical examination • Progressive spread of signs within a region, or to other regions	• EMG evidence of other disease processes that might explain signs of lower motor neuron or upper motor neuron degeneration • Neuroimaging evidence of other disease processes that might explain observed clinical and EMG signs

Abbreviation: EMG = electromyography.

6–2: bulbar, cervical, thoracic, and lumbosacral. Because the progressive spread of signs from region to region is so critically important in the diagnosis of ALS, the El Escorial WFN conference provided guidelines based on topographic criteria to establish the diagnosis with varying degrees of certainty (Table 6–3). Finally, establishing the diagnosis of ALS is a multistep process, as delineated in Table 6–4. It begins with the history and physical examination, moves on to a variety of laboratory studies, and is considered complete when re-evaluation indicates progression.

DISEASES CONSIDERED IN THE DIFFERENTIAL DIAGNOSIS OF ALS

Because ALS may disturb the structure and function of the upper and lower motor neurons—elements crucial to motor control—its manifestations vary. Symptoms and signs of

Table 6–2. **THE FOUR REGIONS ASCERTAINED IN THE DIAGNOSIS OF ALS**

Region	Specific Muscle Groups
Bulbar	Jaw, face, palate, tongue, larynx
Cervical	Neck, arm, hand, diaphragm
Thoracic	Back, abdomen
Lumbosacral	Back, abdomen, leg, foot

ALS are encountered in a large and varied group of disorders, both neurologic and systemic. Thus, in clinical practice, the differential diagnosis of ALS is extensive. In Table 6–5, the differential diagnosis of ALS is reviewed on the basis of the anatomy of the nervous system and therefore a heterogeneous group of disorders is considered: those characterized by pathologic changes in anterior horn cells, corticospinal tracts, or both; and others in which the pathologic alteration occurs outside of the central nervous system in a variety of areas including muscle, the neuromuscular junction, and peripheral nerve tissue.

Disorders of Muscle Tissue

IDIOPATHIC INFLAMMATORY MYOPATHY

The inflammatory myopathies are immune-mediated diseases classified according to one of three types: polymyositis, dermatomyositis, and inclusion body myositis (IBM).[28] In all three, weakness is prominent. Polymyositis is characterized by the subacute onset of proximal muscle and neck flexor weakness; dysphagia occurs in about 30% of cases. Dermatomyositis is similar with regard to the distribution of weakness but produces a coexisting rash that is erythematous, scaling, sometimes pruritic, and distributed over sun-exposed areas of the face, chest, and back. Extramuscular abnormalities include cardiac conduction defects and interstitial pul-

Table 6–3. **LEVELS OF CERTAINTY IN THE CLINICAL DIAGNOSIS OF ALS ACCORDING TO THE WORLD FEDERATION OF NEUROLOGY GUIDELINES**

Level of Certainty	Characteristic Features
Suspected ALS	Only lower motor neuron signs in two or more regions
Possible ALS	• Upper motor neuron and lower motor neuron signs are in only one region; or,
	• Upper motor neuron signs alone are present in two or more regions; or,
	• Lower motor neuron signs are rostral to upper motor neuron signs
	• Special cases:* Monomelic ALS, progressive bulbar palsy without spinal upper motor neuron and/or lower motor neuron signs, primary lateral sclerosis without spinal lower motor neuron signs
Probable ALS	Upper and lower motor neuron signs in at least two regions; although the regions may be different, some upper motor neuron signs must be above the lower motor neuron signs
Definite ALS	• Upper motor neuron as well as lower motor neuron signs in the bulbar region and at least two other spinal regions; or,
	• Upper motor neuron and lower motor neuron signs in three spinal regions

*Lower motor neuron or upper motor neuron signs develop over time to meet criteria for probable ALS; or, probable ALS may be confirmed at autopsy by specific lower and upper motor neuron neuropathologic findings.

Table 6–4. **STEPS IN THE DIAGNOSIS OF ALS SUGGESTED BY WORLD FEDERATION OF NEUROLOGY GUIDELINES**

Steps	Rationale
1. History, physical examination	• Ascertain clinical findings that may suggest level of certainty of diagnosis
2. EMG examination	• Ascertain findings that confirm lower motor neuron degeneration in clinically involved regions
	• Identify lower motor neuron degeneration in clinically uninvolved regions
	• Exclude other disorders
3. Neuroimaging	• Ascertain findings that may exclude other disease processes
4. Clinical laboratory examinations	• Ascertain possible ALS-related syndromes*
5. Neuropathologic examinations	• Ascertain findings that may confirm or exclude sporadic ALS, ALS-related syndromes, ALS variants
6. Repetition of clinical and EMG examinations (6 months apart)	• Ascertain evidence of progression

*See Chapter 7.
Abbreviation: EMG = electromyography.

Table 6–5. **THE DIFFERENTIAL DIAGNOSIS OF ALS CLASSIFIED BY ANATOMY OF THE NERVOUS SYSTEM**

Anatomic Site	Possible Disorder
Muscle	Idiopathic inflammatory myopathy (especially IBM), distal myopathy, nemaline myopathy, isolated neck extensor myopathy, metabolic myopathy, oculopharyngeal dystrophy
Neuromuscular junction	MG, Lambert-Eaton myasthenic syndrome
Roots, plexus, nerve	Radiculopathy, diabetic polyradiculoneuropathy, infectious polyradiculopathy, plexopathies, mononeuropathies, motor neuropathies
Anterior horn cells	Spinal muscular atrophy, BSN, monomelic amyotrophy, paraneoplastic motor neuronopathy, progressive post-polio muscular atrophy, hexosaminidase deficiency
Spinal cord	Spondylotic myelopathy, syringomyelia, MS, adrenomyeloneuropathy, vitamin B_{12} deficiency, familial spastic paraparesis, HTLV-1 myelopathy
Central nervous system	Parkinson's disease, Creutzfeldt-Jakob disease, multisystem atrophy, Huntington's disease, brain-stem stroke, brain-stem glioma, foramen magnum tumors
Systemic disorders	Hyperthyroidism, hyperparathyroidism

Abbreviations: BSN = bulbospinal neuronopathy, HTLV-1 = human T-lymphotropic virus type 1, IBM = inclusion body myositis, MG = myasthenia gravis, MS = multiple sclerosis.

monary fibrosis. About 15% of patients have an underlying neoplasm, and about 20% of patients have an associated collagen-vascular disorder.

In both polymyositis and dermatomyositis, the examination reveals proximal muscle weakness that ranges from mild to pronounced. Most involved are the neck flexors, shoulder and pelvic girdle muscles, and humeral and femoral muscles. Deep tendon reflexes are usually spared. The muscles may thin somewhat with disuse, but marked muscle atrophy does not occur and no fasciculations exist.

IBM differs somewhat from the other forms in that it tends to occur in persons older than 60 years and is much more indolent. It is also more likely to involve distal muscles, especially the foot extensors and deep finger flexors. It often presents in an asymmetric or focal fashion with selective weakness and

atrophy of the forearm flexors, triceps, biceps, quadriceps, and iliopsas.[28] Rarely, severe, isolated erector spinae–paravertebral muscle paresis may occur.[63] Associated neoplasms and collagen-vascular disorders are unusual. Heart and lung complications have not been described.

For all forms, the diagnosis is established by the clinical features, an elevated serum creatinine kinase (CK) level, abnormal electromyography (EMG) findings, and pathologic findings on muscle biopsy histology.[28] The CK level is increased in 80% to 90% of patients in all three forms but tends to be only mildly increased in IBM. The EMG reveals fibrillation potentials and myopathic motor unit potentials in all three myopathies, whereas in IBM and chronic polymyositis, neurogenic-appearing motor unit potentials are also frequently seen. The muscle biopsy reveals muscle fiber necrosis, regeneration, and inflammatory cell infiltrates in all forms, with rimmed vacuoles in IBM.

ALS and the inflammatory myopathies both produce proximal muscle weakness. The presence of a rash immediately differentiates the proximal weakness of dermatomyositis from proximal weakness that might occur in ALS. Distinguishing polymyositis from ALS is somewhat more difficult, but the weakness of polymyositis is not attended by significant atrophy, fasciculations, or upper motor neuron signs. Nonetheless, early in the course of ALS, fasciculations may be difficult to detect and the overall pattern might be consistent with polymyositis. Electromyography and measurement of CK concentration may be required to make the crucial distinction.

Distinguishing ALS from IBM can be challenging (Table 6–6). These conditions share dysphagia and neck and limb muscle weakness, as well as asymmetric presentation and muscle atrophy. Furthermore, in both conditions, the CK level may be mildly to moderately elevated and EMG shows fibrillation potentials and enlarged motor unit potentials. The similarities, however, end at this point. Although muscle atrophy exists in IBM, fasciculations and upper motor neuron signs do not. Nonetheless, even experienced neurologists occasionally have difficulty distinguishing IBM from the progressive muscular atrophy presentation of ALS. A muscle biopsy may be required to reveal the inflammatory cell infiltrates and rimmed vacuoles of IBM.[86]

DISTAL MYOPATHY

In addition to IBM, other myopathies affect the distal muscles. One of these, found mostly in Sweden, has been designated familial distal myopathy of Welander, named after the neurologist who first clearly described the entity.[145] It is autosomal dominant with an onset usually between the ages

Table 6–6. FEATURES OF MYOPATHIES CONSIDERED IN THE DIFFERENTIAL DIAGNOSIS OF ALS

Disease	CLINICAL AND LABORATORY FEATURES	
	Shared with ALS	**Atypical for ALS**
Inclusion body myositis	Asymmetric and focal weakness, atrophy; creatinine kinase level elevation; neurogenic electromyography	No fasciculations; no upper motor neuron signs* Biopsy: vacuolar myopathy
Distal myopathy	Distal muscle weakness, atrophy	Biopsy: vacuolar myopathy
Myotonic dystrophy	Distal muscle weakness, atrophy	Multisystem involvement; clinical and electrical myotonia; biopsy: ringbinden, internalized nuclei
Adult nemaline myopathy	Limb weakness, atrophy; head drop	Biopsy: atrophic fibers with rods
Isolated neck extensor myopathy	Head drop, fibrillation potentials in cervical paraspinals	No progression or spread of weakness
Metabolic myopathies	Limb weakness and wasting	Biopsy: evidence for glycogen or lipid storage
Oculopharyngeal dystrophy	Bulbar symptoms and signs	Ophthalmoparesis; Biopsy: vacuoles in atrophic fibers; filamentous inclusions

*Fasciculations and upper motor neuron signs are absent in all myopathic disorders

of 40 and 60 years. Hand involvement, marked by weakness and clumsiness of fine movements, tends to antedate weakness of foot and anterior tibial muscles. Reports of another familial distal myopathy in other parts of the world have indicated that weakness is more likely to begin in the feet and become generalized. A sporadic form of distal myopathy has been described in this country.[89]

The examination discloses features seen in ALS (see Table 6–6): weakness and wasting of intrinsic muscles of the hands and feet, muscles of the anterior leg compartments, and the finger and wrist extensors, with preservation, early in the course, of tendon reflexes and sensation. Laboratory findings of "myopathic changes" on EMG and muscle biopsy analysis that reveals vacuolation help to establish the correct diagnosis.[77]

MYOTONIC DYSTROPHY

Myotonic dystrophy is another disorder that produces generalized weakness with a distal predominance and leads to muscle loss that in isolation might suggest a denervating disorder like ALS. The presence of facial weakness, dysphagia, and rarely, respiratory involvement[64] are additional features that may lead the clinician to consider ALS. The extramuscular systemic manifestations, typical facial features, and presence of grip, percussion, and electrical myotonia, however, distinguish it from ALS (see Table 6–6). If doubt persists, a muscle biopsy of myotonic dystrophy reveals architectural changes such as ringbinden and sarcoplasmic masses, as well as prominent type I fiber atrophy and a profusion of internalized nuclei; these are features unlikely to be found in ALS. The diagnosis of myotonic dystrophy may also be confirmed by demonstrating an abnormal expansion of the cytosine-thymine-guanine repeat of the myotonic dystrophy gene on chromosome 19.

If the clinician suspects myotonic dystrophy but the abnormal expansion is not present, then consideration should be given to the more benign autosomal-dominant myopathy known as proximal myotonic myopathy, or PROMM.[113] PROMM presents in adult life (fifth to eighth decades) with proximal muscle and anterior neck muscle weakness and thus might lead a clinician to consider the diagnosis of ALS. As in classic myotonic dystrophy, however, in PROMM there is a consistent association with cataracts, and the EMG reveals myotonic discharges, features not seen in ALS.

NEMALINE MYOPATHY

Nemaline myopathy can present in infancy, childhood, and, rarely, in adulthood. Most patients with the late-onset form develop a limb girdle syndrome in the fifth or sixth decade of life.[106] Pelvic girdle and proximal leg muscles are more involved than shoulder girdle and proximal arm muscles. In some patients, neck extensor weakness is severe, and lumbar lordosis is prominent because of truncal weakness. The CK level is usually normal, so this condition could be mistaken for ALS (see Table 6–6). Muscles supplied by cranial nerves are spared, however, and the EMG findings are generally consistent with a myopathy, although neurogenic features have been reported.[20] Most importantly, the muscle biopsy specimen generally reveals myopathic changes in fiber size, fiber degeneration, and an abundance of rod bodies, especially in the smaller fibers.[40]

ISOLATED NECK EXTENSOR MYOPATHY

Isolated neck extensor muscle weakness is a newly recognized myopathy that affects older individuals in the sixth to eighth decades of life.[72,136] Weakness progresses for a variable period of time—weeks to months—and then stabilizes. The CK is typically normal, and the EMG discloses fibrillation potentials with short-duration motor unit potentials in cervical paraspinal muscles. Cervical MRI of cervical paraspinals shows edema-like changes and atrophy, and muscle biopsy demonstrates nonspecific myopathic features. The presentation of neck weakness (head drop) in older adults with fibrillation potentials on EMG raises the possibility of ALS, but the isolated nature and benign course distinguish it clearly from ALS.

METABOLIC MYOPATHIES

These conditions, which are usually autosomal recessive, present in childhood or adolescence and include disorders of glycogen and lipid metabolism. They can manifest initially in adult life, albeit rarely. (Also included in the category of metabolic myopathy are the mitochondrial disorders, but because of prominent ocular involvement, they are rarely confused with ALS.)

Acid maltase deficiency, a lysosomal glycogen-storage disease, can present in the fourth or fifth decade of life with slowly progressive weakness and wasting of limb muscles and respiratory muscle compromise.[71] The CK level is elevated, and EMG may show neuropathic features. Therefore, this disease could stimulate the progressive muscular atrophy presentation of ALS. The EMG, however, typically discloses myotonic discharges, especially in paraspinal muscles, and muscle-biopsy analysis reveals a vacuolar myopathy with a severe reduction in acid maltase level.

Other glycogen-storage diseases include McArdle's disease (caused by myophosphorylase deficiency) and phosphofructokinase deficiency, both of which cause defects in the glycolytic pathway and usually present with a syndrome of muscle aches, cramps, pain, and myoglobinuria. Rarely, however, they present with weakness and wasting in adults but without exercise intolerance, suggesting an acquired late-onset myopathy like polymyositis.[32,41] This presentation might also superficially mimic the progressive muscular atrophy presentation of ALS, but laboratory studies (failure of serum lactate level to rise on a forearm exercise test and glycogen accumulation found on muscle-biopsy specimen) should point to the correct diagnosis of a glycogen-storage disease.

Another metabolic myopathy is debrancher enzyme deficiency. It usually begins in infancy and is characterized by hepatomegaly, growth retardation, fasting hypoglycemia, and cirrhosis. The disease also has been recognized as a cause of slowly progressive weakness in adults. Rarely, wasting and weakness in this condition may resemble disease of the lower motor neuron system.[34]

Muscle carnitine deficiency is a rare lipid metabolism disorder that usually presents during childhood or in the early teenage years as progressive proximal and distal weakness. Rarely, it may cause a late-onset myopathy with neuropathic features on the EMG.[88] Therefore, this condition could be considered in the differential diagnosis of the lower motor neuron form of ALS.

OCULOPHARYNGEAL DYSTROPHY

Oculopharyngeal dystrophy (OPD) is a rare autosomal-dominant disorder (chromosomal location unknown) that affects predominantly French-Canadian and Spanish-American peoples. Affected family members generally develop progressive ptosis and dysphagia in the fifth or sixth decade of life.[93] As the disease progresses, weakness involves the extraocular, facial, and limb muscles in a bilateral and symmetric fashion. The dysphagia can become severe and lead to oropharyngeal or nasopharyngeal regurgitation, choking, and aspiration. Palatal and laryngeal weakness leads to dysphonia.

OPD can simulate the progressive bulbar palsy form of ALS if the ocular features are minimal or mild and the familial nature of the condition is not known. In some cases, dysphagia precedes ptosis, thereby obscuring the diagnosis of OPD. Further, distinguishing between ALS and OPD is difficult because the CK level is usually normal or mildly elevated in both disorders. Another confounding factor is the EMG result of increased insertional activity in the form of positive waves and fibrillation potentials in OPD;[24] this finding is similar to findings in ALS, although fasciculations do not occur in OPD (see Table 6–6). A muscle biopsy specimen is helpful in making the diagnosis of OPD in patients without characteristic ptosis and ophthalmoparesis because it reveals small angulated fibers, rimmed vacuoles, motheaten fibers, rare fiber degeneration, and intranuclear, 9- to 10-nm filamentous inclusions seen on electron microscopy.[141] Recent work, however, has found prominent neurogenic features on muscle histology in some patients and families, suggesting that OPD is most appropriately considered a syndrome with differing pathogenetic mechanisms.[54]

Disorders of the Neuromuscular Junction

MYASTHENIA GRAVIS

Myasthenia gravis (MG) is an autoimmune disease in which antibodies are directed against acetylcholine receptors of the neuromuscular junction and lead to their depletion, resulting in the clinical hallmark of myasthenia, that is, fatigable muscle weakness.[37] The disorder occurs in all age groups but has a somewhat greater incidence in younger women and in older men. In its most common presentation, muscles supplied by cranial nerves (especially ocular muscles) are affected so that patients present with ptosis and diplopia as well as dysarthria, dysphagia, and chewing difficulty. Rarely, patients present with limb girdle muscle weakness and fatigability without bulbar muscle involvement.

The classification of MG, based on the distribution and severity of weakness, includes two major categories, a purely ocular form and a generalized form.[37] The generalized form is subdivided into mild, moderate, and severe types. Myasthenic crisis occurs in the severe generalized type and includes respiratory compromise.

The physical examination discloses a pure motor syndrome with weakness ranging from mild weakness localized to the ocular muscles to severe, generalized weakness including the respiratory muscles. Deep tendon reflexes are usually normal, and there are no pathologic reflexes. Although muscles are weak, they are not atrophic and have no fasciculations. In some particularly severe and longstanding cases, muscles may thin somewhat from disuse, but true neurogenic atrophy does not occur.

Although ocular symptoms and fatigability make the diagnosis of MG easy in most patients, in some, ptosis and diplopia may be absent, and the disease may present with a variety of symptoms, including dysarthria, dysphagia, drooling, and head drop secondary to weakness of the neck extensors. These features are reminiscent of the progressive bulbar palsy form of ALS. Indeed, we have, on occasion, experienced considerable difficulty in differentiating the bulbar presentation of MG from a progressive bulbar palsy form of ALS (Table 6–7). Edrophonium testing and repetitive nerve stimulation might show positive results in both disorders, and in 10% of patients with MG, autoantibodies to the acetylcholine receptor cannot be demonstrated. Therefore, these diagnostic modalities may not distinguish between the two conditions. Another confounding factor is the rare involvement in ALS of cranial nuclei responsible for extraocular movement, so that the occurrence of an eye movement disorder is not absolute evidence against ALS.[97] In MG, however, one would not expect to see atrophy or fasciculations of bulbar muscles, nor should the examiner detect a pathologically brisk jaw reflex, all of which are features of ALS. In ALS, EMG of weak bulbar muscles should disclose fibrillation and fasciculation potentials, findings that would not ordinarily be expected in MG (although fibrillation potentials may be found in longstanding and severe MG). Additionally, autoantibodies to the acetylcholine receptor are present in almost 90% of patients with generalized MG but are absent in ALS.

Table 6–7. FEATURES OF NEUROMUSCULAR JUNCTION DISORDERS CONSIDERED IN THE DIFFERENTIAL DIAGNOSIS OF ALS

| Disease | CLINICAL AND LABORATORY FEATURES | |
	Shared with ALS	Atypical for ALS
Myasthenia gravis	Bulbar symptoms and signs, head drop, respiratory compromise	No fasciculations, no upper motor neuron signs,* ptosis, ophthalmoparesis, positive acetylcholine receptor antibody
Lambert-Eaton myasthenic syndrome	Limb weakness, low motor amplitudes on motor conduction studies	High likelihood of associated neoplasm or connective tissue disease, strength and tendon reflex augmentation after exercise, postactivation facilitation on electromyography

*Fasciculations and upper motor neuron signs are absent in disorders of the neuromuscular junction.

LAMBERT-EATON MYASTHENIC SYNDROME

In Lambert-Eaton myasthenic syndrome (LEMS), antibodies are directed against voltage-gated calcium channels on the motor axon terminal of the neuromuscular junction.[144] Loss of calcium channels leads to failure of acetylcholine release induced by nerve action potentials, and thus muscle weakness develops. LEMS usually occurs as a paraneoplastic syndrome in association with small-cell lung cancer, typically in elderly male smokers, but it also can develop in the absence of cancer as a manifestation of autoimmunity, typically in women.

The clinical hallmark of the illness is limb girdle muscle weakness, sometimes accompanied by autonomic symptoms such as dry eyes, dry mouth, impotence, and constipation.[98] In contrast to MG, weak muscles strengthen with repetitive contraction. Mild cranial nerve findings such as ptosis and ophthalmoparesis may be seen, but prominent involvement of muscles supplied by cranial nerves, as occurs in MG, is unusual. Physical examination reveals weakness without significant atrophy and no fasciculations. Deep tendon reflexes may be attenuated or lost but reappear after brief, maximal voluntary muscular contraction. Particularly in patients with an underlying neoplasm, there may be an associated sensory neuropathy that is a manifestation of another paraneoplastic disorder, subacute sensory neuronopathy. Nerve condition studies show very low initial motor amplitudes that increase by more than 200% after a brief (15-second) period of exercise.[98]

Limb girdle weakness is one clinical feature shared by both ALS and LEMS. In ALS, one would also expect to see muscle atrophy and fasciculations, hyperreflexia and spasticity, or both. In the early stages, however, the diagnosis of ALS may not be clear because these features may be subtle or not evident (see Table 6–7). Two other features that are characteristic of LEMS more clearly differentiate it from ALS: an increase in muscle strength with repetitive use and autonomic dysfunction. EMG is a powerful diagnostic tool if the distinction between the two disorders remains difficult on clinical grounds; although low motor amplitudes may be evoked in both disorders, a significant percentage of postactivation facilitation is highly characteristic and specific for LEMS and is not seen in ALS. Another point of distinction is that the fibrillation and fasciculation potentials seen on EMG that are typical of ALS are never encountered in LEMS (see Chapter 5).

Disorders of Nerve Roots, Plexuses, and the Peripheral Nerves

RADICULOPATHY

Both cervical and lumbosacral radiculopathies are common problems in clinical practice.[23] Nerve roots may be compromised by either disc herniation or joint narrowing caused by osteoarthritis and degenerative joint disease. In the cervical area, the most commonly encountered radiculopathies are at C6 and C7; radiculopathies at C5 and C8 are less common, together amounting to 20% to 25% of cases. As classically described, radiculopathy has a triad of symptoms: pain, paresthesias, and weakness.

Depending on which nerve root is compromised, the examination will disclose different patterns of sensory and motor deficits (Table 6–8). In C6 radiculopathy, sensory loss is most pronounced to pinprick in the C6 dermatome; biceps and brachioradialis reflexes are attenuated. Weakness may be found in one or more C6-supplied muscles such as the infraspinatus or supraspinatus, deltoid, biceps, or brachioradialis. In C7 radiculopathy, sensory loss occurs in the C7 dermatome, the triceps reflex is usually reduced or absent, and one or more of the C7-supplied muscles, such as the triceps and wrist flexor and extensor muscles, are found to be weak. C5 radiculopathy gives rise to weakness, sensory loss in the C5 dermatome, and reflex changes fairly similar to those found in C6 radiculopathy. In C8 radiculopathy, sensory loss occurs in C8 dermatome and weakness is seen in the C8-supplied muscles, including the finger extensors and hand intrinsic muscles supplied by the ulnar and median nerves.

In the lumbosacral region, the most commonly encountered radiculopathies are at L5 and S1. In L5 radiculopathy, there may be

Table 6–8. **RADICULOPATHIES CONSIDERED IN THE DIFFERENTIAL DIAGNOSIS OF ALS**

Radiculopathy	Muscles Weakened	Classic Presentation
C6	Spinati, deltoid, serratus anterior, biceps	Shoulder girdle weakness, atrophy
C7	Triceps, flexors and extensors of wrist	Arm and forearm weakness
C8	Finger extensors, hand intrinsics	Clumsy, atrophic hand
L4	Hip flexors, quadriceps, thigh adductors	Knee buckling (instability)
L5	Tibialis anterior and posterior, glutei, hamstrings	Footdrop
S1	Gastrocnemius, foot intrinsics, glutei, hamstrings	Calf and foot atrophy

sensory loss in the L5 dermatome and weakness of one or more of the L5-supplied muscles: the extensor hallucis longus, tibialis anterior, tibialis posterior, hamstrings, and glutei. S1 radiculopathy produces sensory loss in the S1 dermatome, and the ankle reflex is typically diminished or lost. Weakness may be found in S1-supplied muscles, including the long flexors of the toes, the gastrocnemius and soleus, the hamstrings, and the glutei. In the less commonly encountered L4 radiculopathy, sensory loss occurs in the L4 dermatome, along with attenuation or loss of the knee jerk and weakness in L4-supplied muscles such as the iliopsoas, quadriceps, and thigh adductors.

The diagnosis of radiculopathy rests on the clinical features and is supported by nerve root compression demonstrated on CT myelography or MRI. EMG has an important role in revealing acute and chronic denervation changes in paraspinal muscles and in the limb muscles served predominantly by single roots. The EMG features (distribution of fibrillation potentials) are relatively stereotyped for C5, C7, and C8 radiculopathies, whereas C6 radiculopathy has the most variable presentation; in half the patients the findings are similar to C5 radiculopathy, whereas in the other half, they are identical to C7 radiculopathy.[82]

Because radiculopathy is typically associated with pain and numbness, it is not often mistaken for ALS. Rarely, however, patients with ALS complain of thoracic radicular symptoms, possibly secondary to paraspinal weakness resulting in increased thoracic kyphosis and producing traction on the thoracic roots.[95] In some instances, however, pain and numbness are only minor features or are absent, and weakness may be the major manifestation of the nerve root disorder. Therefore, radiculopathies must be considered in the differential diagnosis of any patient presenting with focal weakness of the lower motor neuron type. For example, footdrop, a common presentation of ALS, could also be caused by an L5 radiculopathy, and hand clumsiness, another presentation of ALS, could be a manifestation of a C8 radiculopathy. The differentiation between ALS and radiculopathy is aided enormously by imaging and EMG studies. MRI of the cervical or lumbosacral spine will disclose nerve root compromise in the case of significant radiculopathy but should be unremarkable in ALS; EMG will reveal changes restricted to a single segment or to contiguous nerve root levels in radiculopathy, whereas such changes should be widespread in ALS (Table 6–9).

DIABETIC POLYRADICULONEUROPATHY

An important nonstructural polyradiculoneuropathy is associated with diabetes. The usual presentation is anterior thigh pain and dysesthesias with weakness, reflecting major involvement of the upper lumbar roots. The onset is usually fairly abrupt, with symptoms

Table 6–9. **FEATURES OF RADICULOPATHIES AND PLEXOPATHIES CONSIDERED IN THE DIFFERENTIAL DIAGNOSIS OF ALS**

Disease	CLINICAL AND LABORATORY FEATURES	
	Shared with ALS	Atypical for ALS
Cervical or lumbosacral radiculopathy	Asymmetric arm or leg weakness, atrophy; neurogenic EMG; fasciculations*	No upper motor neuron signs,[†] segmental pain, numbness, and reflex loss; MRI: nerve root compression
Diabetic polyradiculo-neuropathy	Asymmetric lower extremity weakness; atrophy	Pain, sensory loss; EMG: polyneuropathy
Brachial plexus neuropathy	Asymmetric upper extremity weakness; atrophy	Limited distribution; pain; variable sensory loss
Idiopathic lumbosacral plexopathy	Asymmetric lower extremity weakness; atrophy	Limited distribution; pain; variable sensory loss

*Fasciculations are present (often infrequent and scattered) in these disorders.
[†]Upper motor neuron signs are absent in disorders of the nerve roots and plexuses.
Abbreviation: EMG = electromyography.

developing over days to weeks. The major features are asymmetric weakness of muscles served by the L2–4 roots (the iliopsoas, quadriceps, and thigh adductors), reduced or absent patellar reflex, and mild impairment of sensation over the anterior thigh. As time passes, "territorial spread" may occur,[7] a term that describes proximal, distal, or contralateral involvement as the polyradiculoneuropathy evolves. The condition may worsen steadily or in a stepwise fashion. The interval between onset and peak of the disease averages about 6 months (range, 2 weeks to 18 months).[6] At its peak, weakness varies in severity and extent from mild (with slight, unilateral thigh weakness) to a profound degree of bilateral leg weakness in the territories of the L2–S2 nerve roots. Rarely, territorial spread is so extensive that it involves cervical roots and leads to profound generalized weakness, a condition termed *diabetic cachexia.*

Although the full-blown syndrome with its rapid onset of pain and sensory symptoms is quite distinct from ALS, in some patients sensory symptoms are minimal or absent, so that diabetic polyradiculoneuropathy may resemble the progressive muscular atrophy form of ALS (see Table 6–9). In most patients, however, blood sugar or glycosylated hemoglobin levels are increased, and electrodiagnostic testing discloses a polyradiculoneuropathy with sensory involvement.

METASTATIC POLYRADICULOPATHY

Many types of neoplasms are known to spread to the leptomeninges, including leukemias, lymphomas, melanoma, and breast, lung, and gastric tumors. The clinical features of metastatic polyradiculopathy may include radicular pain, dermatomal sensory loss, areflexia, and weakness of the lower motor neuron type. When the distribution of sensory and motor deficits is widespread, the disorder may simulate a sensorimotor polyneuropathy. In rare instances, sensory symptoms and signs are slight or absent, and the clinical syndrome may resemble the progressive muscular atrophy form of ALS. In most patients, however, metastatic polyradiculopathy is associated with clinical features such as confusion, headache, and cranial neuropathies; the brain MRI discloses hydrocephalus and enhancement of the leptomeninges; and the CSF is abnormal, with elevated protein, pleocytosis, and cytology positive for malignant cells.

INFECTIOUS POLYRADICULOPATHY

A number of infectious diseases affect the nerve roots. In all instances, strong clues suggest a disorder that prominently involves sensory as well as motor fibers. We discuss only syphilitic, Lyme, and zoster infections because they are treatable and can present in atypical fashion, raising the possibility of the progressive muscular atrophy presentation of ALS.

The most common form of neurosyphilis is tabes dorsalis that begins as a spirochete meningitis. After 10 to 20 years of infection, damage to the dorsal roots is severe and extensive. This damage produces characteristic symptoms and signs, including lightning pains, ataxia, and bladder disturbance. The anterior roots may also be involved, leading to muscle weakness and atrophy. An abnormal cerebrospinal fluid (CSF) profile, characterized by pleocytosis, elevated protein level, and abnormal serology, combined with the presence of serum antibodies specific for *Treponema pallidum,* establishes the correct diagnosis. Rarely, syphilis causes a reversible progressive muscular atrophy syndrome, which is probably mediated by a subacute ischemic (arteritic) meningomyelopathy.[2]

Lyme polyradiculopathy caused by the spirochete *Borrelia burgdorferi* is transmitted by the tick *Ixodes dammini*. Nerve root abnormalities occur in both early and late stages of the disease. Clinical features of nerve root involvement include severe radicular pain followed by weakness, sensory loss, and hyporeflexia in the territory of the involved nerve roots.[84] The diagnosis is supported by abnormal CSF (elevated protein, normal glucose, lymphocytic pleocytosis), selective concentration of the antibody to *B. burgdorferi* in CSF, and EMG evidence of radiculoneuropathy. This acute clinical presentation, combined with an active CSF profile, is easily distinguished from ALS. Even in its chronic form (neuroborreliosis), Lyme radiculoneuropathy produces a mainly sensory syndrome resembling a toxic-metabolic polyneuropathy, not a motor syndrome that could be confused with progressive muscular atrophy.[84] A rare late manifestation of Lyme disease is a leukoencephalitis that produces progressive weakness and spasticity.[133] Superficially, it could resemble primary lateral sclerosis or the upper motor neuron form of ALS, except that urinary incontinence usually accompanies it, the serum serology is positive, and the CSF is abnormal as in the acute form.

Herpes zoster is known best as the cause of a common, painful vesicular eruption occurring in a segmental or radicular distribution. A small percentage of patients develop segmental motor weakness.[140] The interval between skin eruption and paralysis is about 2 weeks, with a range of 1 day to 5 weeks. Weakness peaks within hours or days and usually does not spread to muscles served by unaffected segments.

PLEXOPATHIES

Brachial Plexus Neuropathy (Parsonage Turner Syndrome)

Brachial plexus neuropathy (BPN), also known as cervicobrachial neuralgia or neuralgic amyotrophy, is thought to have an inflammatory-immune pathogenesis.[135] It is generally heralded by severe pain in the shoulder girdle region, and 2 to 3 days after the onset of discomfort, arm weakness typically develops.[23] On examination, weakness is found in the muscles of the shoulder girdle, including the spinati, serratus, and biceps, and over a period of weeks rather marked muscle atrophy may occur. Deep tendon reflexes are often attenuated in the affected limb. Sensory examination may show mild and variable sensory loss. Slow resolution of symptoms and signs characterizes the natural history of this disorder.

The diagnosis of BPN is established by the presence of focal, nonprogressive limb weakness and is supported by EMG findings that reveal neurogenic changes in the territory of the brachial plexus. The condition is bilateral in about one-third of patients, but the involvement may be mild and subclinical in one limb. Because of the severe pain and focal weakness, the condition suggests radiculopathy, so imaging studies of the neck are often done to exclude the possibility of nerve root compromise. Patients with this condition are otherwise healthy and have no other risk factors for a brachial plexopathy such as a history of cancer or previous radiation to the plexus.

Both ALS and BPN may cause focal limb weakness, muscle atrophy, and fasciculations (see Table 6–9). We have on occasion seen patients referred for ALS diagnosis who actually have this benign condition. Favoring a diagnosis of BPN is the severe pain that frequently precedes the development of weakness. Some patients with ALS do develop severe shoulder pain, but their pain usually occurs late in the disorder and stems largely from a pericapsulitis in a weak and atrophic limb. In contrast to ALS, weakness in BPN ceases to progress after onset, and upper motor neuron signs never appear. When faced with a patient presenting with weakness restricted mainly to one arm, the clinician must always consider BPN before attributing the weakness to ALS.

Idiopathic Lumbosacral Plexopathy

Like its counterpart in the upper limb, idiopathic lumbosacral plexopathy may be heralded by pain. By definition, patients have no risk factors for a plexopathy (underlying neoplasm, prior radiation therapy, or anticoagulation treatment).[23] Like BPN, this condition is thought to be immune-mediated, although definite proof is lacking. A few days after the onset of pain, weakness develops in the territory of the lumbosacral plexus, most often affecting muscles served by branches of the lumbar plexus. Weakness of hip flexion and adduction results, with attenuation or loss of the knee jerk reflex. As in BPN, the natural history of this disorder is a slow resolution of muscle strength.

Imaging studies of the lumbosacral spine and pelvis can help to establish a diagnosis of idiopathic lumbosacral plexopathy by excluding compressive radiculopathy or a structural plexopathy. The EMG will reveal acute and chronic neurogenic changes in the lumbosacral plexus territory. The condition occurs unilaterally, but in rare instances, evidence exists for subclinical involvement on the contralateral side. In contrast to ALS, however, no neurogenic changes should be observed in the arms.

Because it presents with focal lower extremity weakness, atrophy, and sometimes fasciculations, lumbosacral plexopathy can be confused with the progressive muscular atrophy presentation of ALS (see Table 6–9). In the latter condition, however, pain is unusual, sensory symptoms are minor and infrequent, and weakness increases and spreads rather than slowly improving. Furthermore, the EMG findings in lumbosacral plexopathy are usually restricted to one leg, or occasionally to both legs and paraspinal muscles, unlike the widespread neurogenic changes that are characteristic of ALS.

MOTOR NEUROPATHIES

Most neuropathies seen in everyday clinical practice involve sensory as well as motor fibers. On occasion, however, patients are encountered with peripheral nerve disorders in which motor manifestations predominate or are the sole manifestation. Such pure motor symptoms and signs may prompt consideration of ALS.

Mononeuropathies

The more frequently encountered mononeuropathies of the arm involve the radial, ulnar, and median nerves; those in the leg involve the femoral, obturator, sciatic, and peroneal nerves. The diagnosis of a mononeuropathy is strongly suggested by the history and physical findings and is supported by EMG abnormalities. Nerve conduction studies reveal that conduction velocity slows across entrapment sites, and that motor and sensory amplitudes diminish. EMG shows acute and chronic neurogenic changes in muscles served by the involved nerve.

Because most mononeuropathies encountered in everyday practice are characterized by weakness associated with sensory changes, we do not generally consider them in the differential diagnosis of ALS. When the mononeuropathies have little or no sensory accompaniment or when pure motor branches are involved, however, the resulting muscle weakness and wasting may mimic the progressive muscular atrophy presentation of ALS with a unilateral and focal onset (Tables 6–10 and 6–11). We should also note that focal neuropathies not uncommonly coexist with ALS.[76] In the following paragraphs, some of these mononeuropathies are discussed, including ulnar mononeuropathies, the anterior interosseous nerve syndrome, the posterior interosseus nerve syndrome, and deep peroneal mononeuropathy.[14,134]

The ulnar nerve may be compressed distally at the level of the wrist as it passes through the canal of Guyon. Several patterns of motor and sensory loss may result, depending on exactly where the nerve is compressed.[101] The most common form is purely motor, with involvement of the ulnar nerve

Table 6–10. MONONEUROPATHIES CONSIDERED IN THE DIFFERENTIAL DIAGNOSIS OF ALS

Mononeuropathy	Muscles Weakened (Selected)	Classic Presentation
Ulnar (canal of Guyon)	Hand interossei	Claw hand
Anterior interosseus	Flexor pollicis longus, flexor digitorum (I & II)	Weak pinch
Posterior interosseus	Wrist and finger extensors	Wrist drop
Peroneal (deep branch)	Tibialis anterior, peronei, extensor hallucis longus, extensor digitorum brevis	Footdrop

just after the cutaneous branch diverges. In this distal ulnar mononeuropathy, the ulnar-supplied hand intrinsic muscles show weakness (with variable sparing of the abductor digiti minimi), but sensation is normal. An ulnar motor mononeuropathy may also result from ulnar nerve entrapment at the elbow, presumably because sensory fibers traversing unaffected nerve fascicles are spared.

An important median mononeuropathy involves the anterior interosseous nerve. When this nerve is compromised, a pure motor syndrome (Kiloh-Nevin) follows, which is characterized by weakness of the flexor pollicis longus and the flexor digitorum profundus in digits 2 and 3.[146] Patients with this mononeuropathy cannot flex the distal phalanges of the thumb and index finger and suffer no sensory loss.

When the posterior interosseus nerve, a

Table 6–11. FEATURES OF MOTOR NEUROPATHIES CONSIDERED IN THE DIFFERENTIAL DIAGNOSIS OF ALS

Disease	CLINICAL AND LABORATORY FEATURES	
	Shared with ALS	Atypical for ALS
Motor mononeuropathy	Purely motor, focal weakness, wasting; fasciculations*	No upper motor neuron signs;[†] highly restricted involvement; EMG: mononeuropathy
Motor neuropathy and paraproteinemia	Polyneuropathic pattern of weakness and wasting	Multisystem involvement (POEMS syndrome), sclerotic bony lesions; EMG: demyelinating polyneuropathy;
Multifocal motor neuropathy	Purely motor, asymmetric, weakness, wasting, fasciculations	Protracted course; EMG: conduction block; high titers of autoantibodies to gangliosides[‡]
Porphyric neuropathy	Generalized weakness and wasting	Acute neuropathy (arms > legs) with encephalopathy; autonomic dysfunction; EMG: sensory fiber involvement; urine and blood positive for porphobilinogen
Metal-induced motor neuropathy	Muscle weakness and atrophy (wrist drop in lead intoxication)	Systemic features: anemia and basophilic stippling in lead intoxication; psychosis and ataxia in mercury intoxication

*Fasciculations, usually scattered and infrequent, are seen in all of the motor neuropathies.
[†]Upper motor neuron signs are not a feature of any of the motor neuropathies listed in this table.
[‡]Elevated titer of antibody is found in 50–60 % of patients with multifocal motor neuropathy.
Abbreviations: EMG = electromyography, POEMS = polyneuropathy, organomegaly, endocrinopathy, monoclonal gammopathy, and skin changes.

major branch of the radial nerve, is compromised, patients develop wrist and finger drop because of weakness of the wrist and finger extensors. Further, all muscles supplied by the radial nerve in the forearm distal to the supinator (but sometimes including it) show weakness without sensory loss.

When the deep branch of the common peroneal nerve is involved, the clinical picture includes weakness of the foot and toe dorsiflexors. Sensory symptoms are unusual despite the presence of sensory fibers supplying the skin between the first and second toes.

Motor Neuropathy and Paraproteinemia

Paraproteinemias, in the form of monoclonal gammopathies, may be associated with peripheral neuropathies that are characterized by axonal degeneration, segmental demyelination, or both.[73] Some of these disorders, such as the peripheral neuropathy associated with osteosclerotic myeloma, are predominantly motor in expression, strongly resemble chronic inflammatory demyelinating polyneuropathy, and could raise the possibility of the progressive muscular atrophy form of ALS. The monoclonal protein in these patients is typically lambda light chain with immunoglobulin G or A heavy chain. Skeletal survey establishes the diagnosis in that it reveals a small number of bony lesions (totally sclerotic or mixed sclerotic and lytic). Often these patients develop one or more of the following extra–peripheral-nerve manifestations: organomegaly, endocrinopathy, hypertrichosis, digital clubbing, or gynecomastia.

The fully developed syndrome has therefore been designated POEMS (polyneuropathy, organomegaly, endocrinopathy, monoclonal gammopathy, and skin changes). There is often prominent weight loss and patients develop a gaunt appearance that may be reminiscent of ALS. In up to half the reported cases there is papilledema. Tumoricidal radiation of the solitary bony lesions, surgical excision, or both may lead to substantial improvement in both neurologic and nonneurologic features.[15] In most patients, electrodiagnostic studies help to distinguish this disorder from lower motor neuron involvement in ALS by revealing a large-fiber sensorimotor polyneuropathy with marked slowing of conduction velocities (see Table 6–11).[73] Also helpful in separating this motor neuropathy from ALS is the CSF protein level, which usually exceeds 100 mg/dL.

Sometimes it may be difficult clinically to distinguish a peripheral neuropathy from a disorder of the anterior horn cell. For example, Rowland and colleagues[118] described a patient with macroglobulinemia and widespread weakness with fasciculations who was thought to have progressive spinal muscular atrophy. Further studies disclosed an elevated CSF protein concentration and slowing of motor nerve conduction velocities. Postmortem examination showed a predominantly motor, demyelinating radiculoneuropathy with central chromatolysis. Although the association of paraprotein with such peripheral motor nerve disorders is well established, paraproteinemia also is found in 9% of patients with acquired disorders of the anterior horn cell; these disorders often include upper motor neuron signs, leading to a clinical picture that qualifies as ALS per se.[149]

Multifocal Motor Neuropathy with Conduction Block

Multifocal motor neuropathy (MMN) with conduction block[110] primarily affects men at a relatively young age (less than 45 years old) and usually presents as a slowly progressive, painless, remarkably focal weakness and amyotrophy involving the small hand muscles. Weakness typically begins unilaterally, progresses for a number of years, and then appears in the contralateral limb. Clinical deficits correspond to individual peripheral nerves and remain extremely restricted in their anatomic distribution for years.[102] An acute presentation of MMN with conduction block following *Campylobacter jejuni* enteritis has also been described.[147]

Examination shows marked atrophy of the intrinsic hand and forearm muscles; the humeral and shoulder girdle muscles are less frequently affected. Lower extremity weakness is infrequent. Rarely the cranial nerves are involved.[69] Fasciculations and cramps are common, and myokymia is seen occasionally.[102] Deep tendon reflexes may be attenuated, especially in weak limbs, but occasionally they are normally active or unexpectedly brisk for the degree of muscle atrophy and weakness.[79] Most remarkable is the preservation of normal sensation, even in regions where muscles are markedly atrophic. Electrodiagnostic studies show that motor axons are primarily involved: conduction block is found along focal segments of peripheral nerves that are not usually subject to compression or entrapment. Low-amplitude sensory potentials may be seen, but there is no conduction block in sensory fibers.[102] The EMG generally discloses fibrillation potentials, scattered fasciculation potentials and grouped repetitive discharges, and remodeled motor unit potentials.

An intriguing finding has been the presence of elevated titers of antibodies to the GM1 ganglioside in 50% of 60% of patients.[108] In one patient, a portion of nerve obtained at exploratory surgery revealed demyelination and onion bulb formation.[70] Animal studies have determined that serum antibodies from patients with this syndrome bind to the nodes of Ranvier.[123] It is arguable that the antibodies have a pathogenic role and are responsible for focal areas of demyelination.

The pure motor involvement of this syndrome certainly resembles the weakness produced by the lower motor neuron form of ALS (see Table 6–11). Indeed, occasional patients, qualifying for the diagnosis of ALS with definite or probable upper motor neuron signs, may have multifocal motor conduction block, suggesting that peripheral nerves may be implicated in addition to the central nervous system in some patients with ALS.[150] Thus, the two disorders may overlap; MMN and conduction block cannot always be readily distinguished from ALS. Most patients with MMN have a long and slowly progressive, relatively benign course, however, with the pathology mainly involving the upper extremity nerves. This pattern differs from the usual course of ALS, which, even in the presence of conduction blocks, has a relatively rapid tempo and generalized distribution of weakness and muscle atrophy.[79]

Recognizing MMN is important because in some patients it appears to be treatable. Even if the weakness has been present for many years, the condition may respond to cyclophosphamide;[45,108] the potential side effects of this agent, however, have prompted a search for other therapies. There is minimal if any response to corticosteroids and plasma exchange is not helpful, but treatment with human immune globulin appears promising.[25,69] Unlike cyclophosphamide, the effi-cacy of treatment with this modality does not seem to require that anti-GM$_1$ antibody titers fall.[138] Of note, patients with ALS have received human immune globulin but have not shown a beneficial response.[31]

A distal lower motor neuron syndrome has also been described that resembles MMN except that conduction block is not found.[109] As in MMN, most of these patients have high titers of serum immunoglobulin M anti-GM1 antibodies. In early stages it may resemble the progressive muscular atrophy form of ALS because of asymmetric distal weakness in a hand or foot in the face of preserved reflexes. Distinguishing the syndrome from ALS, however, is slow progression, lack of very brisk reflexes, normal bulbar function, and response in some patients to immunosuppression.[108]

A third lower motor neuron syndrome involves proximal muscles, often remains confined mainly to one or two extremities over periods of at least 3 to 5 years, is associated with high titers of antibodies to asialo-GM1, and does not demonstrate conduction block.[109] It is reasonably considered in the differential diagnosis of ALS, but excluded by its relatively benign clinical features and lack of development of upper motor neuron signs.

Chronic Inflammatory Demyelinating Polyneuropathy

Chronic inflammatory demyelinating polyneuropathy (CIDP) is a disorder that slowly progresses for two or more months, in either a stepwise or continuous fashion, and is sometimes marked by relapses and remissions.[5] It is characterized by symmetric weakness involving proximal and distal muscles of arms and legs, sensory loss, and areflexia, features that help to separate it from ALS. Further clarifying the distinction between CIDP and ALS are both the raised CSF protein concentration and pattern of acquired demyelination noted on EMG in the former.[5] Some patients with CIDP present with signs not too dissimilar from those of MMN, that is, multifocal weakness with little or no sensory involvement,[83] and both disorders may show sural nerve biopsy evidence of demyelination and remyelination.[26,83] The exact relationship of this multifocal motor variant of CIDP to MMN with conduction block is uncertain.[103] Separating the two conditions on a case-by-case basis may be difficult. Patients with the multifocal CIDP variant tend to have attenuated reflexes, sensory symptoms, and in most instances lack antibodies to GM1 ganglioside. Also, CIDP usually responds to treatment with prednisone, plasmapheresis, or intravenous gamma globulin,[39,108] in contrast to the more limited responsiveness of MMN.

Guillain-Barré Syndrome

This polyneuropathy is the most common cause of acute paralysis in North America. It is an immune-mediated disorder that encompasses several pathophysiologic patterns including disorders in which the immune attack is on Schwann cells and axonal constituents, but the most prevalent form is primarily demyelinating.[51] In most instances, it evolves rapidly over days, or a little more slowly over 1 to 6 weeks, until patients reach the nadir of their clinical course. In the typical case, Guillain-Barré syndrome is never confused with ALS. The polyneuropathy is heralded by paresthesias followed by symmetric weakness, which begins in distal muscles and ascends quickly to the trunk and arms, and is characterized by hypo- or areflexia. In almost 25% of patients, respiratory failure necessitates ventilatory assistance. On occasion, the disorder presents with few if any sensory symptoms or signs and with asymmetric weakness, simulating the progressive muscular atrophy presentation of ALS, or with multiple cranial nerve palsies, simulating the progressive bulbar palsy presentation of ALS. Unlike ALS, however, the CSF profile in Guillain-Barré syndrome is abnormal, characterized by an elevated protein level with no or minimal pleocytosis. Except for the less common motor axonal forms, its EMG features are usually characteristic of acquired demyelination and show little overlap with ALS, revealing long distal latencies, dispersed motor responses, slowed conduction velocities, absent or prolonged late responses, and conduction block.[3]

Porphyric Neuropathy

Peripheral neuropathy, usually associated with an acute porphyric attack, is encountered in the hepatic porphyrias, which include acute intermittent porphyria, variegate porphyria, and hereditary coproporphyria. Attacks are generally characterized by autonomic disturbances, including abdominal pain, nausea, vomiting, severe constipation, tachycardia, labile blood pressure, orthostatic hypotension, and micturition difficulty. More severe attacks are followed by progressive motor neuropathy, encephalopathy with seizures, or both.

Certain factors may precipitate attacks, including drugs (e.g., barbiturates, sulfonamides), alcohol, female sex hormones, and a negative caloric balance during a febrile illness. The common link among these factors appears to be the ability to induce hepatic delta-aminolevulinic acid synthase. This is the rate-limiting enzyme in heme biosynthesis, so induction leads to the overproduction and oversecretion of porphobilinogen and delta-aminolevulinic acid.

The neuropathy is predominantly motor and is characterized by weakness that develops over days to weeks.[12] The arms tend to be affected before the legs, and proximal muscles may be preferentially involved. The weakness may be asymmetric or generalized, followed in severe cases by a flaccid quadriplegia with respiratory failure. Muscle wasting occurs fairly rapidly. Tendon reflexes tend to be diminished or absent, but ankle jerks are often retained. Sensory impairment may occur in a distal stocking–glove distribution or may affect the trunk and proximal limbs. Cranial nerve involvement also occurs.

The main biochemical hallmark of the attack is marked elevation of delta-aminolevulinic acid and porphobilinogen levels in the blood and urine. Nerve conduction studies show low-amplitude motor responses and borderline-slow conduction velocities; sensory action potentials are also reduced in amplitude or are absent. The main morphologic feature of nerve biopsy tissue is axonal degeneration.

The rapid onset, the association with autonomic disturbances and encephalopathy, the lack of upper motor neuron features, and the sensory abnormalities generally allow the clinician to distinguish porphyric neuropathy from ALS (see Table 6–11).

Toxic Neuropathy

In adults, lead intoxication gives rise to symptoms and signs of a predominantly motor neuropathy characterized by wrist and finger drop with few or no sensory manifestations.[13] Less commonly, footdrop and weakness of the proximal arm muscles and shoulder girdle group occurs. Although this distribution may suggest the lower motor neuron involvement seen in ALS, the presence of anemia and basophilic stippling of red-cell precursors in the bone marrow and a "lead line" along the gingival margin are helpful clinical clues (see Table 6–11). Blood lead levels generally exceed 70 mg/dL (μmol/L). More reliable indicators of lead toxicity include elevated urinary lead and coproporphyrin levels.

Mercury intoxication produces a variety of neurologic complications that include psychosis, ataxia, parkinsonism, and motor neuropathy. Rarely, the clinical features resemble the lower neuron involvement of ALS.[1]

Dapsone, used primarily to treat leprosy, dermatitis herpetiformis, and other skin disorders, produces a predominantly motor polyneuropathy characterized by progressive muscle weakness and wasting, most often involving distal muscles of the extremities.[52] Paresthesias without objective sensory changes may be present. The recovery that predictably takes place after the drug is discontinued separates this disorder from ALS.

Disorders of Anterior Horn Cells

SPINAL MUSCULAR ATROPHIES

Because these genetically determined disorders usually develop in infancy, childhood, or adolescence, neurologists do not usually consider them in the differential diagnosis of ALS, a condition typically associated with later adult life. However, the recognition of juvenile-onset ALS cases, and the occurrence of spinal muscular atrophy (SMA) in adults lead us to a brief review of these important conditions.

Whereas all SMAs are characterized pathologically by degeneration of anterior horn cells and clinically by muscle weakness and atrophy, they can be classified into four major types, based on their ages of onset and rates of progression.[19] Type I (Werdnig-Hoffmann disease) manifests before 6 months of age and is marked by profound hypotonia, generalized weakness, and areflexia. More than 95% of patients die by 2 years of age from recurrent respiratory infections. The mildest childhood form, designated type III (Kugelberg-Welander disease), has a variable age of onset between 18 months and 17 years (although some patients present in young adult life) and is characterized by slowly progressive, symmetric weakness and atrophy predominantly affecting the legs. Survival to adulthood is common, often with the ability to walk retained. An intermediate form, type II, falls between types I and III in terms of severity, with onset before 18 months, inability ever to stand, and death occurring sometime after age 2 (although some patients have prolonged survival into adult life[121]). All three childhood forms are inherited in autosomal-recessive fashion and arise from mutations at the identical disease locus, an example of allelic heterogeneity.[47]

Typical sporadic ALS may occur before age 20 years but it is exceedingly rare in this age group.[94] Although its age of onset may overlap with type III SMA, its rapid course and upper motor neuron features separate it easily from SMA. Another form of juvenile ALS is chronic, develops in patients between the ages of 3 and 25, progresses very slowly, and appears in most cases to be autosomal recessive.[10] Although it shares features with type III SMA, prominent upper motor neuron signs distinguish juvenile ALS from SMA.

Type IV, adult-onset SMA, is relatively benign compared with the childhood-onset types, with many patients reporting apparent temporary arrest in the progression of muscle weakness.[107] The age of onset ranges between 15 and 50 years (median, 37), with very slow progression of symmetric proximal weakness over decades, often with the ability to walk retained even 20 years after diagnosis. The inheritance of type IV SMA is heterogenous, with autosomal-recessive, autosomal-dominant, and X-linked recessive modes described. For several reasons, type IV SMA can be mistaken for familial ALS (Table 6–12). This is because familial ALS is characterized by a relatively young age of onset (less than 50 years) in some families, an autosomal-dominant pattern of inheritance, and an initial progressive muscular atrophy presentation.[92] However, its usual rapid progression, asymmetry, appearance of upper motor neuron signs, and early appearance of bulbar signs are inconsistent with SMA and should point to a diagnosis of familial ALS.[107]

Table 6–12. **FEATURES OF ANTERIOR HORN CELL DISORDERS CONSIDERED IN THE DIFFERENTIAL DIAGNOSIS OF ALS**

	CLINICAL AND LABORATORY FEATURES	
Disease	**Shared with ALS**	**Atypical for ALS**
Spinal muscular atrophy	Weakness, atrophy, fasciculations*	Absence of upper motor neuron signs;† protracted course, young adult age of onset
Bulbospinal muscular atrophy	Bulbar and limb weakness, atrophy, fasciculations	Gynecomastia; expanded cytosine-adenine-guanine (CAG) repeat; reduced or absent sensory nerve action potentials
Monomelic amyotrophy	Focal upper limb weakness, atrophy	Young adult age of onset; ceases to progress after 2 years; relatively benign electromyography
Motor neuronopathy and lymphoma	Subacute, painless, asymmetric weakness, atrophy and fasciculations	Associated lymphoma; high cerebro-spinal fluid protein level; paraproteinemia
Progressive post-polio muscular atrophy	Weakness, atrophy	History of poliomyelitis; very slow progression
Hex A deficiency–related muscular atrophy	Weakness, atrophy, fasciculations	Young age of onset; protracted disease course; tremor; cognitive impairment; reduced Hex A in serum and leukocytes

*Fasciculations are a feature of all the anterior horn cell disorders listed in this table.

†Upper motor neuron signs are not found in these disorders, with the exception of rare cases of paraneoplastic motor neuronopathy and Hex A deficiency–related muscular atrophy.

Abbreviation: Hex A = hexosaminidase A.

Rarely, adult-onset, dominantly inherited (scapuloperoneal) SMA behaves like ALS in that it progresses rapidly and leads to death from respiratory failure.[65] Evidence of corticospinal tract dysfunction is absent both clinically and at postmortem examination, however, distinguishing it from familial ALS.

As we have seen, the SMAs with childhood and adult onset most commonly cause symmetric, proximal muscle weakness and atrophy. Involvement of distal muscles as a manifestation of hereditary SMA is unusual, but many families and patients have now been studied and the findings are well delineated.[56] The condition resembles the type I (demyelinating) and type II (axon-loss) forms of hereditary sensorimotor neuropathy (HMSN)[58] except that arm weakness is uncommon, tendon reflexes are relatively preserved, and sensory examinations (clinical and neurophysiologic) are normal. The early age of onset (in most patients, the first, second, or third decade) and long benign course easily differentiate this condition from ALS. We should also note that rarely one encounters patients with features of HMSN II who have associated upper motor neuron signs in the form of hyperactive reflexes and Babinski signs.[58] The major feature of this syndrome, however, is a polyneuropathy causing mild slowing of motor conduction and reduced or absent sensory action potentials, findings not seen in ALS.

X-LINKED BULBOSPINAL NEURONOPATHY (KENNEDY'S DISEASE)

Bulbospinal neuronopathy (BSN) is an X-linked disorder that was first described in 1968.[74] It results in slowly progressive, symmetric, proximal muscle weakness; cramps; and atrophy without upper motor neuron features. Weakness involves limb, face, and bulbar muscles; distal muscles are affected later. Fasciculations are prominent in perioral facial muscles and the tongue. Deep tendon reflexes are depressed or absent. In more than 50% of patients, signs of partial androgen deficiency like gynecomastia and infertility accompany the generalized muscle atrophy. Testosterone levels are normal. Onset occurs between the ages of 15 and 60 years, with most patients becoming symptomatic in the third or fourth decade of life. Patients with an earlier onset progress more rapidly and have more widespread and severe weakness than patients with a later onset. Female carriers may have subclinical phenotypic expression manifested by electrodiagnostic abnormalities.[128]

Several interesting laboratory features are peculiar to this illness and help support its diagnosis. Although BSN is not a disease of muscle per se, the serum CK level tends to be elevated to a higher degree than would be expected in neurogenic disorders. In fact, muscle biopsy specimens often disclose fairly vigorous muscle degeneration and regeneration. Electrodiagnostic studies show evidence of a lower motor neuron disorder: a combination of fibrillation and fasciculation potentials and remodeled motor unit potentials are seen on EMG, and nerve conduction studies show attenuated motor responses. In addition, sensory potentials are reduced or even absent, suggesting involvement of either sensory axons or dorsal root ganglia neurons.[100] Indeed, this sensory involvement in the presence of a predominantly motor syndrome led Harding and colleagues[59] to designate the disorder as BSN.

The genetic basis of this disorder has been more clearly delineated in the last few years with the recognition that BSN is one of a growing number of conditions that are associated with an unstable trinucleotide repeat.[131] The cytosine-adenine-guanine (CAG) repeat sequence is expanded in the androgen receptor gene of patients with BSN. Unaffected individuals have 11 to 33 CAG repeats in the first exon; individuals with this disorder have 40 to 62 CAG repeats. The amplification occurs within the translated portion of the androgen receptor gene but outside its receptor-binding domain. It has been proposed that the mutation in BSN causes toxic effects on motor neurons by enhancing the androgen receptor's function.[18] Other mutations in the androgen receptor cause partial or full loss of receptor activity and are manifested clinically as androgen in-

sensitivity (testicular feminization) but are not associated with neurologic symptoms.[18] The length of the CAG-trinucleotide repeats correlates inversely with age of onset (increasing length associated with a younger age of onset).[36] Although the disease severity in some disorders characterized by an unstable trinucleotide repeat increases with longer repeats, this may not be the case with BSN.[112]

In some patients, establishing the diagnosis of BSN may be difficult on the basis of clinical assessment and the usual laboratory studies alone. X-linked BSN may occur in a patient without affected male relatives, gynecomastia may be absent, and sensory potentials may be normal on electrodiagnostic studies. In these instances, the condition is easily confused with the progressive muscular atrophy form of ALS in a young person (see Table 6–12). To further complicate the issue, a slowly progressive, relatively benign disorder highly analogous to BSN with spinal and bulbar lower motor neuron signs but with a normal trinucleotide repeat has also been described.[66] Because of this difficulty in diagnosis, we now analyze the number of CAG repeats in younger male patients presenting with lower motor neuron signs, especially if bulbar muscle involvement is prominent.

BENIGN MONOMELIC AMYOTROPHY

Benign monomelic amyotrophy (BMA), a sporadic disorder, presents with focal weakness involving a single limb and affects men five times more frequently than women. Most patients have been described in reports from Japan[60] and India.[127] The age of onset is between 15 and 30 years. Most often, involvement begins in the hand intrinsic muscles and the C8–T1 myotomes, then spreads centripetally for 1 to 2 years to involve the forearm flexors and extensors.[129] Despite marked forearm muscle atrophy, the brachioradialis tends to be spared.[35] After this slow progression, the condition usually stabilizes. Deep tendon reflexes in the affected limb are usually normal or reduced. Increased reflex activity is found occasionally in the lower extremity of the affected side;[60,111] pathologic reflexes and increased tone are not encountered, and sensation is usually normal. Muscles supplied by cranial nerves are spared, and respiratory function is unaffected.

Routine nerve conduction studies are generally normal except for the presence of low motor amplitudes when recording from atrophic hand muscles. Modest reductions in sensory potentials are found in 30% of cases. EMG reveals fibrillation potentials and positive sharp waves in less than half the patients, whereas recruitment is invariably reduced in a pattern corresponding to the areas of weakness and atrophy.[35] The EMG of muscles in the limb that appears to be uninvolved typically discloses chronic neurogenic changes of motor unit remodeling, suggesting more widespread involvement than is apparent clinically. Imaging of the cervical spine in some cases discloses focal atrophy of the cervical spinal cord.[35] One postmortem study of a patient with monomelic amyotrophy of 23 years' duration found marked atrophy of the cervical anterior roots and anterior horn cells.[60]

Although few patients develop ALS in their third decade and enter a period of relative clinical stability, this pattern is much more consistently seen in BMA. Nevertheless, differentiating BMA from a focal onset of progressive muscular atrophy may be difficult, especially in cases in which tendon reflexes are retained (see Table 6–12). Indeed, in the early stages, it may be impossible to make a definitive diagnosis of BMA. EMG testing may be helpful because in BMA, fibrillation potentials and positive waves are sparse in comparison with classic ALS. An MRI of the cervical spine may be useful because the presence of cord atrophy supports the diagnosis of BMA. In the final analysis, however, the diagnosis of BMA is established most firmly when a young man has clinical and electrodiagnostic evidence of stable lower motor neuron signs that have been restricted to a single limb for at least 2 years.

MOTOR NEURONOPATHY AND LYMPHOMA

Motor neuron disease as a remote but rare effect of lymphoma has been known for many years[119] and was designated by Schold and colleagues[124] as subacute motor neuronopathy. The neurologic disorder is an ex-clusively motor syndrome; sensory symptoms and signs are minimal. It is generally characterized by subacute, progressive, painless, often patchy and asymmetric weakness of the lower motor neuron type, with greater involvement of the legs than the arms.[124] Some patients with lymphoma, however, have definite or probable upper motor neuron signs and qualify for the diagnosis of ALS[150] (see Table 6–12); this combination of upper and lower motor neuron signs in the setting of lymphoma may represent a disorder with a pathogenesis different from the motor neuronopathy described by Schold's group. This ALS-like syndrome in the company of a lymphoma is often accompanied by paraproteinemia, increased CSF protein level, and CSF oligoclonal bands, suggesting that an immunologic disorder has a mediating role.[150] Therefore, when a patient presenting with progressive muscular atrophy or ALS has a paraproteinemia, we analyze the CSF and consider a bone marrow examination if the CSF protein is elevated or if we find oligoclonal bands. When ALS is combined with lymphoma, almost half the reported cases have improved or were stable for long periods of time.[150] The finding of lymphoma therefore provides a target for immunosuppressive therapy.[120]

POST-POLIO SYNDROME

Charcot first described this condition over 100 years ago, and it is now recognized as a cause of slowly progressive weakness in survivors of the major epidemic of poliomyelitis in the 1950s, affecting between 250,000 and 300,000 people.[68] The major neurologic manifestations are weakness, atrophy, fasciculations, and cramps, which together have been designated progressive post-poliomyelitis muscular atrophy (PPMA) (see Chapter 17).

On average, PPMA has its onset 36 years after the acute polio infection (range, 8 to 71 years). Weakness develops in both previously affected and unaffected muscles, but the affected muscles tend to be more involved.[27] The distribution of new weakness appears to correlate with the severity of paralysis at the time of acute poliomyelitis. Weakness tends to develop insidiously, without apparent antecedent. The course of PPMA is slowly progressive with periods of stabilization; on average, strength declines at a rate of 1% per year.[29]

Except for an occasional patient with a Babinski sign, upper motor neuron signs are not a feature of PPMA.[27] In addition to limb muscle weakness, other neurologic symptoms include respiratory insufficiency from progressive respiratory muscle weakness, dysarthria, and dysphagia.[130] Sleep apnea may also be a neurologic complication and is more likely to be found in patients with prior bulbar poliomyelitis who required ventilatory support.[68]

A variety of other clinical features of PPMA have been described.[27,68] Fatigue occurs in 75% of these patients and can be severe, even without much weakness or wasting. Patients also require more sleep, and develop dizziness, syncope, and headache. Coolness and color changes may also occur in the affected extremities, suggesting involvement of the sympathetic nervous system; possibly these symptoms relate to prior damage of the intermediolateral cell column during the acute infection. Musculoskeletal problems are also prominent in many patients, with joint instability as a major feature. Joint pain may be accompanied by chronic back and neck strain. Indeed, generalized pain and tenderness, nonrestorative sleep, fatigue, and morning stiffness, qualifying for the diagnosis of the fibromyalgia syndrome, occur in about 10% of patients.[143]

EMG studies in patients with prior polio both with and without new weakness disclose motor unit potentials of increased amplitude and duration and reduced recruitment.[29] Evidence of new denervation in the form of fibrillation potentials and positive sharp waves is seen to a varying degree and does not appear to distinguish symptomatic from asymptomatic patients. Fasciculations are seen frequently in all patients. Muscle biopsy discloses fiber-type grouping, indicating denervation and reinnervation, and myopathic changes, believed to be secondary to the longstanding neurogenic process, are often striking.[38] Patients with PPMA have small, angulated fibers suggesting active denervation, but such features also are found in asymptomatic patients with prior poliomyelitis.[29] Thus, no diagnostic test finding can be considered pathognomonic for PPMA.[68]

In general, the clinical and laboratory data support the view that PPMA is a result of new or possibly continuing instability of previously damaged motor units. The cause of PPMA is not entirely clear, but the current hypothesis is that the process involves a loss or dropout of axon terminals from reinnervated motor units that is engendered by one or more conditions: motor unit exhaustion, persistent viral infection, or immune-mediated mechanisms.[29]

Because ALS shares clinical, EMG, and morphologic features with PPMA, one might anticipate some difficulty in differentiating one condition from the other (see Table 6–12). Further, in rare instances, ALS per se occurs in patients with a history of poliomyelitis.[115] Nonetheless, very slowly progressive weakness without upper motor neuron signs in a patient with a history of acute poliomyelitis strongly supports the diagnosis of PPMA.

HEXOSAMINIDASE DEFICIENCIES ASSOCIATED WITH MOTOR NEURON DISORDERS

The lysosomal enzyme *N*-acetyl-b-hexosaminidase (Hex) is dimeric and comprises two major isozymes, acidic Hex A and basic Hex B.[75] Hex A is composed of alpha and beta subunits, whereas Hex B is composed of only beta subunits. The role of Hex A, acting in concert with a small transport protein (a GM2 activator) is to degrade (hydrolyze) GM2 ganglioside, which is highly concentrated in neuronal membranes. The best-known hexosaminidase deficiency is Tay-Sachs disease, most prevalent in Ashkenazi Jews, which results from a severe alpha-subunit mutation and leads to complete absence of the alpha polypeptide, and hence a severe deficiency of Hex A. Accumulation of GM2 ganglioside in neuronal lysosomes results in a profound encephalopathy with myoclonic seizures, macular cherry-red spots, and death before the age of 5 years.

In the last 25 years, it has become recognized that Hex-A deficiency underlies a group of recessively inherited progressive neurologic diseases and may begin in infants or adults.[67] The described conditions include late infantile or juvenile encephalopathy, juvenile- or adult-onset spinocerebellar ataxia, and (most germane to this discussion) syndromes resembling ALS and spinal muscular atrophy.[90] These latter conditions first present in childhood to the fifth decade of life and are characterized by alpha-subunit mutations that result in low levels of residual Hex-A activity, preventing the overwhelming neurodegenerative manifestations of infantile Tay-Sachs disease.[75] Patients with motor neuron syndromes are usually compound heterozygotes with one severe (Tay-Sachs–like) alpha-subunit mutation and a second, less severe mutation.[75] Adult-onset motor neuron disease can also be a presentation of a beta-subunit mutation.[22]

Although spinal muscular atrophy caused by Hex-A deficiency may superficially resemble sporadic progressive muscular atrophy, certain clues point to the enzyme deficiency (see Table 6–12).[90] These include onset of weakness at a young age, a long disease course, prominent muscle cramps, postural and action tremor, mental changes that include dementia and affective disorders, CT or MRI evidence of cerebellar atrophy, nerve conduction studies revealing peripheral sensory nerve involvement, and complex repetitive discharges seen on EMG. A definitive laboratory diagnosis may be established when Hex-A activity is markedly reduced in serum or leukocytes.

Spinal Cord Disorders

SPONDYLOTIC MYELOPATHY

Spondylotic myelopathy is a common problem in clinical practice. Because of degenerative joint disease at the level of the cervical spine, spinal cord compression with or without nerve root compromise may occur. Patients usually have a predisposition for this syndrome because of a congenitally narrow cervical spinal canal. With aging and its attendant wear and tear, osteophyte development and thickening of the posterior longitudinal ligament further compromise the spinal canal. Neck pain is a common clinical feature, and patients with coexisting radiculopathy also have typical radicular pain. Lhermitte's sign may be present. The usual features of this myelopathy are gait disorder because of leg spasticity, difficulty controlling the urinary sphincter, and numbness in the feet and legs. If a radiculopathy exists, then the expected symptoms of nerve root compromise will be seen as well.

The signs of cervical myelopathy include spasticity in the legs, lower extremity hyperreflexia, and Babinski signs. There may also be associated sensory findings, especially vibration and position abnormalities, because of posterior column involvement. Spasticity and marked proprioceptive loss contribute to the gait abnormality, giving it a spastic-ataxic quality. Although this description of spondylotic myelopathy suggests it can be clearly distinguished from the pure motor syndrome of ALS, in some cases neck ache is either absent or minimal, sphincter abnormalities are not present, and few if any sensory signs are found. Isolated spondylotic myelopathy thus can simulate the upper motor neuron features of ALS. If there is a coexisting radiculopathy with minimal pain and sensory symptoms, the resulting clinical syndrome of spondylotic myelopathy with radiculopathy can produce lower motor neuron features in the arms and upper motor neuron features in the legs almost exactly simulating ALS (Table 6–13).[148] Occasionally, spondylotic narrowing at C3–C4 and C5–C6 leads to painless hand muscle wasting and weakness in the absence of radiculopathy per se, perhaps by causing venous congestion and hypoxia of central gray matter at C7–T1 spinal segments.[132]

When faced with lower motor neuron findings in the arms (or hands) with or without upper motor neuron findings in the legs, it behooves the neurologist to consider the possibility of spondylotic myelopathy, even in the absence of pain and sensory loss. An MRI of the cervical spine should be performed to rule out this treatable degenerative disorder.

SYRINGOMYELIA

Most often syringomyelia is a developmental disorder characterized by the presence of an abnormal cavity because of dilatation of the central canal of the spinal cord. The cavity originates in the midcervical region but may extend upward into the medulla (producing syringobulbia) or downward into the thoracic and lumbar regions. Many cases occur in association with craniovertebral ab-

Table 6–13. **FEATURES OF MYELOPATHIES CONSIDERED IN THE DIFFERENTIAL DIAGNOSIS OF ALS**

Disease	CLINICAL AND LABORATORY FEATURES	
	Shared with ALS	**Atypical for ALS**
Spondylotic myelopathy	Lower motor neuron signs in the arms, upper motor neuron signs in the legs	Neck pain and stiffness, proprioceptive loss in the legs, sphincter disturbance
Syringomyelia	Weakness, atrophy, fasciculations in hand; upper motor neuron findings in the legs	Dissociated sensory loss in upper cervical segment, associated Chiari malformation, young age of onset, MRI positive for syrinx
Multiple sclerosis	Progressive spastic paraparesis	Visual, ocular, sensory, cerebellar and sphincter symptomatology; MRI positive for white matter disease; oligoclonal bands in CSF
Adrenoleukodystrophy	Progressive spastic paraparesis; distal muscle weakness	Sensory loss; impotence, sphincter disturbance; X-linked, peripheral neuropathy; low serum sodium; increased plasma very long chain fatty acids
Subacute combined degeneration	Progressive spastic paraparesis	Numbness and tingling in hands and feet; disturbed mentation; megaloblastic anemia; glossitis; depressed serum B_{12} level
Familial spastic paraplegia	Progressive spastic weakness in the legs	Very slow progression; absence of bulbar or respiratory involvement; absence of lower motor neuron signs; urinary incontinence
HTLV-1 associated myelopathy	Slowly progressive spastic paraparesis	Urinary frequency and urgency; rarity of lower motor neuron signs; CSF pleocytosis and raised protein; MRI: demyelination
Human immunodeficiency virus (HIV) myelopathy	Upper and lower motor neuron signs	Peripheral neuropathy (axon loss); clinical signs of acquired immunodeficiency syndrome

Abbreviation: HTLV-1 = human T-lymphotropic virus type 1.

normalities, most commonly the Arnold-Chiari malformation.[85] This cavity enlarges slowly over many years, first interrupting the decussating second-order neurons that convey pain and temperature sensation and then expanding to involve the anterior horn cells in the lower cervical segments and sometimes the more laterally situated corticospinal tracts.

The clinical syndrome resulting from syringomyelia is characterized by mixed sensory and motor features.[87] As classically described, there is dissociated sensory loss (loss of pain and thermal sense with preservation of the sense of touch) in a fairly symmetric distribution involving the lower, mid, and upper cervical segments (C8 and T1 up to C4 and C3). This involvement translates to sensory loss over the neck, shoulders, and arms in a so-called capelike distribution. Damage to the ventral portion of the central gray regions leads to lower motor neuron signs: weakness, atrophy, and fasciculations of the intrinsic hand muscles. Loss of tendon reflexes in the arms invariably occurs. Upper motor neuron signs in the lower extremities occur with extension of the cavity to the corticospinal tracts. Syringobulbia may lead to palatal and vocal cord paralysis, dysarthria, nystagmus, tongue weakness, and Horner's syndrome.

The relatively young age of onset (mean of 26 years old), long duration of disease (mean of 14 years), and presence of prominent sensory signs (and neck pain)[87] ensure that syringomyelia is unlikely to be confused with ALS (see Table 6–13). Syringomyelia, however, may progress rapidly and manifest primarily with prominent motor findings,[85,87] leading the clinician to consider ALS. Any doubt about the diagnosis is dispelled by MRI scanning, which is the best method of visualizing syrinx length and diameter.[49]

MULTIPLE SCLEROSIS

In this inflammatory, demyelinating disorder of central nervous system white matter, most patients become symptomatic between the ages of 20 and 40 years. Regions of the nervous system most often affected include the periventricular white matter, the optic nerves, the white matter tracts of the brain stem and cerebellum, and the posterior and lateral columns of the spinal cord. In the classic relapsing and remitting form of multiple sclerosis (MS), visual, ocular, sensory, cerebellar, and sphincter disturbances create a clinical picture that bears little resemblance to the pure motor syndrome caused by ALS.

In a small subset of patients with MS, particularly in individuals more than 50 years old, the disorder presents and evolves as a slowly progressive spastic paraparesis with severe weakness of the upper motor neuron type. Because these patients may have few if any sensory symptoms or signs, the diagnosis of ALS may be considered (see Table 6–13). Similarly, occasional MS patients have pseudobulbar palsy that simulates bulbar ALS. Some patients with MS have lower motor signs such as loss of deep tendon reflexes and amyotrophy;[96] these signs are probably explained by the presence of lesions or plaques in root entry and exit zones, respectively. Another subset of patients has intrinsic hand muscle atrophy that appears neurogenic, but in fact is related to disuse secondary to disease of the central pathways.[43] In these patients, diagnostic uncertainty can usually be resolved with laboratory studies that are characteristically positive in MS and normal in ALS. In MS, MRI studies of the spinal cord and brain generally disclose areas of T2 brightening, and the CSF often has oligoclonal bands and an elevated gamma globulin fraction of the total protein.

ADRENOLEUKODYSTROPHY

Adrenoleukodystrophy is a severe X-linked childhood disturbance with an onset between the ages of 4 and 8 years, adrenal insufficiency, progressive mental and psychologic deterioration, and quadriparesis. It is a peroxisomal disorder caused by a genetic defect in beta oxidation of saturated very long chain fatty acids that leads to their accumulation in a variety of tissues. A relatively mild "spinal-neuropathic" form designated as *adrenomyeloneuropathy* is found in adult men and is characterized by progressive spastic paraparesis with a mild peripheral neuropathy. A chronic nonprogressive spinal cord disorder has also been described in heterozygous women. Adrenomyeloneuropathy presents in the second to third decades of life with progressive spastic paraparesis, distal muscle weakness and sensory loss, impotence, and sphincter disturbances.[50] Because the sensory, autonomic, and sphincter disturbances may be relatively mild, and the motor component of this syndrome (upper motor neuron signs of weakness and spasticity) may be striking, the disorder can resemble ALS (see Table 6–13). Most patients, however, do have some degree of peripheral neuropathy, and nerve conduction studies disclose reduced motor conduction velocities. Additional important diagnostic information may be obtained from a sural nerve biopsy specimen, which reveals loss of myelinated fibers, small onion bulbs, and characteristic lipid clefts in the Schwann cell cytoplasm, the so-called lamellar lipid inclusions.[14] A laboratory chemistry clue is the presence of low sodium and elevated potassium concentrations, reflecting atrophy of the adrenal gland. Diagnosis can be established by demonstrating increased levels of very long chain fatty acids in the plasma of patients and heterozygous carriers.[91]

SUBACUTE COMBINED DEGENERATION OF THE SPINAL CORD

This disorder is but one manifestation of vitamin B_{12} deficiency. Because B_{12} has a key role in DNA synthesis, B_{12} deficiency leads to abnormalities associated with rapid cell division, including megaloblastic anemia, glossitis, and hypospermia. The neurologic manifestations include mental signs, visual impairment, peripheral neuropathy, and myelopathy.[8]

The first symptoms of spinal cord dysfunction are usually numbness and tingling in the feet and hands, which reflect abnormalities in the posterior columns. If the condition continues untreated, limb stiffness and weakness, particularly of the legs, develops as a result of corticospinal tract involvement. Ultimately, well-recognized upper motor neuron signs such as spasticity, hyperreflexia, clonus, and Babinski responses evolve.

Although ALS and subacute combined degeneration share upper motor neuron features, the latter disease generally features prominent sensory signs as well as manifestations referable to other neural systems. Nonetheless, even in patients who have few or no sensory symptoms, we generally obtain a vitamin B_{12} level to exclude an unusual presentation (primarily or exclusively motor manifestations) of subacute combined degeneration (see Table 6–13).

FAMILIAL SPASTIC PARAPLEGIA

Another condition that might superficially resemble the upper motor neuron features of ALS is familial spastic paraplegia. The condition is usually autosomal dominant, but occasional families with recessive inheritance are described, and onset may be at any age from childhood to late adult life.[55] In adults, this disorder usually presents between the third and fifth decades and typically progresses very slowly as patients develop progressive spastic weakness that begins in the legs. Involvement of the arms usually is slight, but occasionally some stiffness and clumsiness in hand movements exists. Tendon reflexes are brisk, and plantar responses are extensor. Distal amyotrophy can occur, but it is a variable and late manifestation of the condition.

When family history is not available and onset is in later life, differentiating familial spastic paraplegia from ALS can pose a diagnostic challenge. However, the long clinical course, absence of bulbar or respiratory involvement, absence of prominent lower motor neuron findings, presence of urinary symptoms, and mild but definite sensory findings help to separate this condition from ALS (see Table 6–13).

TROPICAL SPASTIC PARAPARESIS OR HTLV-1–ASSOCIATED MYELOPATHY

This chronic myelopathy associated with human T-lymphotropic virus type 1 (HTLV-1) typically presents during the third or fourth decade of life with a slowly progressive spastic paraparesis.[46] It is most commonly encountered in Japan, the Caribbean basin, parts of South America, and West Africa, but isolated cases have occurred in the southeastern United States and many other locations. The condition is acquired through blood transfusions, sexual contact, intravenous drug use, and vertical transmission from mother to fetus.[46] The clinical features are primarily upper motor neuron in type and characterized by leg weakness, paraparesis or paraplegia with brisk reflexes, clonus, and Babinski signs. Urinary frequency and urgency are common. Although patients describe paresthesias and dysesthesias, only mild sensory signs of decreased vibratory sensation and minor impairment of pinprick or light touch are found, and a thoracic sensory level is uncommon.[46] Therefore, because the features are overwhelmingly motor, this myelopathy can simulate a slowly evolving upper motor neuron presentation of ALS, or it can resemble primary lateral sclerosis. In most patients, muscle atrophy and fasciculations are absent, reflecting the sparing of anterior horn cells noted on pathologic examination.[125] However, cases of HTLV-1 myelopathy with upper and lower motor neuron features resembling ALS have been described,[78] albeit rarely (see Table 6–13).

Laboratory abnormalities[46] help to distinguish this chronic, progressive myelopathy from ALS: the diagnosis of HTLV-1–associated myelopathy can be established with the detection of serum and CSF anti–HTLV-1 antibodies. About 50% of patients have a mild lymphocytic pleocytosis and an elevation of the CSF protein. The MRI generally shows evidence of demyelination; the somatosensory evoked potentials indicate posterior column dysfunction even when sensory findings are mild or absent, and urodynamic studies show a spastic bladder.

HUMAN IMMUNODEFICIENCY VIRUS MYELOPATHY

The myelopathy associated with human immunodeficiency virus (HIV) infection is usually seen in the later stages of the disease when acquired immunodeficiency syndrome is well established. It is characterized by a gait disorder with sensory complaints, sphincter disturbances, and brisk reflexes. The disorder is likely to be mediated by cytokines, including tumor necrosis factor.[126] Although lower motor neuron features have been described in the setting of HIV infection, most of these patients have had a diffuse axonopathy,[48,62] not ALS per se (see Table 6–13). Moreover, some investigators have retrospectively screened their patients with ALS for antibodies to retroviruses, including HIV and HTLV-1, and these results have been uniformly negative.[30] A notable exception was a 26-year-old man with classic, rapidly progressive ALS after seroconversion to HIV-positive status[61] who had lower and upper motor neuron signs in the limbs and bulbar muscles. Although the disorder fulfilled all the clinical criteria for ALS, the diagnosis was not confirmed pathologically. With the information collected thus far, we agree with the prevailing opinion that concurrent ALS and HIV infection is likely to be incidental.[80]

Other Disorders of the Central Nervous System

PARKINSON'S DISEASE

This well-known disorder of movement and posture typically begins in the sixth and seventh decades of life, although development of symptoms in the fourth and fifth decades is not uncommon. Parkinson's disease often begins with muscle soreness and

cramping and, therefore, neuromuscular clinicians and rheumatologists may be asked for an opinion at a relatively early stage of the illness when the classic hallmarks of parkinsonism are not yet present. The clinical hallmarks are rigidity, bradykinesia, postural instability, and tremor. The presentation is often unilateral. In the fully developed form of Parkinson's, the elderly patient with a shuffling and festinating gait, rest tremor, and cogwheel rigidity is rarely mistaken to have ALS. However, at an earlier stage and in patients without tremor, features of parkinsonism may raise the possibility of ALS. For example, a combination of drooling and monotonous, hypophonic, dysarthric speech may suggest bulbar musculature involvement that is seen commonly in ALS. In some patients with Parkinson's disease, although the Babinski response cannot be elicited, reflexes may be rather brisk; in combination with increased tone, this bradykinetic, rigid syndrome may be mistaken for the spasticity of ALS. We have on a number of occasions encountered patients in whom Parkinson's disease simulated ALS. There are also reports of patients with concurrent, sporadic parkinsonism and ALS (without evidence of a generalized motor systems degeneration).[16] The distinction, however, between ALS and Parkinson's disease is usually clear because symptoms of the latter generally respond to L-dopa, and, in contrast to ALS, no abnormalities are found on nerve conduction studies or EMG in patients with the movement disorder.

MULTISYSTEM ATROPHY

A number of conditions are characterized by degeneration of neurons belonging to a variety of neural systems. Because anterior horn cells can be involved, we briefly discuss olivopontocerebellar atrophy, Machado-Joseph or Azorean disease, striatonigral degeneration, and Shy-Drager syndrome. All share a relative absence of tremor, rigidity, a tendency to fall early in the course, autonomic dysfunction, poor or no response to L-dopa, and a steady and sometimes rapid downhill course.[105]

In olivopontocerebellar atrophy, some patients develop muscular weakness and atrophy resembling the lower motor neuron form of ALS. The presence of cerebellar ataxia and parkinsonian features are incompatible with ALS and point to the diagnosis of olivopontocerebellar atrophy, with its much wider involvement. In Machado-Joseph disease, the spasticity and distal amyotrophy that may occur suggest ALS, but progressive ataxia with eye-movement weakness, nystagmus, eyelid retraction, and extrapyramidal manifestations generally marks the condition as a familial multisystem degeneration. Although clinical signs and pathologic features of upper and lower motor neuron involvement may occur in Shy-Drager syndrome,[137] the overwhelming clinical manifestation is autonomic disturbance characterized by urinary bladder dysfunction, postural dizziness and syncope, impotence, and decreased sweating. Features of parkinsonism and cerebellar degeneration also are prominent.

CREUTZFELDT-JAKOB DISEASE

Creutzfeldt-Jakob disease is a rare, transmissible neurodegenerative disorder (incidence, one case per 1 million population) with onset usually in the fifth to seventh decade of life. It is most often sporadic, but in about 15% of patients, the condition is familial. The clinical features include a rapidly progressive dementia associated with myoclonus, extrapyramidal, pyramidal, and cerebellar signs. Cortical blindness often occurs, and many patients have a typical startle response. The electroencephalogram shows periodic generalized sharp-and-slow wave complexes occurring at a frequency of about one per second.

Creutzfeldt-Jakob disease is unlikely to masquerade as ALS because prominent lower motor neuron signs are uncommon in the former, and when they occur it is usually late in the course of the disease, when the other features are already well established.[122] Patients presenting with dementia and prominent amyotrophy early in the course of Creutzfeldt-Jakob disease were at one time thought to have an "amyotrophic" or corticopallidospinal form of the disease.[4] A careful review of these cases, however, reveals that they lack the typical time course, pathologic features, and transmissibility of typical Creutzfeldt-Jakob disease and are more appropriately considered variants of ALS.[122]

HUNTINGTON'S DISEASE AND NEUROACANTHOCYTOSIS

Typically, Huntington's disease rarely poses a problem in differential diagnosis. From time to time, however, a patient is encountered who has no documentable family history and no features of dementia; they may present in mid-adult life with progressive rigidity rather than choreiform movements. In combination with poorly articulated speech, the overall syndrome may resemble the slowness and stiffness reminiscent of upper motor neuron findings seen in ALS. In these patients, however, imaging studies of the brain (disclosing a flattened or concave appearance of the caudate nuclei in Huntington's disease) and EMG (normal in Huntington's disease) help to distinguish between these two diseases. Of interest, a patient has been described with Huntington's disease who also had ALS.[11]

Neuroacanthocytosis is a movement disorder that resembles Huntington's disease.[114] It is characterized by familial chorea, dystonia, parkinsonism, orofacial dyskinesias, dysarthria, dysphagia, and intellectual impairment. Acanthocytes are seen on a peripheral blood film. In contrast to Huntington's disease, the CK level may be elevated, and the EMG may disclose chronic neurogenic features that suggest involvement of the lower motor neurons. Indeed, pathologic studies reveal neuronal loss in the anterior horns. The many extrapyramidal findings in neuroacanthocytosis, however, generally overwhelm the neurogenic features and leave no doubt about the diagnosis.

CEREBROVASCULAR DISEASE

Patients who have had multiple lacunar infarctions may present with spastic dysarthria, abulia, and bilateral pyramidal signs that may be mistaken for a primarily upper motor neuron presentation of ALS. The possibility of misdiagnosis is increased because involvement of sensory or cerebellar pathways may be slight or nonexistent. Helping to distinguish this form of vascular disease (the lacunar state) from ALS, however, is a disturbance of affect in the former with marked emotional lability, a moderate degree of dementia, a history of hypertension, and CT or MRI evidence for prior lacunar infarction in subcortical white matter and the brain stem.

We hasten to add, however, that emotional lability may be prominent in bulbar ALS, and the distinction between bulbar ALS and cerebrovascular disease may not always be immediately clear. Indeed, we have seen several patients originally diagnosed as having brainstem stroke who actually had ALS.

BRAIN-STEM GLIOMA

In most instances, brain-stem glioma is a tumor of childhood, with 80% of affected individuals presenting before the age of 21. It generally produces a complex syndrome of cranial nerve palsies, hemiparesis, gait ataxia, sensory disturbances, and gaze disorders. Rarely, however, the tumor arises for the first time in later adult life and may present with signs of corticobulbar and corticospinal dysfunction in the absence of disturbance referable to other neural systems within or traversing the brain stem. Such an unusual presentation could suggest ALS, but an MRI study of the brain and brain stem should lead to the correct diagnosis of a glioma. Also, in the case of glioma, an EMG may disclose facial myokymia, a feature not associated with ALS.

TUMORS OF THE FORAMEN MAGNUM

Although suboccipital or posterior cervical pain is usually the first and most prominent complaint associated with tumors in the foramen magnum, patients may present with bibrachial paresis and, in particular, wasting of the small muscles of the hands as a false localizing sign.[139] Cranial nerve signs may also develop as a result of intracranial extension, so that patients may have a combination of dysphagia, dysphonia, and dysarthria. Taken together, these lower motor neuron features suggest the progressive bulbar palsy form of ALS. Imaging studies of the brain stem, however, with particular attention to the foramen magnum, will generally reveal that the cause of such findings is structural rather than degenerative as in ALS.

Systemic Disorders

HYPERTHYROIDISM

The neurologic manifestations of hyperthyroidism are many and varied, including alterations in mental status, convulsions, abnormal movements such as tremor and chorea, ophthalmic disturbances, weakness, atrophy, and fasciculations.[142] In addition, patients with hyperthyroidism commonly have brisk deep tendon reflexes, and some may have frank evidence for corticospinal tract dysfunction with spasticity and Babinski signs.[44] Patients with hyperthyroidism thus may develop a combination of weakness and upper motor neuron signs that resembles ALS. Of course, most patients with hyperthyroidism have evidence of diffuse toxic goiter, anxiety, and insomnia that will differentiate it from ALS. It is important to note, however, that in older patients hyperthyroidism may be manifested by apathy and depression, the so-called apathetic hyperthyroidism. A low level of thyroid-stimulating hormone certainly suggests that an upper motor syndrome is being caused by hyperthyroidism.

HYPERPARATHYROIDISM

Neurologic manifestations in hyperparathyroid disease are generally related to hypercalcemia, hypophosphatemia, and an elevated parathyroid hormone level, and consist of alterations in mental status such as lethargy, confusion, and ultimately coma.[142] When hypercalcemia is not severe or acute, however, weakness and fatigability may be presenting symptoms of primary hyperparathyroidism. Infrequently, patients develop signs of a myopathy.[81] Rarely, hyperparathyroidism and ALS occur concurrently in the same patient, raising the possibility that the high level of parathyroid hormone contributes to the development of the motor neuron syndrome.[104] Hypercalcemia and raised levels of parathyroid hormone, however, should help to distinguish between this endocrinopathy and ALS.

THE DIFFERENTIAL DIAGNOSIS OF SYMPTOMS AND SIGNS IN ALS

Now that we have reviewed the diseases that should be considered in the differential diagnosis of ALS, it is useful to review also the differential diagnosis of the cardinal presenting symptoms of ALS (Table 6–14), and the classic presentations of ALS (Table 6–15).

Table 6–14. **THE DIFFERENTIAL DIAGNOSIS OF SYMPTOMS IN ALS**

Symptoms	Disease(s)
Dysarthria, dysphagia	Inflammatory myopathy, oculopharyngeal dystrophy, myasthenia gravis, bulbospinal neuronopathy, foramen magnum tumor, brain-stem tumor, stroke, Parkinson's disease
Dyspnea	Myasthenia gravis, Guillain-Barré syndrome, bulbospinal neuronopathy, post-polio progressive muscular atrophy, acid maltase deficiency, high cervical cord lesion
Head drop	Myasthenia gravis, inflammatory myopathy, nemaline myopathy, isolated neck extensor myopathy, Parkinson's disease
Upper limb weakness, clumsiness	Inclusion body myositis, mononeuropathy, multifocal motor neuropathy, brachial plexus neuropathy, cervical radiculopathy, benign monomelic amyotrophy, syringomyelia
Lower limb weakness, clumsiness	Inclusion body myositis, mononeuropathy, lumbosacral plexopathy, lumbosacral radiculopathy, diabetic polyradiculo-neuropathy
Fasciculations	Multifocal motor neuropathy, radiculopathy, bulbospinal neuronopathy, spinal muscular atrophy, benign monomelic amyotrophy, benign fasciculations
Cramps	Metabolic myopathy, radiculopathy, progressive post-polio muscular atrophy, bulbospinal neuronopathy, metabolic disorders,* electrolyte imbalance

*Pregnancy, uremia, hypothyroidism, hypoadrenalism.[81]

The diagnostic approaches discussed in this chapter, differential diagnosis by disease entity and by key symptoms and signs, are complementary and provide the clinician with a framework for the diagnostic evaluation of patients suspected of having ALS. Using the foundation of differential diagnosis developed in this chapter, we describe in the next chapter the many laboratory investigations that may be needed in this group of patients.

SUMMARY

There are several forms of motor neuron disease, each with a distinctive presentation: bulbar muscle weakness is the major finding in progressive bulbar palsy; limb muscle atrophy and fasciculations are the hallmarks of progressive muscular atrophy; hyperreflexia with spasticity are key features of primary lateral sclerosis; lower and upper motor neuron signs are found together in bulbar and spinal regions in ALS. These presentations may be seen in a wide variety of neurologic and systemic disorders, and therefore each presentation is associated with many and varied differential diagnostic possibilities. As a result, the process of differential diagnosis is complex and challenging.

Progressive bulbar palsy prompts the clinician to consider myasthenia gravis, oculopharyngeal dystrophy, foramen magnum tumor, brain-stem stroke, and Parkinson's disease. A presentation of progressive muscular atrophy may resemble the weakness encountered in myopathies, polyradiculoneuropathies, motor neuropathies, and a varied

Table 6–15. **THE DIFFERENTIAL DIAGNOSIS OF ALS CLASSIFIED BY CLINICAL PRESENTATION**

Clinical Presentation	Differential Diagnosis
Progressive bulbar palsy	Myasthenia gravis, bulbospinal neuronopathy, MS, foramen magnum tumor, cerebrovascular disease, syringobulbia, brain-stem glioma
Progressive muscular atrophy	Inclusion body myositis, mononeuropathy, multifocal motor neuropathy, CIDP, brachial or lumbar plexopathy, diabetic polyradiculoneuropathy, syphilitic meningomyelopathy, spinal muscular atrophy, bulbospinal neuronopathy, benign monomelic amyotrophy, motor neuronopathy with lymphoma, post-polio progressive muscular atrophy, Hex-A deficiency motor neuronopathy
Progressive spastic paraparesis	MS, cervical spondylotic myelopathy, syringomyelia, adrenoleukodystrophy, subacute combined degeneration, familial spastic paraparesis, HTLV-1 myelopathy, HIV myelopathy, Parkinson's disease, multisystem atrophy, Huntington's disease, hyperthyroidism, hyperparathyroidism

Abbreviations: CIDP = chronic inflammatory demyelinating polyneuropathy, Hex-A = hexosaminidase, HIV = human immunodeficiency virus, HTLV-1 = human T-lymphotropic virus type 1, MS = multiple sclerosis.

group of anterior horn cell disorders, such as spinal muscular atrophy, bulbospinal neuronopathy, benign monomelic amyotrophy, progressive postpoliomyelitis muscular atrophy, and Hex-A-deficiency–related muscular atrophy. Primary lateral sclerosis leads the neurologist to consider disorders of the spinal cord, including spondylotic myelopathy, multiple sclerosis, familial spastic paraparesis, and retroviral myelopathy. Unfortunately, the clinical presentation of ALS is rarely produced by a process other than motor neuron disease, but it is important to consider spondylotic myelopathy with radiculopathy, and a variety of rare conditions, such as Hex-A-deficiency–related motor neuron involvement, hyperthyroidism with weakness and hyperreflexia, and syphilitic radiculomyelopathy.

REFERENCES

1. Adams, CR, Ziegler, DK, and Lynn, JT: Mercury intoxication simulating amyotrophic lateral sclerosis. JAMA 250:642–643, 1983.
2. Alaoui-Faris, M El, Medejel, A, Zemmouri, K, et al: Le syndrome de sclérose latérale amyotrophique d'origine syphilitique. Étude de 5 cas. Rev Neurol (Paris) 146:41–44, 1990.
3. Albers, JW and Kelly, JJ: Acquired inflammatory demyelinating polyneuropathy: Clinical and electrodiagnostic features. Muscle Nerve 12:435–451, 1989.
4. Allen, IV, Dermott, E, Connolly, JH, et al: A study of a patient with the amyotrophic form of Creutzfeldt-Jakob disease. Brain 94:715–724, 1971.
5. Barohn, RJ, Kissel, JT, Warmolts, JR, et al: Chronic inflammatory polyradiculopathy: Clinical characteristics, course, and recommendations for diagnostic criteria. Arch Neurol 46:878–884, 1989.
6. Barohn, RJ, Sahenk, Z, Warmolts, JR, et al: The Bruns-Garland syndrome (diabetic amyotrophy). Revisited 100 years later. Arch Neurol 48:1130–1135, 1991.
7. Bastron, JA and Thomas, JE: Diabetic polyradiculopathy: Clinical and electromyographic findings in 105 patients. Mayo Clin Proc 56:725–732, 1981.
8. Beck, WS: Cobalamin and the nervous system. N Engl J Med 318:1752, 1988.
9. Belsh, JM and Schiffman, PL: Misdiagnosis in patients with amyotrophic lateral sclerosis. Arch Intern Med 150:2301–2305, 1990.
10. Ben Hamida, M, Hentati, F, and Ben, Hamida, C: Hereditary motor system diseases. (Chronic juvenile amyotrophic lateral sclerosis). Conditions combining a bilateral pyramidal syndrome with

limb and bulbar amyotrophy. Brain 113:347–363, 1990.

11. Blin, O, Samuel, D, Guieu, R, et al: Sclérose latérale amyotrophique familiale associée àune chorée de Huntington avec élévation du taux d'aspartate dans le liquide céphalo-rachidien. Rev Neurol (Paris) 148:144–146, 1992.

12. Bonkowsky, HL and Schady, W: Neurologic manifestations of acute porphyria. Sem Liver Dis 2:108–124, 1982.

13. Boothby, JA, deJesus, PV, and Rowland, LP: Reversible forms of motor neuron disease. Lead "neuritis." Arch Neurol 31:18–23, 1974.

14. Bosch, EP and Mitsumoto, H: Disorders of peripheral nerves. In Bradley, WG, Daroff, RB, Fenichel, GM, and Marsden, CD (eds): Neurology in Clinical Practice. Butterworth-Heinemann, Boston: 1996, pp 1881–1952.

15. Bosch, EP and Smith, BE: Peripheral neuropathies associated with monoclonal proteins. Med Clin North America 77:125–139, 1993.

16. Brait, K, Fahn, S, and Schwarz, GA: Sporadic and familial parkinsonism and motor neuron disease. Neurology 23:990–1002, 1973.

17. Brooks, BR: El Escorial World Federation of Neurology criteria for the diagnosis of amyotrophic lateral sclerosis. J Neurol Sci 124 (suppl):96–107, 1994.

18. Brooks, BP and Fischbeck, KH. Spinal and bulbar muscular atrophy: A trinucleotide repeat expansion neurodegenerative disease. Trends Neurosci 18:459–461, 1995.

19. Brown, RH: Inherited motor neuron diseases: recent progress. Semin Neurol 13:365–368, 1993.

20. Brownell, AKW, Gilbert, JJ, Shaw, DT, et al: Adult onset nemaline myopathy. Neurology 28:1306–1309, 1978.

21. Brunberg, JA, McCormick, WF, and Schoshet, SS: Type II glycogenolysis: An adult with diffuse weakness and muscle wasting. Arch Neurol 25:171–178, 1971.

22. Cashman, NR, Antel, J, Hancock, LW, et al: N-Acetyl-β-hexosaminidase β locus defect and juvenile motor neuron disease: A case study. Ann Neurol 19:568–572, 1986.

23. Chad, DA: Disorders of roots and plexuses. In Bradley, WG, Daroff, RB, Fenichel, GM, and Marsden, CD (eds): Neurology in Clinical Practice. Butterworth-Heinemann, Boston: 1996, pp 1853–1880.

24. Chad, DA, and Drachman, DA: Progressive external ophthalmoplegia. In Vinken, PJ, Bruyn, GW, Klawans, HL, et al (eds): Handbook of Clinical Neurology, Vol 60. Elsevier Science BV, Amsterdam: 1991, pp. 47–59.

25. Chaudhry, V, Corse, AM, Cornblath, D, et al: Multifocal motor neuropathy: Response to human immune globulin. Ann Neurol 33:237–242, 1993.

26. Corse, AM, Chaudhry, V, Crawford, TO, et al: Sural nerve pathology in multifocal motor neuropathy. Ann Neurol (abstract) 34:268, 1993.

27. Cwik, VA and Mitsumoto, H: Postpoliomyelitis syndrome. In Smith RA (ed): Handbook of Amyotrophic Lateral Sclerosis. Marcel Dekker, New York, 1992, pp 77–91.

28. Dalakas, MC: Polymyositis, dermatomyositis and inclusion-body myositis. N Engl J Med 325:1487–1498, 1991.

29. Dalakas, M, Elder, G, Hallett, M, et al: A long-term follow-up study of patients with post-poliomyelitis neuromuscular symptoms. N Engl J Med 314:959–963, 1986.

30. Dalakas, MC and Pezeshkpour, GH: Neuromuscular diseases associated with human immuno deficiency virus infection. Ann Neurol 23(suppl): S38–S48, 1988.

31. Dalakas, MC, Stein, DP, Otero, C, et al: Effect of high-dose intravenous immunoglobulin on amyotrophic lateral sclerosis and multifocal motor neuropathy. Arch Neurol 51:861–864, 1994.

32. Danon, MJ, Servidei, S, Dimauro, S, et al: Late onset muscle phosphofructokinase deficiency. Neurology 38:956–960, 1988.

33. Deyo, RA, Loeser, JD, and Bigos, SJ: Herniated lumbar intervertebral disc. Ann Intern Med 112:598–603, 1990.

34. Dimauro, S, Hartwig, GB, Hayes, A, et al: Debrancher deficiency: Neuromuscular disorder in five adults. Ann Neurol 5:422–436, 1979.

35. Donofrio, PD: Monomelic amyotrophy. Muscle Nerve 17:1129–1134, 1994.

36. Doyu, M, Sobue, G, Mukai, E, et al: Severity of X-linked recessive bulbospinal neuronopathy correlated with size of the tandem CAG repeat in androgen receptor gene. Ann Neurol 32:707–710, 1992.

37. Drachman, DB: Myasthenia gravis. N Engl J Med 330:1797–1810, 1994.

38. Drachman, DB, Murphy, SR, Nigam, MO, et al: "Myopathic" changes in chronically denervated muscle. Arch Neurol 16:14–24, 1967.

39. Dyck, PJ, Litchy, WJ, Kratz, KM, et al: A plasma exchange versus immune globulin infusion trial in chronic inflammatory polyradiculoneuropathy. Ann Neurol 36:838–845, 1994.

40. Engel, AG: Late onset rod myopathy (a new syndrome?): Light and electron microscopic observations in two cases. Mayo Clin Proc 41:713–741, 1966.

41. Engel, WK, Eyerman, EL, and Williams, AG: Late onset type of skeletal muscle phosphorylase deficiency. A new familial variety with completely and partially affected subjects. N Engl J Med 268:135–137, 1963.

42. Fischbeck, KH: The mechanism of myotonic dystrophy. Ann Neurol 35:255–256, 1994.

43. Fisher, M, Long, RR, and Drachman, DA: Hand muscle atrophy in multiple sclerosis. Arch Neurol 40:811–815, 1983.

44. Fisher, M, Mateer, JE, Ullrich, I, et al: Pyramidal tract deficits and polyneuropathy in hyperthyroidism. Combination clinically mimicking amyotrophic lateral sclerosis. Am J Med 78:1041–1044, 1985.

45. Feldman, EL, Bromberg, MB, Albers, JW, et al: Immunosuppressive treatment in multifocal motor neuropathy. Ann Neurol 30:397–401, 1991.

46. Gessain, A and Gout, O: Chronic myelopathy associated with human T-lymphotropic virus type I (HTLV-I). Ann Intern Med 117:933–946, 1992.

47. Gilliam, TC, Brzustowicz, LM, Castilla, LH, et al: Genetic homogeneity between acute and chronic forms of spinal muscular atrophy. Nature 345:823–825, 1990.

48. Goldstein, JM, Azizi, SA, Booss, J, et al: Human im-

munodeficiency virus-associated motor axonal polyradiculoneuropathy. Arch Neurol 50:1316–1319, 1993.

49. Grant, R, Hadley, DM, Macpherson, P, et al: Syringomyelia: cyst measurement by magnetic resonance imaging and comparison with symptoms and disability. J Neurol Neurosurg Psychiatry 50:1008–1014, 1987.

50. Griffin, JW, Goren, E, Schaumberg, H, et al: Adrenomyeloneuropathy: A probable variant of adrenoleukodystrophy. Neurology 27:1107–1113, 1977.

51. Griffin, JW, Li, CY, Ho, TW, et al: Pathology of the motor-sensory axonal Guillain-Barré syndrome. Ann Neurol 39:17–28, 1996.

52. Gutmann, L, Martin, JD, and Welton, W: Dapsone motor neuropathy—An axonal disease. Neurology 26:514–516, 1976.

53. Hader, WJ, Rozdilsky, B, and Nair, CP: The concurrence of multiple sclerosis in amyotrophic lateral sclerosis. Can J Neurol Sci 13:66–69, 1986.

54. Hardiman, O, Halperin, JJ, Farrell, MA, et al: Neuropathic findings in oculopharyngeal muscular dystrophy. SA report of seven cases and a review of the literature. Arch Neurol 50:481–488, 1993.

55. Harding, AE: Hereditary "pure" spastic paraplegia: a clinical and genetic study of 22 families. J Neurol Neurosurg Psychiatry 44:871–883, 1981.

56. Harding, AE and Thomas, PK: Hereditary distal spinal muscular atrophy. A report on 34 cases and a review of the literature. J Neurol Sci 45:337–348, 1980.

57. Harding, AE and Thomas, PK: The clinical features of hereditary motor and sensory neuropathy types I and II. Brain 103:259–280, 1980.

58. Harding, AE and Thomas, PK: Peroneal muscular atrophy with pyramidal features. J Neurol Neurosurg Psychiatry 47:168–172, 1984.

59. Harding, AE, Thomas, PK, Baraitser, M, et al: X-linked recessive bulbospinal neuronopathy: A report of ten cases. J Neurol Neurosurg Psychiatry 45:1012–1019, 1982.

60. Hirayama, K, Tomonaga, M, Kitano, K, et al: Focal cervical poliopathy causing juvenile muscular atrophy of distal upper extremity: A pathological study. J Neurol Neurosurg Psychiatry 50:285–290, 1987.

61. Hoffman, PM, Festoff, BW, Giron, LT, et al: Isolation of LAV HTLV-III from a patient with amyotrophic lateral sclerosis [letter]. N Engl J Med 313:324–325, 1985.

62. Huang, PP, Chin, R, Song, S, et al: Lower motor neuron dysfunction associated with human immuno deficiency virus infection. Arch Neurol 50:1328–1330, 1993.

63. Hund, E, Heckl, R, Goebel, HH, et al: Inclusion body myositis presenting with isolated erector spinae paresis. Neurology 45:993–994, 1995.

64. Jammes, Y, Pouget, J, Grimaud, C, et al: Pulmonary function and electromyographic study of respiratory muscles in myotonic dystrophy. Muscle Nerve 8:595–605, 1985.

65. Jansen, PH, Jootsen, MG, Jaspar, HHJ, et al: A rapidly progressive autosomal dominant scapuloperoneal form of spinal muscular atrophy. Ann Neurol 20:538–540, 1986.

66. Jöbsis, GJ, Louwerse, ES, de Visser, M, et al: Differential diagnosis in spinal and bulbar muscular atrophy clinical and molecular aspects. J Neurol Sci 129(S):56–57, 1995.

67. Johnson, WG: The clinical spectrum of hexosaminidase deficiency diseases. Neurology 31:1453–1456, 1981.

68. Jubelt, B and Cashman, NR: Neurological manifestations of the post-polio syndrome. CRC Crit Rev Neurobiol 3:199–220, 1987.

69. Kaji, R, Shibasaki, H, and Kimura, J: Multifocal demyelinating motor neuropathy: Cranial nerve involvement and immunoglobulin therapy. Neurology 42:506–509, 1992.

70. Kaji, R, Oka, N, Tsuji, T, et al: Pathological findings at the site of conduction block in multifocal motor neuropathy. Ann Neurol 33:152–158, 1993.

71. Karpati, G, Carpenter, S, Eisen, A, et al: The adult form of acid maltase (a-1, 4-glucosidase) deficiency. Ann Neurol 1:276–280, 1977.

72. Katz, JS, Wolfe, GI, Burns, DK, et al: Isolated neck extensor myopathy: A common cause of dropped head syndrome. Neurology 46:917–921, 1996.

73. Kelly, JJ: Peripheral neuropathies associated with monoclonal proteins: A clinical review. Muscle Nerve 8:138–150, 1985.

74. Kennedy, WB, Alter, M, and Sung, JG: Report of an X-linked form of spinal muscular atrophy. Neurology 18:671–680, 1968.

75. Kolodny, EH: The GM2 gangliosidoses. In Rosenberg, RN, Prusiner, SB, DiMauro, S et al (eds): The Molecular and Genetic Basis of Neurological Disease. Butterworth-Heinemann, Boston, 1992, pp 531–540.

76. Kothari, MJ, Rutkove, SB, Logigian, EL, et al: Coexistent entrapment neuropathies in patients with amyotrophic lateral sclerosis. Neurology 45:A447–448, 1995.

77. Kratz, R and Brooke, MH: Distal myopathy. In Vincken, PJ and Bruyn, GW (eds): Handbook of Clinical Neurology. North-Holland, Amsterdam, 1980, pp 471–483.

78. Kuroda, Y and Sugihara, H: Autopsy report of HTLV-I-associated myelopathy presenting with ALS-like manifestations. J Neurol Sci 106:199–205, 1991.

79. Lange, DJ, Trojaborg, W, Latov, N, et al: Multifocal motor neuropathy with conduction block: Is it a distinct clinical entity? Neurology 42:497–505, 1992.

80. Lange, DJ: AAEM minimonograph #41: Neuromuscular diseases associated with HIV-1 infection. Muscle Nerve 17:16–30, 1994.

81. Layzer, RB: Neuromuscular manifestations of systemic disease. FA Davis, Philadelphia, 1985, pp 112–115.

82. Levin, KH, Maggiano, HJ, and Wilbourn, AJ: Cervical radiculopathies: comparison of surgical and EMG localization of single-root lesions. Neurology 46:1022–1025, 1996.

83. Lewis, RA, Sumner, AJ, Brown, MJ, et al: Multifocal demyelinating neuropathy with persistent conduction block. Neurology 32:958–964, 1982.

84. Logigian, EL, and Steere, AC: Clinical and electrophysiologic findings in chronic neuropathy of Lyme disease. Neurology 42:303–311, 1992.

85. Logue, V, and Edwards, MR: Syringomyelia and its surgical treatment—An analysis of 75 patients. J Neurol Neurosurg Psychiatry 44:273–284, 1981.

86. Lotz, BP, Engel, AG, Nishimo, H, et al: Inclusion body myositis. Brain 112:727–742, 1989.

87. Mariani, C, Cislaghi, MG, Barbieri, S, et al: The natural history and results of surgery in 50 cases of syringomyelia. J Neurol 238:433–438, 1991.

88. Marksbury, WR, McQuillen, MP, Procobis, TG, et al: Muscle carnitine deficiency. Association with a lipid myopathy, vacuolar neuropathy, and vacuolate leukocytes. Arch Neurol 31:320–324, 1974.

89. Miller, RG, Blank, K, and Layzer, RB: Sporadic distal myopathy with early adult onset. Ann Neurol 5:220–227, 1979.

90. Mitsumoto, H, Sliman, RJ, Schafer, IA, et al: Motor neuron disease in adult hexosaminidase A deficiency in two families: Evidence for multisystem degeneration. Ann Neurol 17:378–385, 1985.

91. Moser, HW, Moser, AB, Frayer, KF, et al: Adrenoleukodystrophy: Increased plasma content of saturated very long chain fatty acids. Neurology 31:1241–1249, 1981.

92. Mulder, DW, Kurland, LT, Offord, KP, et al. Familial adult motor neuron disease: Amyotrophic lateral sclerosis. Neurology 36:511–517, 1986.

93. Murphy, SF and Drachman, DB: The oculopharyngeal syndrome. JAMA 203:99–104, 1968.

94. Nelson, JS and Prensky, AL: Sporadic juvenile amyotrophic lateral sclerosis. A clinicopathological study of a case with neuronal cytoplasmic inclusions containing RNA. Arch Neurol 27:300–306, 1972.

95. Newman, DS, Aggarwal, SK, and Silbergleit, R: Thoracic radicular symptoms in amyotrophic lateral sclerosis. J Neurol Sci 129(S):38–41, 1995.

96. Noseworthy, JH and Heffernan, LPM: Motor radiculopathy—An unusual presentation of multiple sclerosis. Can J Neurol Sci: J 207–209, 1980.

97. Noseworthy, JH, Rae-Grant, AD, and Brown, WF: An unusual subacute progressive motor neuronopathy with myasthenia-like features. Can J Neurol Sci 15:304–309, 1988.

98. O'Neil, JH, Murray, NMF, and Newsome-Davis, J: The Lambert-Eaton myasthenic syndrome: A review of 50 cases. Brain 111:577–596, 1988.

99. O'Reilly, DF, Brazis, PW, and Rubino, FA: The misdiagnosis of unilateral presentation of amyotrophic lateral sclerosis. Muscle Nerve 5:724–726, 1982.

100. Olney, RK, Aminoff, MJ, and So, YT: Clinical and electrodiagnostic features of X-linked recessive bulbospinal neuronopathy. Neurology 41:823–828, 1991.

101. Olney, RK and Hanson, M: Ulnar neuropathy at or distal to the wrist. Muscle Nerve 11:828, 1988.

102. Parry, GJ: AAEM Case Report #30: Multifocal motor neuropathy. Muscle Nerve 19:269–276, 1996.

103. Parry, GJ and Sumner, AJ: Multifocal motor neuropathy. Neurol Clin 10:671–684, 1992.

104. Patten, BM, and Pages, M: Severe neurological disease associated with hyperparathyroidism. Ann Neurol 15:453–456, 1984.

105. Paulson, GW and Aotsuka, A: Parkinsonian syndromes. Semin Neurol 13:359–364, 1993.

106. Paulus, W, Peiffer, J, Becker, I, et al: Adult-onset rod disease with abundant internuclear rods. J Neurol 235:343–347, 1988.

107. Pearn, JH, Hudgson, P, and Walton, JN: A clinical and genetic study of spinal muscular atrophy of adult onset. The autosomal recessive form as a discrete disease entity. Brain 101:591–606, 1978.

108. Pestronk, A: Invited review: Motor neuropathies, motor neuron disorders, and antiglycolipid antibodies. Muscle Nerve 14:927–936, 1991.

109. Pestronk, A, Chaudhry, V, Feldman, EL, et al: Lower motor neuron syndromes defined by patterns of weakness, nerve conduction abnormalities and high titers of anti-glycolipid antibodies. Ann Neurol 27:316–326, 1990.

110. Pestronk, A, Cornblath, DR, Ilyas, AA, et al: A treatable multi-focal motor neuropathy with antibodies to GM 1 ganglioside. Ann Neurol 24:73–78, 1988.

111. Pilgaard, S: Unilateral juvenile muscular atrophy of upper limbs. Acta Orthop (Scand)39:327–331, 1968.

112. Pioro, EPJ, Kant, J, and Mitsumoto, H: Disease expression in a Kennedy's disease kindred is unrelated to CAG tandem repeat size in the androgen receptor gene: Characterization in a symptomatic female. [abstract]. Ann Neurol 36:318, 1994.

113. Ricker, K, Koch, MC, Lehmann-Horn, F, et al: Proximal myotonic myopathy. Clinical features of a multisystem disorder similar to myotonic dystrophy. Arch Neurol 52:25–31, 1995.

114. Rinne, JO, Daniel, SE, Scaravilli, F, et al: The neuropathological features of neuroacanthocytosis. Mov Disord 9:297–304, 1994.

115. Roos, R, Viola, MV, Wollmann, R, et al: Amyotrophic lateral sclerosis with antecedent poliomyelitis. Arch Neurol 37:312–313, 1980.

116. Rowland, LP: Diverse forms of motor neuron diseases. In Rowland, LP (ed): Advances in Neurology, Vol 36, Human Motor Neuron Diseases. Raven Press, New York, 1982.

117. Rowland, LP: Ten central themes in a decade of ALS research. In Rowland, LP (ed): Advances in Neurology, Vol 56, Amyotrophic Lateral Sclerosis and Other Motor Neuron Diseases. Raven Press, New York, 1991.

118. Rowland, LP, Defendini, R, Sherman, WH, et al: Macroglobulinemia with peripheral neuropathy simulating motor neuron disease. Ann Neurol 11:532–536, 1982.

119. Rowland, LP and Schneck, SA: Neuromuscular diseases associated with malignant neoplastic diseases. J Chronic Dis 16:777–795, 1963.

120. Rowland, LP, Sherman, WH, Latov, N, et al: Amyotrophic lateral sclerosis and lymphoma: Bone marrow examination and other tests. Neurology 42:1101–1102, 1992.

121. Russman, BS, Iannacone, ST, Buncher, CR, et al: Spinal muscular atrophy: New thoughts on the pathogenesis and classification schema. J Child Neurol 7:347–353, 1992.

122. Salazar, AM, Masters, CL, Gajdusek, C, et al: Syndromes of amyotrophic lateral sclerosis in dementia: Relation to transmissable Creutzfeldt-Jacob disease. Ann Neurol 14:17–26, 1983.

123. Santoro, M, Thomas, F, Fink, M, et al: IgM deposits at nodes of Ranvier in a patient with amyotrophic lateral sclerosis, anti-GM1 antibodies, and multifocal conduction block. Ann Neurol 28:373–377, 1990.

124. Schold, SC, Cho, ES, Somasundaram, M, et al: Subacute motor neuronopathy: A remote effect of lymphoma. Ann Neurol 5:271–287, 1979.

125. Shibasaki, H, Endo, C, Kuroda, Y, et al: Clinical picture of HTLV-I associated myelopathy. J Neurol Sci 87:15–24, 1988.

126. Simpson, DM and Tagliati, M: Neurologic manifestations of HIV infection. Ann Intern Med 121:769–785, 1994.

127. Singh, N, Sachdev, K, and Susheela, AK: Juvenile muscular atrophy localized to arms. Arch Neurol 37:297–299, 1980.

128. Sobue, G, Doyu, M, Kachi, T, et al: Subclinical phenotypic expressions in heterozygous females of X-linked recessive bulbospinal neuronopathy. J Neurol Sci 117:74–78, 1993.

129. Sobue, I, Saito, N, Iida, M, et al: Juvenile type of distal and segmental muscular atrophy of upper extremities. Ann Neurol 3:429–432, 1978.

130. Sonies, BC and Dalakas, MC: Dysphagia in patients with the post-polio syndrome. N Engl J Med 324:1162–1167, 1991.

131. Spada, ARL, Wilson, EM, Lubahn, DB, et al: Androgen receptor gene mutations in X-linked spinal and bulbar muscular atrophy. Nature 352:77–79, 1991.

132. Stark, RJ, Kennard, C, and Swash, M: Hand wasting in spondylotic high cord compression: An electromyographic study. Ann Neurol 9:58–62, 1981.

133. Steere, AC: Lyme disease. N Engl J Med 321:586–596, 1989.

134. Stewart, JD: Focal peripheral neuropathies, ed 2. Raven Press, New York, 1993.

135. Suarez, GA, Giannini, C, Bosch, EP, et al: Immune brachial plexus neuropathy: Suggestive evidence for an inflammatory-immune pathogenesis. Neurology 46:559–561, 1996.

136. Suarez, GA and Kelly, JJ: The dropped head syndrome. Neurology 42:1625–1627, 1992.

137. Sung, JH, Mastri, AR, and Segal, E: Pathology of Shy-Drager syndrome. J Neuropathol Exp Neurol 38:353–368, 1979.

138. Tan, E, Lynn, J, Amato, AA, et al: Immunosupressive treatment of motor neuron syndromes. Attempts to distinguish a treatable disorder. Arch Neurol 51:194–200, 1994.

139. Taylor, AR and Byrnes, DP: Foramen magnum and high cervical cord compression. Brain 97:473–480, 1974.

140. Thomas, JE, Howard, FM: Segmental zoster paresis—A disease profile. Neurology 22:459–466, 1972.

141. Tome, FMS and Fardeau, M: Nucelar inclusions in oculopharyngeal dystrophy. Acta Neuropathol 49:85–87, 1980.

142. Tonner, DR and Schlechte, JA: Neurologic complications of thyroid disease and parathyroid disease. Med Clin North Am 77:251–263, 1993.

143. Trojan, DA and Cashman, NR: Fibromyalgia is common in a postpoliomyelitis clinic. Arch Neurol 52:620–624, 1995.

144. Vincent, A, Lang, B, and Newsom-Davis, J: Autoimmunity to the voltage gated calcium channel underlies the Lambert-Eaton myasthenic syndrome, a paraneoplastic disorder. Trends Neurol Sci 12:496–502, 1989.

145. Welander, L: Myopathia distalis tarda hereditaria. Acta Med Scand 141:(suppl 265):1–124, 1951.

146. Wertsch, JJ: Anterior interosseus nerve syndrome. Muscle Nerve 15:977, 1992.

147. White, JR, Sachs, GM, and Gilchrist, JM: Multifocal motor neuropathy with conduction block and Campylobacter jejuni. Neurology 46:562–563, 1996.

148. Wilkinson, M: Cervical spondylosis. Its early diagnosis and treatment. WB Saunders, Philadelphia, 1971.

149. Younger, DS, Rowland, LP, Latov, N, et al: Motor neuron disease in amyotrophic lateral sclerosis: Relation of high CSF protein content to paraproteinemia and clinical syndromes. Neurology 40:595–599, 1990.

150. Younger, DS, Rowland, LP, Latov, N, et al: Lymphoma, motor neuron disease and amyotrophic lateral sclerosis. Ann Neurol 29:78, 1991.

CHAPTER 7

DIAGNOSTIC INVESTIGATION FOR ALS

ELECTROMYOGRAPHIC EVALUATION
NEUROIMAGING STUDIES
CLINICAL LABORATORY STUDIES
ALS-Related Syndromes
Influence of Clinical Presentation on Test
   Selection
ROLE OF MUSCLE BIOPSY

When a patient is suspected to have ALS, the clinician who takes responsibility for making the diagnosis is pulled by two competing impulses. First is the desire to establish a diagnosis without undue delay and provide the patient with a clear and compassionate explanation of the nature and course of the illness. Establishing a diagnosis in this fashion is important, so that the patient and family can adjust to the new reality and plan for the future. Second is the equally powerful need to question the diagnosis of ALS, not accepting it until all other possibilities have been excluded. The first approach may leave patient and family feeling that not everything was done to identify a treatable process, and that an opportunity for treatment, albeit remote, was missed. The second approach may take many weeks or even months to complete, as isolated laboratory abnormalities are pursued with increasingly expensive and complex tests.[2] Like most neurologists, it is our practice to incorporate aspects of both approaches. When we are strongly considering a diagnosis of ALS, we

ask ourselves if the findings the patient exhibits could *reasonably* be explained by any other disease process.

In the sections that follow, we will present our approach to the diagnostic investigation of the patient suspected to have ALS. The framework for our discussion is the motor neuron disease classification that includes ALS, bulbar palsy, progressive muscular atrophy, and primary lateral sclerosis. Before committing ourselves to the diagnosis of motor neuron disease, however, we view these subtypes more generically, according to their clinical presentations, with the potential for a diverse set of causes.

We employ four major categories of laboratory assessment when evaluating patients suspected to have ALS or an ALS subtype: electrodiagnostic (primarily electromyographic [EMG]) studies (see Chapter 5), neuroimaging tests (see Chapter 8), clinical laboratory studies, and muscle biopsy interpretation. The rationale for each category of testing is outlined in Table 7–1.

ELECTROMYOGRAPHIC EVALUATION

In virtually all patients presenting with motor neuron disease, we perform an EMG after completion of the history and physical examination. In ALS, we expect the EMG to reveal a characteristic pattern of normal sensory conduction studies, essentially normal

Table 7–1. **STEPS IN DIAGNOSTIC EVALUATION WHEN ALS IS SUSPECTED**

Investigation	Rationale and Points to Consider
Electromyography	Confirm lower motor neuron involvement.
	• Are there features of denervation and reinnervation?
	• Is the process generalized or is it focal?
	• Is there conduction block?
	• Are sensory fibers involved?
	• Is there a decremental motor response?
	• Is there postactivation facilitation?
Neuroimaging of brain and spinal cord	Confirm normal anatomy and examine for motor pathway abnormalities seen in ALS.
	• Is there structural pathology of brain, brain stem, cervicomedullary junction, spinal cord, or nerve roots?
Clinical laboratory studies	Confirm normal results.
	• Is there evidence for treatable or reversible disorders of a metabolic, autoimmune, neoplastic, infectious, or vasculitic nature?
Muscle biopsy	Confirm denervation and reinnervation.
	• Is there evidence for inflammatory, metabolic, genetic, or toxic myopathy?

motor conduction studies (although motor amplitudes are often reduced) and needle examination findings of fibrillation and fasciculation potential activity with evidence of motor unit potential remodeling in a wide distribution (see Chapter 5). We use the EMG to search for specific abnormalities that are recognizable neurophysiologic signatures of disorders that may at times mimic ALS, but in contrast to ALS are treatable, self-limited, or reversible. These disorders have been described in Chapter 6 and can be grouped according to clinical presentation— whether they most closely resemble the syndrome of bulbar palsy, progressive muscular atrophy, or primary lateral sclerosis. Tables 7–2, 7–3, and 7–4 summarize the EMG results considered characteristic or pathognomonic of these different disorders.

NEUROIMAGING STUDIES

Even when the EMG results strongly support a diagnosis of ALS, it is our practice to seek assurance that no structural abnormali-

Table 7–2. **ELECTROMYOGRAPHIC TESTS USED IN THE DIFFERENTIAL DIAGNOSIS OF BULBAR PALSY**

Differential Diagnosis	Electromyographic Test	Results
Myasthenia gravis	Repetitive nerve stimulation	Decremental response
	Single-fiber study	Increased jitter
Inflammatory myopathy	Needle electromyography	Fibrillation potentials, myopathic motor units, early recruitment

Table 7–3. **ELECTROMYGORAPHIC TESTS USED IN THE DIFFERENTIAL DIAGNOSIS OF PROGRESSIVE MUSCULAR ATROPHY**

Differential Diagnosis	Electromyographic Test	Results
Lambert-Eaton myasthenic syndrome	Stimulation after brief isometric contraction	Postactivation facilitation
	Single-fiber study	Increased jitter
Inclusion body myositis	Needle electromyography	Mixed neurogenic and myopathic features
Motor mononeuropathy	Motor and sensory nerve conduction	Slowed conduction velocity, focal conduction block, prolonged distal latency
	Needle electromyography	Highly focal acute and chronic neurogenic features
Multifocal motor neuropathy	Motor nerve conduction	Conduction block
Brachial or lumbosacral plexopathy	Sensory nerve conduction	Reduced sensory potentials
	Needle electromyography	Restricted distribution of acute and chronic neurogenic features
Diabetic polyradiculopathy	Nerve conduction studies	Features of a sensorimotor polyneuropathy
	Needle electromyography	Acute and chronic neurogenic features, predominantly in lumbosacral segments
Bulbospinal neuronopathy	Sensory nerve conduction	Reduced or absent sensory responses
Hexosaminadase-A-deficiency motor neuronopathy	Sensory nerve conduction	Reduced sensory responses
	Needle electromyography	Complex repetitive discharges

Table 7–4. **ELECTROMYOGRAPHIC TESTS USED IN THE DIFFERENTIAL DIAGNOSIS OF PRIMARY LATERAL SCLEROSIS**

Differential Diagnosis	Electromyographic Test	Results
Spondylotic myelopathy	Needle electromyography	Acute and chronic neurogenic features in the cervical segments, with sparing of lumbosacral segments
Syringomyelia	Needle electromyography	Acute and chronic neurogenic features in the cervical segments, with sparing of lumbosacral segments
Adrenoleukodystrophy	Motor and sensory nerve conduction	Features of a polyneuropathy

ty exists that might even remotely explain a combination of upper and lower motor neuron findings. Therefore, despite clinical features of ALS and confirmatory EMG evidence of involvement of the lower motor neurons, we proceed with imaging studies (usually MRI) of that portion of the CNS implicated by the physical examination and EMG evaluation to affirm the anatomic integrity of the brain stem and cervical spinal cord. Neuroimaging is especially important in patients presenting with features of a motor neuron disease subtype but without all the classic signs of ALS per se (Table 7–5). For example, in patients presenting with bulbar palsy, the brain MRI scan is critical in identifying possible multiple sclerosis, brain-stem glioma, or brain-stem vascular disease. For patients with progressive muscular atrophy, an MRI scan of the brain and spinal cord may provide a clue to pathology involving multiple nerve roots, such as neoplastic polyradiculopathy; and in a patient with features of primary lateral sclerosis, the MRI may have an important role in supporting the diagnosis of myelopathies caused by spondylosis or retroviral infection. In ALS or other motor neuron disease subtypes, MRI scans of the brain and spinal cord should be normal or show only mild abnormalities without definite evidence of brain-stem, spinal cord, or nerve root pathology (see Chapter 8).

CLINICAL LABORATORY STUDIES

We then turn to the clinical laboratory for a variety of studies. We use laboratory studies for two major reasons. Because ALS is not known to be mediated by conventional or well-established infectious, inflammatory, immunologic, toxic, or metabolic mechanisms, we expect clinical laboratory studies to be normal. Indeed, by definition, *normal results* from a variety of tests *support* the diagnosis of ALS.[2] Second, in the few weeks after initially examining a patient we suspect may have ALS, we strive to find an alternate diagnosis, using our clinical judgment and experience to identify laboratory abnormalities that might explain upper or lower motor neuron findings, or both. This approach forces us to cast a wide net and use various laboratory tests as we ascertain the overall health of our patients and search for treatable conditions (Table 7–6).

Table 7–5. **NEUROIMAGING PERFORMED FOR DIFFERENTIAL DIAGNOSIS IN PATIENTS PRESENTING WITH MOTOR NEURON DISEASE ALS SUBTYPES**

Clinical Presentation	Diagnostic Consideration	MRI Findings
Bulbar palsy	Foramen magnum tumor	Mass lesion at craniocervical junction
Bulbar palsy	Multiple sclerosis	Abnormal T2 brightening in periventricular white matter
Bulbar palsy	Brain-stem glioma	Swollen pons with abnormal signal
Bulbar palsy	Brain-stem vascular disease	Lacunar infarction in brain stem
Progressive muscular atrophy	Neoplastic polyradiculopathy	Hydrocephalus, nodular enhancement of ventricles, sulci, and meninges
Primary lateral sclerosis	Spondylotic myelopathy	T2 brightening in spinal cord; spinal stenosis
Primary lateral sclerosis	Retroviral myelopathy	T2 brightening in spinal cord

Table 7–6. **ROUTINE CLINICAL LABORATORY TESTING FOR SUSPECTED ALS**

- Complete blood count, platelet count, Westergren sedimentation rate, prothrombin time, urinalysis
- Electrolytes (Na, K, Cl, CO_2, Ca, Mg, PO_4), glucose, blood urea nitrogen, creatinine, liver function tests
- Serum VDRL
- Chest roentenogram
- Creatine kinase
- Thyroid studies (T_4, T_3, thyroid-stimulating hormone)
- Assessment of stool for occult blood
- Screening for connective tissue diseases (antinuclear antibody, rheumatoid factor, complement)
- Serum protein electrophoresis, serum immunoelectrophoresis with immunofixation
- Antineural antigen testing (GM1, asialo-GM1)

ALS-Related Syndromes

It is also helpful to consider clinical laboratory evaluation in the context of disorders associated with the various clinical presentations of a motor neuron disease (see Chapter 6). The World Federation of Neurology research group[4] has designated these disorders as ALS-related syndromes. These syndromes "have unique laboratory-defined or epidemiologically defined features which are time-linked to the development of the ALS phenotype."[4] They include ALS-related syndromes associated with paraproteinemia, anti-GM$_1$ antibodies, lymphoma, endocrinopathies, infections, toxins, ischemia, and cervical spondylosis.

Paraproteinemia-associated motor neuropathy presents as a progressive muscular atrophy; the key laboratory abnormality is a monoclonal gammopathy. The motor neuron disorder associated with anti-GM1 antibodies may present as either progressive muscular atrophy or ALS and is characterized by highly elevated titers of anti-GM1 antibodies. Lymphoma-associated motor neuronopathy presents as progressive muscular atrophy and is marked by abnormalities including lymphadenopathy (noted on chest roentgenogram); monoclonal gammopathy (detected by serum immunoelectrophoresis with immunofixation); increased cerebrospinal fluid (CSF) protein, oligoclonal bands, or both; and an abnormal bone marrow biopsy. Endocrinopathy-associated motor neuron disease may present as progressive muscular atrophy, progressive bulbar palsy, or ALS. Abnormalities may include a reduced thyroid-stimulating hormone and high T_4 levels consistent with hyperthyroidism, or high serum calcium, low serum phosphate, and high alkaline phosphatase levels consistent with hyperparathyroidism.[13] Motor neuron disease associated with infection may present as either primary lateral sclerosis or ALS and is characterized by CSF pleocytosis and specific serologic abnormalities, such as antiretroviral antibodies, or positive CSF syphilis reactivity (VDRL). Toxin-associated motor neuron disease presents as progressive muscular atrophy and is diagnosed when levels of lead or mercury in serum and urine are also elevated. The clinical and laboratory features of brain-stem ischemia and cervical spondylosis are described in Chapter 6.

If treatment is instituted to correct the laboratory abnormality and clinical improvement occurs, then the designation "ALS-related syndrome" is valid. For example, testing for serum and urine paraproteins and anti-ganglioside antibodies is especially important in the patient with a progressive muscular atrophy presentation because positive results may be markers of an underlying lymphoma, in which motor neuron disease may be a paraneoplastic syndrome,[14] or of immune-mediated motor neuron syndromes,[1] which may be reversible with immunotherapy. On the other hand, if clinical findings persist and worsen despite correction of the laboratory abnormalities, the patient is considered to have sporadic ALS.

In our clinic practice, virtually all patients evaluated for ALS are tested with the many and varied clinical laboratory studies listed in Table 7–6. The more closely the clinical features resemble classic ALS, the less likely we are to carry out additional or specialized laboratory evaluations (Table 7–7). In general, we reserve these tests for the patient whose motor neuron disease clinical presentation is atypical by virtue of age (less than 40 years, older than 70 years), positive family history of a CNS disorder, features of an accompanying systemic disease (neoplastic, infectious, endocrine), or involvement of portions of the nervous system in addition to upper and lower motor neurons.

In the setting of one or more of these atypical features, we are usually willing to perform a lumbar puncture because this test is well tolerated, has virtually no serious morbidity, and can reveal evidence of treatable autoimmune, infectious, inflammatory, neoplastic, and paraneoplastic disorders. (The CSF is usually normal in ALS, although 33% of patients with pathologically confirmed ALS have elevated CSF protein levels [>45 mg/dL];[11] values in excess of 75 mg/dL are

Table 7–7. **INDICATIONS FOR SPECIAL LABORATORY TESTING FOR SUSPECTED ALS**

Test	Indication
CSF examination	Young age of onset (<40 yr)
	Clinical evidence of infectious disease
	Clinical suspicion of meningeal metastases
	Clinical suspicion of multiple sclerosis
	Features of chronic neuropathy
Bone marrow examination	Clinical suspicion of lymphoma
	Monoclonal gammopathy
	Elevated CSF protein
	CSF oligoclonal bands
Anti-Hu antibody measurement	Multiple neural systems involved
	Suspicion of paraneoplastic syndrome
Leukocyte hexosaminidase A assay	Young age of onset (<40 yr)
	Mental changes
	Cramps
	Sensory neuropathy
Test for cytosine-adenine-guanine repeat in androgen receptor gene (X chromosome)	Young age of onset (< 40 yr)
	Gynecomastia
	Sensory neuropathy
	Cerebellar ataxia
Anti-HIV antibody measurement	Risk factors for HIV
Anti-HTLV-1 antibody measurement	Risk factors for tropical spastic paraparesis
Serum very long chain fatty acids	Young age of onset (< 40 yr)
	Polyneuropathy (axon-loss)
	Adrenal insufficiency
Serum parathyroid hormone assay	Serum chemistry profile suggesting hyperparathyroidism

Abbreviations: CSF = cerebrospinal fluid, HIV = human immunodeficiency virus, HTLV-1 = human T-lymphotropic virus type 1.

occasionally encountered.[8,11] Patients with ALS rarely have mild pleocytosis or oligoclonal bands.[11]) The possibility of lymphoma is strengthened by findings of elevated CSF protein and oligoclonal bands;[14] in the setting of these abnormalities, bone marrow biopsy is indicated. In view of the 5% incidence of lymphoma in patients with motor neuron disease, and the 50% chance of improvement with treatment of the lymphoma, bone marrow examination has been recommended for all patients with ALS.[12] We reserve anti-Hu antibody testing for those patients in whom the clinical presentation is associated with some other neurologic abnormality (such as change in mentation, sensory signs, or cerebellar abnormalities), because the anti-Hu antibody is more accurately regarded as a marker for diffuse encephalomyelitis, rather than for a selective disorder of motor neurons.[5] Serum parathyroid hormone is measured only if electrolyte concentrations suggest hyperparathyroidism (hypercalcemia, hypophosphatemia).[12] Leukocyte hexosaminadase A is measured in patients with earlier onset, slowly progressive ALS, or progressive muscular atrophy.[9] Genetic testing for bulbospinal muscular atrophy is undertaken in younger men presenting with bulbar palsy or progressive muscular atrophy phenotypes with slow progression.[3] Evidence of human T-lymphotropic virus type 1 infection is sought in patients with

a slowly progressive primary lateral sclerosis.[6] Last, evidence of adrenoleukodystrophy should be sought in younger men with a chronic primary lateral sclerosis, especially if a mild peripheral neuropathy exists.[7,10]

Influence of Clinical Presentation on Test Selection

Although most patients undergo the same battery of routine diagnostic studies irrespective of presenting motor neuron disease features (see Table 7–6), our choice of tests is influenced by the patient's specific clinical presentation. For example, bulbar palsy triggers a search for myasthenia gravis, inflammatory myopathy, and possibly bulbospinal neuronopathy (Table 7–8). Patients presenting with progressive muscular atrophy are likely to undergo tests for disorders that include diabetes, myopathy, metal toxicity, paraproteinemia, and lymphoma (Table 7–9). A primary lateral sclerosis presentation is likely to prompt measurements of vitamin B_{12} and thyroid function, and indirect tests of parathyroid function (Table 7–10).

ROLE OF MUSCLE BIOPSY

In the investigation of ALS, the muscle biopsy has diminished in importance in the

Table 7–8. CLINICAL LABORATORY TESTING FOR DIFFERENTIAL DIAGNOSIS OF BULBAR PALSY

Differential Diagnosis	Clinical Laboratory Tests	Results
Myasthenia gravis	Anti-acetylcholine receptor antibody assay	Positive
Inflammatory myopathy	Serum creatine kinase	Elevated (nl, 0.17–1.5 μkat/L [10–90 U/L])*
Bulbospinal neuronopathy	Serum creatine kinase	Elevated (nl, 0.17–1.5 μkat/L [10–90 U/L])*
	Assay for expanded cytosine-adenine-guanine repeat on X chromosome	Positive
Multiple sclerosis	Cerebrospinal fluid examination	Increased IgG (nl, 0.01–0.014 g/L [1–1.4 mg/dL]); oligoclonal bands present (nl, absent)

*SI units (Système International d'Unités) appear first; traditional units appear after SI units.
Abbreviation: nl = normal.

Table 7–9. **PROGRESSIVE MUSCULAR ATROPHY PHENOTYPE—CLINICAL LABORATORY TESTING BASED ON DIFFERENTIAL DIAGNOSIS**

Differential Diagnosis	Clinical Laboratory Tests	Results
Myopathy	Serum creatine kinase	Elevated (nl, 0.17–1.5 μkat/L [10–90 U/L])*
Multifocal motor neuropathy	ELISA for anti-GM1 ganglioside antibody	Positive and elevated (>1:3200)
Paraproteinemic motor neuropathy	Serum immunoelectrophoresis with immunofixation	Monoclonal gammopathy
Vasculitic mononeuritis multiplex	Westergren sedimentation rate	Elevated (nl, 1–7 mm/h)
	Antinuclear antibody	Positive
	Antineutrophil cytoplasmic antibodies	Positive (rising titers)
	C3	Reduced (nl, 0.55–1.2 g/L [55–120 mg/dL])*
Toxic motor neuropathy	Screen for heavy metals	Increased serum lead level (nl, <1.0 μmol/L [<20 μg/dL],* and increased blood zinc protoporphyrin level (nl, <40 μg/mL);† increased blood mercury level (nl, <2 μg/dL),† increased urine levels (nl, <10 μg/L)†
Diabetic polyradiculoneuropathy	Fasting and 2-h post-prandial glucose	Elevated (nl, 4.2–6.4 mmol/L [75–115 mg/dL]; nl, <7.8 mmol/L [<140 mg/dL], respectively)*
	Glycosylated hemoglobin (HgB A$_1$C)	Elevated (nl, 4%–7%)
Infectious polyradiculopathy	Serum antibodies vs. *Borrelia burgdorferi*	Positive
	Serum and cerebrospinal fluid VDRL titer	Positive
	Anti-human immunodeficiency virus antibodies	Positive
	Cerebrospinal fluid examination	Elevated protein (nl, 0.2–0.5 g/L [20–50 mg/dL])*
		Pleocytosis (nl, <5 WBC/mm^3)
Bulbospinal neuronopathy	Serum creatine kinase	Elevated (nl, 0.17–1.5 μkat/L [10–90 U/L])*
	Assay for expanded cytosine-adenine-guanine repeat on X chromosome	Positive
Hexosaminidase A deficiency neuronopathy	Hexosaminadase A leukocyte assay	Reduced

*SI units (Système International d'Unités) appear first; traditional units appear after SI units.
†Only traditional units noted.
Abbreviations: ELISA = enzyme-linked immunosorbent assay, nl = normal, WBC = white blood cells.

Table 7–10. **CLINICAL LABORATORY TESTING FOR DIFFERENTIAL DIAGNOSIS OF PRIMARY LATERAL SCLEROSIS**

Differential Diagnosis	Clinical Laboratory Tests	Results
Subacute combined degeneration	Serum vitamin B_{12}	Reduced (nl, 148–443 pmol/L [200–600 pg/mL])*
Multiple sclerosis	Cerebrospinal fluid examination	Increased IgG (nl, 0.01–0.014 g/L [1–1.4 mg/dL]); oligoclonal bands present (nl, absent)
Hyperthyroid myelopathy	Thyroid-stimulating hormone	Reduced (nl, 0.4–5 mU/L [0.4–5 μU/mL])*
Hyperparathyroid myelopathy	Plasma calcium	Increased (nl, 2.2–2.6 mmol/L [9–10.5 mg/dL])
	Serum phosphorus	Decreased (nl, 1.0–1.4 mmol/L [3–4.5 mg/dL])*
	Parathyroid hormone	Increased (nl, 210–310 pg/mL)†
Paraneoplastic encephalomyelitis	Anti-Hu antibodies	Positive
Retroviral myelitides	Serum viral antibodies (HIV, HTLV-1)	Positive
	Cerebrospinal fluid examination	Elevated protein (nl, 0.2–0.5 g/L [20–50 mg/dL]);* pleocytosis (nl, <5 WBC/mm^3)
Adenoleukodystrophy	Serum very long chain fatty acids	Increased

*SI units (Système International d'Unités) appear first; traditional units appear after SI units.
†Only traditional units noted.
Abbreviations: HIV = human immunodeficiency virus, HTLV-1 = human T-lymphotropic virus type 1, WBC = white blood cells.

last 10 to 20 years as noninvasive electrodiagnostic, neuroimaging, and clinical laboratory studies have evolved into highly sensitive diagnostic tools. Nonetheless, over the last three decades, neurologists have gained a wealth of experience in interpreting muscle biopsy specimens from ALS patients, and we have developed a clear picture of the histologic features expected in ALS. In the early stages of the disease, disseminated, small, angulated atrophic fibers of both type I and type II indicate denervation (Fig. 7–1). Typically, these fibers react intensely (staining dark) with the oxidative enzyme reaction (reduced nicotine adenine dinucleotide tetrazolium reductase, also designated NADH dehydrogenase). Fiber-type grouping, in which a normal mosaic pattern of type I and II fibers is replaced by separate groups of normally sized type I or type II fibers, indicates compensatory reinnervation. In the later stages of the disease, small-group atrophy (small groups of atrophic fibers of the same type scattered throughout the biopsy specimen) indicates continuing denervation after reinnervation. Another sign of denervation followed by reinnervation is the target fiber (Fig. 7–2). This fiber stains with NADH dehydrogenase in a three-zone fashion: a lightly staining central region, a darkly staining intermediate zone, and a normally staining periphery. Longstanding denervation is suggested by clumps of pyknotic nuclei (groups of atrophic fibers that have almost disappeared, leaving residual nuclei). On occasion, in patients whose course is slowly progressive, secondary myopathic changes occur, including muscle fiber hypertrophy, fiber splitting, fiber degeneration and regeneration, inflammatory infiltrates, and endomysial fibrosis.

Although today the muscle biopsy is used infrequently to provide morphologic evidence in support of an ALS diagnosis, occasionally some combination of clinical findings, EMG features, and clinical laboratory studies leads us to question whether a myo-

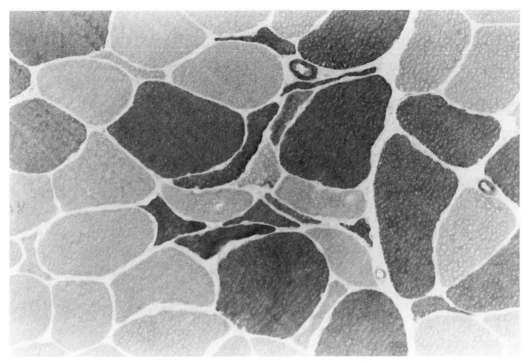

Figure 7–1. Muscle biopsy showing early denervation. There are small groups of angulated, atrophic muscle fibers of both histochemical types. Type II fibers are darkly staining, and type I fibers are lightly staining. ATPase (pH 9.4) ×215 (before reduction). (Courtesy of TW Smith, MD, University of Massachusetts Medial Center.)

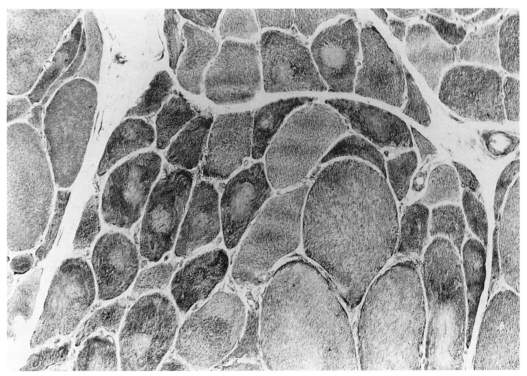

Figure 7–2. Muscle biopsy showing chronic denervation and reinnervation. There are small, angulated, darkly staining muscle fibers, many of which contain small targets. Scattered hypertrophic muscle fibers are also present. NADH-TR ×215 (before reduction). (Courtesy of TW Smith, MD, University of Massachusetts Medical Center.)

131

Table 7–11. **CLINICAL AND LABORATORY FEATURES THAT PROMPT A MUSCLE BIOPSY IN THE DIAGNOSIS OF ALS**

- Muscle weakness with few or no fasciculations.
- No upper motor neuron signs.
- Elevated creatine kinase level (nl, 0.17–1.5 μkat/L [10–90 U/L]).*
- Electromyography discloses myopathic features or myotonic discharges.
- Family history is positive for, or raises the possibility of, a myopathy.
- Patient is younger than expected (<40 yr) for the diagnosis of ALS.
- Patient has exercise-induced muscle cramping.

*SI units (Système International d'Unités) appear first; traditional units appear after SI units.
Abbreviation: nl = normal.

pathic disorder might be presenting as ALS, especially if the presentation is progressive muscular atrophy (Table 7–11). In such an instance, we perform a muscle biopsy to provide histologic evidence for a specific myopathy (Table 7–12). To enhance the possibility of correctly identifying the muscle pathology, the muscle chosen should be moderately weak (graded 4 on the Medical Research Council scale), but not paralyzed or severely weakened, because in minimally functioning muscles, muscle fibers may be replaced by fat and connective tissue, and the biopsy specimen may therefore retain few if any diagnostic features.

SUMMARY

When evaluating a patient with features of motor neuron disease, our main goal is ac-

curate diagnosis. We must confirm a strong index of suspicion for the diagnosis of ALS with characteristic EMG findings, normal neuroimaging studies, and normal clinical laboratory tests.

The diagnosis of ALS is a multistep process that begins with history taking and physical examination. After this key first step, experienced clinicians are usually able to classify the patient's motor neuron disease features as ALS, bulbar palsy, progressive muscular atrophy, or primary lateral sclerosis. The second step involves EMG examination to confirm lower motor neuron degeneration in clinically involved areas and to identify lower motor neuron degeneration in clinically uninvolved regions (and to exclude other neuropathic disorders simulating motor neuron disease). The third step requires neuroimaging studies to exclude disease processes that disturb normal structure and function of the

Table 7–12. **DIAGNOSTIC IMPLICATIONS OF HISTOLOGIC FINDINGS OF MUSCLE BIOPSY FOR ALS**

Histologic Feature	Diagnostic Implication
Lymphocytic infiltration (inflammation) (perivascular and endomysial)	Inflammatory myopathy
Inflammation plus vacuolated fibers (rimmed vacuoles)	Inclusion body myositis
Muscle fiber necrosis and regeneration; no inflammation	Toxic myopathy
Rimmed vacuoles in angulated fibers; no inflammation	Oculopharyngeal dystrophy
Excess of internalized nuclei; ring fibers	Myotonic dystrophy
Rod bodies in atrophic fibers	Nemaline myopathy (adult onset)
Vacuolated muscle fibers	Metabolic myopathy (e.g., acid maltase deficiency, carnitine deficiency)

nervous system and that might provide an alternate explanation for the motor findings. The fourth step is clinical laboratory testing. The variety and breadth of our testing is determined by two factors: the clinical signs and symptoms of the motor neuron disease and the extent to which the clinical features are atypical for ALS.

We perform routine laboratory testing on virtually all patients, searching for some clue to a systemic disorder like neoplasia, infection, vasculitis, endocrinopathy, or autoimmune diathesis that might conceivably explain the abnormal motor findings and be treatable. These tests assess hematologic status, erythrocyte sedimentation rate, renal and liver function, and endocrine function, and evaluate for autoimmune disorders and for abnormal serum immunoglobulin profiles. The choice of certain tests may be influenced by the presenting features of the motor neuron disease. When presentations are atypical, we perform additional tests, usually including CSF examination, sometimes muscle biopsy, and often genetic, metabolic, and immunologic tests to detect a condition masquerading as ALS.

REFERENCES

1. Apostolski, S and Latov, N: Clinical syndromes associated with anti-GM$_1$ antibodies. Semin Neurol 13:264–268, 1993.
2. Bradley, WG: Amyotrophic lateral sclerosis: The diagnostic process. In Mitsumoto, H and Norris, FH (eds): Amyotrophic Lateral Sclerosis. A Comprehensive Guide to Management. Demos, New York, 1994, pp 21–28.
3. Brown, RH: Inherited motor neuron diseases: Recent progress. Semin Neurol 13:365–368, 1993.
4. Brooks, BR: El Escorial World Federation of Neurology criteria for the diagnosis of amyotrophic lateral sclerosis. J Neurol Sci 124(suppl):96–107, 1994.
5. Dalmau, J, Graus, F, Rosenblum, MK, et al: Anti-Hu-associated paraneoplastic encephalomyelitis/sensory neuronopathy. A clinical study of 71 patients. Medicine 71:59–72, 1992.
6. Gessain, A and Gout, O: Chronic myelopathy associated with human T-lymphotropic virus type I (HTLV-I). Ann Intern Med 117:933–946, 1992.
7. Griffin, JW, Goren, E, Schaumberg, H, et al: Adrenomyeloneuropathy: A probable variant of adrenoleukodystrophy. Neurology 27:1107–1113, 1977.
8. Guiloff, RJ, McGregory, B, Thompson, E, et al: Motor neurone disease with elevated cerebrospinal fluid protein. J Neurol Neurosurg Psychiatry 43:390–396, 1980.
9. Mitsumoto, H., Sliman, RJ, Schafer, IA, et al: Motor neuron disease in adult hexosaminidase A deficiency in two families; Evidence for multisystem degeneration. Ann Neurol 17:378–385, 1985.
10. Moser, HM, Moser, AB, Frayer, KF, et al: Adrenoleukodystrophy: Increased plasma content of saturated very long chain fatty acids. Neurology 31:1241–1249, 1981.
11. Norris, FH, Burns, W, U, KS, et al: Spinal fluid cells and protein in amyotrophic lateral sclerosis. Arch Neurol 50:489–491, 1993.
12. Rowland, LP, Sherman, MD, Latov, N, et al: Amyotrophic lateral sclerosis and lymphoma: Bone marrow examination and other diagnostic tests. Neurology 42: 1101–1102, 1992.
13. Tonner, DR and Schlechte, JA: Neurologic complications of thyroid and parathyroid disease. Med Clin North Am 77:251–263, 1993.
14. Younger, DS, Rowland, LP, Latov, N, et al: Lymphoma, motor neuron diseases, and amyotrophic lateral sclerosis. Ann Neurol 29:78–86, 1991.

CHAPTER 8

NEUROIMAGING

modalities in studying patients suspected of having ALS are included in a policy statement by the World Federation of Neurology in their El Escorial criteria for the diagnosis of amyotrophic lateral sclerosis.[17] The statement outlines specific findings required for the diagnosis of ALS and those that are inconsistent with it (Tables 8–1 and 8–2).

Anatomic changes in the brains and spinal cords of patients with ALS that probably represent neurodegeneration can be identified by CT, and particularly by MRI, because of their ability to reveal parenchymal detail. Some of these neuroimaging changes, such as increased signal along the corticospinal tract on T2-weighted and proton density MRI (see below), are relatively specific for ALS.

Denervation in skeletal muscles of patients with ALS has also been detected by CT.[38] MRI of tongue musculature in patients with ALS has been reported to have characteristic

The major use of neuroimaging in evaluating patients with suspected ALS has been to identify conditions that produce upper motor neuron and lower motor neuron signs mimicking this motor neuron disease. A variety of imaging modalities are available. Of these, the most clinically useful are CT, including postmyelography CT, and MRI. They are now more frequently the first line of neuroimaging techniques used to study suspected ALS, having supplanted the older techniques of plain film x-ray, spinal myelography, and angiography, although the latter two are still used in certain circumstances. The appropriate uses of these neuroimaging

Table 8–1. NEUROIMAGING FEATURES THAT *SUPPORT* THE DIAGNOSIS OF ALS

- Minimal or no bony abnormalities of the skull or spinal canal evident on **plain x-rays.**
- Minimal or no abnormalities on **MRI** of the head or spinal cord without compression of spinal cord or nerve roots.
- Minimal or no abnormalities on **myelography** of the spinal cord with postmyelography CT showing no spinal cord or root compression.

Source: From El Escorial World Federation of Neurology criteria for the diagnosis of amyotrophic lateral sclerosis. J Neurol Sci 124(suppl):96–107, 1994, with permission.

Table 8–2. **NEUROIMAGING FEATURES *INCONSISTENT* WITH THE DIAGNOSIS OF ALS**

- Significant bony abnormalities evident on **plain x-rays** of the skull or spinal canal that might explain the clinical findings
- Significant abnormalities of the head or spinal cord evident on **MRI,** suggesting intraparenchymal processes or arteriovenous malformations; compression of the brain stem, cranial nerves, spinal cord, or spinal nerve roots by bony abnormalities, tumors, etc.
- Significant abnormalities of the spinal cord evident on **myelography** with or without **CT** or on CT alone, suggesting the lesions noted above
- Significant abnormalities of the spinal cord evident on **angiography,** suggesting arteriovenous malformations

Source: From El Escorial World Federation of Neurology criteria for the diagnosis of amyotrophic lateral sclerosis. J Neurol Sci 124(suppl):96–107, 1994, with permission.

changes in size, shape, position, and internal structure that are more severe than would be suspected clinically.[11] These findings are discussed further in Chapter 23 in relation to speech dysfunction.

Special neuroimaging techniques that have been used to study brain abnormalities in patients with ALS include positron-emission tomography (PET) and single-photon-emission computed tomography (SPECT), which provide metabolic information, and proton magnetic resonance spectroscopy (^{1}H-MRS), a modification of MRI that allows in vivo measurement of certain neurochemicals. Although studies with these modalities in ALS have been limited, they have provided novel information and may become useful in the clinical workup of such patients. In the future, the statement by the World Federation of Neurology in their El Escorial criteria for the diagnosis of amyotrophic lateral sclerosis[17] that "there are no neuroimaging tests which confirm the diagnosis of ALS" may then require revision.

In this chapter, we discuss the roles of common neuroimaging modalities, including myelography, CT, and MRI, in the investigation of patients with ALS. These modalities are used primarily to identify diseases that cause ALS-like symptoms and signs. However, MRI can reveal abnormalities that support the diagnosis of ALS. We also highlight some important findings from ALS research using the nuclear medicine techniques of PET and SPECT, as well as ^{1}H-MRS.

NEUROIMAGING AND CONDITIONS RESEMBLING ALS

Several radiologically identifiable lesions can produce symptoms and signs that are virtually indistinguishable from the various forms of ALS. Many are discussed in Chapters 4, 6, and 7, and others are listed in Table 8–3.

The spinal cord is frequently the site of such lesions, which can be compressive,[45] demyelinating, ischemic, or inflammatory (Table 8–4). Spondylotic stenosis of the cervical spinal cord frequently causes deficits resembling ALS by producing myelopathy alone or in combination with radiculopathy (Fig. 8–1). Similar clinical presentations can result from spinal cord compression due to either intradural or extradural tumors (Fig. 8–2). In the absence of neck or limb pain, these lesions may elude diagnosis until neuroimaging is performed. Lesions within the spinal cord (e.g., syringomyelia) can result in muscle weakness and atrophy at the level of the lesion and spasticity below it (Fig. 8–3). Other regions in the CNS where lesions can produce ALS-like clinical findings include the junction of the brain stem and spinal cord (the craniocervical or cervcomedullary junction)[41] (Fig. 8–4), the lower brain stem (the pons and medulla) (Fig. 8–5), and the cerebral hemispheres (the parasagittal cortex or multifocally in the subcortical white matter) (Fig. 8–6) (Table 8–5).

The prompt identification of treatable

Table 8–3. **RADIOLOGICALLY IDENTIFIABLE LESIONS PRODUCING ALS-LIKE CONDITIONS**

Lesion	Type of ALS
Multiple-level radiculopathies (cervical, lumbosacral, or both) (e.g., spondylosis, carcinomatous meningitis)	Generalized ALS (LMN-predominant)
Radiculomyelopathy (e.g., intradural and extradural spinal cord tumors)	
Syringomyelia	
Cervical myelopathy	Generalized ALS (UMN-predominant)
Multiple sclerosis	Generalized ALS (UMN-predominant) ± bulbar involvement
Craniocervical junction (e.g., foramen magnum lesion, syringobulbia, syringomyelia, Chiari malformation)	Bulbar-onset ALS
Parasagittal intracranial lesions (e.g., meningioma, vascular malformation)	Lower-extremity onset

Abbreviations: LMN = lower motor neuron, UMN = upper motor neuron.

causes is essential. However, the presence of a condition causing ALS-like symptoms does not exclude the coexistence of true ALS. This is particularly true for cervical spondylotic radiculomyelopathy, which, like ALS, tends to occur more frequently with increasing age. The co-occurrence of both conditions in an elderly individual, therefore, would not be uncommon.[41] A general approach to the routine neuroimaging investi-

Table 8–4. **SPINAL CORD LESIONS PRODUCING AN ALS-LIKE CONDITION: LIKELIHOOD OF DETECTION BY IMAGING MODALITIES**

Spinal Cord Lesion	MODALITY		
	X-ray Myelography	CT (with or without Myelography)	MRI
Adrenomyeloneuropathy	—	—	+
Foramen magnum lesion	±	+	+
Infectious conditions*			
HIV-associated myelopathy	—	—	+
HTLV-1–associated myelopathy	—	—	+
Syphilitic meningitis	—	±	+
Multiple sclerosis	—	—	+
SCD of the spinal cord	—	—	+
Spondylotic myelopathy	+	+	+
Syringomyelia	±	+	+
Tumor (intradural or extradural)	+	+	+
Vascular anomaly	±	±	+[†]

*Abnormality may be seen better after metrizamide (CT) or gadolinium (MRI) enhancement.
[†]MR angiography or arterial angiography may detect some vascular anomalies better than MRI.
Abbreviations: + = detected, ± = possibly detected, — = not detected, HIV = human immunodeficiency virus, HTLV-1 = human T-lymphotropic virus type 1, SCD = subacute combined degeneration.

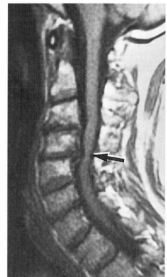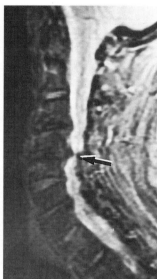

Figure 8–1. Cervical spinal cord compression is seen predominantly at the C3-4 and C4-5 intervertebral levels (arrows) on T1-weighted (*Left*) and T2-weighted (*Right*) MRI in a 55-year-old man. This patient's clinical features of proximal arm weakness and muscle atrophy as well as spasticity of legs and distal arm muscles resembled classic ALS until MRI revealed spondylomyeloradiculopathy.

gation of patients with suspected ALS was presented in Chapter 7. A discussion of potentially treatable conditions that should be included in the differential diagnosis of ALS can be found in Chapter 6.

CENTRAL NERVOUS SYSTEM ATROPHY IN ALS

Cerebral Atrophy

Varying degrees of cortical atrophy have been described in postmortem studies of the brains of ALS patients,[7,39] but only a few neuroimaging studies have systematically compared the frequency of cerebral atrophy in ALS patients with age-matched controls. An early CT study comparing the brains of 50 patients with various forms of ALS and 50 control subjects with unrelated neurologic problems revealed cortical atrophy in 64% of individuals with ALS and in only 12% of controls.[57] Of the 35 patients with classic ALS or bulbar ALS, approximately 75% had cortical atrophy; it was seen in 44% of those with upper motor neuron–predominant ALS ($n = 9$) but in 16% of those with lower motor neuron–predominant ALS ($n = 6$). Men were twice as likely as women to develop cortical atrophy. This observation may in part be due to the higher number of male patients in this study ($n = 34$) because the mean age was similar in both groups (approximately 57 years). The atrophy was usually bilateral, multifocal, and mild to moderate in degree but did not

Table 8–5. **BRAIN LESIONS PRODUCING AN ALS-LIKE CONDITION: LIKELIHOOD OF DETECTION BY IMAGING MODALITIES**

	MODALITY		
Brain Lesion	**CT (with or without contrast)**	**MRI**	**Angiogram**
Intracranial tumor (e.g., parasagittal meningioma)	+	+	±
Multiple sclerosis	±	+	—
Vascular anomaly (e.g., AVM)	±	+*	±

*MR angiography may detect some vascular anomalies better than MRI.
   Abbreviations: + = detected, ± = possibly detected, — = not detected, AVM = arteriovenous malformation.

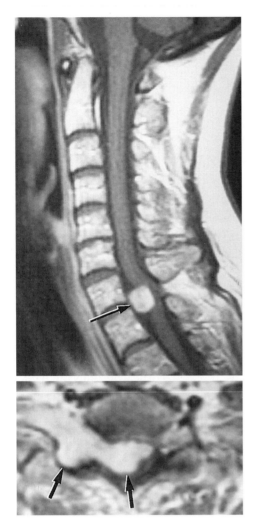

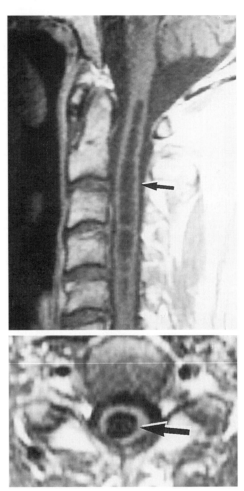

Figure 8–2. Atrophy and weakness of intrinsic hand muscles unilaterally and progressive leg spasticity in a 65-year-old man is found to result from a gadolinium-enhancing tumor compressing the spinal cord at the C7–C8 level, as seen by sagittal T1-weighted MRI (arrow at top). A transverse view at this level reveals a "dumbbell-shaped" intradural neurinoma of the nerve root invading the spinal canal (arrows at bottom) to severely compress the spinal cord.

Figure 8–3. Syringomyelia of the cervical spinal cord (arrows) in a 49-year-old woman, revealed with T1-weighted MRI in the sagittal (*Top*) and coronal (*Bottom*) planes. This patient had weakness and atrophy of intrinsic hand muscles initially thought to represent lower motor neuron–predominant ALS.

correlate with the duration of disease. The parietal cortex was predominantly affected (50%), followed by the insular (38%), frontal (32%), and temporal (20%) cortices. These regions contribute in varying degrees to the corticospinal tract.[59]

In another study, CT and MRI were performed annually to document the progression of cerebral atrophy in relation to the presence of upper and lower motor neuron dysfunction, ophthalmoplegia, dementia, and the need for assisted ventilation.[31] Atrophy appeared first in the frontal and anterior temporal lobes, then in the precentral gyrus, and finally in the postcentral gyrus, cingulate gyrus, and corpus callosum. Although the severity of cerebral atrophy did not correlate with disease duration or severity, atrophy progressed most rapidly in patients with early-onset respiratory failure and with se-

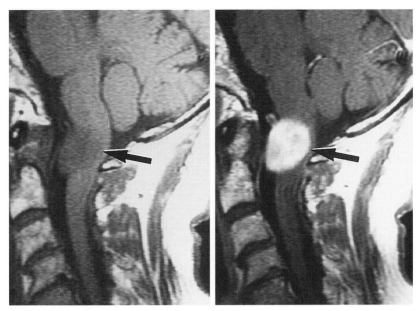

Figure 8–4. A meningioma of the foramen magnum (arrow) in a 63-year-old woman, seen with sagittal MRI before (*Left*) and after (*Right*) gadolinium enhancement, compresses the cervicomedullary junction to produce spasticity and weakness of the arms and legs.

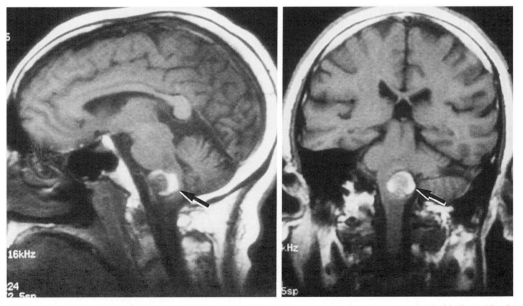

Figure 8–5. Gadolinium-enhanced MRI in sagittal (*Left*) and coronal (*Right*) views shows a spherical lesion with a hyperintense rim (arrows) compressing the medulla in a 55-year-old hypertensive man with progressive dysphagia and dysarthria that resembled bulbar-onset ALS. Arterial angiography confirmed a partially thrombosed aneurysm of the posterior inferior cerebellar artery.

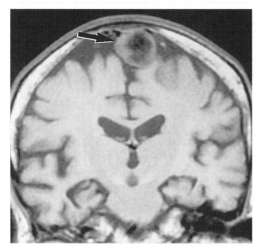

Figure 8–6. A gadolinium-enhancing meningioma arising from the falx cerebri is seen on coronal MRI (arrow) compressing the parasagittal motor cortex of a 60-year-old woman who had progressive leg weakness mimicking ALS.

vere ophthalmoplegia. Those few patients surviving 10 to 20 years without assisted ventilation had virtually no cerebral atrophy.

In contrast, other studies using either CT[19] or MRI[12] found no significant difference in the incidence of brain atrophy between patients with motor neuron disease or typical ALS and age-matched controls.

Spinal Cord Atrophy

Compared to CT, MRI provides much better resolution of images of spinal cord parenchyma,[30,66] and a few studies have described the MRI appearance of the spinal cord in patients with motor neuron disease.[5,10,18,71,72] However, spinal cord atrophy has been rarely reported in motor neuron disease. A 51-year-old woman with bulbar-onset ALS and prominent upper motor neuron signs also had mild atrophy (a flattening of the ventral and lateral aspects) of the cervical spinal cord.[18] The spinal cord atrophy, however, was minor compared to a hyperintensity seen on the T2-weighted MRI in the region of the lateral and ventral corticospinal tracts. Such corticospinal tract hyperintensity has been described primarily intracranially and is discussed below.

Monomelic amyotrophy (benign focal

amyotrophy, juvenile amyotrophy of the distal arms) is a slowly progressive, relatively benign form of focal motor neuron disease. Although differentiation from ALS should be relatively easy over time, monomelic atrophy may resemble the early stages of juvenile-onset ALS. Pathologically, anterior horn cells, usually in the lower cervical spinal cord, degenerate with resulting spinal cord atrophy. MRI has revealed focal atrophy in the lower cervical spinal cord in some patients with this condition.[5] Monomelic amyotrophy is described in Chapter 6.

HYPERINTENSE MAGNETIC RESONANCE SIGNALS IN THE CORTICOSPINAL TRACTS

Any condition resulting in corticospinal tract degeneration will potentially produce a hyperintensity (increased signal) on T2-weighted MRI[13,27,37,49] or hypodensity on CT.[32] Although this finding is not pathognomonic of ALS, its occurrence in the appropriate clinical setting and without other radiologic abnormalities makes the diagnosis very likely.

Hyperintense Intracranial Signals

As MRI is used more frequently to visualize the CNS of patients with ALS, abnormalities not previously detected by CT are being identified. The first MRI report of increased signal intensity in the subcortical white matter of two patients with ALS appeared in 1988.[20] This hyperintensity, seen on T2-weighted MRI, could be traced from beneath the primary motor cortex, through the centrum semiovale, the posterior limb of the internal capsule, and the cerebral peduncles into the pons. Fibers that follow this trajectory comprise the corticospinal (or pyramidal) tract,[24,37,58] which degenerates in the brains of ALS patients[7,64] (see Chapter 11). A combined neuroimaging and pathologic study showed that the hyperintensity corresponded to the demyelination and degeneration of large-caliber corticospinal tract fibers.[77] Degeneration of the large-caliber corticospinal tract fibers in ALS produces hyperintense signals both within the internal capsule and out-

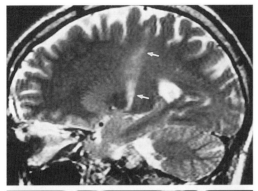

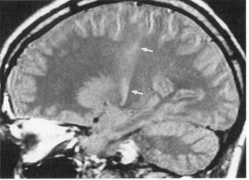

Figure 8–7. Parasagittal T2-weighted (*Top*) and proton density–weighted (*Bottom*) MR brain images of a 35-year-old man with ALS show the infrequently seen signal hyperintensity along the corticospinal tract (arrows).

side it in the subcortical white matter (corona radiata, centrum semiovale) and lower brain stem.[12,26,31,46,60,77]

Several MRI studies have confirmed the occurrence of similar T2-weighted hyperintensities of the corticospinal tract in 17% to 67% (median 40%) of patients with ALS.* One report even noted its occurrence in all of 16 patients with ALS undergoing MRI.[62] This relatively high percentage may be a reflection of the patient population studied, because we have detected such corticospinal tract hyperintensities in only 15% to 20% of the approximately 350 newly diagnosed ALS patients we see yearly. Similar changes have been observed in patients with familial ALS[40] or primary lateral sclerosis (PLS).[44] Figure 8–7 illustrates this abnormal hyperintensity along the pyramidal tracts in a T2-weighted MRI of a patient with ALS.

Compared to ALS patients with no MRI ab-

normalities, those with corticospinal tract hyperintensities on T2-weighted images tended to be more often female,[†] younger,[‡] with prominent upper motor neuron features (e.g., spasticity, hyperreflexia; Babinski reflex),[29,73] and have a shorter duration of disease[12,46,53,73] that may be more rapidly progressive.[12,20] Analysis of pooled data from such studies revealed no statistically significant differences between the two groups for most of these features. However, ALS patients with corticospinal tract hyperintensities were significantly ($p < 0.001$, t test assuming unequal variances) younger (50.7 ± 11.0 years, mean ± SD, $n = 42$) than those without such MRI abnormalities (59.0 ± 10.7 years $n = 74$). Although younger patients with ALS are probably more likely to undergo MRI and therefore more apt to have corticospinal tract hyperintensities identified, they may represent a subgroup with earlier onset ALS. Three of the four (three females, one male) ALS patients in whom we have seen this MRI abnormality were in their thirties and had symptoms for 6 to 8 months before presentation; two were initially thought to have multiple sclerosis because of the predominance of upper motor neuron signs.

A small region of hyperintensity in the posterior limb of the internal capsule detected by T2-weighted MRI has been described in 53% to 76% (median 57%) of normal individuals.[12,49,62,77] It probably represents the aggregated, thickly myelinated, large-diameter axons of the normal corticospinal tract in this location[77] and is not noted outside of the internal capsule. When visible in normal persons, the hyperintensity is relatively faint on T2-weighted images and is not seen on proton-density MRI[12,49,62,77] (Fig. 8–8). For this reason, proton-density-weighted MRI sequences are more specific than T2-weighted sequences in revealing the abnormal hyperintensities in the corticospinal tracts of ALS patients.

Hyperintense Spinal Cord Signals

A hyperintense signal in the corticospinal tract of the spinal cord on a T2-weighted MR

---

*References 1, 12, 29, 31, 46, 53, 60, 73, 77.

[†]References 1, 12, 29, 31, 46, 53, 60, 62, 73.
[‡]References 1, 12, 29, 31, 46, 53, 73.

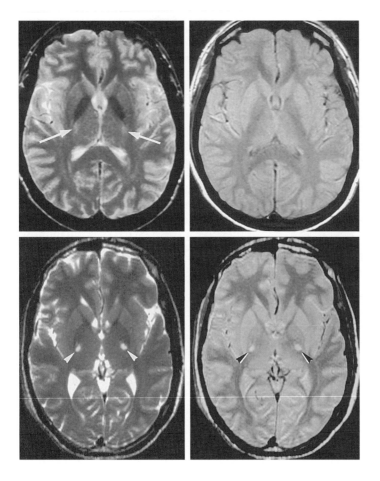

Figure 8–8. Faint hyperintensities in the posterior limb of the internal capsule (arrows) occasionally seen in normal individuals on T2-weighted MRI (*Top Left*) but not on proton density–weighted MRI (*Top Right*) in the transverse plane. This is in contrast to prominent hyperintensities seen here on both T2-weighted (*Bottom Left*) and proton density–weighted (*Bottom Right*) sequences (arrowheads) in the ALS patient of Fig. 8–7.

image has been reported in only six patients with ALS, all of whom also had intracranial hyperintensities.[10,18,60,71,72] The relative infrequency of this change in the spinal cord may represent either a technical limitation of MRI detection or an actual difference in corticospinal tract pathology at this level. As with intracranial corticospinal tract hyperintensities, those in the spinal cord seem to result from axonal degeneration and demyelination.[42,71,72]

HYPOINTENSE MAGNETIC RESONANCE SIGNALS IN THE NEOCORTEX

Another abnormality detected by T2-weighted MRI in the brains of ALS patients, less common than corticospinal tract hyper-intensity, is hypointensity (a diminished signal) of the superficial neocortex, primarily in the precentral gyrus bilaterally.[12,18,28,53] This ribbon-like hypointensity, which has also been reported along the surface of the primary sensory cortex or premotor cortex,[53] is sharply contrasted by the hyperintense signal of cerebrospinal fluid in the adjacent sulci (Fig. 8–9). Neuronal degeneration and the accumulation of a paramagnetic substance is likely the pathologic cause of the diminished T2-weighted signal because postmortem examination of some of these brains has revealed iron-laden astrocytes and macrophages in the precentral cortex.[28,53]

Patients with this MRI abnormality have typical ALS,[28,53] although their clinical progression may be slower than in patients with no cortical hypointensity.[12] Similar neocortical hypointensity has been seen in the pari-

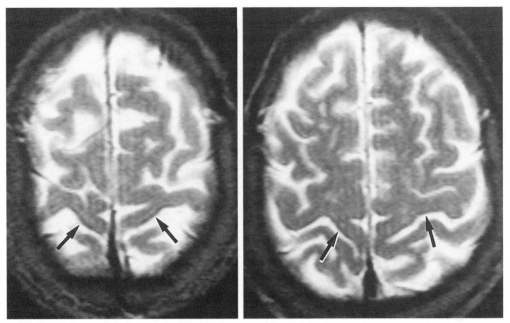

Figure 8–9. The relatively rarely seen thin ribbon-like band of hypointensity (arrows) is noted on T2-weighted MRI along the precentral gyrus (primary motor cortex) at two transverse levels of a 54-year-old man with ALS.

etal cortex of up to 50% of patients with Alzheimer's disease[15,22] and even in patients with nonspecific neurologic complaints.[28] Nevertheless, a diminished signal in the primary motor cortex on T2-weighted MR images of patients presenting with the features of ALS suggests this diagnosis. Some patients with ALS show both cortical hypointensity and corticospinal tract hyperintensity.[12]

BRAIN HYPOMETABOLISM IN ALS

Cerebral blood flow and metabolism can be determined with the nuclear medicine techniques of PET and SPECT. Patients with motor neuron disease, particularly ALS, have abnormal cerebral blood flow, and therefore diminished neuronal metabolism, primarily in sensorimotor regions.* These metabolic abnormalities in the brains of ALS patients have not usually been accompanied by pathology visible on CT or MRI.[14,23,33–35,43]

ALS patients with neuropsychologic evidence of clinical or subclinical dementia have cerebral blood flow abnormalities in extramotor regions that are detected by PET[34,36,42,43,70] and by SPECT.[1,51,54,73,76] Although these techniques have been used only in the research of motor neuron disease, PET or SPECT or both could potentially assist in the clinical diagnosis of ALS, particularly in cases associated with dementia.

Positron-Emission Computed Tomography

The results of PET studies in ALS patients have been inconsistent, in part because of differing techniques but also because of differences in data analysis. Although different radiolabeled isotopes, such as [^{18}F]2-fluoro-2-deoxy-D-glucose (FDG)[21,55] or oxygen 15 gas ([15]O$_2$),[36,70] and oxygen 15–labeled carbon dioxide (C[15]O$_2$), have been used in various studies, this difference in isotopes is not likely responsible for the discrepancies. In addition to measuring patients at rest, studies in which imaging was performed

*References 14, 23, 26, 33–35, 36, 42, 43, 70

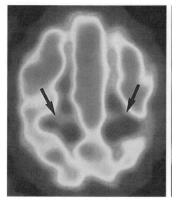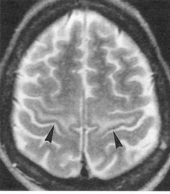

Figure 8–10. Positron emission tomography shows diminished metabolism of [^{18}F]2-fluoro-2-deoxy-D-glucose in the subcortical frontoparietal regions (arrows) from a 55-year-old woman with ALS (*Left*). The equivalent brain level on T2-weighted MRI (*Right*) reveals diffuse hyperintensity in her white matter of the precentral gyrus (primary motor cortex) (arrowheads) at the origin of the corticospinal tract.

while patients performed certain motor functions have provided information on the dynamic state of brain activation in ALS. Figure 8–10 shows diminished FDG uptake in the subcortical region of the primary motor cortex of a patient with ALS who also had corticospinal tract hyperintensity on T2-weighted MRI.

PET STUDIES AT REST

The earliest PET studies at rest revealed a widespread decrease in brain glucose metabolism, especially in the motor-sensory cortex and basal ganglia, when ALS patients were compared to age-matched normal volunteers. Decreased metabolism correlated with the length of disease, the presence of upper motor neuron signs, and the extent of clinical deterioration. Metabolic activity was normal in the cerebellum.[14,23] In contrast, another PET study of patients with ALS showed statistically significant abnormalities only if results were not corrected for multiple comparisons.[25] Significant decreases in metabolism were present in the right precentral gyrus, the bilateral heads of the caudate nucleus, the dentate region of the cerebellum, and the right superior lobule of the cerebellum. Paradoxically, the metabolic rate was increased in the frontal white matter.

PET studies of FDG metabolism in ALS patients with frontal lobe neuropsychologic dysfunction or dementia have revealed statistically significant abnormalities. Compared to normal controls, patients had hypometabolism in the frontal, frontobasal, and superior parieto-occipital cortices, but not in the cerebellum.[43] The abnormalities were

not correlated with the duration or severity of disease. These abnormalities, however, again became statistically nonsignificant when the analysis was adjusted for multiple comparisons. In contrast, another study[42] revealed significant hypometabolism in the frontal (superior and inferior) and temporal (superior and mesial) cortical regions of demented ALS patients when compared to nondemented ALS patients. The reduction remained significant regardless of the method of statistical analysis. This study emphasized that the regional distribution of hypometabolism in ALS patients with dementia is opposite that of patients with Alzheimer's dementia, in which FDG uptake is low in the parietal cortex and relatively normal in the frontal lobes.[42]

PET studies using $^{15}O_2$ and $C^{15}O_2$ have also revealed diminished cerebral blood flow and cerebral metabolic rate of oxygen in ALS patients with progressive dementia. Abnormalities have been most prominent in the bilateral media frontal cortex, the temporal cortex, and the bilateral thalamus.[36,70] Dysfunction of these brain areas was believed to be related to the dementia. Unexpectedly, and of uncertain importance, blood flow, but not oxygen metabolism, was significantly lower in the cerebellum of ALS patients with dementia.[70]

The possibility that ALS may share a common pathogenesis with idiopathic parkinsonism[9] and the finding of diminished 6-fluorodopa uptake in patients with longstanding Guamanian ALS,[65] prompted a 6-fluorodopa PET study in patients with sporadic ALS with no extrapyramidal signs.[67] Compared to age-matched controls, the ALS patients showed a small but progressive fall of striatal 6-fluorodopa uptake, which worsened with longer duration of disease.

PET STUDIES WITH ACTIVATION

PET studies (using $^{15}O_2$ and $C^{15}O_2$) of patients with motor neuron disease performing movements with a joystick after baseline measurements made at rest have revealed unique abnormalities in regional cerebral blood flow and oxygen metabolic rate.[33–35] In addition to confirming reduced cerebral blood flow in several sensorimotor and motor association cortical regions at rest, freely selected joystick movements resulted in marked increases in blood flow to the *ipsilateral* anterior cingulate cortex as well as to the contralateral anterior insula, ventral primary sensorimotor, ventral premotor, and parietal association cortical regions.[35] These findings suggest cortical reorganization and abnormal recruitment of nonprimary motor areas as a result of motor neuron loss. Stereotyped movements in these ALS patients revealed impaired activation in frontal lobe regions, suggesting underlying frontal lobe cognitive deficits, even though none of the patients were clinically demented. Neuropsychologic testing of similar nondemented ALS patients in a related PET study found that those with abnormal self-generated motor tasks had markedly impaired activation in cortical regions not giving rise to the corticospinal tract.[34]

Activation PET studies have uncovered abnormalities in cortical function of five patients with *lower* motor neuron–predominant ALS, even when no abnormalities were detectable at rest.[33] During joystick movement, these patients had significantly ($p < 0.001$) enhanced cerebral blood flow in the anterior insular cortex bilaterally when compared to five unaffected individuals or to six patients with classic ALS. Abnormal activation of this perisylvian area was thought to reflect recruitment of an accessory sensorimotor area in response to limb weakness.[33]

Single-Photon-Emission Computed Tomography

Unlike PET studies, SPECT studies do not measure cerebral blood flow, although values in ALS patients have been expressed relative to cerebellar blood flow,[68,69,75,76] which should remain constant.[14,23] Advantages of SPECT over PET include stable and less expensive radiochemicals and the need for less expensive hardware, which is more accessible and requires less complex technical support. ^{123}I-iodoamphetamine (IMP) and [99mTc]-d,l-hexamethyl-propylene-amine-oxime (HMPAO)[52,75] are two radiochemicals used in SPECT studies of patients with ALS.[1,51,54,61,68,73,76] Because SPECT is being used regularly in many nuclear medicine departments to study patients with various problems, it may become useful in the workup of patients with suspected ALS—for example, in differentiating ALS from other conditions that do not produce cortical abnormalities, such as cervical spondylotic radiculomyelopathy.[1,73]

Regional cerebral hypoperfusion has been detected by SPECT in patients with various forms of ALS, some with dementia. Most[76] but not all[73,76] patients with typical ALS who were not demented had hypoperfusion of motor and premotor areas. All patients with ALS-related dementia had hypoperfusion, particularly in regions anterior and inferior to the primary motor cortex. No SPECT abnormalities were detected in patients with lower motor neuron–predominant ALS, although those with mild or borderline dementia had hypoperfusion of motor and premotor regions.[73,76] A recent SPECT study examining a possible association between classic ALS, ALS with frontotemporal dementia, and dementia alone found statistically significant hypoperfusion in the inferofrontal and temporal areas of all groups, particularly in the patients with dementia.[68] Based on these and the accompanying behavioral findings, the authors suggested that classic ALS, ALS-dementia complex, and frontotemporal dementia comprise a continuum of a common pathology.

NEURONAL DYSFUNCTION AND MAGNETIC RESONANCE SPECTROSCOPY

^{1}H-MRS is a modification of MRI that allows noninvasive assessment of specific chemical pathologies in various tissues in vivo.[4,6] It has been used to measure and mon-

itor the evolution of neuronal-axonal damage in the brains of patients with multiple sclerosis,[3] stroke,[2,8,16] HIV-associated cognitive impairment,[48] Alzheimer's disease,[47] and ALS.[56] In the latter study, no brain abnormalities were seen on MRI.[56]

The most prominent signal in the water-suppressed proton spectra of normal brain is produced by N-acetyl (NA) groups, mainly from N-acetylaspartate (NAA) and less from N-acetylaspartyl glutamate (NAAG). Although their metabolic roles are unclear, these compounds are localized to neurons and their processes[50,63] and are not present in mature glial cells.[74] Thus, the NAA resonance can be used as a marker of neuronal (including axonal and dendritic) integrity. Another prominent signal detected on brain ^{1}H-MRS comes from creatine and phosphocreatine (Cr), compounds involved in energy metabolism that remain stable and are distributed relatively evenly in all cells throughout the brain. A decrease in the resonance intensity of NAA relative to Cr can therefore provide an index of neuronal loss or dysfunction as shown in a patient with ALS (Fig. 8–11).

A ^{1}H-MRS study of patients with various forms of motor neuron disease revealed evidence of neuronal loss or damage in the neo-cortex and subjacent white matter in patients with classic ALS and ALS with prominent lower motor neuron signs but probable upper motor neuron signs (ALS–PUMNS). No abnormalities were detected in the cortex of patients with spinal muscular atrophy (SMA) or in the anterior premotor region of patients with ALS.[56] Compared with healthy controls, the decrease of NAA/Cr ratios was most significant in patients with ALS in the primary motor and sensory cortices, but it was also present in the posterior premotor and superior parietal gyrus–precuneate regions (Fig. 8–12). The fact that the NAA/Cr ratio was normal in all regions measured in SMA patients suggests that the abnormalities reflected a pathologic process specific to the upper motor neuron. NAA/Cr ratios tended to be slightly more abnormal in patients with classic ALS than in those with ALS–PUMNS, again paralleling the more prominent upper motor neuron deficit that occurs in classic ALS.[78] Repeat ^{1}H-MRS of one ALS–PUMNS patient whose clinical condition deteriorated markedly over 8 months showed a further reduction of NAA/Cr values, consistent with progressive neuronal dysfunction or loss. Although used now only for research, in vivo ^{1}H-MRS of specific CNS regions in patients

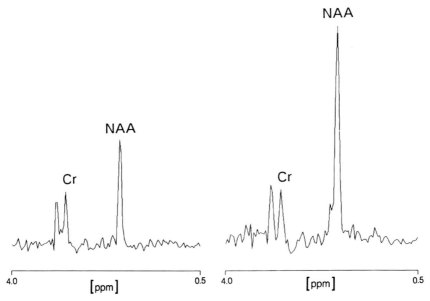

Figure 8–11. Proton MR spectroscopy of the primary motor cortex shows an N-acetylaspartate (NAA) signal that is lower, relative to creatine (Cr), in a patient with upper motor neuron–predominant ALS (*Left*) than in a healthy age-matched volunteer (*Right*). (Adapted from Pioro et al.,[56] p 1935, 1994.)

Figure 8–12. Scatterplot of individual *N*-acetylaspartate/creatine ratios in various cortical regions from patients with classic ALS (*n* = 12) compared to the means from healthy age-matched controls (*n* = 10); bars represent standard errors of means. Statistically significant decreases in the ratios of patients occur in the primary motor and sensory cortices. Significantly low values are also noted in the posterior parietal cortex and in the premotor region posteriorly but not anteriorly. Statistical analysis was by Wilcoxon rank sum test. (Data from Pioro et al.,[56] pp 1933–1938, 1994.)

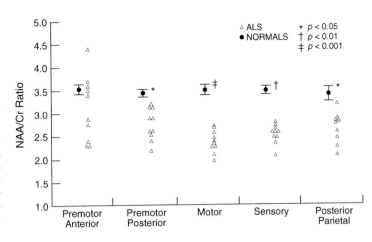

with various forms of ALS may assist in the clinical diagnosis, monitor neuronal degeneration, and even contribute to understanding its pathogenesis.

SUMMARY

Neuroimaging of patients with suspected ALS is performed primarily to exclude diseases that can resemble it. Various pathologies affecting the brain—and particularly the spinal cord—can resemble ALS. The most useful techniques for these investigations are CT, CT myelography, and MRI. Angiography and MR angiography are reserved for investigation of vascular malformations. Radiologic identification of treatable conditions mimicking ALS is essential, although ALS can coexist with other pathologies.

Cortical and spinal cord atrophy have been seen on CT and MRI in some patients with ALS. Cortical atrophy is more frequent in ALS patients than in age-matched controls, although it occurs in a minority of patients. Although the sensorimotor cortex is primarily affected, the severity and distribution of cortical atrophy is not clearly related to the severity or type of neurologic deficit, including dementia. Spinal cord atrophy has been rarely reported in ALS; it is probably more frequent in motor neuron diseases where lower motor neurons are predominantly affected, such as monomelic amyotrophy.

T2-weighted MRI studies have documented that a range of ALS patients have hyper-intense signals along the intracranial course of their corticospinal tracts in the subcortical white matter of the motor cortex, centrum semiovale, corona radiata, posterior limb of the internal capsule, or brain stem. These changes tend to occur in younger female patients who have a shorter duration of disease with prominent upper motor neuron involvement. Similar hyperintensities have been reported in the corticospinal tract of the spinal cord. As in the brain, these hyperintensities are probably caused by demyelination and degeneration of descending axons. A ribbon-like hypointensity of the motor cortex has also been seen on T2-weighted MRI in some ALS patients. It may occur in combination with hyperintensity of the corticospinal tract. Accumulation of iron in astrocytes and macrophages has been suggested as the cause of the cortical hypointensity. Although neither hyperintensity of the corticospinal tract nor cortical hypointensity is pathognomonic of ALS, the presence of either in the appropriate clinical setting and the absence of other radiographic abnormalities make the diagnosis likely.

The nuclear medicine techniques of PET and SPECT have been used in ALS for research rather than assisting in diagnosis. Although results have varied, they have generally revealed hypometabolism in sensorimotor and frontal areas of ALS patients, most consistently in those with upper motor neuron deficits, dementia, or both. These findings have often been made in nondemented ALS patients in whom brain CT and MRI showed no abnormalities. Activation PET studies and some SPECT studies have even revealed abnormalities in cerebral regions of patients who only had lower motor neuron deficits. ^{1}H-MRS is a neuroimaging modality related to MRI that has revealed neuronal dysfunction or loss in sensorimotor areas of patients with classic ALS but not in those with SMA.

As further experience is acquired in the MRI recognition of specific changes in ALS, and as the imaging modalities of PET, SPECT, and ^{1}H-MRS are increasingly applied to studying ALS patients, this disease may be diagnosed more rapidly and with greater assurance.

REFERENCES

1. Abe, K, Fujimura, H, Toyooka, K, et al: Single photon emission computed tomographic investigation of patients with motor neuron disease. Neurology 43:1569–1573, 1993.
2. Arnold, DL, Matthews, PM, Francis, GS, et al: Proton magnetic resonance spectroscopic imaging for metabolic characterization of metabolic plaques. Ann Neurol 31:235–241, 1992.
3. Arnold, DL, Matthews, PM, Tampieri, D, et al: Magnetic resonance imaging and spectroscopy show specific diagnostic abnormalities in the MELAS syndrome [abstract]. Proc Soc Magn Res Med 2:912, 1991.
4. Bachelard, H and Badar-Goffer, R: NMR spectroscopy in neurochemistry. J Neurochem 61:412–429, 1993.
5. Biondi, A, Dormont, D, Weitzner, I Jr, et al: MR imaging of the cervical cord in juvenile amyotrophy of distal upper extremity. AJNR 10:263–268, 1989.
6. Bottomley, PA: Human in vivo NMR spectroscopy in diagnostic medicine: Clinical tool or research probe. Radiology 170:1–15, 1989.
7. Brownell, B, Oppenheimer, DR, and Hughes, JT: The central nervous system in motor neuron disease. J Neurol Neurosurg Psychiatry 33:338–357, 1970.
8. Bruhn, H, Frahm, J, Gyngell, ML, et al: Cerebral metabolism in man after acute stroke: new observations using localized proton NMR spectrosocopy. Magnetic Reson Med 9:126–131, 1989.
9. Calne, DB, Eisen, A, McGeer, E, et al: Alzheimer's disease, Parkinson's disease, and motor neuron disease: Abiotrophic interaction between aging and environment? Lancet 2:1067–1070, 1986.
10. Carvlin, MJ, Fielding, R, Rajan, SS, et al: MR imaging appearance of amyotrophic lateral sclerosis: Results of a high resolution study of spinal cord specimens [abstract]. Radiology 173(P)suppl:84, 1989.
11. Cha, CH and Patten, BM: Amyotrophic lateral sclerosis: Abnormalities of the tongue on magnetic resonance imaging. Ann Neurol 25:468–472, 1989.
12. Cheung, G, Gawal, MJ, Cooper, PW, et al: Amyotrophic lateral sclerosis: Correlation of clinical and MR imaging findings. Radiology 194:263–270, 1995.
13. Cobb, SR and Mehringer, CM: Wallerian degeneration in a patient with Schilder disease: MR imaging demonstration. Radiology 162:521–522, 1987.
14. Dalakas, MC, Hatazawa, J, Brooks, RA, et al: Lowered cerebral utilization in amyotrophic lateral sclerosis. Ann Neurol 22:580–586, 1987.
15. Drayer, BP: Imaging of the aging brain, Part II. Pathologic conditions. Radiology 166:797–806, 1988.
16. Duijn, JH, Matson, GB, Maudsley, AA, et al: Proton magnetic spectroscopic imaging of human brain infarction. Radiology 183:711–718, 1992.
17. El Escorial World Federation of Neurology criteria for the diagnosis of amyotrophic lateral sclerosis. J Neurol Sci 124(suppl):96–107, 1994.
18. Friedman, DP and Tartaglino, LM: Amyotrophic lateral sclerosis: Hyperintensity of the corticospinal tracts on MR images of the spinal cord. Am J Radiol 160:604–606, 1993.
19. Gallassi, R, Montagna, P, Morreale, A, et al: Neuropsychological, electroencephalogram and brain computed tomography findings in motor neuron disease. Eur Neurol 29:115–120, 1989.
20. Goodin, DS, Rowley, HA, and Olney, RK: Magnetic resonance imaging in amyotrophic lateral sclerosis. Ann Neurol 23:418–420, 1988.
21. Greenberg, JH, Reivich, M, Alavi, A, et al: Metabolic mapping of functional activity in human subjects with the [^{18}F]-fluorodeoxyglucose technique. Science 212:678–680, 1981.
22. Hallgren, B and Sourander, P: The non-haemin iron in the cerebral cortex in Alzheimer's disease. J Neurochem 5:307–310, 1960.
23. Hatazawa, J, Brooks, RA, Dalakas, MC, et al: Cortical motor-sensory hypometabolism in amyotrophic lateral sclerosis: A PET study. J Comput Assist Tomogr 12:630–636, 1988.
24. Hirayama, K, Tsubaki, T, Toyokura, Y, et al: The representation of the pyramidal tract in the internal capsule and basis pedunculi. Neurology 12:337–342, 1962.
25. Hoffman, JM, Mazziotta, JC, Hawk, TC, et al: Cerebral glucose utilization in motor neuron disease. Arch Neurol 49:849–854, 1992.
26. Ikeda, K, Mitsumoto, H, Antar, M, et al: Imaging in motor neuron disease [letter]. Neurology 44:1186–1187, 1994.
27. Inoue, Y, Matsumura, Y, Fukuda, T, et al: MR imaging of wallerian degeneration in the brainstem: Temporal relationships. AJNR 11:897–902, 1990.
28. Ishikawa, K, Nagura, H, Yokota, T, et al: Signal loss in the motor cortex on magnetic resonance images in amyotrophic lateral sclerosis. Ann Neurol 33:218–222, 1993.
29. Iwasaki, Y, Kinoshita, M, Ikeda, K, et al: MRI in patients with amyotrophic lateral sclerosis: Correlation with clinical features. Int J Neurosci 59:253–258, 1991.
30. Karnaze, MG, Gado, MH, Sartor, KJ, et al: Comparison of MR and CT myelography in imaging the cervical and thoracic spine. AJNR 8:983–989, 1987.
31. Kato, S, Hayashi, H, and Yagishita, A: Involvement of the frontotemporal lobe and limbic system in amyotrophic lateral sclerosis: As assessed by serial computed tomography and magnetic resonance imaging. J Neurol Sci 116:52–58, 1993.
32. Kazui, S, Kuriyama, Y, Sawada, T, et al: Very early

demonstration of secondary pyramidal tract degeneration by computed tomography. Stroke 25:2287–2289, 1994.

33. Kew, JJM, Brooks, DJ, Passingham, RE, et al: Cortical function in progressive lower motor neuron disorders and amyotrophic lateral sclerosis: A comparative PET study. Neurology 44:1101–1110, 1994.

34. Kew, JJM, Goldstein, LH, Leigh, PN, et al: The relationship between abnormalities of cognitive function and cerebral activation in amyotrophic lateral sclerosis. A neuropsychological and positron emission tomography study. Brain 116:1399–1423, 1993.

35. Kew, JJM, Leigh, PN, Playford, ED, et al: Cortical function in amyotrophic lateral sclerosis. A positron emission tomography study. Brain 116:655–680, 1993.

36. Kitamura, S, Taji, N, Komiyama, T, et al: A case of motor neuron disease with dementia—cerebral blood flow and cerebral oxygen metabolism. Clin Neurol 32:57–61, 1992.

37. Kuhn, MJ, Johnson, KA, and Davis, KR: Wallerian degeneration: Evaluation with MR imaging. Radiology 168:199–202, 1988.

38. Kuther, G, Rodiek, SO, and Struppler, A: CT-scanning of skeletal muscles in amyotrophic lateral sclerosis. Adv Exp Med Biol 209:143–148, 1987.

39. Lawyer, T and Netsky, MG: Amyotrophic lateral sclerosis. A clinicoanatomic study of 53 cases. Arch Neurol Psychiatry 69:171–192, 1953.

40. Lazzarino, LG and Nicolai, A: MRI findings in a patient with a familial form of motor neuron disease. Acta Neurol 13:25–30, 1991.

41. Lee, KS and Kelly, DL Jr: Amyotrophic lateral sclerosis and severe cervical spondylotic myelopathy in a patient with a posterior fossa arachnoid cyst: Diagnostic dilemma. South Med J 80:1580–1583, 1987.

42. Levine, RL, Brooks, BR, Matthews, CG, et al: Frontotemporal hypometabolism in amyotrophic lateral sclerosis-dementia complex: preliminary observations. J Neuroimag 3:234–241, 1993.

43. Ludolph, AC, Langen, KJ, Regard, M, et al: Frontal lobe function in amyotrophic lateral sclerosis: a neuropsychologic and positron emission tomography study. Acta Neurol Scand 85:81–89, 1992.

44. Martí-Fàbregas, J and Pujol, J: Selective involvement of the pyramidal tract on magnetic resonance imaging in primary lateral sclerosis. Neurology 40:1799–1800, 1990.

45. Miska, RM, Pojunas, KW, and McQuillen, MP: Cranial magnetic resonance imaging in the evaluation of myelopathy of undetermined etiology. Neurology 37:840–843, 1987.

46. Mitsui, Y, Tajahashi, M, Nakamura, Y, et al: Studies on motor neuron disease with cranial magnetic resonance imaging. Clin Neurol 32:469–473, 1992.

47. Meyerhoff, DJ, MacKay, S, Bachman, L, et al: Reduced brain N-acetylaspartate suggests neuronal loss in cognitively impaired human immunodeficiency virus-seropositive individuals: In vivo ^{1}H magnetic resonance spectroscopic imaging. Neurology 43:509–515, 1993.

48. Meyerhoff, DJ, MacKay, RDS, Grossman, N, et al: Effects of normal aging and Alzheimer's disease on cerebral ^{1}H metabolites [abstract]. Proc Soc Magn Reson Med 1:1931, 1992.

49. Mirowitz, S, Sartor, K, Gado, M, et al: Focal signal-intensity variations in the posterior internal capsule: normal MR findings and distinction from pathological findings. Radiology 172:535–539, 1989.

50. Moffett, JR, Namboodiri, MAA, Cangro, CB, et al: Immunohistochemical localization of N-acetylaspartate in rat brain. Neuroreport 2:131–134, 1991.

51. Neary, D, Snowden, JS, Mann, DMA, et al: Frontal lobe dementia and motor neuron disease. J Neurol Neurosurg Psychiatry 53:23–32, 1990.

52. Neirinckx, RD, Canning, LR, Piper, IMN, et al: Technetium-99m d,l-HMPAO: A new radiopharmaceutical for SPECT imaging of regional cerebral blood perfusion. J Nucl Med 28: 191–202, 1987.

53. Oba, H, Araki, T, Ohtomo, K, et al: Amyotrophic lateral sclerosis: T2 shortening in motor cortex at MR imaging. Radiology 189:843–846, 1993.

54. Okuda, B, Kawabata, K, Tachibana, H, et al: Three-dimensional display using ^{123}I-IMP in a case of motor neuron disease with dementia. Jap J Psychiatry 47:599–602, 1993.

55. Phelps, ME, Huang, SG, and Hoffman, EJ: Tomographic measurement of local cerebral glucose metabolic rate in humans with (F-18) 2 fluoro-2-deoxy-D-glucose: Validation of method. Ann Neurol 18:60–67, 1979.

56. Pioro, EP, Antel, JP, Cashman, NR, et al: Detection of cortical neuron loss in motor neuron disease by proton magnetic resonance spectroscopic imaging in vivo. Neurology 44:1933–1938, 1994.

57. Poloni, M, Mascherpa, C, Faggi, L, et al: Cerebral atrophy in motor neuron disease evaluated by computed tomography. J Neurol Neurosurg Psychiatry 45:1102–1105, 1982.

58. Ross, ED: Localization of the pyramidal tract in the internal capsule by whole brain dissection. Neurology 30:59–64, 1980.

59. Russell, JR and DeMyer, W: The quantitative cortical origin of pyramidal axons of Macaca rhesus. Neurology 11:96–108, 1961.

60. Sales Luís, ML, Hormigo, A, et al: Magnetic resonance imaging in motor neuron disease. J Neurol 237:471–474, 1990.

61. Sawada, H, Udaka, F, Kishi, Y, et al: Single photon emission computed tomography in motor neuron disease with dementia. Neuroradiology 30:577–578, 1988.

62. Segawa, F: MR findings of the pyramidal tract in ALS. Clin Neurol 33:835–844, 1993.

63. Simmons, ML, Frondoza, CG, and Coyle, JT: Immunocytochemical localization of N-acetyl-aspartate with monoclonal antibodies. Neuroscience 45: 37–45, 1991.

64. Smith, MC: Nerve fibre degeneration in the brain in amyotrophic lateral sclerosis. J Neurol Neurosurg Psychiatry 23:269–282, 1960.

65. Snow, BJ, Peppard, RF, Guttman, M, et al: Positron emission tomographic scanning demonstrates a presynaptic dopaminergic lesion in Lytico-Bodig. Arch Neurol 47:870–874, 1990.

66. Sze, G: MR imaging of the spinal cord: current status and future advances. Am J Radiol 159:149–159, 1992.

67. Takahashi, H, Snow, BJ, Bhatt, MH, et al: Evidence for a dopaminergic deficit in sporadic amyotrophic lateral sclerosis on positron emission scanning. Lancet 342:1016–1018, 1993.

68. Talbot, PR, Goulding, PJ, Lloyd, JJ, et al: Inter-relation between "classic" motor neuron disease: neuropsychological and single photon emission computed tomography study. J Neurol Neurosurg Psychiatry 58:541–547, 1995.

69. Talbot, PR, Lloyd, JJ, Snowden, JS, et al: The choice of reference region in the quantification of SPECT in primary degenerative dementia. Eur J Nucl Med 21:503–508, 1994.

70. Tanaka, M, Kondo, S, Hirai, S, et al: Cerebral blood flow and oxygen metabolism in progressive dementia associated with amyotrophic lateral sclerosis. J Neurol Sci 120:22–28, 1993.

71. Terao, S, Sobue, G, Yasuda, T, et al: Magnetic resonance imaging of spinal pyramidal tract degeneration in amyotrophic lateral sclerosis. J Neurol 242:178–183, 1995.

72. Terao, S, Sobue, G, Yasuda, T, et al: The corticospinal tract lesion of amyotrophic lateral sclerosis—magnetic resonance imaging of the spinal cord. Clin Neurol 34:865–869, 1994.

73. Udaka, F, Sawada, H, Seriu, N, et al: MRI and SPECT findings in amyotrophic lateral sclerosis. Demonstration of upper motor neurone involvement by clinical neuroimaging. Neuroradiology 34:389–393, 1992.

74. Urenjak, J, Williams, SR, Gadian, DG, et al: Specific expression of N-acetylaspartate in neurons, oligdendrocyte-Type-2 astrocyte progenitors, and immature oligodendrocytes in vitro. J Neurochem 59:55–61, 1992.

75. Waldemar, G, Hasselbalch, SG, Andersen, AR, et al: [^{99m}Tc]-d,l-HMPAO and SPECT of the brain in normal aging. J Cereb Blood Flow Metab 11:508–521, 1991.

76. Waldemar, G, Vorstrup, S, Jensen, TS, et al: Focal reductions of cerebral blood flow in amyotrophic lateral sclerosis: A [^{99m}Tc]-d,l-HMPAO SPECT study. J Neurol Sci 107:19–28, 1992.

77. Yagashita, A, Nakano, I, Oda, M, et al: Location of the corticospinal tract in the internal capsule at MR imaging. Radiology 191:455–460, 1994.

78. Younger, DS, Rowland, LP, Latov, N, et al: Motor neuron disease and amyotrophic lateral sclerosis: Relation of high CSF protein content to paraproteinemia and clinical syndromes. Neurology 40:595–599, 1990.

CHAPTER 9

COURSE AND PROGNOSIS

Charcot[13] described the prognosis of ALS most explicitly in his lectures: "The prognosis, up to the present, is of the gloomiest. There does not exist, so far as I am aware, a single example of a case where, the group of symptoms just described having existed, recovery followed. Is this doom final? The future alone can decide." Charcot's statement probably holds true even today; however, in the past several decades, the study of the course and prognosis of ALS has expanded enormously.

In clinical neurology, a major task is to give patients an accurate prognosis. Particularly for those who have a disease like ALS, for which specific treatments are lacking, prognostic evaluation becomes imperative.[32] Furthermore, prognostic information is helpful in making treatment decisions, particularly with regard to withholding or withdrawing care from terminally ill patients.[5] In the past several years, obtaining accurate data on the natural history of ALS has become an essential part of effective therapeutic trials (see Chapter 20).

PRECLINICAL STAGES

Swash and Ingram[60] raised an important issue regarding the preclinical stages of ALS that can help explain the disease course and prognosis. They suggested that ALS probably begins a long time, months or even years, before it manifests clinically. Before any clinical sign of muscle atrophy appears in ALS, it is estimated that more than 30% of motor neurons are probably destroyed.[67] Based on extensive correlation between clinical and pathologic changes in patients who had acute poliomyelitis, Sharrard[55] concluded that muscle weakness in those who survived poliomyelitis may not be detected until more than 50% of motor neurons are lost. When muscle weakness is detected by manual muscle strength testing (4 of 5 on the Medical Research Council [MRC] scale[38]), as many as 80% of motor neurons may be lost in patients who survived acute poliomyelitis.[55] McComas[36] had an unusual opportunity to study the number of motor units in the hypothenar muscles in a patient 9 months before ALS onset. The number was normal in this presymptomatic stage, whereas 3 months after the onset of symptoms, it had fallen to 40% of normal. Therefore, a substantial

151

number of motor neurons can be lost before any clinical signs develop.

Further electrophysiologic analyses have provided more insight into the preclinical course of ALS.[4] Uninvolved or only slightly involved muscles may be suitable for studying the preclinical stages. The maximum motor unit voltage (not compound motor action potentials but the voltage equivalent to fiber density) in only slightly affected muscles is three to four times larger than that in the corresponding muscles of normal controls, suggesting that vigorous reinnervation compensates for the progressive denervation occurring in the early stages of the disease, until the motor unit loss reaches about 50%.[20,23] The twitch force of slightly affected muscles is also significantly greater in patients with ALS than that of the corresponding muscles in controls. In these muscles, the motor unit is markedly enlarged, resulting in increased twitch force.[17] Similarly, muscle strength on the MRC scale may even increase while reinnervation initially compensates for motor neuron loss and before weakness develops because reinnervation can no longer offset loss.[62]

Single-fiber[54,58,61,62] and macro[54] electromyography (EMG) studies, which evaluate the size and innervation of motor units (see Chapter 5), also show that many motor units undergo extensive reinnervation in ALS. Motor unit loss occurs at a uniform rate, very rapidly in the preclinical stages and slowly in the late stages.[9,10,14,36] Bradley[4] believes that the degree of reinnervation in ALS is similar to that found in chronic neuromuscular diseases such as spinal muscular atrophy and Charcot-Marie-Tooth disease. In contrast, Swash and Schwartz[62] do not think that it increases to the degree seen in other chronic denervating conditions. Regardless, the balance between neuronal loss and reinnervation probably determines the duration of the preclinical stage and the disease course.

Swash and Ingram[60] discussed two cases that raised an intriguing issue as to what represents the preclinical stages. One patient was a 42-year-old army officer who could not pass an annual physical because he lacked strength but who did pass after exercise training. Every year for the next 6 years he needed extra training to pass the annual physical; then, progressive generalized weakness developed that turned into typical ALS. The second was a 34-year-old policeman who developed recurrent spontaneous limb weakness followed by improvement each time for 5 years before ALS finally developed. Both patients had similar and unusual preclinical presentations of ALS. Further detailed clinical and electrophysiologic studies on such patients, although rarely feasible and often obtained serendipitously, should provide crucial information about the natural history of ALS.

NATURAL HISTORY

The ideal study of prognosis would examine the natural history of a condition from its biologic start to its end without interventions that could influence outcome. Such a study is improbable in neurodegenerative disorders because the time of onset is unknown and various diagnostic and therapeutic maneuvers are applied during the course of such diseases in most patients. Once a treatment comes to be considered as "standard therapy" (like levodopa-carbidopa for Parkinson's disease), the study of natural history and prognosis becomes impossible.[55] In ALS, riluzole is likely to become a standard therapy.

A natural history study in ALS begins usually at diagnosis. Using uniform diagnostic criteria and measurement techniques is imperative to develop reliable natural history data and permit comparisons among studies. Analysis of how ALS symptoms develop and how muscle strength and motor function deteriorate during the course of the disease is the primary concern.

Only in the last several years has the natural history of ALS been investigated prospectively. Brooks and colleagues[8] analyzed the evolution of symptoms as a function of the site of onset in 702 patients with ALS. The sites of onset are classified as arm, leg, or bulbar. Figure 9–1 shows the natural history when contralateral leg, ipsilateral arm, contralateral arm, and bulbar symptoms begin in those with leg onset. The accrual of symptoms in the opposite leg was faster than in other regions, and contralateral arm accrual was slower than in the contralateral leg and ipsilateral arm. Bulbar symptom accrual was

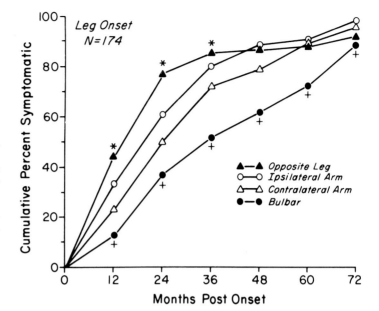

Figure 9–1. In patients with leg-onset ALS, symptoms accrue in the opposite leg, ipsilateral and con-tralateral arms, and bulbar mus-cles. The opposite leg is affected in the shortest interval, whereas the bulbar muscles take the longest in-terval. (From Brooks, BR, et al: De-sign of clinical therapeutic trials in amyotrophic lateral sclerosis. In Rowland, LP (ed): Amyotrophic Lateral Sclerosis and Other Motor Neuron Disease. Adv Neurol 56: 526, 1991, with permission.)

slowest. In those with arm onset, symptoms in the opposite arm developed faster than in any other region (Fig. 9–2). Comparison of Figures 9–1 and 9–2 shows that bulbar symp-tom accrual in patients with arm onset was significantly faster than that in patients with leg onset at 2, 3, and 4 years of disease. Fig-ure 9–3 shows bulbar symptom accrual in pa-tients with limb onset ALS. In patients with arm onset, bulbar-symptom accrual was sig-nificantly faster than in those with leg onset. Neuronal degeneration appears to develop within contiguous areas more quickly than it does between noncontiguous areas.[8] The pattern also suggests that rostral-caudal in-volvement is faster than caudal-rostral spread,

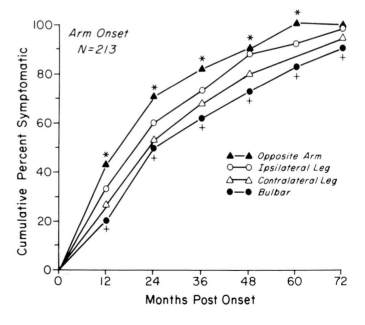

Figure 9–2. In patients with arm-onset ALS, symptom accrual occurs first in the opposite arm, then in the ipsilat-eral and contralateral legs, and last in the bulbar muscles. (From Brooks, BR, et al: Design of clinical therapeutic tri-als in amyotrophic lateral sclerosis. In Rowland, LP (ed): Amyotrophic Lat-eral Sclerosis and Other Motor Neu-ron Disease. Adv Neurol 56:527, 1991, with permission.)

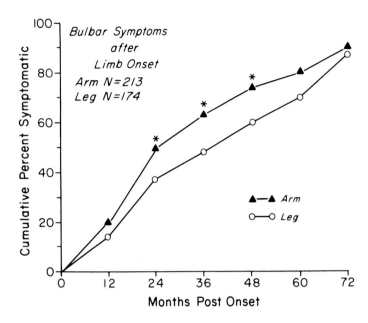

Figure 9–3. In patients with bulbar-onset ALS, symptom accrual begins in the arms earlier than in the legs. (From Brooks, BR, et al: Design of clinical therapeutic trials in amyotrophic lateral sclerosis. In Rowland, LP (ed): Amyotrophic Lateral Sclerosis and Other Motor Neuron Disease. Adv Neurol 56:527, 1991, with permission.)

supporting the idea that axonal transport might be involved in the development of neuronal degeneration in ALS.[6] In analyzing gender effects, arm involvement after bulbar onset is more rapid in men than in women in the first 3 years of diagnosis.[8] This difference suggests that gender might affect the pattern of neuronal degeneration.[7,25]

Quantitative natural history data have been extensively accumulated primarily by three research teams.[8,42,47] Because ALS causes progressive muscle weakness and deterioration of motor function, quantitative techniques have been developed to measure such changes.[2,42] The methods and reliability of these techniques are fully reviewed in Chapter 20. Munsat and colleagues[2,42] developed isometric muscle strength testing (maximum voluntary isometric contraction) and quantitative motor function testing. They computed the z-scores, normalized with data from the ALS population, a process that not only allows data to be easily compared among different muscles but also allows multiple strength and motor function measurements to be combined as a megascore. The motor function in ALS declines linearly and symmetrically.[42] Age at onset and rate of deterioration are not correlated. Further studies confirmed that deterioration is strikingly linear.[45] Deterioration rates in arm and leg strength are highly correlated in

individual patients, but the rates range widely among patients.[45] Ringel and colleagues[47] found a highly variable rate of decline in muscle strength among patients. The rate of decline does not differ with sex and gender. Decline of pulmonary function is associated most closely with death.

Analyzing the Wisconsin ALS Database, Brooks et al.[7] found more complex changes in the muscle strength of ALS patients. Arm and leg megascores do not decline linearly over time in all patients, and may have an inflection point at the beginning of isometric strength loss after prolonged periods of stable strength. Such variability appears to occur more frequently during the first year after ALS is diagnosed. Furthermore, strength may transiently increase for variable periods of up to a few months. A second inflection point may occur when the muscles are weakest because muscle strength changes very little, and functioning muscles are lost for testing in these stages. However, the overall slope of the loss of arm or leg strength for their population of ALS patients is best described by a linear relationship. It seems unlikely that the slope can be predicted for the rest of the course by a linear regression line that is based on the analysis of these quantitative measurements for only several months[11] (ALS ciliary neurotrophic factor [CNTF] Treatment Study Groups, unpublished observation).

DISEASE DURATION

The duration of disease in ALS is defined as the interval between the onset of symptoms and death. In clinical practice, the *mean* disease duration is widely used to describe the prognosis of a disease. Theoretically, it should be used only when the data are normally distributed. If the distribution is not uniform, the *median* duration provides a more accurate description because it eliminates the effects of outliers. Table 9–1 summarizes the results of recent clinical epidemiology studies in ALS, which indicate that the mean duration ranges from 27 to 43 months, whereas the median duration ranges from 23 to 52 months. The range reflects the shortest and longest survival time in the patient sample in a particular study.

In contrast to the duration of the disease, the survival rate may be a better indicator of prognosis because it gives probability of survival at the time of study (or diagnosis). It can also provide the probability of survival at various years after onset. Table 9–1 shows the 5-year survival rate ranging from 9% to 40%, with an arithmetic average of 25%. The 10-year-survival rates provide information about the proportion of long-survival cases. Figure 9–4 shows several representative Kaplan-Meier survival curves of patients with ALS. The number of surviving patients decreases first rapidly, then more slowly. The Kaplan-Meier analysis estimates the number of patients alive at various times after an event, such as after the onset of ALS.[29]

FACTORS INFLUENCING PROGNOSIS

Several standard demographic characteristics, as well as factors specific to ALS, have been analyzed extensively to determine prog-

Table 9–1. **PROGNOSTIC STUDIES IN ALS***

Investigator	Study Location	Study Period	Patients (n)	DURATION OF DISEASE (MONTHS)			5-yr Survival (%)	10-yr Survival (%)
				Median	Mean	Range		
Mulder et al.[41]	USA	1954–76	100	—	—	—	20	10
Mackay[34]	USA	?–1962	70	—	36	3–156	—	—
Juergens et al.[28]	USA	1925–77	35	23	—	10–120	9	—
Kristensen et al.[30]	Denmark	1948–75	118	31	—	—	19	8
Mukai et al.[40]	Japan	1951–82	273	—	34	—	—	—
Gubbay et al.[22]	Israel	1959–75	318	36	—	—	39	16
Uebayashi et al.[66]	Japan	1960–80	768	—	—	—	13	—
Granieri et al.[21]	Italy	1964–82	72	—	—	—	40	—
Rosati et al.[48]	Italy	1965–74	64	—	29	—	—	—
Li et al.[31]	England	1965–82	98	—	31	—	—	—
Kondo et al.[29]	Japan	1966	379	—	42	4–464	20	8
Jokelainen et al.[27]	Finland	1969–73	157	—	32	—	—	—
Norris et al.[44]	USA	1970–86	708	37	37	5–390	—	—
López-Vega et al.[33]	Spain	1974–85	42	—	27	—	18	—
Smith et al.[56]	USA	1976–86	166	—	36	12–216	39	13
Scarpa et al.[51]	Italy	1976–86	51	25	29	5–90	24	—
Caroscio et al.[12]	USA	1978–82	388	52	—	6–192	—	—
Tysnes et al.[64]	Norway	1978–88	70	28	—	—	37	—
Eisen et al.[18]	Canada	1985–91	138	—	43	—	—	—
Ringel et al.[47]	USA	1989–91	48	48	—	—	—	—

*Studies are listed in chronological order from the oldest study done.

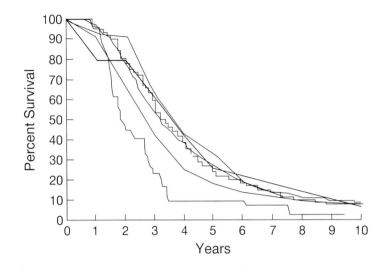

Figure 9–4. A composite figure of survival curves that have been reported in various studies.[21,22,28,30,41,44,56] The shortest survival curve was derived from a study done in Rochester, Minnesota (Juergens, et al.[28]). In most studies, 50% survival ranges from 2 to 4 years after the onset of illness. Approximately 10% or so of patients survive beyond 10 years.

Table 9–2. FACTORS THAT MAY SUGGEST A BETTER PROGNOSIS OF ALS

Age
Younger patients (age <35–40 yr)

Type of ALS
Spinal (arm or leg) onset
Progressive muscular atrophy type
Primary lateral sclerosis type
Nonfamilial form*

Pulmonary Function
No dyspnea at onset
Slow deterioration of pulmonary function

Electrophysiology
Normal compound action potentials on EMG†
No decremental responses on repetitive stimulation on EMG

Severity and Duration of Disease
Less severe involvement at diagnosis
A long interval from onset to diagnosis (or ALS clinic visit)
Having survived more than 46 months after onset

Other Factors
Absent or less widespread fasciculations
Psychologically well
Normal serum chloride levels

---

*Certain SOD mutations are associated with a markedly prolonged disease course (see Chapter 10).
†EMG = electromyography.

nosis. Table 9–2 summarizes the results; the details are discussed below.

Age

A younger age of onset is associated with a better prognosis in all studies except two.[1,24,33,64,65] The differences in prognosis between younger and older patients are statistically significant. These differences are seen in disease duration,[12,44,48] 5-year survival rate,[49,66] 50% survival rate,[47] and expected survival period[18] (Fig. 9–5).

Gender

Most studies show that prognosis does not differ according to gender. In the studies that did find differences, the results conflict. For example, two studies found that women with ALS lived longer than men.[12,27] According to one Japanese study,[40] women below age 39 years survived significantly longer compared with men of the same age. In a Spanish study,[33] when men were analyzed separately, those less than 60 years old lived longer than those over 69; however, this trend disappeared when men and women were analyzed together, and no differences were found when women alone were analyzed. Other studies show that men live longer than women.[44,56] Such contradictory data suggest

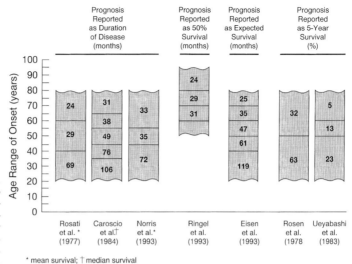

Figure 9–5. Relationship between age of onset and prognosis for ALS is shown. All the studies consistently show that the older the age of onset, the poorer the prognosis. Wavy ends of each column represent no set limit for either older age group above the line or younger age group below the line.

that gender probably does not influence prognosis.

Type of ALS

The prognosis of bulbar-onset ALS (probably including progressive bulbar palsy, which is exceedingly rare) is poor compared with the spinal-onset type (Table 9–3). On the other hand, several studies show no differences in survival rate and duration between bulbar- and spinal-onset ALS.[12,33,48,51]

Among the subsets of ALS, primary lateral sclerosis has the best prognosis, followed by progressive muscular atrophy (Table 9–4). Survival is longer in cases with a mainly spastic form than in those with marked atrophy.[65] The duration of familial ALS is probably shorter than that of sporadic ALS (see Chapter 10). Strong et al.[57] reviewed the world literature and found the median duration of familial ALS to be 24 months, which is shorter than any duration estimated for sporadic ALS (see Table 9–1). Several individual studies for disease duration in familial ALS show contradictory results, most likely caused by different sampling in these studies.[44,49,65]

Table 9–3. **PROGNOSIS OF ALS: SPINAL ONSET VS. BULBAR ONSET**

Investigators	Spinal Onset	Bulbar Onset
Five-Year Survival Rate		
Tysnes et al.[64]	37%	9%*
Rosen et al.[49]	44%	14%*
Mean Duration of Disease		
Jokelainen et al.[27]	34 mo	25 mo
Kristensen et al.[30]	36 mo	24 mo
Gubbay et al.[22]	38 mo	26 mo
Mackay[34]	Spastic form: 36 mo Paretic form: 33 mo	Spastic form: 24 mo Paretic form: 17 mo
Tysnes et al.[65]	26 mo	12 mo

*Statistically significant differences ($p < 0.01$)

Table 9–4. **PROGNOSIS OF DIFFERENT SUBTYPES OF ALS**

Authors	Survival Measure	Sporadic ALS	Familial ALS	PMA	PLS
Norris et al.[44]	Mean (mo)	37	43	159	224
Smith et al.[56]	Mean (mo)	36	23	41	—
Li et al.[31]	Mean (mo)	31	13	—	—
Strong et al.[57]	Median (mo)	—	24	—	—
Granieri et al.[21]	5-yr survival (%)	37	64	—	—

Abbreviations: PMA = progressive muscular atrophy, PLS = primary lateral sclerosis.

Pulmonary Impairment

Those with dyspnea at disease onset have a modest but statistically significant shorter disease duration.[47] At the same time, the evaluation of pulmonary function during the disease course may be more helpful in predicting the overall prognosis of ALS than other function tests.[1,52] A specific analysis of this issue showed a statistically significant correlation between decline in pulmonary function and a poor prognosis.[7,24] Ringel and colleagues[47] conducted a large natural history study (see Chapter 20) and confirmed that among all variables tested during the course of ALS, a decline in pulmonary function (as determined by forced vital capacity) best predicts a poor prognosis. Similarly, when the Appel score is used, respiratory subscore significantly correlated with survival.[24]

Electrophysiologic Changes

A reduction in compound motor action potentials (CMAP) is well correlated with a poor prognosis.[15] One of our studies also showed that reduced CMAP in the most affected extremity alone or in all extremities combined was significantly associated with shortened survival and an increase in functional disability. The rate of CMAP reduction over the follow-up period also was related to the degree of functional disability.[39] That CMAP decreases in response to repetitive stimulation is well known in patients with ALS (see Chapter 5), and in fact the greater the decrease, the poorer the prognosis.[3] The combination of a reduction in CMAP and a decremental response on repetitive nerve stimulation increases the accuracy in predicting the prognosis of ALS.[15]

Severity and Duration of the Disease

In general, severe clinical involvement at diagnosis is a reliable predictor of a rapidly progressive clinical course.[15] A recent clinical study with ciliary neurotrophic factor (CNTF) confirmed that severe ALS correlated with a poor prognosis in patients who were assigned to a placebo group: patients with ALS who died during the clinical study had a lower ALS functional rating scale score and reduced muscle strength as measured by maximum voluntary isometric contraction testing at entry into the study.[1] In another study, a monthly decline of more than 3.3 on the Appel ALS score corresponded to a shorter survival.[24]

A short interval between symptom onset and diagnosis correlated with increased disability scores[39] and poor prognosis.[65] On the other hand, our study indicated that a longer delay from onset of symptoms to diagnosis was associated with less disability and longer survival. We suspect the reason for this correlation is that the longer the interval is from onset to diagnosis, the milder the disease. On the other hand, patients who seek medical attention soon after symptoms begin tend to have a rapid course and severe neurologic involvement.[26,39] A recent study in a large population of patients with ALS confirmed that those who visited the ALS clinic more than 12 months after the onset of the illness had significantly longer survival.[24] Comparing the survival (duration of disease) between incidence cases (patients entering the study within 1 year of onset) and prevalence cases (patients entering the study more than 1 year after onset), survival was significantly longer in the prevalence cases, suggesting that they are a part of a preselected group because patients with a rapid course or who had already died would not be included.[47]

Another interesting point regarding the duration of ALS is that the predicted life expectancy decreases in the first 46 months after diagnosis but then increases. This pattern suggests that those who survive the first 46 months are likely to survive longer.[29] Whether this is a result of unknown defense mechanism(s) that become effective in the later stages of disease, or whether two distinct types of ALS exist, remains to be determined.

Psychological Factors

Psychological factors have been examined for influence on the outcome of chronic diseases.[16,46] McDonald and colleagues[37] first analyzed the correlation between the psychological status of patients with ALS and outcome. They used 10 independent instruments for assessment of status in 138 patients and followed them for an average of 3.5 years after the initial assessment. The assessment instruments all used numerical scoring systems, with higher scores indicating better psychological well-being. Only 32% of patients with high scores died during the follow-up period, whereas 82% of those with low scores died in the same period, a statistically significant difference. The analysis of confounding factors, such as length of illness and disease severity, showed that psychological distress had a greater risk of mortality. This study certainly suggests we need to broaden our view of ALS and go beyond physical factors to include the psychological dimension.[37]

Other Factors

In the pseudoneuritic form of ALS (see Chapters 4 and 5), in which motor weakness begins in the territory of a major peripheral nerve, disease duration has been found to be longer than in the typical spinal form of ALS,[48,51,66] but the differences are not statistically significant in any studies.

Fasciculations may be an important prognostic factor. One study[44] found that absence of fasciculations at onset correlated with longer survival, and another study[56] showed that the fewer the number of extremities having fasciculations, the longer the duration of ALS. However, this finding has not been confirmed by other investigators.[66]

Dementia, sensory symptoms, and vesicorectal dysfunction appear to have no prognostic influence in patients with ALS.[66] Esophagostomy or gastrostomy also had no effects on the duration of ALS.[56] Recently, however, percutaneous endoscopic gastrostomy tube feeding was found to be associated with longer survival.[35] An intriguing correlation between a high cerebrospinal fluid protein level and a shortened duration of ALS has been reported by Uebayashi et al.,[66] but another study found no such relationship.[65]

The ALS CNTF Treatment Study (ACTS) Group[1] recently reported that a low serum chloride level was significantly associated with poor prognosis in patients who were randomized into the placebo groups in their clinical trials. Particularly, a sudden decline of serum chloride concentration occurred 3 to 4 months prior to death. Such an abrupt change in the rate of decline in serum chloride level clearly reflects a metabolic compensation for the chronic respiratory acidosis that occurs in the terminal stages of ALS.

CASES WITH A PROLONGED COURSE

Swank and Putnum[59] pointed out that occasionally in patients with typical ALS, the disease ceases to progress or progresses very slowly. They found that 5% to 10% of patients with ALS were long survivors, living from 5 to 11 years after diagnosis. Such figures are well within the range of 10-year survival rates reported by others (see Table 9–1). Mulder and Howard[41] initially suspected that those who were diagnosed with ALS and survived for long periods were wrongly diagnosed. Furthermore, in some of these survivors as the diseases progressed, features of upper motor neuron involvement disappeared and lower motor neuron signs predominated. However, autopsy findings resembled those in patients who died after a shorter, more typical course. Therefore, Mulder and Howard[41] concluded that the duration of illness alone could not distinguish between typical and protracted forms of ALS. In fact, patients who survive for more than 10 years may not be all that rare. We have followed patients who had a protracted course but were not certain about the diagnosis of ALS; we designated their condition as "atypical" ALS. This patient population requires further investigation to characterize this aspect of ALS.

According to the two largest epidemiologic studies, the two longest documented durations of ALS are 32 years[44] and 39 years.[43] In fact, Norris[43] used the term "benign" ALS to describe such protracted cases, although he did not believe the terminology was accurate. In these patients, the annual decline of the Norris score (see Chapter 20) is 1 or 2 at most, and the disease progresses very slowly, yet the overall functional impairment is still severe. Of 613 patients with sporadic ALS, progression ceased in 28 male patients for at least 5 years.[44] Mulder and Howard[41] suggested that a patient's disease "resistance" might influence the course of ALS. Whether patients with a more benign course have more reinnervation activity or other moderating influences is a particularly crucial question in understanding ALS prognosis.[60]

"REVERSIBLE" ALS

Patients have been described who presented with ALS-like features and subsequently improved.[59] One such patient developed ALS but progressed minimally over 6 years, then suddenly deteriorated with generalized fasciculations and died within 2 years. Whether this patient's initial course represented the preclinical stages of ALS[60] or was the initial phase of protracted ALS is an interesting question. Mulder and Howard[41] reported a 49-year-old surgeon who developed weakness in the left arm followed by weakness in the left leg along with fasciculations. Tendon reflexes were brisk except for left biceps and brachioradialis reflexes, which were diminished. The Hoffmann reflex was posi-

tive only on the right, and he had no Babinski signs. EMG showed denervation, reduced numbers of motor units, an abnormal recruitment pattern, increased motor unit amplitudes, and a few fasciculations in affected, weak muscles. However, the patient gradually improved his muscle strength over several months, and re-examination after 6 years showed nearly normal muscle strength.

Similar cases with recovery or improvement from motor neuron disease also have been reported.[19,50] More recently, Tucker and colleagues[63] reported four cases and reviewed the topic in detail. Interestingly, all cases reported to date[19,41,50,63] are characterized by predominantly lower motor neuron signs, although in some patients reflexes are brisk but not pathologic. No patient had spasticity or bulbar symptoms. Based on the El Escorial World Federation of Neurology diagnostic criteria,[68] these cases probably are not ALS. Identifying and understanding similar cases of this "reversible" ALS syndrome is an important task for clinical neurologists.

PROGNOSTICATION

Although many factors that influence the prognosis of ALS (see Table 9–2) are now identified, providing an accurate prognosis to an individual patient is improbable because too many patients with ALS share these factors.[44] Furthermore, no factors appear to be distinctive enough to predict whether the course will be prolonged or "reversed." Such an event is unpredictable and exceedingly rare. Diagnostic criteria vary between previous studies, and thus identified prognostic factors may not be applicable to all patients. Tysnes and colleagues[65] were probably the first to use prognostic factors to predict the course of ALS. They selected the three strongest prognostic factors: type of ALS, period from onset to diagnosis, and extent of motor neuron involvement (upper motor neuron, lower, or mixed involvement). Their predictive rule assigned 8 of 11 patients (73%) to the correct prognostic group. Further natural history studies using uniform diagnostic criteria are essential for predicting prognosis in the future.

SUMMARY

Accurate knowledge of the course and prognosis of ALS is crucial for better understanding of the disease process and for discussing the prognosis of ALS with patients and their families. This chapter reviewed the clinical course of ALS, including the preclinical stages, natural history, duration, and prognosis.

Information concerning the preclinical course is largely speculative, but motor neuron loss probably begins long before the disease manifests clinically. Electrophysiologic studies done in the early stages of ALS, particularly in uninvolved extremities, suggest that reinnervation is active and probably offsets initial motor neuron loss until reinnervation can no longer compensate. The degree of this reinnervation may determine the disease course in the preclinical and early stages. However, what determines the degree of reinnervation is unknown.

The natural history of ALS begins at clinical recognition. How ALS symptoms develop from the onset suggests that the neuronal degeneration spreads in the contiguous areas and that rostral-caudal extension appears to be faster than caudal-rostral. Quantitative muscle strength testing and motor function testing indicate that muscle strength and motor function in ALS decline linearly; possible exceptions are the early and end stages of the illness.

The duration of ALS has been extensively investigated. A significant proportion of ALS patients may live beyond 5 years after onset. Better prognosis appears to be associated with young age at onset, spinal onset, predominantly upper or lower motor neuron involvement, absent or slowly progressive pulmonary impairment, fewer fasciculations, a long interval from onset to diagnosis, milder muscle involvement at diagnosis, normal CMAPs on EMG, and psychologic well-being. Nevertheless, accurate prognosis in an individual patient is not probable. Unusual cases of protracted course of ALS and several cases of patients who improved spontaneously from motor neuron disease or ALS have been reported. In patients with a lengthy course, questions concerning reinnervation and moderating influences need to be investigated. Those patients in whom the disease reversed may not have had true ALS.

REFERENCES

1. ALS CNTF Treatment Study (ACTS) Group: Prognostic indicators of survival in amyotrophic lateral sclerosis [abstract]. Neurology 46:A208, 1996.
2. Andres, PL, Finison, LJ, Conlon, T, et al: Use of composite scores (megascores) to measure deficit in amyotrophic lateral sclerosis. Neurology 38:405–408, 1988.
3. Bernstein, LP and Antel, JP: Motor neuron disease: Decremental responses to repetitive nerve stimulation. Neurology 31:202–204, 1981.
4. Bradley, WG: Recent views on amyotrophic lateral sclerosis with emphasis on electrophysiological studies. Muscle Nerve 10:490–502, 1987.
5. Brody, B: Ethical issues raised by the clinical use of prognostic information. In Evans, RW, Baskins, DS, and Yatsu, FM (eds): Prognosis of Neurological Disorders. Oxford University Press, New York, 1992, pp 3–11.
6. Brooks, BR: The role of axonal transport in neurodegenerative disease spread: A meta-analysis of experimental and clinical poliomyelitis compares with amyotrophic lateral sclerosis. Can J Neurol Sci 18:435–438, 1991.
7. Brooks, BR, Lewis, D, Rawling, J, et al: The natural history of amyotrophic lateral sclerosis. In Williams, AC (ed): Motor Neuron Disease. Chapman & Hall Medical, London, 1994, pp 131–169.
8. Brooks, BR, Sufit, RL, DePaul, R, et al: Design of clinical therapeutic trails in amyotrophic lateral sclerosis. In Rowland, LP (ed): Amyotrophic Lateral Sclerosis and Other Motor Neuron Disease. Adv Neurol 56, Raven Press, New York, 1991, pp 521–546.
9. Brown, WF: Functional compensation of human motor units in health and disease. J Neurol Sci 20:199–209, 1973.
10. Brown, WF and Jaatoul, N: Amyotrophic lateral sclerosis. Arch Neurol 30:242–248, 1974.
11. Bryan, WW, Barohn, RJ, Murphy, JR, et al: Placebo versus natural history in an ALS clinical trial [abstract]. Neurology 45(suppl 4):A280–281, 1995.
12. Caroscio, JT, Mulvihill, MN, Sterling, R, et al: Amyotrophic lateral sclerosis. Its natural history. Neurol Clin 5:108, 1987.
13. Charcot, JM: Lectures on the diseases of the nervous system. Sigerson, S, (ed, trans). Hafner, New York, 1962.
14. Dantes, M and McComas, AJ: The extent and time course of motoneuron involvement in amyotrophic lateral sclerosis. Muscle Nerve 14:416–421, 1991.
15. Daube, JR: Electrophysiologic studies in the diagnosis and prognosis of motor neuron disease. Neurol Clin 3:473–493, 1985.
16. Dean, C and Surtees, PG: Do psychological factors predict survival in breast cancer? J Psychosom Res 33:561–569, 1989.
17. Dengler, R, Konstanzer, MD, Küther, G, et al: Amyotrophic lateral sclerosis: Macro-EMG and twitch

forces of single motor units. Muscle Nerve 13:545–550, 1990.

18. Eisen, A, Schulzer, M, MacNeil, M, et al: Duration of amyotrophic lateral sclerosis is age dependent. Muscle Nerve 16:27–32, 1993.

19. Engel, WK, Hogenhuis, LAH, Collis, WJ, et al: Metabolic studies and therapeutic trials in amyotrophic lateral sclerosis. In Norris, FH and Kurland LT (eds): Motor Neuron Diseases: Research on Amyotrophic Lateral Sclerosis and Related Disorders. Grune & Stratton, New York, 1969, pp 199–213.

20. Erminio, F, Buchthal, F, and Rosenfalk, P: Motor unit territory and muscle fiber concentration in paresis due to peripheral nerve injury and anterior horn cell involvement. Neurology 9:657–671, 1959.

21. Granieri, E, Carreras, M, Tola, R, et al: Motor neuron disease in the province of Ferrara, Italy, in 1964–1982. Neurology 38:1604–1608, 1988.

22. Gubbay, SS, Kahana, E, Zilber, N, et al: Amyotrophic lateral sclerosis. A study of its presentation and prognosis. J Neurol 232:295–300, 1985.

23. Hansen, S and Ballantyne, JP: A quantitative electrophysiological study of motor neurone disease. J Neurol Neurosurg Psychiatry 41:773–783, 1978.

24. Haverkamp, LJ, Appel, V, and Appel, SH: Natural history of amyotrophic lateral sclerosis in a database population. Validation of a scoring system and a model for survival predication. Brain 118:707–719, 1995.

25. Heitzman, D, Wilbourn, A, and Mitsumoto, H: A retrospective study examining the clinical and electrodiagnostic features of patients with bulbar-onset amyotrophic lateral sclerosis [abstract]. Neurology 45(suppl 4):A447, 1995.

26. Jablecki, CK, Berry, C, and Leach, J: Survival prediction on amyotrophic lateral sclerosis. Muscle Nerve 12:833–841, 1989.

27. Jokelainen, M: Amyotrophic lateral sclerosis in Finland. 2. Clinical characteristics. Acta Neurol Scand 56:194–204, 1977.

28. Juergens, SM, Kurland, LT, Okazaki, H, et al: ALS in Rochester, Minnesota. Neurology 30:463–470, 1980.

29. Kondo, K and Hemmi, I: Clinical statistics in 515 fatal cases of motor neuron disease. Neuroepidemiology 3:129–148, 1984.

30. Kristensen, O and Melgaard, B: Motor neuron disease. Prognosis and Epidemiology. Acta Neurol Scand 56:299–308, 1977.

31. Li, T-M, Alberman, E, and Swash, M: Comparison of sporadic and familial disease amongst 580 cases of motor neuron disease. J Neurol Neurosurg Psychiatry 51:778–784, 1988.

32. Longstreth, WT Jr, Koepsel, TD, Melson, LM, et al: Prognosis: Keystone of clinical neurology. In Evans, RW, Baskin, DS, and Yatsu, FM (eds): Prognosis of Neurological Disorders. Oxford University Press, New York, 1992, pp 29–44.

33. López-Vega, JM, Calleja, J, Combarros, O, et al: Motor neuron disease in Cantabria. Acta Neurol Scand 77:1–5, 1988.

34. Mackay, RP: Course and prognosis in amyotrophic lateral sclerosis. Arch Neurol 8:17–27, 1963.

35. Mazzini, L, Corra, T, Zaccala, M, et al: Percutaneous endoscopic gastrostomy and enteral nutrition in amyotrophic lateral sclerosis. J Neurol 242:695–698, 1995.

36. McComas, AJ: Neuromuscular Function and Disorders. Butterworth, London, 1977.

37. McDonald, ER, Wiedenfeld, SA, Hillel, A, et al: Survival in amyotrophic lateral sclerosis. Arch Neurol 51:17–23, 1994.

38. Medical Research Council. Aid to the investigation of peripheral nerve injuries. War Memorandum, ed 2 (revised). His Majesty's Stationary Office, London, 1943, pp 11–46.

39. Mitsumoto, H, Schwartzman, M, Levin, KH, et al: Electromyographic (EMG) changes and disease progression in ALS [abstract]. Neurology 40(suppl 1):318, 1990.

40. Mukai, E, Sakakibara, T, and Sobue, I: The relationship between prognosis and sex and age at onset in amyotrophic lateral sclerosis. Clin Neurol 24:679–685, 1984.

41. Mulder, DW and Howard, FM: Patient resistance and prognosis in amyotrophic lateral sclerosis. Mayo Clin Proc 51:537–541, 1976.

42. Munsat, TL, Andres, PL, Finison, L, et al: The natural history of motoneuron loss in amyotrophic lateral sclerosis. Neurology 38:409–413, 1988.

43. Norris, FH: Amyotrophic lateral sclerosis: The clinical disorder. In Smith RA (ed): Handbook of Amyotrophic Lateral Sclerosis. Marcel Dekker, New York, 1992, pp 3–38.

44. Norris, F, Shepherd, R, Denys, E, et al: Onset, natural history and outcome in idiopathic adult motor neuron disease. J Neurol Sci 118:48–55, 1993.

45. Pradas, J, Finison, L, Andres, PL, et al: The natural history of amyotrophic lateral sclerosis and the use of natural history controls in therapeutic trials. Neurology 43:751–755, 1933.

46. Ragland, DR and Brand, RJ: Type A behavior and mortality from coronary heart disease. N Engl J Med 318:65–69, 1988.

47. Ringel, SP, Murchy, JR, Alderson, MK, et al: The natural history of amyotrophic lateral sclerosis. Neurology 43:1316–1322, 1993.

48. Rosati, G, Pinna, L, Granieri, E, et al: Studies on epidemiological, clinical, and etiological aspects of ALS disease in Sardinia, Southern Italy. Acta Neurol Scand 55:231–244, 1977.

49. Rosen, AD: Amyotrophic lateral sclerosis. Clinical features and prognosis. Arch Neurol 35:638–642, 1978.

50. Rowland, LP: Motor neuron diseases: The clinical syndromes. In Mulder, DW (ed): The Diagnosis and Treatment of Amyotrophic Lateral Sclerosis. Houghton Mifflin, Boston, 1988, pp 7–33.

51. Scarpa, M, Colombo, A, Panzetti, P, et al: Epidemiology of amyotrophic lateral sclerosis in the province of Modena, Italy. Influence of environmental exposure to lead. Acta Neurol Scand 77:456–460, 1988.

52. Schiffman, PL and Belsh, JM: Pulmonary function at diagnosis of amyotrophic lateral sclerosis. Chest 103:508–513, 1993.

53. Schwartz, MS and Swash, M: Pattern of involvement in the cervical segments in the early stage of motor neurone disease: A single fibre EMG study. Acta Neurol Scand 65:424–431, 1982.

54. Selby, G: Clinical features. In Stern, GM (ed): Parkinson's Disease. Johns Hopkins University Press, Baltimore, 1990, pp 333–388.

55. Sharrard, WJW: The distribution of the permanent paralysis in the lower limb in poliomyelitis; a clinical and pathological study. J Bone Joint Surg 37b:540–548, 1955.

56. Smith, LD, Kenney, CE, Ringel, SP, et al: Motor neuron disease in the Rocky Mountain region. West J Med 148:430–432, 1988.

57. Strong, MJ, Hudson, AJ, and Alvord, WG: Familial amyotrophic lateral sclerosis 1850–1989: A statistical analysis of the world literature. Can J Neurol Sci 18:45–58, 1991.

58. Stålberg, E and Sanders, DB: Neurophysiological studies in amyotrophic lateral sclerosis. In Smith, RA (ed): Handbook of Amyotrophic Lateral Sclerosis. Marcel Dekker, New York, 1992, pp 209–235.

59. Swank, RL and Putnam, TJ: Amyotrophic lateral sclerosis and related conditions. Arch Neurol Psychiatry 49:151–177, 1943.

60. Swash, M and Ingram, D: Preclinical and subclinical events in motor neuron disease. J Neurol Neurosurg Psychiatry 51:165–168, 1988.

61. Swash, M and Schwartz, MS: A longitudinal study of changes in motor units in motor neuron disease. J Neurol Sci 56:185–197, 1982.

62. Swash, M and Schwartz, MS: Staging motor neurone disease: Single fibre EMG studies of asymmetry, progression and compensatory reinnervation. In Rose, FC (ed): Research Progress in Motor Neuron Disease. Pitman, London, 1984, pp 123–140.

63. Tucker, T, Layzer, RB, Miller, RG, et al: Subacute, reversible motor neuron disease. Neurology 41:1541–1544, 1991.

64. Tysnes, O-B, Vollset, SE, and Aarli, JA: Epidemiology of amyotrophic lateral sclerosis in Hordaland County, western Norway. Acta Neurol Scan 83:280–285, 1991.

65. Tysnes, O-B, Vollset, SE, Larsen, JP, et al: Prognostic factors and survival in amyotrophic lateral sclerosis. Neuroepidemiology 13:225–235, 1994.

66. Uebayashi, Y: Epidemiological investigation of motor neuron disease in the Kii Peninsula, Japan and on Guam: The significance of long survival cases. Wakayama Med Rep 23:13–27, 1980.

67. Wohlfart, G: Collateral reinnervation in partially denervated muscle. Neurology 8:175–180, 1958.

68. World Federation of Neurology Research Group on Neuromuscular Diseases Subcommittee on Motor Neuron Disease: El Escorial World Federation of Neurology criteria for the diagnosis of amyotrophic lateral sclerosis. J Neurol Sci 124(suppl):96–107, 1994.

CHAPTER 10

FAMILIAL ALS

FAMILIAL ALS THAT MIMICS SPORADIC
  ALS
AUTOSOMAL-DOMINANT FAMILIAL ALS
Cu, Zn Superoxide Dismutase (*SOD1*) Gene
  Mutation
Non-*SOD1*-Linked Familial ALS
AUTOSOMAL-RECESSIVE FAMILIAL ALS
Autosomal-Recessive *SOD1* Mutation
Chronic Juvenile ALS (2q33-q35-Linked)
Non-*SOD,* Non-2q33-q35-Linked Recessive
  ALS
THE ALS PHENOTYPE IN OTHER
  HEREDITARY DISEASES
Hexosaminidase-A Deficiency
Machado-Joseph Disease
Polyglucosan Body Disease
Disinhibition-Dementia-Parkinsonism-
  Amyotrophy Complex
GENETIC COUNSELING

Familial ALS (FALS) constitutes approximately 5% to 10% of all ALS cases.[28] FALS differs from sporadic ALS in several ways, including occurring equally in males and females, having a younger age of onset, and lower-extremity onset occurring more often (see Chapter 1).[29,49,53] However, these clinical features per se are not specific enough to distinguish FALS from sporadic ALS (see Chapters 4 and 6). (Certain neuropathologic features may also be characteristic of FALS but are not pathognomonic, as discussed in Chapter 11.) The identification of at least one additional family member with ALS in successive generations is essential for establishing the diagnosis of FALS.[36] The World Federation of Neurology El Escorial diagnos-

tic criteria for ALS are applicable for the diagnosis of both sporadic and familial ALS.[51,55]

The recent discovery of the Cu, Zn superoxide dismutase (*SOD1*) gene mutation in a subset of patients with FALS[12,42] has greatly influenced ALS research, management, and genetic counseling. Nevertheless, the *SOD1* mutation accounts for only about 15% of all cases of FALS.[42,46] The genetic abnormalities have not been identified in the remaining patients with FALS. Therefore, neurologists have to rely on clinical and family histories to distinguish most patients with FALS from those with apparently sporadic disease. Table 10–1 lists several forms of

Table 10–1. **DIFFERENTIAL
DIAGNOSES AND CLASSIFICATION
OF FAMILIAL ALS AND HEREDITARY
ALS PHENOTYPES**

"Sporadic-appearing" ALS
Autosomal-dominant FALS
  SOD1 mutations
  Non-*SOD1* FALS
Autosomal-recessive FALS
  Recessive *SOD1* mutation
  Chronic juvenile ALS (2q33-q35-linked)
  Non-*SOD1*, non-2q33-q35-linked recessive ALS
ALS phenotypes in other hereditary diseases
  Hexosaminidase-A deficiency
  Spinocerebellar ataxia, Machado-Joseph disease
  Polyglucosan body disease
  Disinhibition-dementia-parkinsonism-amyotrophy
    complex

Abbreviation: *SOD1* = superoxide dismutase-1.

FALS and the ALS phenotypes appearing in hereditary neurodegenerative disorders. This chapter reviews the potential difficulties in identifying FALS; the types of FALS, including the forms with *SOD1* mutations; and genetic counseling.

FAMILIAL ALS THAT MIMICS SPORADIC ALS

Patients are diagnosed as having sporadic ALS when there is no definite family history of ALS. Unless patients know that one or more family members have been affected by ALS, a perfunctory review of the family history may miss FALS.[53] In many families, members live in different parts of the country, and thus a complete and accurate family history may be difficult to ascertain. In such situations, a case of FALS might be easily mistaken

for sporadic ALS. In a study by Williams et al.[54] an initial assessment of family history identified FALS in 8% (4/50) of ALS patients. Further investigations, including additional family history from other family members, review of death certificates and medical records, revealed two additional FALS cases (4%) and an additional two cases that were considered probable FALS. His study indicates that the frequency of FALS is probably underestimated.[54] Therefore, a detailed family history, review of death certificates and medical records, and a genealogic study by family members who can undertake such responsibility may be crucial to identify FALS.

Figure 10–1 illustrates hypothetical pedigrees that explain some potential pitfalls and difficulties in identifying FALS. Pedigrees A through D represent typical families in which affected members are diagnosed with sporadic ALS. In pedigrees A and B, no parents

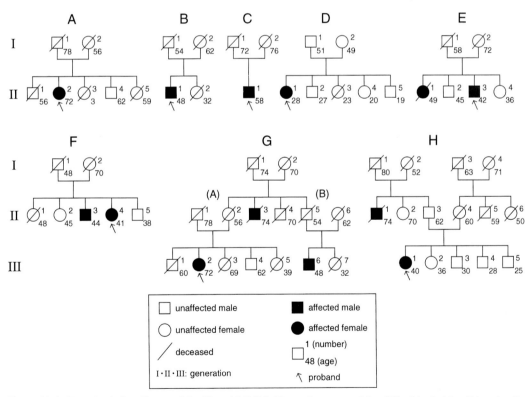

Figure 10–1. Hypothetical pedigrees of families with FALS, illustrating some of the difficulties in identifying the disease. Pedigrees A through D represent typical families in which affected members are misdiagnosed with sporadic ALS. Pedigree G illustrates the situation in which apparently unrelated families (pedigrees A and B) are later found to be related, revealing that FALS is the correct diagnosis for affected members in A and B. Pedigrees E, F, and H show small aggregations of cases that are likely to be FALS, probably with a diminished penetrance.

are living. Some family members (pedigree A, II-3 and pedigree B, II-2) died at an early age, possibly before FALS could manifest. Pedigree C is too small to identify any familial nature of the disease. Pedigree D is somewhat different from the earlier pedigrees because only one 28-year-old individual (II-1) is diagnosed as having ALS. It is possible that she may, in fact, have FALS because the young age of onset is atypical for sporadic ALS, and some of her siblings may be in the preclinical stages of FALS. Concurrently, her relatively young parents may be in the preclinical stages of FALS. Full ascertainment of this family should include a detailed family history of the parents' siblings and the grandparents' families. Clinicians also need to be aware that apparently unrelated families may actually be part of a larger family.[17,47] Pedigree G illustrates just such an example: pedigrees A and B were later found to be related members of G. A detailed family history reveals that II-3 of pedigree G died of ALS. In this way, II-2 of pedigree A (now III-2 of pedigree G) and II-1 of pedigree B (now III-6 of pedigree G) are diagnosed as having FALS. II-2 and II-5 of pedigree G must be the obligate carriers of the FALS gene.

Occasionally a small aggregation of family members with ALS occurs, as illustrated in pedigrees E and F. Does such an aggregation result from chance alone, recessive inheritance, or dominant inheritance with low penetrance? Because ALS is responsible for approximately 1 in 800 of all deaths, chance alone is unlikely to account for the observed aggregation in these families.[53] Unless there is consanguinity between parents, autosomal-recessive inheritance is also unlikely in these pedigrees. Both parents in pedigrees E and F are deceased, and it is always possible that if they had lived longer, the disease may have been expressed. Although one cannot establish definitively the inheritance pattern in pedigrees E and F, autosomal-dominant inheritance appears to be most likely. Families having an aggregation of two or more ALS cases may well represent fragmented pedigrees that belong to a larger FALS pedigree.[53,54]

Pedigree H represents another type of familial aggregation involving two individuals in two consecutive generations but who are not offspring of first-degree relatives with ALS. ALS occurred in the proband III-1 and an uncle of the proband, II-1. The proband's father, II-3, is probably a carrier who is in the preclinical stage. Other siblings of the 40-year-old proband III-1 are likely to have preclinical FALS also. Unless a detailed family history is available, FALS can be easily missed in this type of pedigree.

Pedigrees E though H have a pattern suggesting autosomal-dominant inheritance with diminished penetrance, as implied in pedigrees G and H. The average ages of onset in these families are comparable to those in sporadic motor neuron disease. Low penetrance appears to be related to a higher average age at disease onset (pedigree G), so abnormal-gene carriers have an increased likelihood of dying from other causes before developing motor neuron disease. When penetrance is low, the family history may be insufficient for diagnosis of FALS or a determination of "no family history" may be made, and thus an individual with ALS may be mistakenly considered to have sporadic disease.

Although lack of a complete family history is a major reason FALS is underestimated,[54] genetically determined ALS may be expressed in what appears to be a sporadic form. Possible explanations for this lack of familial aggregation are listed in Table 10–2.[46] Even if the disease is transmitted by an autosomal-dominant gene, the disease may manifest in only a small proportion of patients if gene penetrance is low.[5,17] If ALS is caused by oligogenic inheritance, that is, disease expression that requires the combination of certain responsible genes, it may appear to

Table 10–2. **REASONS FOR A LACK OF FAMILIAL AGGREGATION IN FAMILIAL ALS**

- Modified autosomal-dominant inheritance (diminished penetrance)
- Other modes of inheritance
    Oligogenic
    Multigenic
    Recessive
    Mitochondrial
    New mutation or other genetic change
- Gene-environment interactions
- Common environmental exposure

be sporadic because not all the oligogenic genes are expressed in all the family members. Similarly, if the ALS is caused by multigenic genes, it is manifested in a limited number of patients.[17] The genetic predisposition to a disease is thought to reflect the cumulative effect of genetic variation at several and many loci, each with a small effect on phenotype.[17]

When a hereditary disease is expressed in only one member of the immediate family or in a very few members of a remote kindred, the gene may be recessive. However, the lack of consanguinity in the parents of most patients who develop sporadic ALS speaks against recessive inheritance in the majority of FALS cases. Another unlikely possibility is mitochondrial inheritance. Although mitochondrial inheritance may be one of multiple genetic factors involved in ALS, it is unlikely because ALS is not maternally inherited. Also, the sudden appearance of a rare disease can be caused by a spontaneous genetic event, such as mutation. New mutations of *SOD1* have been claimed in several independent families, in which other family members were apparently not affected by ALS,[22–24] but detailed DNA studies were not performed in these members.

Expression of ALS can be the result of genetic and environmental interactions. A multifactorial threshold model suggests that environmental triggers of disease are most likely to have a major impact on genetically predisposed individuals.[17] Searching for environmental triggers of multifactorial disease should be most fruitful when the search focuses on those at highest risk. Identifying these individuals should aid in determining the environmental components in multifactorial illnesses[17] (see Chapter 2).

ALS and various types of spinal muscular atrophy have been reported in the same pedigrees.[4,26,43,52] Because neuropathologic studies were not available in these cases, it is uncertain whether these motor neuron diseases are not simply atypical FALS. It is also possible that the interaction between genetic susceptibility and environmental factors results in ALS in some and spinal muscular atrophy in other members of these families.[17]

Genetic susceptibility is also suspected in ALS, dementia, and Parkinson's disease. The risk for dementia was higher in the relatives of patients with FALS or sporadic ALS than in other families without ALS.[32] The risk of Parkinson's disease is higher in relatives of patients with FALS than in relatives of patients with sporadic ALS.[32] Such findings suggest that these three conditions may share the same genetic susceptibility. Another intriguing finding is that five of 356 patients with sporadic ALS had an allelic variant of C-terminal with a slightly larger molecular size, and repeated amino acid profile Lys-Ser-Pro has been identified.[15] This revealed a 1 or 34 codon deletion in these five patients. Such molecular variation in a small proportion of patients with sporadic ALS may explain different genetic susceptibilities in patients who develop sporadic ALS,[15] but this mutation has not been confirmed by other investigators.[52a]

AUTOSOMAL-DOMINANT FAMILIAL ALS

Most FALS is autosomal-dominantly inherited. Age appears to be the defining characteristic of autosomal-dominant FALS. According to Williams et al.,[54] the age of onset is 47.5 ± 12.9 years in FALS patients ($n = 43$) with strong aggregation (if each affected individual has an affected parent). On the other hand, 59 ± 12.3 years ($n = 33$) is the average age of onset when aggregation is weak, that is, when ALS is found in the siblings only. This trend is also confirmed by other reports.[29,49,53] The weak aggregation is produced by the death of carriers of an FALS gene from common conditions associated with aging before they develop symptomatic ALS.

Cu, Zn Superoxide Dismutase (*SOD1*) Gene Mutation

Only 2 years after a large collaborative study group for FALS in the United States identified a linkage to a region on chromosome 21 (q22.1-22.2),[10,47] Rosen and colleagues, the same collaborative group,[42] found mutations in the *SOD1* gene. Nearly 50 different *SOD1* missense mutations have been identified in families with ALS.[2,3,12,20,25,38,46]

It is estimated that approximately 15% of all FALS cases are caused by *SOD1* mutations; the inheritance pattern is autosomal-dominant.

SOD1 is a cytosolic metalloenzyme containing tightly bound copper and zinc atoms; it converts superoxide anion ($O_2 \cdot ^-$) to hydrogen peroxide and oxygen. Other *SOD* enzymes are mitochondrial *SOD* (*SOD2*) and serum *SOD* (*SOD3*). The mechanisms underlying motor neuron degeneration in the setting of the *SOD1* mutations has been extensively investigated in the past few years[8,11] (see Chapter 12). The gene encoding the *SOD1* protein consists of 5 exons and 153 codons.[44] Some of the well-recognized missense mutations are depicted in Figure 10–2. The most common mutation, constituting more than 40% of all mutations, occurs at exon 1 in codon 4. In this mutation, the middle position cytosine (C), of the guanine-cytosine-cytosine code for alanine, is replaced with thymine (T), resulting in GTC to encode valine. This change is represented as Ala4→Val or A4V.[25,42] Other mutations are Glu100→Gly and Gly85→Arg,[25] involving only three families. Ile 113→Thr is the next most frequent type of mutation after A4V.[45]

Figure 10–3 shows the typical FALS pedigree with an *SOD1* mutation. A new *SOD1* mutation found in this pedigree also has been reported.[12] This FALS phenotype is characterized by a predominance of lower motor neuron signs over upper motor neuron signs. The mother (II-1) of the proband, who declined a neurologic examination, reportedly has had gait problems. An *SOD1* gene analysis study identified her to be the abnormal gene carrier.

Extensive studies of patients with *SOD1* mutations show that the disease has 90%

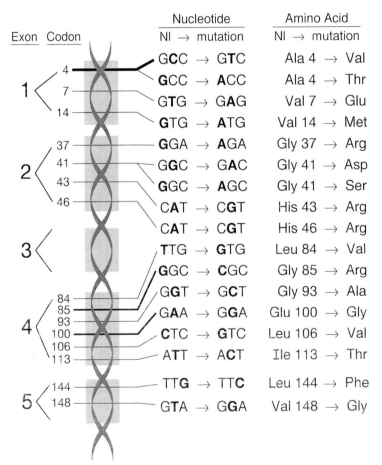

Figure 10–2. Schematic presentation of superoxide dismutase 1 (*SOD1*) gene consisting of 5 exons. The sites of identified mutations are grouped by codon number. The mutation at codon 4 (the thickest line) indicates the most frequently encountered mutation, and two thicker lines at codons 85 and 100 indicate mutations that occur more frequently than others. Bases: A = adenine; C = cytosine; G = guanine; and T = thymine. Boldface letters indicate the site of missense mutation; Nl = normal.

Exon	Codon	Nucleotide Nl → mutation	Amino Acid Nl → mutation
1	4	GCC → GTC	Ala 4 → Val
	4	GCC → ACC	Ala 4 → Thr
	7	GTG → GAG	Val 7 → Glu
	14	GTG → ATG	Val 14 → Met
2	37	GGA → AGA	Gly 37 → Arg
	41	GGC → GAC	Gly 41 → Asp
	43	GGC → AGC	Gly 41 → Ser
	46	CAT → CGT	His 43 → Arg
		CAT → CGT	His 46 → Arg
3		TTG → GTG	Leu 84 → Val
		GGC → CGC	Gly 85 → Arg
4	84	GGT → GCT	Gly 93 → Ala
	85	GAA → GGA	Glu 100 → Gly
	93	CTC → GTC	Leu 106 → Val
	100	ATT → ACT	Ile 113 → Thr
	106		
	113		
5	144	TTG → TTC	Leu 144 → Phe
	148	GTA → GGA	Val 148 → Gly

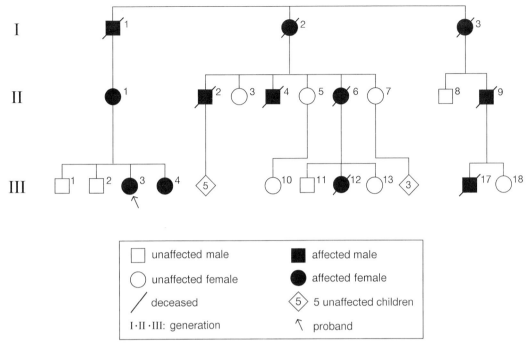

Figure 10–3. A typical pedigree of *SOD1*-linked familial ALS. The proband is a 42-year-old woman (arrow) who has had predominantly lower motor neuron signs and hyperreflexia for 3 years. Her mother, an obligate gene carrier who declined physical examination, underwent an *SOD1* gene study that confirmed she is affected. A new *SOD1* mutation in this pedigree has been reported.[12]

penetrance at age 70, so penetrance is clearly age-related[46] (Teepu Siddique, MD, Northwestern University, Chicago, personal communication, 1996). However, recent reports suggest that the Ile113→Thr mutation may have a markedly reduced penetrance.[24,50] Age of onset is essentially identical in all types of *SOD1* mutations[25] (Fig. 10–4A). The mean age at onset of *SOD*-linked FALS is 47.6 ± 13.7 years (n = 158), which is considerably younger than that of sporadic ALS[29,49,53] (see Chapter 2). The most common mutation, Ala4→Val, is characterized by the shortest disease duration (approximately 1 year),[25,41] whereas the mean duration of all FALS cases is 3.5 ± 4.6 years in one study[25] and 2.5 ± 1.9 years in another study.[41] In other mutations, such as Ala4→Thr and His43→Arg, disease duration also is short, being approximately 1 year. In contrast, the Glu100→Gly mutation is associated with a prolonged disease duration (5.1 ± 3.3 years) (Fig. 10–4B). The mutations in exon 2, such as Gly37→Arg and His46→Arg, have an average disease course of 17 to 18 years.[25]

Therefore, the specific type of *SOD1* mutation determines disease duration and provides important prognostic information for patients with *SOD1*-linked FALS.

Most testing for *SOD1* gene mutation is still performed at the two major ALS genetic research laboratories: the laboratories of Robert Brown, MD, at Massachusetts General Hospital, Boston, and of Teepu Siddique, MD, at Northwestern University, Chicago, but such studies may now be arranged through commercial laboratories, who will contract with a research laboratory. The decision to order this molecular genetic study should be made with care because the test is laborious and has potential ethical implications.

Table 10–3 lists the indications for *SOD1* genetic studies. The test should be ordered to identify *SOD1* mutations in patients who are diagnosed or strongly suspected to have FALS. A negative result only indicates that the patient does not have an *SOD1* mutation and obviously does not address the question of whether the patient has FALS. When the

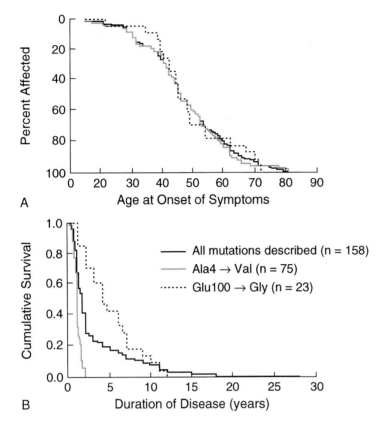

A

B

Figure 10–4. (*Top*) Kaplan-Meier curves for patients with point mutations in *SOD1* (in years). Age of onset is identical in different mutations. (*Bottom*) Kaplan-Meier survival function for patients with point mutations in *SOD1*. The curve shows that virtually all patients with the Ala4→Val mutations died within 2 years of symptom onset (mean 1.0 year), whereas 75% of patients with the Glu100→Gly were alive 2 years after onset of symptoms. The 50% survival of all patients with any *SOD1* mutation is approximately 2 years, and the mean duration of disease is 3.5±4.6 years (Redrawn from Juneja T,[25] page 56, used with permission of Lippincott Raven Publishers.)

ALS is clinically atypical and FALS is suspected, as shown in Figure 10–1, pedigree D, or when the family history is very limited (pedigree C), an *SOD1* genetic study can be performed. A negative result does not exclude the possibility of FALS that is not linked to an *SOD1* mutation.

SOD1 genetic testing can be used for genetic counseling in families in which *SOD1* mutations are already established. Neurologists ordering such tests should be aware that a presymptomatic diagnosis of FALS is likely to be extremely distressing to those with the mutation, so expert genetic counseling before and after testing is essential.[5,17]

Table 10–3. INDICATIONS FOR *SOD1* MOLECULAR STUDIES IN PATIENTS WITH ALS

Necessary

- When the patient has familial ALS and testing for an *SOD1* mutation has not been performed.
- When a potential aggregation of patients is found in the family, as shown in Fig. 10–2, pedigrees E through H.

Optional

- When a full family history is not available, as seen in Fig. 10–1, pedigrees B and C, particularly when the patient is unusually young.
- Presymptomatic testing of family members of the patient with FALS with an *SOD1* mutation who are determined to know their own *SOD1* genetic status.

Non-*SOD1*-Linked Familial ALS

The rest of autosomal-dominant FALS, probably more than 80% of patients with FALS, have autosomal-dominant, non-*SOD1*-related FALS. Until the genes responsible for these non-*SOD1*-linked FALS cases are identified, we will not know the molecular cause of most autosomal-dominant FALS cases. Further gene linkage studies of many FALS families are essential.[9,16,47] If patients give consent to molecular genetic studies, DNA samples from patients with FALS and their family members should be banked for future analyses. Large American and European FALS collaborative study groups have been established to accomplish this genetic research.[9,10,45,51]

AUTOSOMAL-RECESSIVE FAMILIAL ALS

Autosomal-Recessive *SOD1* Mutation

One of the *SOD* mutations, Asp90→Ala, has been known for some time in American patients.[46] However, it was recently reported as a recessive form in a Scandinavian population.[1] An identical mutation found in Belgium was clinically expressed in patients who were heterozygous for this mutation and thought to have sporadic ALS.[39] Why the same mutation is expressed in homozygous patients in one population and in heterozygous patients in another population is unknown.[39,48] Careful DNA studies of all involved family members appear to be crucial in resolving such questions.

Chronic Juvenile ALS (2q33-q35-Linked)

A motor neuron disease syndrome characterized by upper motor neuron signs, muscle atrophy, generalized fasciculations, bulbar and pseudobulbar signs, and normal sensory findings has been reported predominantly in Tunisians.[6] This autosomal-recessive condition, named chronic juvenile ALS, has a mean age of onset of 12.1 years with a range from 3 to 25 years. Recent genetic studies have located a linkage to chromosome 2q33-q35.[18] The disease progresses slowly for many years.

Non-*SOD,* Non-2q33-q35-Linked Recessive ALS

There are likely to be rare recessive forms of ALS that have eluded our recognition, es-pecially in cases in which knowledge of the family history is limited, as discussed above (see Fig. 10–1).

THE ALS PHENOTYPE IN OTHER HEREDITARY DISEASES

Clinical features suggesting ALS, or at least an ALS phenotype, can be found in several hereditary disorders. In none of these disorders, however, does the ALS phenotype appear to be the sole manifestation of the disease. Instead, it is one of multiple manifestations of disease affecting the CNS.

Hexosaminidase-A Deficiency

Adult-onset, hexosaminidase-A deficiency is caused by a missense mutation involving the α subunit of hexosaminidase-A encoded on chromosome 15q. Multiple point mutations have been reported. For example, the homozygous mutation Gly269→Ser occurs in both Ashkenazi-Jewish and non-Jewish populations with this disorder. However, a compound heterozygote mutation involving the same Gly269→Ser in one allele and an unidentified mutation in the α subunit in the other allele have been found only in the non-Jewish population.[37] The phenotypic expression of this motor neuron disease ranges from spinal muscular atrophy[21] to a juvenile ALS phenotype.[35] In most cases of adult-onset hexosaminidase-A deficiency, motor neuron disease is only one aspect of a multisystem disorder (see Chapter 6).

Machado-Joseph Disease

As described in Chapter 6, the main clinical feature of autosomal-dominant Machado-Joseph disease is spinocerebellar ataxia. However, the neurologic manifestations may vary markedly and include generalized dystonia, external ophthalmoplegia, proptosis, pyramidal signs, distal amyotrophy, bulbar palsy, and other brain-stem signs, and fasciculations. An ALS phenotype can also be found in some patients with Machado-Joseph disease.[27,33] An abnormal expansion of a cytosine-adenine-guanine trinucleotide repeat has been found on chromosome 14q32.1.[34]

Polyglucosan Body Disease

Polyglucosan body disease is probably an autosomal-recessive disorder. Axons and neural sheath cells contain periodic acid-Schiff positive polyglucosan bodies (see Chapter 11). These patients develop progressive upper motor neuron and lower motor neuron signs, marked sensory loss, and neurogenic bladder.[40] No genetic analyses have been performed. The condition is rare and poorly understood.

Disinhibition-Dementia-Parkinsonism-Amyotrophy Complex

An autosomal-dominant disease characterized clinically by progressive "childish" disinhibited behavior, dementia, parkinsonian extrapyramidal manifestations, amyotrophy, and fasciculations has been reported.[31] Autopsy studies showed widespread neuronal loss in the substantia nigra, cerebral cortex, and anterior horn of the spinal cord; also, extensive spongy degeneration in the temporal and frontal lobes is highly characteristic. The disease appears linked to chromosome 17q21-23.[31] The name proposed for this disease is Wilhelmsen-Lynch disease.[14]

GENETIC COUNSELING

Genetic counseling must be offered to patients with FALS and their family members. Because of the serious nature of the disease and the enormous negative impact on patients and their families, the diagnosis of FALS must be established with caution. When FALS is autosomal-dominant, it is also crucial to determine if it is caused by an SOD1 mutation (see Table 10–3). Such information is essential before accurate genetic counseling can be provided.[7] The American Society of Human Genetics defines genetic counseling as:[13]

A communication process which deals with the human problems associated with the occurrence, or the risk of occurrence, of a genetic disorder in a family. This process involves an attempt by one or more appropriately trained persons to help the individual or family to:

(1) comprehend the medical facts, including the diagnosis, probable course of the disorder, and the available management;
(2) appreciate the way heredity contributes to the disorder, and the risk of recurrence in specified relatives;
(3) understand the alternatives for dealing with the risk of recurrence;
(4) choose the course of action which seems to them appropriate in view of their risk, their family goals, and their ethical and religious standards, and to act in accordance with that decision; and
(5) make the best possible adjustment to the disorder in an affected family member and/or to the risk of recurrence of that disorder.

Genetic counseling for patients with FALS and their families is particularly difficult because ALS is in almost all cases an inexorably progressive disease without cure. If patients are young and wish to have a family, genetic counseling with regard to childbearing becomes important. The chance that children with an affected parent have inherited the FALS gene is 50%. Their options are to not have children, to have one child or two children, to disregard the risk completely, or to examine alternatives such as adoption.[17] At present, a prenatal diagnostic test for SOD1 mutation is not available (Teepu Siddique, MD, Northwestern University, personal communication, 1996). In female patients who have elected to have children, uneventful pregnancies and deliveries have been reported.[30] However, the complex nature of this disease, particularly the progressive neurologic deterioration and shorter life expectancy, may make child-rearing arduous. When considering whether to start a family, patients with ALS and their spouses need to consider carefully the increased burdens children will bring and that, unless the surviving parent remarries, they will be raised by only one parent.

The diagnosis of FALS also has a great impact on the unaffected siblings and the children of patients. In a family with FALS that has a well-established autosomal-dominant inheritance, the probability that siblings and

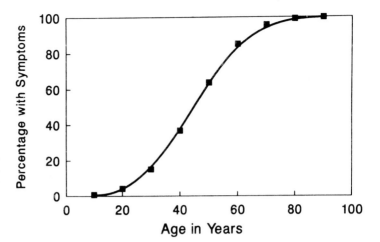

Figure 10–5. Age curve showing percentage of FALS patients with onset of symptoms at various ages ($n = 55$). (From Siddique, T: Molecular genetics of familial amyotrophic lateral sclerosis. In Rowland, LP [ed]: Amyotrophic Lateral Sclerosis and Other Motor Neuron Disease. Adv Neurol 56:228, 1991, with permission.)

children will develop FALS is 50%. The probability that a carrier of the mutated gene will develop the disease increases with age[45] (Fig. 10–5).

The greatest issue in genetic counseling at present is presymptomatic diagnosis.[7] *SOD1* gene tests will become progressively more simple and widely available for family members. However, the psychologic and ethical impact is a major challenge because the diagnosis of FALS means a progressive, paralyzing disease that may evolve over just a few years. If otherwise healthy individuals are given a presymptomatic diagnosis of FALS, they may greatly fear the later appearance of FALS to the extent that the fear itself becomes debilitating. According to the experience of patients with Huntington's disease and their families, those with a presymptomatic diagnosis can develop a disturbed perception of the self that may be associated with depression and risk of suicide.[5,19] Furthermore, a positive presymptomatic diagnosis not only has a psychologic impact on the individual but also affects insurance coverage, employment, and perception of the person by family and peers. These and other unforeseen social and ethical issues will be raised as molecular diagnostic tests become available for FALS and other diseases.

Individuals who want to know their *SOD1* gene status must receive thorough genetic counseling before the test is performed. Despite careful counseling, many individuals experience great psychologic stress. Presymptomatic individuals who are found to

have the *SOD1* mutation often start looking for signs of the disease (Teepu Siddique, MD, and Jocelyn Kaplan, MA, genetic counselor, Northwestern University, personal communication, 1996). Such behavioral patterns have occurred in families with Huntington's disease, and in the immediate family members of patients with FALS, even if they do not know if they are affected. Unexpectedly, family members of the patients with *SOD1*-linked FALS who are found to have no *SOD1* mutation also experience psychological distress. They appear to undergo a difficult psychological adjustment involving survivor's guilt, owing to the fact that they do not have to worry about FALS (Jocelyn Kaplan, MA, personal communication, 1996). Genetic counselors thus must work closely with neurologists to provide optimal counseling for families in which FALS may exist. A special guide and instructions are available from FALS genetic centers for neurologists and genetic counselors who are not familiar with genetic counseling for FALS.

SUMMARY

Patients are diagnosed as having FALS rather than sporadic ALS when a definite family history of ALS exists. FALS is believed to account for only 5% to 10% of all ALS patients, but for several reasons, this figure may be an underestimate: (1) a perfunctory taking of the family history may miss a history of ALS in other family members; (2) the patient may lack information about ALS in the family; and (3) even in families with aggregation of cases, insufficient information about the extended family may lead to a diagnosis of sporadic ALS. A detailed family history, review of death certificates and medical records, and a genealogic study by family members are essential. FALS can be mistaken for sporadic ALS for other, less common reasons, including low penetrance of autosomal-dominant inheritance, control of ALS expression by oligogenic or multigenic genes, and recessive inheritance. Interaction between genetic predisposition and environmental factors also may affect FALS expression.

Dementia and Parkinson's disease appear to occur with FALS or sometimes sporadic ALS, suggesting that FALS, dementia, and Parkinson's disease all share a common genetic defect. ALS also occurs in families with a history of spinal muscular atrophy; some of these cases may be atypical FALS. Finally, sporadic ALS itself may have a genetic component.

The clinical features of FALS and sporadic ALS are the same, with the exception that the age of onset in FALS is much earlier. Most FALS cases have autosomal-dominant inheritance; recessive inheritance appears to be rare. The only genetic defects identified thus far involve missense mutation in the *SOD1* gene: about 15% of all FALS cases have such a mutation, and nearly 50 *SOD1* mutations have been identified. The type of mutation appears to determine the duration of disease. Patients with the most common *SOD1* mutation, Ala4→Val at codon 4 in axon 1, have the shortest duration, about 1 year. Some mutations are associated with a markedly prolonged duration of the disease.

Several unusual hereditary neurodegenerative disorders may produce an ALS phenotype as part of a multisystem degeneration and thus should be considered in the differential diagnosis of FALS. These include hexosaminidase-A deficiency, Machado-Joseph disease, polyglucosan body disease, and disinhibition-dementia-parkinsonism-amyotrophy complex.

For *SOD1* mutation, genetic testing is available and should be given to patients who clearly have FALS or who have ALS that occurs in an aggregation in the family, clinically atypical ALS, or what appears to be sporadic ALS with an incomplete family history. The decision to have children may be a major issue, especially given the young age of onset. Genetic counseling is equally important for siblings and the children of patients as for the patients, and when *SOD1* mutation is involved, presymptomatic testing of the family members can be done. However, one must remember that the psychologic and emotional impact of such a diagnosis in otherwise healthy people may be much greater than anticipated. Thorough and experienced genetic counseling is essential before the testing and long after the results are given.

REFERENCES

1. Andersen, PM, Nilsson, P, Ala-Hurula, V, et al: Amyotrophic lateral sclerosis associated with homozygosity for an Asp90Ala mutation in CuZn-superoxide dismutase. Nature Gen 10:61–66, 1995.
2. Aoki, M, Abe, K, Houi, K, et al: Variance of age at onset in a Japanese family with amyotrophic lateral sclerosis associated with a novel Cu/Zn superoxide dismutase mutation. Ann Neurol 37:676–679, 1995.
3. Aoki, M, Ogasawara, M, Matsubara, Y, et al: Familial amyotrophic lateral sclerosis (ALS) in Japan associated with H46R mutation in Cu/Zu superoxide dismutase gene: A possible new subtype of familial ALS. J Neurol Sci 126:77–83, 1994.
4. Appelbaum, JS, Roos, RP, Salazar-Grueso, EF, et al: Intrafamilial heterogeneity in hereditary motor neuron disease. Neurology 42:1488–1492, 1992.
5. Baraitser, M: The Genetics of Neurological Disorders. Oxford, London, 1985, pp 230–237.
6. Ben Hamida, M, Hentati, F, and Ben Hamida, C: Hereditary motor system diseases (chronic juvenile amyotrophic lateral sclerosis). Brain 113:347–363, 1990.
7. Bird, TD and Bennett, RL: Why do DNA testing? Practical and ethical implications of new neurogenetic tests. Ann Neurol 38:141–146, 1995.
8. Borchelt, DR, Lee, MK, Slunt, HS, et al: Superoxide dismutase 1 with mutations linked to familial amyotrophic lateral sclerosis possesses significant activity. Proc Nat Acad Sci 91:8292–8296, 1994.
9. Brown, RH, Horvitz, HR, Rouleau, GA, et al: Gene linkage in familial amyotrophic lateral sclerosis: A progress report. Adv Neurol 56:215–226, 1991.
10. Conneally, PM: A first step toward a molecular genetic analysis of amyotrophic lateral sclerosis. N Engl J Med 324:1430–1432, 1991.
11. Deng, H-X, Hentati, A, Trainer, JA, et al: Amyotrophic lateral sclerosis and structural defects in Cu/Zn superoxide dismutase. Science 261:1047–1051, 1993.
12. Deng, H-X, Tainer, JA, Mitsumoto, H, et al: Two novel SOD1 mutations in patients with familial amyotrophic lateral sclerosis. Hum Mol Genet 4:1113–1116, 1995.

13. Epstein, CJ: Genetic counseling. Am J Hum Genet 27:240–242, 1975.

14. Fahn, S, Mayeux, R, and Rowland, LP: A new eponym: Wilhelmsen-Lynch disease. Neurology 44:1980, 1994.

15. Figlewicz, DA, Krizus, A, Martinoli, MG, et al: Variants of the heavy neurofilament subunit are associated with the development of amyotrophic lateral sclerosis. Hum Mol Genet 3:1757–1761, 1994.

16. Figlewicz, DA and Rouleau, GA: Familial disease. In Williams AC (ed): Motor Neuron Disease. Chapman & Hall Medical, London, 1994, pp 427–450.

17. Gelehrter, TD and Collins, FS: Principles of Medical Genetics. Baltimore: Williams & Wilkins, Baltimore, 1990, pp 27–65.

18. Hentati, A, Bejaoui, K, Pericak-Vance, MA, et al: Linkage of recessive familial amyotrophic lateral sclerosis to chromosome 2q33-q35. Nature Genet 7:425–428, 1994.

19. Hersch, S, Jones, R, Koroshetz, W, et al: The neurogenetics genie: Testing for the Huntington's disease mutation. Neurology 44:1369–1373, 1994.

20. Hirano, M, Fujii, J, Hagai, Y, et al: A new variant Cu/Zn superoxide dismutase (Val^7→Glu) deduced from lymphocyte mRNA sequences from Japanese patients with familial amyotrophic lateral sclerosis. Biochem Biophys Res Comm 204:572–577, 1994.

21. Johnson, WG, Wigger, HJ, Karp, HR, et al: Juvenile spinal muscular atrophy: A new hexosaminidase deficiency phenotype. Ann Neurol 11:11–16, 1982.

22. Jones, CT, Brock, DJH, Chancellor, AM, et al: Cu/Zn superoxide dismutase (SOD1) mutations and sporadic amyotrophic lateral sclerosis. Lancet 342:1050–1051, 1993.

23. Jones, CT, Shaw, PJ, Chari, G, et al: Identification of a novel exon 4 SOD1 mutation in a sporadic amyotrophic lateral sclerosis patient. Mol Cell Prob 8:329–330, 1994.

24. Jones, CT, Swinger, RJ, and Brock, DJH: Identification of a novel SOD1 mutation in an apparently sporadic amyotrophic lateral sclerosis patient and the detection of Ile113Thr in three others. Hum Mol Genet 3:649–650, 1994.

25. Juneja, T, Pericak-Vance, MA, Laing, NG, et al: Prognosis in familial ALS: Progression and survival in patients with glu100gly and ala4val mutations in Cu,Zn superoxide dismutase. Neurology 48:55–57, 1997.

26. Kaeser, HE and Wurmser, P: Atrophie pseudomyopathique de type Kugelberg-Welander et sclerose laterale amyotrophique. Rev Neurol (Paris) 118:554–555, 1968.

27. Kinoshita, A, Hayashi, MN, Oda, M, et al: Clinicopathological study of the peripheral nervous system in Machado-Joseph disease. J Neurol Sci 130:48–58, 1995.

28. Kurland, LT and Mulder, DW: Epidemiologic investigations of amyotrophic lateral sclerosis. Familial aggregation indicative of dominant inheritance. Neurology 5:182–196, 1955.

29. Li T-M, Alberman, E, and Swash, M: Comparison of sporadic and familial disease amongst 580 cases of motor neuron disease. J Neurol Neurosurg Psychiatry 51:778–784, 1988.

30. Lupo, VR, Rusterholz, JH, Reichert, JA, et al: Amyotrophic lateral sclerosis in pregnancy. Obstet Gynecol 82:682–685, 1993.

31. Lynch, T, Sano, M, Marder, KS, et al: Clinical characteristics of a family with chromosome 17-linked disinhibition-dementia-parkinsonism-amyotrophy complex. Neurology 44:1878–1884, 1994.

32. Majoor-Krakauer, D, Ottman, R, Johnson, WG, et al: Familial aggregation of amyotrophic lateral sclerosis, dementia, and Parkinson's disease: Evidence of shared genetic susceptibility. Neurology 44:1872–1877, 1994.

33. Martin, J-J, Van Regemorter, N, Krols, L, et al: On an autosomal dominant form of retinal-cerebellar degeneration: An autopsy study of five patients in one family. Acta Neuropathol 88:277–286, 1994.

34. Matilla, T, McCall, A, Subramony, SH, et al: Molecular and clinical correlations in spinocerebellar ataxia Type 3 and Machado-Joseph disease. Ann Neurol 38:68–72, 1995.

35. Mitsumoto, H, Sliman, RJ, Schafer, IA, et al: Motor neuron disease and adult hexosaminidase-A deficiency in two families: Evidence for multisystem degeneration. Ann Neurol 17:378–385, 1985.

36. Mulder, DW, Kurland, LT, Offord, KP, et al: Familial adult motor neuron disease: Amyotrophic lateral sclerosis. Neurology 36:511–517, 1986.

37. Navon, R, Kolodny, EH, Mitsumoto, H, et al: Ashkenazi-Jewish and non-Jewish adult G_{M2} gangliosidosis patients share a common genetic defect. Am J Hum Genet 46:817–821, 1990.

38. Rainero, I, Pinessi, L, Tsuda, T, et al: SOD1 missense mutation in an Italian family with ALS. Neurology 44:347–349, 1994.

39. Robberecht, W, Aguirre, T, van den Bosch, L, et al: D90A heterozygosity in the SOD1 gene is associated with familial and apparently sporadic amyotrophic lateral sclerosis. Neurology 47:1336–1339, 1996.

40. Robitaille, Y, Carpenter, S, Karpati, G, et al: A distinct form of adult polyglucosan body disease with massive involvement of central and peripheral neuronal processes and astrocytes. A report of four cases and a review of the occurrence of polyglucosan bodies in other conditions such as LaFora's disease and normal aging. Brain 103:315–336, 1980.

41. Rosen, DR, Bowling, AC, Patterson, D, et al: A frequent ala 4 to val superoxide dismutase-1 mutation is associated with a rapidly progressive familial amyotrophic lateral sclerosis. Hum Mol Genet 3:981–987, 1994.

42. Rosen, DR, Siddique, T, Patterson, D, et al: Mutations in Cu/Zn superoxide dismutase gene are associated with familial amyotrophic lateral sclerosis. Nature 362:59–62, 1993.

43. Shaw, PJ, Ince, PG, Goodship, J, et al: Adult-onset motor neuron disease and infantile Werdnig-Hoffmann disease (spinal muscular atrophy type 1) in the same family. Neurology 42:1477–1480, 1992.

44. Sherman, L, Dafni, N, Leiman-Hurwitz, J, et al: Nucleotide sequence and expression of human chromosome 21-encoded superoxide dismutase mRNA. Proc Nat Acad Sci 80:5465–5469, 1983.

45. Siddique, T: Molecular genetics of familial amyotrophic lateral sclerosis. In Rowland, LP (ed): Amyotrophic Lateral Sclerosis and Other Motor Neuron Disease. Adv Neurol 56, Raven Press, New York, 1991, pp 521–546.

46. Siddique, T and Deng, H–X: Genetics of amyotrophic lateral sclerosis. Hum Mol Genet 5:1465–1470, 1996.

47. Siddique, T, Figlewicz, DA, Pericak-Vance, MA, et al: Linkage of a gene causing familial amyotrophic lateral sclerosis to chromosome 21 and evidence of genetic-locus heterogeneity. N Engl J Med 324:1381–1384, 1991.

48. Själander, A, Backman, G, Deng, H-X, et al: The D90A mutation results in a polymorphism of Cu,Zn superoxide dismutase that is prevalent in northern Sweden and Finland. Hum Mol Gent 4:1105–1108, 1995.

49. Strong, MJ, Hudson, AJ, and Alvord, WG: Familial amyotrophic lateral sclerosis, 1850–1989: A statistical analysis of the world literature. Can J Neurol Sci 18:45–58, 1991.

50. Suthers, G, Laing, N, Wilton, S, et al: "Sporadic" motoneuron disease due to familial SOD1 mutation with low penetrance. Lancet 344:1773, 1994.

51. Swash, M and Leigh, N: Criteria for diagnosis of familial amyotrophic lateral sclerosis. Neuromusc Disord 2:7–9, 1992.

52. Tonali, P and Anepeta, L: Osservazione di un caso di sclerosi laterale amiotrofica e di due casi di amiotrofia prossimale spinale infantile in una stessa famiglia. Riv Neurol 41:196–217, 1971.

52a. Vechio, JD, Bruijn, LI, Xu, Z, et al: Sequence variants in human neurofilament proteins: Absence of linkage to familial amyotrophic lateral sclerosis. Ann Neurol 40:603–610, 1996.

53. Williams, DB: Familial amyotrophic lateral sclerosis. In Smith, RA (ed): Handbook of Amyotrophic Lateral Sclerosis. Marcel Dekker, New York, 1992, pp 39–63.

54. Williams, DB, Floate, DA, and Leicester, J: Familial motor neuron disease: Differing penetrance in large pedigrees. J Neurol Sci 86:215–230, 1988.

55. World Federation of Neurology Subcommittee on Neuromuscular Diseases: El Escorial World Federation of Neurology criteria for the diagnosis of amyotrophic lateral sclerosis. J Neurol Sci 124(suppl): 96–107, 1994.

PART 3

Pathology and Pathogenesis

CHAPTER 11

NEURO-PATHOLOGY

In the past two decades, descriptive neuropathology has expanded our knowledge of ALS, particularly with regard to endemic ALS, the parkinsonism-dementia complex of Guam, and familial ALS (FALS) (see Chapter 1). Recently, investigational postmortem ultrastructural and immunocytochemical studies have defined several critical histopathologic features that provide clues to the pathogenesis of ALS. Knowledge of the descriptive neuropathology of ALS is essential in comprehending the clinical features of the disease, and knowledge of investigational neuropathology is important in understanding the pathogenesis of ALS. In this chapter, we will discuss basic neuropathology of ALS following the World Federation of Neurology diagnostic criteria[150] and touch on recent advances in the investigational neuropathology.

GROSS PATHOLOGY

Gross examination of the brain and spinal cord does not provide the information needed to confirm a diagnosis of ALS (Table 11–1, section A). Focal atrophy of the primary motor cortex may be easily found in some cases without corresponding atrophy in other cortical regions; however, focal atrophy of the motor cortex may not be apparent even in typical cases of ALS.

In the spinal cord, the affected ventral roots appear gray and thin. Judging atrophy of the ventral roots by comparing them with the dorsal roots requires caution because the ventral roots are normally thinner than the dorsal roots. On cross sections of the spinal cord, the lateral columns may appear gray, which suggests sclerotic changes caused by gliosis.

HISTOPATHOLOGY

To establish a pathologic diagnosis of ALS, light microscopy studies must show loss of giant pyramidal cells in the motor cortex, loss of motor neurons in the spinal cord anterior horn and brain stem, abnormal cellular pathology in these motor neurons, and corticospinal tract involvement at the same level where loss of motor neurons is found (Table 11–1, section B).

179

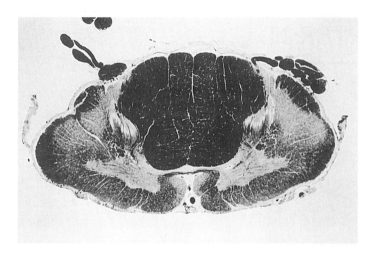

Figure 11–1. Myelin staining of the cervical spinal cord in a patient with ALS shows well-preserved posterior column posterior roots and spinocerebellar tract. There is diffuse pallor of the anterior and lateral columns. Loss of myelin is markedly pronounced in the lateral and anterior corticospinal tracts and anterior roots. (From Hirano, A: Neuropathological aspects of motor neuron disease. In Gourie-Devi, A (ed): Motor Neuron Disease. Global Clinical Patterns and International Research. Oxford & IBH Publishing Co, New Delhi, p 136, 1987, with permission.)

Upper Motor Neuron Involvement

Upper motor neurons by definition include not only neurons in the motor cortex and surrounding cortices but also neurons in the brain stem that exert supranuclear control over the lower motor neurons (see Chapter 2). Histologic abnormalities are predominantly seen in the cerebral cortex. In ALS, large pyramidal motor neurons are diminished in number. The neuronal loss, however, is not confined to the motor cortex—it also involves the surrounding cortices, including the premotor areas, sensory cortex, and temporal cortex. Histometric studies of cortical neurons reveal that neuronal cell bodies atrophy before neuronal death.[72] Golgi stains demonstrate that cortical neurons are sparse and that their dendrites are shortened, fragmented, and disorganized.[36,65,126] Large and small pyramidal cells and the surrounding basket cells show intracellular accumulation of phosphorylated neurofilaments,[140] although such accumulation is seen less frequently than in spinal cord motor neurons. Occasionally, these inclusions are ubiquitinated.[81] These findings suggest not only that the changes found in ALS upper motor neurons differ from those found in other neurodegenerative disorders but also that some changes are similar to those occurring in ALS lower motor neurons.[105,110,116] However, further studies are required to confirm the above findings. Glial cell clusters are also found in the motor cortex. Once they were thought to be unique to ALS,[63,106] but the same changes are now described in other conditions, including aging brains, which suggests they are nonspecific.[140]

Corticospinal Tract Involvement

The corticospinal tracts are abnormal in ALS. Myelin stain of the spinal cord shows typical pallor because of demyelination in the lateral and uncrossed ventral corticospinal tracts (Fig. 11–1). Demyelination is secondary to axonal degeneration of descending large myelinated fibers. Microscopically, gliosis and digested lipid deposits are found. Early myelin breakdown can be shown well with the Marchi method,[131,137] and corticospinal tract involvement can readily be detected below the medulla. Axonal swellings, or spheroids (see below), containing packed neurofilamentous material and other cellular debris are present in the corticospinal tracts, particularly between the internal capsule and the bulbar pyramids.[15,115]

Lower Motor Neuron Involvement

In the spinal cord, loss of large motor neurons in the anterior horn should be clearly identified when confirming the diagnosis of ALS (see Table 11–1). In the lower brain stem, particularly in the hypoglossal nucleus,

Table 11–1. **EL ESCORIAL WORLD FEDERATION OF NEUROLOGY CRITERIA FOR THE DIAGNOSIS OF ALS**

A. GROSS PATHOLOGIC CHANGES

Features That Support the Diagnosis

1. Selective atrophy of the motor cortex
2. Grayness and atrophy of the anterior spinal nerve roots compared with normal roots
3. Grayness of the lateral columns of the spinal cord
4. Atrophy of skeletal muscles

Features That Rule Out the Diagnosis of ALS or Suggest the Presence of Additional Disease

1. Plaques of multiple sclerosis
2. A focal cause of myelopathy

B. LIGHT MICROSCOPIC STUDIES

Features Required for the Diagnosis

1. Some degree of loss of both of the following neuronal systems. Large motor neurons of the anterior horns of the spinal cord and motor nuclei of the brain stem (V motor, VII motor, IX and X somatic motor, and XII); and large pyramidal neurons of the motor cortex, and/or large myelinated axons of the corticospinal tracts.
2. The following cellular pathologic changes in the involved neuronal regions described above: Neuronal atrophy with relative increase in lipofuscin and loss of Nissl substance. There should be evidence of different stages of the process of neuronal degeneration, including the presence of normal-appearing neurons, even in the same region.
3. Evidence of degeneration of the corticospinal tracts at the same level.

Features That Strongly Support the Diagnosis

1. Lack of pathologic change in the motor neurons of cranial nerves III, IV, and VI; the intermediolateral column of the spinal cord; and Onufrowicz nucleus.
2. The occurrence of one or more of the following cellular pathologic changes in the involved neuronal systems described above:
   - Axonal spheroids with accumulation of masses of neurofilaments.
   - Bunina bodies
   - Basophilic cytoplasmic inclusions
   - Nonbasophilic hyaline bodies ("Lewy-body-like structures") seen in hematoxylin and eosin–stained sections.
   - Increased immunocytochemical staining for phosphorylated neurofilaments in perikarya of the motor neurons
   - Ubiquitinated intracytoplasmic inclusions in the motor neurons
   - Atrophy or loss of the arborization of the dendrites of the motor neurons of the anterior horns of the spinal cord and the brain stem motor nuclei.

Features That Are Compatible With and Do Not Exclude the Diagnosis

1. Variable involvement of the Clarke's nucleus and the spinocerebellar tracts, the posterior root ganglia, the posterior columns of the spinal cord, peripheral sensory nerves, the brain stem reticular neurons, the anterolateral columns of the spinal cord, the thalamus, the subthalamic nucleus, and the substantia nigra.

Features That Rule Out the Diagnosis or Suggest the Presence of Additional Disease

1. Major pathologic involvement of other parts of the nervous system, including: cerebral cortex other than the motor cortex, basal ganglia, substantia nigra, cerebellum, cranial nerves II and VIII, and dorsal root ganglia.

Continued on following page

Table 11–1—*continued*

2. The following cellular pathologic changes in the involved neuronal systems described above:
   - Extensive central chromatolysis
   - Extensive active neuronophagia
   - Neurofibrillary tangles
   - The presence of abnormal storage material
   - The presence of significant spongiform change
   - The presence of extensive inflammatory cell infiltration

C. ELECTRON MICROSCOPY STUDIES (Ultrastructural studies are not required for the diagnosis of ALS)

Features That Strongly Support the Diagnosis
1. Accumulation of the interwoven bundles of 10-nm neurofilaments in axonal spheroids or motor neuron perikarya and thicker linear structures associated with dense granules
2. Bunina bodies

Features That Are Compatible With and Do Not Exclude the Diagnosis
1. The presence of intra-axonal polyglucosan bodies

Features That Rule Out the Diagnosis or Suggest the Presence of Additional Disease
1. The presence of significant numbers of definitive viral particles
2. The presence of significant amounts of abnormal storage material
3. Extensive vacuolation of neuronal perikarya

Source: From the World Federation of Neurology Research Group on Neuromuscular Diseases Subcommittee on Motor Neuron Disease: El Escorial World Federation of Neurology criteria for the diagnosis of amyotrophic lateral sclerosis. J Neurol Sci 124(suppl):96–107, 1994, with permission.

large motor neurons are also affected.[4] The pattern of lower motor neuron involvement in the anterior horn is patchy and focal[135] (Fig. 11–2). Histometric studies have shown that large motor neurons are selectively depleted.[*] In these cells, neuronal shrinkage or atrophy precedes neuronal death as in the cortical upper motor neurons.[72] Such shrinkage also involves axons and dendrites, causing marked thinning of neuronal processes.[65,108] In the remaining neurons, an active degenerative process occurs that consists of central chromatolysis (loss of Nissl substance), vacuolation (rare), neuronophagia (rare), and faintly recognizable neuronal cell bodies (ghost cells).[44,49] The RNA content of anterior horn cells is markedly reduced in both histologically normal and abnormal neurons, suggesting that abnormal RNA synthesis precedes the histologic abnormalities.[17,18,84,104] Lipofuscin deposits

*References 37, 59, 71, 104, 133, 142, and 148.

are prominent, but whether such changes are of pathogenic significance remains unclear.[92] In the anterior horn, a diffuse fibrillary gliosis is commonly found and is presumably a response to neuronal loss.[126]

In the following sections, specific abnormalities found in the anterior horn motor neurons are described.

NEUROFILAMENT ABNORMALITIES

Silver impregnation specifically stains the perikaryal neurofilament network, which is abnormal in the anterior horn motor neurons in ALS[31,47] (Fig. 11–3). Immunostaining with monoclonal antibodies reveals that these perikaryal neurofilaments are phosphorylated[87,103,132] and are present in amounts 5 to 10 times that seen in normal motor neurons. Abnormal neurofilament accumulation in the perikaryon occurs in two distinct patterns: homogeneously diffuse accumulation, which is seen in all forms of ALS but most commonly in sporadic ALS, and fo-

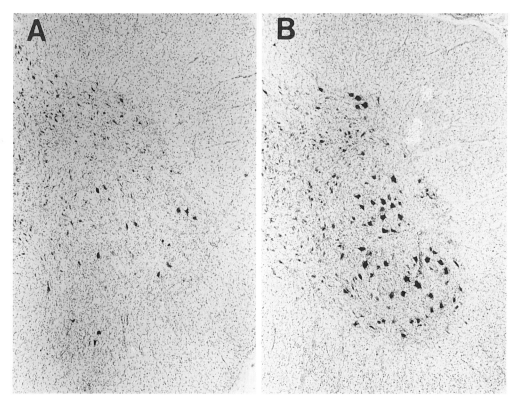

Figure 11–2. (*A*) Nissl staining of the lumbar cord shows a marked loss of large anterior horn cells in a patient with ALS. (*B*) A normal lumbar cord showing a normal number of large anterior horn cells. (From Hirano, A: Neuropathological aspects of motor neuron disease. In Gourie-Devi, A (ed): Motor Neuron Disease. Global Clinical Patterns and International Research. Oxford & IBH Publishing Co, New Delhi, p 136, 1987, with permission.)

cal accumulation in various shapes (such as tubular, round, or cordlike), which characteristically is found in FALS.[53,96]

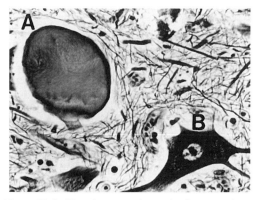

Figure 11–3. Silver impregnation stain shows two large anterior horn cells in a patient with ALS. One motor neuron (*A*) is markedly swollen with packed interwoven neurofilaments. (*B*) A normal anterior horn cell.

AXONAL SWELLING (SPHEROIDS)

Wohlfart[147] first described axonal swelling, referring to the swollen areas as "knobs," and believed that the swelling indicated axonal regeneration. Later, Carpenter[11] established the pathologic significance of axonal swellings in ALS and termed them spheroids, which is the term currently used. They are eosinophilic, usually greater than 20 μm in diameter, and contain packed 10-nm-thick neurofilaments.[47] Some spheroids are clearly located near the cell body, but more often the connection to the cell body cannot be identified.[11,19,45,48] Some are suspected of developing in the dendrites and perhaps in axons distant from the cell body.[48] Inoue and Hirano[59] found that these axonal swellings are present much more frequently in early than in late ALS and in cases with shorter as opposed to longer clinical courses (Fig. 11–4).

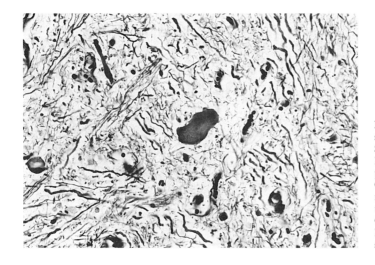

Figure 11–4. A large spheroid is shown in the anterior horn of ALS. Silver impregnation stain. (From Hirano, A: Neuropathological aspects of motor neuron disease. In Gourie-Devi, A (ed): Motor Neuron Disease. Global Clinical Patterns and International Research. Oxford & IBH Publishing Co, New Delhi, p 136, 1987, with permission.)

Spheroids are found in age-matched controls, but they are fewer in number and generally smaller than those found in ALS.[16] Small spheroids (also called *globules*) are nonspecific and seen in other conditions, including the normal aging brain. Spheroids are not found in FALS, and neurofilamentous changes differ from those in sporadic ALS.[47] Like intraneuronal neurofilament accumulations, spheroids are phosphorylated. Because neurofilaments normally are phosphorylated only along the distal axons, the processing and transporting of neurofilaments may be altered in ALS motor neurons. Nevertheless, such findings are not specific for ALS because many other neurologic conditions produce similar phosphorylated neurofilamentous changes in neurons.[87,132] The neurofilamentous accumulations found in ALS structurally resemble those found in experimental models in which slow axonal transport is impaired, suggesting that spheroids in ALS may also result from impaired slow transport or abnormal processing of neurofilaments[15] (Fig. 11–5).

UNIQUE INCLUSION BODIES IN ALS

The perikarya and proximal axons of anterior horn motor neurons have a variety of unique inclusions and related morphologic changes (see Table 11–1). Several types of inclusion bodies in ALS are immunoreactive to ubiquitin.[79] Ubiquitin is a 76-amino-acid protein that is involved in ATP-dependent nonlysosomal proteolysis of abnormal or short-lived proteins.[77] Lewy-body-like hyalin inclusions are usually intensely ubiquitinated, whereas Bunina bodies and spheroids are less reactive.[104] Ubiquitinated inclusions are more frequently found in patients with an aggressive clinical course than those with a slow course, suggesting that ubiquitination is associated with the activity of neuronal degeneration.[129] Although lower motor neuron ubiquitin inclusions are unique to ALS, ubiquitin is also found in Lewy bodies, Pick bodies, and neurofibrillary tangles.[129] Thus, in neurodegenerative disorders, ubiquitination itself may be a nonspecific reaction in neurons carrying intracytoplasmic inclusions.[83] Although Chou[14,15] has presented a theory as to how the inclusions in ALS develop in affected motor neurons, further studies are needed to establish the relationships between these inclusions.[32]

Bunina Bodies. Bunina bodies were originally described in familial ALS,[9] but they are also found in classic sporadic ALS and Guamanian ALS.[45,48] Histologically, they are small, eosinophilic, irregularly shaped, occasionally refractile granules that are 2 to 3 μm in diameter and are only found in the perikaryon. Ultrastructurally, they are electron-dense, amorphous structures surrounded by vesicles, endoplasmic reticulum fragments, lipofuscin granules, and other debris. In the middle of this structure is a clear space loosely filled with filaments that are larger

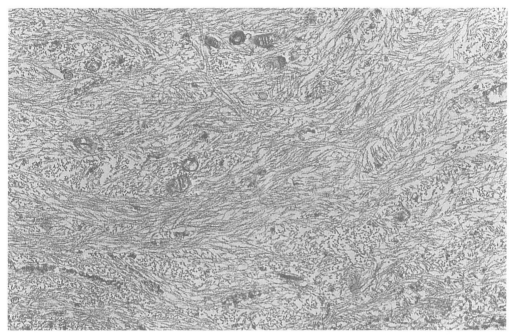

Figure 11–5. Electron micrograph (magnification ×16,000) of a portion of an anterior horn cell of a patient with ALS. Bundle of neurofilaments fills the cytoplasm (spheroid). (From Hirano, A: Neuropathological aspects of motor neuron disease. In Gourie-Devi, A (ed): Motor Neuron Disease. Global Clinical Patterns and International Research. Oxford & IBH Publishing Co, New Delhi, p 136, 1987, with permission.)

than neurofilaments.[38,128,139] Okamoto[112] recently suggested an intriguing relationship between Bunina bodies and Golgi apparatus because cystatin C, which is present mainly in Golgi apparatus, is now found in these inclusions. Bunina bodies, when accompanied by the typical ultrastructural changes described in the previous sections, are highly specific for ALS.[48,112]

Lewy-Body-Like Hyalin Inclusions. Lewy-body-like hyalin inclusions were originally described by Hirano and colleagues[50] in patients with FALS that involved the posterior columns and spinocerebellar tracts. These inclusions measure 7 to 20 μm in diameter; are surrounded by a lighter, slightly basophilic halo; and are found in the soma and proximal axons of anterior horn motor neurons. Since the original description, similar inclusions have also been found in some cases of sporadic ALS. They contain a dense eosinophilic core of granules associated with 15-nm-thick filaments that are not immunoreactive to any cytoskeletal components such as neurofilaments, tubulin, microtubules-associated protein 2, and phosphorylated tau

protein.[104] These inclusions are probably degenerated neurofilaments in the early stages of cellular degeneration.[144] Lewy-body-like inclusion bodies found in ALS indeed resemble the Lewy bodies of Parkinson's disease; however, the differences and similarities are not fully investigated.[67]

Basophilic Inclusions. Basophilic inclusions are found in sporadic juvenile ALS.[14,91,111] These inclusions are globular, irregularly shaped, and sometimes fragmented, measuring approximately 4 to 16 μm in diameter. Electron microscopy reveals 12- to 15-nm-thick filamentous structures associated with granules. These inclusions show occasional granular ubiquitin-immunoreactive deposits.[91]

Skeinlike Inclusions. Another inclusion identified by ubiquitin immunostaining, the skeinlike inclusion, may be specific to ALS.[78,82,93] These inclusions are threadlike linear or tubular structures consisting mainly of filaments and measuring approximately 15 to 25 nm in diameter.[97] They are present exclusively in the major subsets of ALS, that is, the sporadic, familial, and Guamanian types, but not in other motor neuron diseases, such as Werdnig-Hoffmann's disease or juvenile ALS with basophilic inclusions.[88] The role, if any, of this protein in ALS pathophysiology is unclear, although skeinlike inclusions pathogenetically are closely related to Lewy-body-like hyaline inclusions and Bunina bodies.[127] These inclusions may be involved in the proteolysis of abnormally accumulated phosphorylated neurofilaments and other abnormal proteins in diseased cell bodies.[80]

GOLGI APPARATUS FRAGMENTS

The Golgi apparatus plays a central role in processing and transporting plasma membrane, lysosomal, and secretory proteins. Using immunocytochemical staining with antibodies against the Golgi apparatus membrane component, Mourelatos and colleagues[99] reported that in patients with ALS, about 30% of remaining motor neurons contain fragmented Golgi apparatus. The same changes are also found in patients with Guamanian ALS who died after a short course.[100] The Golgi apparatus may fragment early in the pathogenesis of neuronal degeneration.[35] Nevertheless, how specific these changes are for ALS remains to be determined.

POLYGLUCOSAN BODIES

Two types of polyglucosan bodies may be seen in ALS: Lafora bodies and corpora amylacea. Although Lafora bodies are not a feature of ALS pathology, they appear to have been found in some patients. Orthner et al.[118] reported a recessive form of familial ALS, and an autopsy in one patient showed extensive Lafora-body-like inclusions in cortical motor neurons and other neurons. Corpora amylacea were also markedly increased. Robitaille et al.[122] also described four cases of progressive upper and lower motor neuron involvement and marked sensory loss with or without neurogenic bladder and dementia. Autopsy of two patients revealed a profusion of microscopic bodies resembling corpora amylacea or Lafora bodies in the astrocytic and axonal processes in the CNS and peripheral nerves. Polyglucosan bodies immunostain with a heat shock protein, Hsp 72,

but do not stain positively for ubiquitin. On the other hand, corpora amylacea are positive for ubiquitin.[32]

Perivascular Lymphocytic Infiltration

A small number of perivascular lymphocytes have been found in occasional cases of more rapidly advancing sporadic ALS[76] and in cases of FALS.[41] Appel et al.[3] described at autopsy a perivascular lymphocytic infiltration of the spinal cord in 10 of 15 patients with ALS. Other investigators have reported similar lymphocytic infiltration of the spinal cord in patients with ALS.[69,141] The infiltrating lymphocytes are predominantly T lymphocytes.[27,141] Furthermore, immunoglobulin G (IgG) immunoreactivity has been found in both upper and lower motor neurons in ALS.[26,27] Whether such lymphocytic infiltration and IgG immunoreactivity in motor neurons support an autoimmune theory for ALS remains an intriguing question (see Chapter 13).

Ventral Root and Peripheral Nerve Involvement

Histologic analysis at the ventral roots is particularly useful for the investigation of motor neuron disease because these roots contain predominantly motor axons originating from lower motor neurons. (Spinal ventral roots between T1 and L3 contain preganglionic autonomic nerve fibers.) Histometric studies of spinal ventral roots in ALS consistently show that the total number of myelinated fibers is reduced because of selective loss of large myelinated fibers that corresponds to loss of large motor neurons (alpha motor neurons) in the spinal cord anterior horns (see above).[37,59,70,104,133] The number of ventral root large myelinated fibers correlates well to the strength of muscles innervated by the ventral roots.[134] The effects on small myelinated fibers are less clear. Kawamura et al.[70] determined that, like large fibers, the number of small myelinated fibers was decreased in a patient with ALS. In contrast, other studies have found no change in the number of small fibers, which suggests that gamma motor neurons are preserved in ALS.[70,104,133] In another study,[37] however, the number of small fibers was found to be increased, suggesting axonal regeneration. Inoue and Hirano[59] found similar changes but believed that large motor axons atrophy, resulting in the shift to a smaller fiber size. In fact, one case[70] showed an increase of myelinated fibers of intermediate size, supporting the idea that large myelinated fibers atrophied, as occurs in degenerating lower motor neurons that atrophy[72] (see above). Teased nerve fiber preparation reveals a frequency of nerve fibers undergoing axonal degeneration that is out of proportion to the number of remaining motor neurons and chromatolytic neurons,[134] raising the possibility that axonal degeneration may be a primary process (axonopathy) at the ventral root.

Phrenic and hypoglossal nerves provide another unique opportunity to study axonal pathology in the peripheral motor nerves because they have no branches. Detailed morphometric studies in these nerves show loss of large myelinated fibers as seen in the ventral root.[4,7] Bradley and colleagues[7] demonstrated that the number of small myelinated fibers is increased at both the proximal and distal phrenic nerve segments where they studied. They thought that axonal regeneration increases the number of small myelinated fibers, suggesting that it takes place in the nerve segment even proximal to the segment they studied in the phrenic nerve (at the most proximal phrenic nerve segment in the intrathoracic cavity). Primary focal axonopathy may result in axonal regeneration in the proximal phrenic nerve.[7] In comparing the ratio of myelin lamellae to axonal circumference between proximal and distal segments of the phrenic nerves, this study showed a distal axonal atrophy in phrenic motor axons.[7] These studies indicate that motor axons manifest complex histopathology during motor neuron degeneration.

Skeletal Muscles

Skeletal muscles are atrophied as a result of denervation secondary to progressive loss of anterior horn motor neurons. In the early stages of the disease, microscopic examination of skeletal muscles shows scattered atrophic muscle fibers. Histochemical studies show that atrophied muscle fibers are both type I and II, which is consistent with denervation atrophy. Furthermore, nonspecific esterase and NADH-tetrazolium reductase stain small angulated denervated muscle fibers darker than the rest of the muscle fibers, which is helpful in identifying denervation atrophy.[21,60]

In more advanced stages of denervation, small to large collections of denervated fibers, a phenomenon often called group atrophy, are seen.[24] A high density of atrophied fibers may correlate with the degree of clinically apparent muscle weakness and a poor prognosis,[119] although some studies have found no such correlations.[29] Group atrophy results from repeated bouts of denervation followed by reinnervation. Type grouping characterized by aggregation of contiguous muscle fibers of the same fiber type indicates continuous reinnervation and can occur, but it is usually a minor finding, presumably because reinnervation is not robust in ALS. Target or targetoid fibers seen in reinnervated muscle fibers are relatively uncommon in ALS. Secondary myopathic changes such as rounding of fibers, central nucleation, and degeneration and regeneration of muscle fibers are not uncommon and are seen in patients with disease duration of more than 2 years[1] (see Chapter 7).

Spared Motor Neurons

The factors contributing to selective motor neuron involvement in ALS remain to be defined. Recent studies of neuronal calbinden D–28k and parvalbumin show intriguing data.[2,58] According to Alexianu et al.,[58] motor neurons that are vulnerable in ALS do not immunostain with calbinden D-28k or parvalbumin, whereas those that are spared in ALS, including those in the oculomotor, trochlear, abducens, and Onufrowicz nuclei, heavily immunostain. This difference suggests that the level of the calcium-binding proteins may be closely related to the selective vulnerability of motor neurons.

ONUFROWICZ (ONUF'S) NUCLEUS

Motor neurons that belong to the Onufrowicz nucleus, located in the ventral margin of the anterior horn at the second sacral spinal cord level, control striated muscles in the pelvic floor, including the external urethral and anal sphincters.[54] These motor neurons are generally spared in ALS;[86] if any are affected, it is to a very limited degree.[61] Why these neurons are spared in ALS is of great interest.[85] A major question concerns whether Onufrowicz neurons should be classified as somatic motor neurons or autonomic neurons. Immunocytochemical techniques revealed that these neurons have a strong hypothalamic and brain-stem presynaptic influence, supporting the possibility that they are more autonomic than somatic in nature.[34] According to Iwatsubo et al.,[62] all somatic motor neurons but the Onufrowicz, oculomotor, and abducens neurons receive the corticofugal projections, supporting the idea that Onufrowicz neurons are not typical somatic motor neurons.

Ultrastructural morphometry of the presynaptic terminals on Onufrowicz neurons confirms that by definition these neurons are somatic motor neurons.[121] This is clearly inconsistent with the idea that the Onufrowicz nucleus is an extension of the preganglionic parasympathetic nucleus or has intrinsic autonomic properties. Holstege and Tan[54] suggested that "perhaps the Onufrowicz motoneurons should be considered as neither autonomic nor somatic, but as a special class of motoneurons."

Although several investigators have found that the size of Onufrowicz neurons in patients with ALS does not differ from that in healthy controls,[73,121] others have found that the size decreases in ALS.[75] Histopathologically, the motor neurons in the Onufrowicz nucleus undergo changes identical to those described in other lower motor neurons in ALS.[75] However, such histopathology is uncommon, suggesting that Onufrowicz neurons are less vulnerable to the ALS disease process.[74,75,114] As discussed previously, the presence of calcium-binding proteins found in the Onufrowicz neurons may have an important disease-sparing effect in ALS. Further studies are necessary.

MOTOR NUCLEI FOR EXTERNAL OCULAR MUSCLES

Microscopic examination shows that motor neurons remain intact in cranial nerves III, IV, and VI. In a rare case, however, a patient did develop external ophthalmoplegia, and postmortem study showed neuronal loss and gliosis in these motor nuclei.[39] Okamoto and colleagues[113] recently showed that motor neurons of the oculomotor and trochlear nuclei in ALS have occasional inclusion bodies that are characteristic of those found in the affected motor neurons in ALS; this finding suggests that the motor neurons for external ocular muscles are not completely spared. Patients with ALS who survive for long periods because of life-sustaining ventilatory care may develop a predominantly supranuclear ophthalmoplegia.[42] In such patients, autopsy shows lesions not only in the ocular nuclei but also extensively in neurons outside the motor system.[98]

Generally Spared Neuronal Systems

PERIPHERAL SENSORY SYSTEM

Morphologic studies of the peripheral sensory nerves (sural or superficial peroneal nerves) have shown early axonal atrophy, increased secondary demyelination and remyelination, a shift to smaller fiber diameter, and eventual axonal degeneration.[7,22,43] Furthermore, the severity of axonal pathology appears to be correlated with disease duration.[43] Morphometric analyses of dorsal root ganglia cells obtained at autopsy have revealed loss of large ganglion cells, suggesting that sensory neurons are also involved in ALS, but to a much lesser degree than motor neurons.[70] Such sensory involvement is not surprising, given the mild sensory abnormality seen in some patients with ALS (see Chapter 4).

CLARKE'S COLUMNS AND THE SPINOCEREBELLAR TRACTS

In sporadic ALS, Clarke's column neurons may contain spheroid and Bunina bodies—the identical histopathologic changes occurring in anterior horn motor neurons.[5,138] The number of Clarke's neurons clearly is diminished,[6] and immunocytochemical studies show evidence of neuronal degeneration.[146] Degeneration of the spinocerebellar tracts (the ascending tracts of Clarke's column) is a well-recognized neuropathologic feature of familial ALS, although it also has been described in some cases of apparently sporadic ALS.[8,76,137] Such lesions in sporadic ALS, however, are rare.[48,57] Neurons in Clarke's column receive direct input from Ia-afferent fibers in muscle spindles.[124,136] Clarke's column and the spinocerebellar tracts mediate sensory feedback to the cerebellum (see Chapter 3). The functional significance of spinocerebellar tract degeneration is not readily apparent.

OTHER GENERALLY SPARED NEURONAL SYSTEMS

Involvement of the centrum semiovale in ALS is far more extensive than would be expected from primary motor cortex involvement alone, and abnormal histopathologic changes are found in the basal ganglia and substantia nigra in ALS.[8,10,120,131] Posterior column degeneration is rare in sporadic ALS.[48,57] After a comprehensive analysis of the extent of pathologic involvement in motor neuron disease, Brownell et al.[8] concluded that "ALS is merely part of the spectrum of a particular type of multiple system atrophy," but not all investigators share this view.

Some unique cases of sporadic ALS have been reported from Japan that show extensive lesions far beyond the motor system, particularly in patients kept alive on ventilatory support.[127] Such experience poses a question whether the extensive neuronal involvement may simply represent a Japanese variant or a natural history of ALS in any patient kept alive for a long period. However, other patients who were similarly kept alive with a ventilator for an extended period had no such extensive neuronal changes, but typical changes seen in sporadic ALS cases.[40] Thus, long survival alone may not be the cause of the extensive neuropathologic lesion in these patients with ALS. The extent of neuronal involvement in ALS may not be uniform in all patients.[68]

CEREBRAL CORTEX INVOLVEMENT OTHER THAN THE MOTOR CORTEX

A small proportion of patients with otherwise typical ALS develop dementia, as discussed in Chapter 4. The dementia in ALS has several explanations (see Table 4–10), but "presentile dementia with motor neuron disease" originally described by Mitsuyama[94,95] seems to be unique among dementias in ALS. In this form of ALS with dementia, in addition to the histopathologic findings consistent with motor neuron disease, there are mild to moderate, nonspecific degenerative changes, including spongiform changes (status spongiosus) in the superficial layers of the frontotemporal cerebral cortices. The substantia nigra frequently is involved. A number of cases show pathologic features similar to those described by Mitsuyama.[12,55,95,109,145] These patients had no evidence of Pick's disease, Alzheimer's disease, or Creutzfeldt-Jakob disease.

In further immunocytochemical studies of patients with presenile dementia and motor neuron disease, ubiquitin-positive intraneuronal inclusions are found in the frontal and temporal lobes, indicating that ubiquitin-related cytoskeletal abnormalities do occur in neurons outside the motor neuron.[117] After an extensive literature review of ALS cases with associated dementia, parkinsonism, or both, Hudson[57] concluded that all three conditions are part of the same process. Dementia can occur in familial ALS,[28] and rarely, Alzheimer's disease may coincide. Thalamic dementia also has been found in patients with ALS.[20,102] Detailed neuropathologic analysis is thus essential when investigating dementia in patients with ALS.

FAMILIAL ALS

Whereas the clinical examination alone cannot distinguish familial from sporadic ALS,[101] neuropathologic analysis may apparently distinguish between these two conditions:[25,50] the lesions in the posterior columns (the so-called butterfly lesion in the middle root zone) and Clarke's columns, and Lewy-body-like inclusions in anterior horn cells are changes unique to FALS. Hudson[57] showed that 80% of FALS cases have degeneration in the posterior columns, and in half those cases, Clarke's column degeneration exists as well. Based on these histopathologic alterations and disease duration, Horton et al.[56] classified FALS according to three categories: type 1, which is clinically and pathologically indistinguishable from the sporadic form; type 2, which is clinically the same as the sporadic form but pathologically different because of the characteristic pathology in the posterior column and spinocerebellar tracts; and type 3, which is clinically and pathologically identical to type 2 but has a disease duration of more than 10 years. Further histopathologic investigation has shown that spheroids are generally absent in FALS; instead, focal accumulation of phosphorylated neurofilaments appears to be specific for familial cases.[53,96] Recently, consistent involvement of the brain-stem reticular formation, with changes identical to those found in anterior horn cells,[64] or another involvement in substantia nigra,[149] has been reported in FALS. Thus, all current information available suggests that the histopathologic features of FALS vary substantially from case to case, making a uniform description difficult.

In 1993, a large collaborative team[125] discovered varied mutations in the Cu/Zn superoxide dismutase (*SOD1*) gene on chromosome 21, which are now found in approximately 15% of all FALS cases (see Chapter 10). It is essential to clarify whether the histopathologic features of this particular FALS with the *SOD1* mutation is distinct from other forms of FALS.

GUAMANIAN ALS AND PARKINSONISM-DEMENTIA COMPLEX

Hirano and colleagues[46,51,52] established the neuropathologic features of this unique disease, which is endemic on the island of Guam. Similar cases of ALS have also been reported to occur in the Kii peninsula of Japan[13,143] and West New Guinea.[30] The gross pathology shows marked cortical atrophy. The pathognomonic changes include widespread neuronal loss and formation of neurofibrillary tangles in specific areas of the brain—the frontotemporal cortices, striatum, amygdala, hypothalamus, nucleus basalis of Meynert, locus ceruleus, dorsal raphe nucleus, and substantia nigra. These tangles are also found in the spinal cord but predominantly in the posterior horn and rarely in the primary sensory or motor neurons.[89] Ultrastructural analyses show that the tangles consist of approximately 15-nm-thick straight fibrils with a periodicity of approximately 80 nm.[66] Immunocytochemistry analysis indicates that they are phosphorylated and positive for tau protein and ubiquitin, both of which suggest that the tangles in Guamanian ALS, parkinsonism-dementia complex, and Alzheimer's disease resemble each other.[89,90] Also frequently found in anterior horn motor neurons are ubiquitin-immunoreactive filamentous inclusion bodies, Bunina bodies,[90] and, importantly, fragmented Golgi apparatus,[100] all of which are characteristic of other forms of ALS.

A puzzling feature of Guamanian ALS is that an autopsy study done in healthy Chamorros in Guam showed more than 70% of these people had a significant number of neurofibrillary tangles.[13,51] Even more surprisingly, the pathology in 15% of these healthy people with neurofibrillary tangles is indistinguishable from that found in definite parkinsonism-dementia complex. It is conceivable that neurofibrillary tangle formation and neuronal loss may be a basic process of aging in the Chamorro population in general. Conversely, it is possible that a substantial portion of Chamorro people have subclinical or preclinical disease.

The high prevalence of the Guamanian disease in the past and its current rapid disappearance strongly support the speculation that environmental factors play a part in Guamanian ALS.[13,33] To identify a possible explanation for the declining incidence in Guam, the changes in the clinical and neuropathologic features of Guamanian ALS and parkinsonism-dementia complex were investigated.[123] Changes in clinical and neuropathologic features were the same as those seen before the decline. In both conditions, however, an equal increase occurred in age of onset. The duration of disease became shorter in ALS but longer in the parkinsonism-dementia complex.

ALS and parkinsonism-dementia complex

may not be endogenous to the Mariana Islands. Schmitt and colleagues[130] reported cases of ALS, parkinsonism, and dementia with neurofibrillary tangles in a German family who lived in Germany. The Guamanian disease complex also supports the hypothesis that Parkinson's disease, Alzheimer's disease, and ALS may be manifestations of the same disease process.[23]

SUMMARY

An understanding of ALS neuropathology is essential: descriptive neuropathology is crucial for definitive diagnosis, and investigational neuropathology provides intriguing clues to ALS pathogenesis. This chapter reviewed ALS neuropathology according to the World Federation of Neurology diagnostic criteria and discussed investigational neuropathology findings.

Gross pathology may show focal atrophy of the motor cortex and thinning of the ventral roots, but only histopathologic examination provides the diagnostic features of ALS. Loss of upper motor neurons, specifically large pyramidal motor neurons, is a crucial finding. Their descending tracts (the corticospinal tracts) must reveal bilateral degeneration. Another prerequisite for diagnosis is loss of lower motor neurons in the lower brain-stem motor nuclei, the spinal cord anterior horn, or both. Histometric studies show a selective loss of large motor neurons (alpha motor neurons) and correspondingly, a selective loss of large myelinated motor axons in the peripheral nerves. Remaining motor neurons may undergo various degrees of neuronal degeneration, including neuronal atrophy with lipofuscin accumulation and loss of Nissl substance. In particular, anterior horn motor neurons have a unique cellular pathology. Neurofilamentous abnormalities found in both neuron cell bodies and in axons may be a key pathogenetic process in ALS neuronal degeneration. In addition, intracytoplasmic inclusion bodies such as Bunina bodies, and Lewy-body-like hyaline, skeinlike, and basophilic inclusions are found. Most of these inclusions are ubiquitinated, a process of nonlysosomal proteolysis. These changes are not diagnostic but strongly support the diagnosis of ALS. The recent-

ly recognized fragmentation of the Golgi apparatus appears to be specific to ALS. In the CNS, occasional predominantly T-cell lymphocytic infiltration is found in ALS, but the significance of such inflammatory reaction remains unknown. In skeletal muscles, a varying degree of denervation muscle atrophy is present.

In regard to selective vulnerability and resistance, the majority of lower motor neurons are affected, whereas motor neurons controlling ocular muscles and pelvic floor, urinary, and rectal sphincter muscles are spared. The motor system is selectively affected, but the sensory system and spinocerebellar tracts are generally spared. Mechanisms that buffer excess intracellular calcium may play a key role in selective involvement.

Dementia is not part of ALS, but it does occur in a small proportion of patients. It has various histopathologic explanations, but presenile dementia associated with spongiform degeneration in superficial layers of the frontotemporal cerebral cortices appears unique among dementias in ALS.

Familial ALS cannot be distinguished clinically from sporadic ALS; in some of FALS, however, histopathologic analysis shows that the posterior columns and spinocerebellar tracts are frequently involved and that a neurofilamentous pathology exists that differs from that found in sporadic ALS. The extent to which histopathologic changes in FALS are associated with a missense mutation of the *SOD1* gene remains to be determined. The histopathologic characteristics of Guamanian ALS were compared with those of sporadic and FALS.

REFERENCES

1. Achari, AN and Anderson, S: Myopathic changes in amyotrophic lateral sclerosis. Neurology 24:477–481, 1974.
2. Alexianu, ME, Ho, B-K, Mohamed, H, et al: The role of calcium-binding proteins in the selective motoneuron vulnerability in amyotrophic lateral sclerosis. Ann Neurol 36:846–858, 1994.
3. Appel, SH, Englehardt, JI, Garcia, J, et al: Autoimmunity and ALS: A comparison of animal models of immune-mediated motor neuron destruction and human ALS. In Rowland, LP (ed): Amyotrophic Lateral Sclerosis and Other Motor Neuron Diseases. Adv Neurol 56. Raven Press, New York, 1991, pp 405–412.

4. Atsumi, T and Miyatake, T: Morphometry of the degenerative process in the hypoglossal nerves in amyotrophic lateral sclerosis. Acta Neuropathol 73:25–31, 1987.

5. Averback, P and Crocker, P: Abnormal proximal axons of Clarke's neurons in sporadic motor neuron disease. Can J Neurol Sci 8:173–175, 1981.

6. Averback, P and Crocker, P: Regular involvement of Clarke's nucleus in sporadic amyotrophic lateral sclerosis. Arch Neurol 39:155–156, 1982.

7. Bradley, WG, Good, P, Rasool, CG, et al: Morphometric and biochemical studies of peripheral nerves in amyotrophic lateral sclerosis. Ann Neurol 14:267–277, 1983.

8. Brownell, B, Oppenheimer, DR, and Hughes, JT: The central nervous system in motor neurone disease. J Neurol Neurosurg Psychiatry 33:338–357, 1970.

9. Bunina, TL: On intracellular inclusions in familial amyotrophic lateral sclerosis. AH Neuropat Psikhit Korsakov 62:1293–1299, 1962.

10. Burrow, JNC and Blumbergs, PC: Substantia nigra degeneration in motor neurone disease: A quantitative study. Aust NZ J Med 22:469–472, 1992.

11. Carpenter, S: Proximal axonal enlargement in motor neuron disease. Neurology 18:841–851, 1968.

12. Caselli, RJ, Windebank, AJ, Petersen, C, et al: Rapidly progressive aphasic dementia and motor neuron disease. Ann Neurol 33:200–207, 1993.

13. Chen, K and Yase, Y: Parkinsonism-dementia, neurofibrillary tangles, and trace elements in the Western Pacific. Senile Dement Alzh Type, 153–173, 1985.

14. Chou, SM: Pathognomy of intraneuronal inclusions. In Tsubaki, T, Toyokura, Y, (eds): Amyotrophic Lateral Sclerosis. University Park Press, Baltimore, 1978, pp 135–176.

15. Chou, SM: Pathology—light microscopy of amyotrophic lateral sclerosis. In Smith, RA (ed): Handbook of Amyotrophic Lateral Sclerosis. Marcel Dekker, New York, 1992, pp 133–181.

16. Clark, AW, Parhad, IM, Griffin, JW, et al: Neurofilamentous axonal swellings as a normal finding in the spinal anterior horn of man and other primates. J Neuropath Exp Neurol 43:253–262, 1984.

17. Davidson, TJ and Hartmann, HA: Base composition of RNA obtained from motor neurons in amyotrophic lateral sclerosis. J Neuropathol Exp Neurol 40:193–198, 1981.

18. Davidson, T, Hartmann, HA, and Johnson, PC: RNA content and volume of motor neurons in amyotrophic lateral sclerosis: I. The cervical swelling. J Neuropathol Exp Neurol 40:187–192, 1981.

19. Delisle, MB and Carpenter, S: Neurofibrillary axonal swellings and amyotrophic lateral sclerosis. J Neurol Sci 63:241–250, 1984.

20. Deymeer, F, Smith, TW, DeGirolami, U, and Drachman, DA: Thalamic dementia and motor neuron disease. Neurology 39:58–61, 1989.

21. Dubowitz, V, Booke, M, and Neville, HE: Muscle biopsy: A modern approach. WB Saunders, Philadelphia, 1973.

22. Dyck, PJ, Stevens, JC, Mulder, DW, et al: Frequency of nerve fiber degeneration of peripheral motor and sensory neurons in amyotrophic lateral sclerosis. Neurology 25:781–785, 1975.

23. Eisen, A and Calne, D: Amyotrophic lateral sclerosis, Parkinson's disease and Alzheimer's disease: Phylogenetic disorders of the human neocortex sharing many characteristics. Can J Neurol Sci 19:117–120, 1992.

24. Engel, WK and Brooke, MH: Muscle biopsy in ALS and other motor neuron disease. In Norris, FH Jr and Kurland, LT (eds): Motor Neuron Diseases. Grune & Stratton, New York, 1969, pp 154–159.

25. Engel, WK, Kurland, LT, and Klatzo, I: An inherited disease similar to amyotrophic lateral sclerosis with a pattern of posterior column involvement. An intermediate form? Brain 82:203–222, 1959.

26. Engelhardt, JI and Appel, SH: IgG reactivity in the spinal cord and motor cortex in amyotrophic lateral sclerosis. Arch Neurol 47:1210–1216, 1990.

27. Engelhardt, JI, Tajti, J, and Appel, SH: Lymphocytic infiltrates in the spinal cord in amyotrophic lateral sclerosis. Arch Neurol 50:30–36, 1993.

28. Finlayson, MH, Guberman, A, and Martin, JB: Cerebral lesions in familial amyotrophic lateral sclerosis. Acta Neuropathol 26:237–246, 1973.

29. Froes, MMW, Kristmundsdottir, F, Mahon, M, et al: Muscle morphometry in motor neuron disease. Neuropathol Appl Neurobiol 13:405–419, 1987.

30. Gajdusek, DC and Salazar, AM: Amyotrophic lateral sclerosis and parkinsonian syndromes in high incidence among the Auyu and Jakai people of West New Guinea. Neurology 32:107–126, 1982.

31. Gambetti, P, Schecket, G, Ghetti, B, et al: Neurofibrillary changes in human brain. J Neuropathol Exp Neurol 42:69–79, 1983.

32. Garofalo, O, Kennedy, PGE, Swash, M, et al: Ubiquitin and heat shock protein expression in amyotrophic lateral sclerosis. Neuropathol Appl Neurobiol 17:39–45, 1991.

33. Garruto, RM, Yanagihara, R, and Gajdusek, C: Disappearance of high-incidence amyotrophic lateral sclerosis and parkinsonism-dementia on Guam. Neurology 35:193–198, 1985.

34. Gibson, SJ, Polak, JM, Katagiri, T, et al: A comparison of the distributions of eight peptides in spinal cord from normal controls and cases of motor neurone disease with special reference to Onuf's nucleus. Brain Res 474:255–278, 1988.

35. Gonatas, NK, Stiber, A, Mourelatos, Z, et al: Fragmentation of the Golgi apparatus of motor neurons in amyotrophic lateral sclerosis. Am J Pathol 140:731–737, 1992.

36. Hammer, RP, Tomiyasu, U, and Scheibel A: Degeneration of the human betz cell due to amyotrophic lateral sclerosis. Exp Neurol 63:336–346, 1979.

37. Hanyu, N, Oguchi, K, Yanagisawa, N, et al: Degeneration and regeneration of ventral root motor fibers in amyotrophic lateral sclerosis. J Neurol Sci 55:99–115, 1982.

38. Hart, MN, Cancilla, PA, Frommes, S, et al: Anterior horn cell degeneration and Bunina-type inclusions associated with dementia. Acta Neuropathol 38:225–228, 1977.

39. Harvey, DG, Torack, RM, and Rosenbaum, HE: Amyotrophic lateral sclerosis with ophthalmoplegia. Arch Neurol 36:615–617, 1979.

40. Hashizume, Y, Yoshida, M, and Murakami, N: Clinicopathological study of two respirator-assisted

long survival cases of amyotrophic lateral sclerosis. Neuropathology 13:237–241, 1993.

41. Hawkes, CH, Cavanagh, JB, Mowbray, S, et al: Familial motorneuron disease: Report of a family with five post-morten studies. In Rose, FC (ed): Research Progress in Motor Neuron Disease. Pitman Books, London, 1984, pp 405–411.

42. Hayashi, H, Kato, S, Kawada, T, et al: Amyotrophic lateral sclerosis: Oculomotor function in patients in respirators. Neurology 37:1431–1432, 1987.

43. Heads, T, Pollock, M, Robertson, A, et al: Sensory nerve pathology in amyotrophic lateral sclerosis. Acta Neuropathol 82:316–320, 1991.

44. Hirano, A: Neuropathological aspects of motor neuron disease. In Gourie-Devi, A (ed): Motor Neuron Disease. Global Clinical Patterns and International Research. Oxford & IBH Publishing, New Delhi, 1987, pp 131–146.

45. Hirano, A: Cytopathology of amyotrophic lateral sclerosis. Adv Neurol 56:91–101, 1991.

46. Hirano, A, Arumugasamy, N, and Zimmerman, HM: Amyotrophic lateral sclerosis. A comparison of Guam and classical cases. Arch Neurol 16:357–363, 1967.

47. Hirano, A, Donnenfeld, H, Sasaki, S, et al: Fine structural observations of neurofilamentous changes in amyotrophic lateral sclerosis. J Neuropathol Exp Neurol 43:461–470, 1984.

48. Hirano, A, Hirano, M, and Dembitzer, M: Pathological variations and extent of disease process in amyotrophic lateral sclerosis. In Hudson, AJ (ed): Amyotrophic Lateral Sclerosis. University of Toronto Press, Toronto, 1990, pp 166–192.

49. Hirano, A and Iwata, M: Pathology of motor neurons with special reference to amyotrophic lateral sclerosis and related diseases. In Tsubaki, T and Toyokura, Y (eds): Amyotrophic Lateral Sclerosis. University Park Press, Baltimore, 1978, pp 1107–1134.

50. Hirano, A, Kurland, LT, and Sayre, GP: Familial amyotrophic lateral sclerosis. A subgroup characterized by posterior and spinocerebellar tract involvement and hyaline inclusions in the anterior horn cells. Arch Neurol 16:232–243, 1967.

51. Hirano, A, Malamud, N, Elizan, TS, et al: Amyotrophic lateral sclerosis and parkinson-dementia complex of Guam. Further pathologic studies. Arch Neurol 15:35–51, 1966.

52. Hirano, A, Malamud, N, and Kurland, L: Parkinsonism-dementia complex, an endemic disease on the Island of Guam. II Pathological features. Brain 84:662–679, 1961.

53. Hirano, A, Nakano, I, Kurland, T, et al: Fine structural study of neurofibrillary changes in a family with amyotrophic lateral sclerosis. J Neurol 43:471–480, 1984.

54. Holstege, G and Tan, J: Supraspinal control on motoneuron innervating the striated muscles of pelvic floor including urethral and anal sphincters in the cat. Brain 110:1323–1344, 1987.

55. Horoupian, DS, Thal, L, Katzman, R, et al: Dementia and motor neuron disease: Morphometric, biochemical and Golgi studies. Ann Neurol 16:305–313, 1984.

56. Horton, WA, Eldridge, R, and Brody, JA: Familial motor neuron disease. Neurology 26:460–465, 1976.

57. Hudson, AJ: Amyotrophic lateral sclerosis: Clinical evidence for differences in pathogenesis and etiology. In Hudson, A (ed): Amyotrophic Lateral Sclerosis. University of Toronto Press, Toronto, 1990, pp 108–143.

58. Ince, P, Stout, N, Shaw, P, et al: Parvalbumin and calbindin D-28k in the human motor system and in motor neuron disease. Neuropathol Appl Neurobiol 19:291–299, 1993.

59. Inoue, K and Hirano A: Early pathological changes of amyotrophic lateral sclerosis. Autopsy findings of a case of 10 months' duration. Neurol Med 5:448–455, 1979.

60. Iwasaki, Y and Kinoshita, M: Study on the relationship between the musclar pathology and prognosis in motor neuron disease. Jpn J Med 26:335–338, 1987.

61. Iwata, M and Hirano, A: Sparing of the Onufrowicz nucleus in sacral anterior horn lesions. Ann Neurol 4:245–249, 1978.

62. Iwatsubo, T, Kuzuhara, S, Kanematsu, A, et al: Corticofugal projections to the motor nuclei of the brainstem and spinal cord in humans. Neurology 40:309–312, 1990.

63. Kamo, H, Haebara, H, Akiguchi, I, et al: Peculiar patchy astrocytosis in the precentral cortex of amyotrophic lateral sclerosis. Clin Neurol 23:974–981, 1983.

64. Kato, S and Hirano, A: Involvement of the brain stem reticular formation in familial amyotrophic lateral sclerosis. Clin Neuropathol 11:41–44, 1992.

65. Kato, T, Hirano, A, and Donnenfeld, H: A Golgi study of the large anterior horn cells of the lumbar cords in normal spinal cords and in amyotrophic lateral sclerosis. Acta Neuropathol 75:34–40, 1987.

66. Kato, S, Hirano, A, Llena, JF, et al: Ultrastructural identification of neurofibrillary tangles in the spinal cords in Guamanian amyotrophic lateral sclerosis and parkinsonism-demential complex on Guam. Acta Neuropathol 83:277–282, 1992.

67. Kato, T, Katagiri, T, Hirano, A, et al: Lewy body-like hyaline inclusions in sporadic motor neuron disease are ubiquitinated. Acta Neuropathol 77:391–396, 1989.

68. Kato, S, Oda, M, and Hayashi, H: Neuropathology in amyotrophic lateral sclerosis patients on respirators: Uniformity and diversity in 13 cases. Neuropathology 13:229–236, 1993.

69. Kawamata, T, Akitama, H, Yamada, T, et al: Immunologic reactions in amyotrophic lateral sclerosis brain and spinal cord tissue. Am J Pathol 140:691–707, 1992.

70. Kawamura, Y, Dyck, PJ, Shimono, M, et al: Morphometric comparison in the vulnerability of peripheral motor and sensory neurons in amyotrophic lateral sclerosis. J Neuropathol Exp Neurol 40:667–675, 1981.

71. Kawamura, Y, O'Brien, P, Okazaki, H, et al: Lumbar motoneurons of man. II. The number and diameter distribution of large- and intermediate-diameter cytons in "motoneuron columns" of spinal cord of man. J Neuropathol Exp Neurol 36:861–870, 1977.

72. Kiernan, JA and Hudson, AJ: Changes in sizes of cortical and lower motor neurons in amyotrophic lateral sclerosis. Brain 114:843–853, 1991.

73. Kiernan, JA and Hudson, AJ: Changes in shapes of surviving motor neurons in amyotrophic lateral sclerosis. Brain 116:203–215, 1993.

74. Kihira, T, Mizusawa, H, Tada, J, et al: Lewy body-like inclusions in Onuf's nucleus from two cases of sporadic amyotrophic lateral sclerosis. J Neurol Sci 115:51–57, 1993.

75. Kihira, T, Yoshida, S, Uebayashi, Y, et al: Involvement of Onuf's nucleus in ALS. Demonstration of intraneuronal conglomerate inclusions and Bunina bodies. J Neurol Sci 104:119–128, 1991.

76. Lawyer, JR and Netsky, MG: Amyotrophic lateral sclerosis. Arch Neurol Psychiatry 69:171–192, 1953.

77. Leigh, PN: Ubiquitin. In Williams, AC (ed): Motor Neuron Disease. Chapman & Hall Medical, London, 1994, pp 343–370.

78. Leigh, PN, Anderton, BH, Dodson, A, et al: Ubiquitin deposits in anterior horn cell in motor neurone disease. Neurosci Lett 93:197–203, 1988.

79. Leigh, PN, Dodson, A, Swash, M, et al: Cytoskeletal abnormalities in motor neuron disease: An immunocytochemical study. Brain 112:521–535, 1989.

80. Leigh, PN and Garofalo, O: The molecular pathology of motor neuron disease. In Leigh, PN and Swash, M (eds): Motor Neuron Disease. Springer-Verlag, London, 1995, pp 139–161.

81. Lowe, J, Aldridge, F, Lennox, G, et al: Inclusion bodies in motor cortex and brainstem of patients with motor neurone disease detected by immunocytochemical localization of ubiquitin. Neurosci Lett 105:7–13, 1989.

82. Lowe, J, Lennox, G, and Jefferson, D: A filamentous inclusion body within anterior horn neurons in motoneurone disease defined by immunocytochemical localisation of ubiquitin. Neursci Lett 94:203–210, 1988.

83. Lowe, J, Mayer, RJ, and Landon, M: Ubiquitin in neurodegenerative diseases. Brain Pathol 3:55–65, 1993.

84. Mann, DMA and Yates, PO: Motor neurone disease: The nature of the pathogenic mechanism. J Neurol Neurosurg Psychiatry 37:1036–1046, 1974.

85. Mannen, T: Neuropathology of Onuf's nucleus. Rinsho Shinkeigaku (Clin Neurol) 31:1281–1285, 1991.

86. Mannen, T, Iwata, M, Toyokura, Y, et al: Preservation of a certain motoneurone group of the sacral cord in amyotrophic lateral sclerosis: Its clinical significance. J Neurol Neurosurg Psychiatry 40:464–469, 1977.

87. Manneto, V, Sternberger, NH, Perry, G, et al: Phosphorylation of neurofilaments is altered in amyotrophic lateral sclerosis. J Neuropathol Exp Neurol 47:642–653, 1988.

88. Matsumoto, S, Goto, S, Kusaka, H, et al: Ubiquitin-positive inclusion in anterior horn cells in subgroups of motor neuron diseases: A comparative study of adult-onset amyotrophic lateral sclerosis, juvenile amyotrophic lateral sclerosis and Werdnig-Hoffmann disease. J Neurol Sci 115:208-213, 1993.

89. Matsumoto, S, Hirano, A, and Goto, S: Spinal cord neurofibrillary tangles of Guamanian amyotrophic lateral sclerosis and parkinsonism-dementia complex: An immunohistochemical study. Neurology 40:975–979, 1990.

90. Matsumoto, S, Hirano, A, and Goto, S: Ubiquitin-immunoreactive filamentous inclusions in anterior horn cells of Guamanian and non-Guamanian amyotrophic lateral sclerosis. Acta Neuropathol 80:233–238, 1990.

91. Matsumoto, S, Kusaka, H, Murakami, N, et al: Basophilic inclusions in sporadic juvenile amyotrophic lateral sclerosis: An immunocytochemical and ultrastructural study. Acta Neuropathol 83:579–583, 1992.

92. McHolm, GB, Aguilar, MJ, and Norris, FH: Lipofuscin in amyotrophic lateral sclerosis. Arch Neurol 41:1187–1188, 1984.

93. Migheli, A, Autilio-Gambetti, L, Gambetti, P, et al: Ubiquitinated filamentous inclusions in spinal cord of patients with motor neuron disease. Neurosci Lett 114:5–10, 1990.

94. Mitsuyama, Y: Presenile dementia with motor neuron disease in Japan: Clinico-pathological review of 26 cases. J Neurol Neurosurg Psychiatry 47:953–959, 1984.

95. Mitsuyama, Y: Presenile dementia with motor neuron disease. Dementia 4:137–142, 1993.

96. Mizusawa, H, Matsumoto, S, Yen, SH, et al: Focal accumulation of phosphorylated neurofilaments within anterior horn cell in familial amyotrophic lateral sclerosis. Acta Neuropathol 79:37–43, 1989.

97. Mizusawa, H, Nakamura, H, Wakayama, I, et al: Skein-like inclusions in the anterior horn cells in motor neuron disease. J Neuro Sci 105:14–21, 1991.

98. Mizutani, T, Aki, M, Shiozawa, R, et al: Development of ophthalmoplegia in amyotrophic lateral sclerosis during long-term use of respirators. J Neurol Sci 99:311–319, 1990.

99. Mourelatos, Z, Adler, H, Hirano, A, et al: Fragmentation of the Golgi apparatus of motor neurons in amyotrophic lateral sclerosis revealed by organelle-specific antibodies. Proc Nat Acad Sci 87:4393–4395, 1990.

100. Mourelatos, Z, Hirano, A, Rosenquist, AC, et al: Fragmentation of the Golgi apparatus of motor neurons in amyotrophic lateral sclerosis (ALS). Clinical studies in ALS of Guam and experimental studies in deafferented neurons and in beta, beta'-iminodipropionitrile axonopathy. Am J Pathol 144:1288–300, 1994.

101. Mulder, DW, Kurland, LT, Offord, KP, et al: Familial adult motor neuron disease: Amyotrophic lateral sclerosis. Neurology 36:511–517, 1986.

102. Müller, M, Vieregge, P, Reusche, E, et al: Amyotrophic lateral sclerosis and frontal lobe dementia in Alzheimer's disease. Eur Neurol 33:320–324, 1993.

103. Munoz, DG, Greene, C, Perl, DP, et al: Accumulation of phosphorylated neurofilaments in anterior horn motoneurons in amyotrophic lateral sclerosis patients. J Neuropathol Exp Neurol 47:9–18, 1988.

104. Murakami, T: Motor neuron disease: Quantitative morphological and microdensitophotometric studies of neurons of anterior horn and ventral root of cervical spinal cord with special reference to the pathogenesis. J Neurol Sci 99:101–115, 1990.

105. Murayama, S, Bouldin, TW, and Suzuki, K: Immunocytochemical and ultrastructural studies of upper motor neurons in amyotrophic lateral sclerosis. Acta Neuropathol 83:518–524, 1992.

106. Murayama, S, Inoue, K, Kawakami, H, et al: A unique pattern of astrocytosis in the primary motor area in amyotrophic lateral sclerosis. Acta Neuropathol 82:456–461, 1991.

107. Murayama, S, Mori, H, Ihara, Y, et al: Immunocytochemical and ultrastructural studies of lower motor neurons in amyotrophic lateral sclerosis. Ann Neurol 27:137–148, 1990.

108. Nakano, I and Hirano, A: Atrophic cell processes of large motor neurons in the anterior horn in amyotrophic lateral sclerosis: Observation with silver impregnation method. J Neuropath Exp Neurol 46:40–49, 1987.

109. Neary, D, Snowden, JS, Mann, DMA, et al: Frontal lobe dementia and motor neuron disease. J Neurol Neurosurg Psychiatry 53:23–32, 1990.

110. Nihei, K, McKee, AC, and Kowall, NW: Patterns of neuronal degeneration in the motor cortex of amyotrophic lateral sclerosis patients. Acta Neuropathol 86:55–64, 1993.

111. Oda, M, Akagawa, N, Tabuchi, Y, et al: A sporadic juvenile case of the amyotrophic lateral sclerosis with neuronal intracytoplasmic inclusions. Acta Neuropathol 44:211–216, 1978.

112. Okamoto, K: Bunina bodies in amyotrophic lateral sclerosis. Neuropathology 13:193–199, 1993.

113. Okamoto, K, Hirai, S, Amari, M, et al: Oculomotor nuclear pathology in amyotrophic lateral sclerosis. Acta Neuropathol 85:458–462, 1993.

114. Okamoto, K, Hirai, S, Ishiguro, K, et al: Light and electron microscopic and immunohistochemical observations of the Onuf's nucleus of amyotrophic lateral sclerosis. Acta Neuropathol 81:610–614, 1991.

115. Okamoto, K, Hirai, S, Shoji, M, et al: Axonal swellings in the corticospinal tracts in amyotrophic lateral sclerosis. Acta Neuropathol 80:222–226, 1990.

116. Okamoto, K, Hirai, S, Yamazaki, T, et al: New ubiquitin-positive intraneuronal inclusions in the extra-motor cortices in patients with amyotrophic lateral sclerosis. Neurosci Lett 129:233–236, 1991.

117. Okamoto, K, Murakami, N, Kusaka, H, et al: Ubiquitin-positive intraneuronal inclusions in the extramotor cortices of presenile dementia patients with motor neuron disease. J Neurol 239:426–430, 1992.

118. Orthner, H, Becker, PE, and Müller, D: Recessiv erbliche amyotrophische Lateralsklerose mit "Lafora-Körpern." Arch Psychiar Nervenkr 217:387–412, 1973.

119. Patten, BM, Zito, G, and Harati, Y: Histologic findings in motor neuron disease. Arch Neurol 36:560–564, 1979.

120. Pioro, EP, Antel, JP, Cashman, NR, et al: Detection of cortical neuron loss in motor neuron disease by proton magnetic resonance spectroscopic imaging in vivo. Neurology 44:1933–1938, 1994.

121. Pullen, AH, Martin, JE, and Swash, M: Ultrastructure of pre-synaptic input to motor neurons in Onuf's nucleus: Controls and motor neuron disease. Neuropathol Appl Neurobiol 18:213–234, 1992.

122. Robitaille, Y, Carpenter, S, Karpati, G, et al: A distinct form of adult polyglucosan body disease with massive involvement of central and peripheral neuronal processes and strocytes. Brain 103:315–336, 1980.

123. Rodgers-Johnson, P, Garruto, RM, Yanagihara, R, et al: Amyotrophic lateral sclerosis and parkinsonism-dementia on Guam: A 30-year evaluation of clinical and neuropathologic trends. Neurology 36:7–13, 1986.

124. Rosales, RL, Osame, M, Madriaga, EP, et al: Morphometry of intramuscular nerves in amyotrophic lateral sclerosis. Muscle Nerve 11:223–226, 1988.

125. Rosen, DR, Siddique, T, Patterson, D, et al: Mutations in Cu/Zn superoxide dismutase gene are associated with familial mayotrophiclateral sclerosis. Nature 362:59–62, 1993.

126. Rossi, M: Classical pathology. In Williams, AC (ed): Motor Neuron Disease. London, Chapman & Hall Medical, 1994, pp 307–342.

127. Sasaki, S and Maruyama, S: Ultrastructural study of skein-like inclusions in anterior horn neurons of patients with motor neuron disease. Neurosci Lett 147:121–124, 1992.

128. Sasaki, S and Muruyama, S: Ultrastructural study of Bunina bodies in the anterior horn neurons of patients with amyotrophic lateral sclerosis. Neurosci Lett 154:117–120, 1993.

129. Schiffer, D, Autilio-Gambetti, L, Chio, A, et al: Ubiquitin in motor neuron disease: Study at the light and electron microscope. J Neuropathol Exp Neurol 50:463–473, 1991.

130. Schmitt, HP, Emser, W, and Heimes, C: Familial occurrence of amyotrophic lateral sclerosis, parkinsonism, and dementia. Ann Neurol 16:642–648, 1984.

131. Smith, MC: Nerve fibre degeneration in the brain in amyotrophic lateral sclerosis. J Neurol Neurosurg Psychiatry 23:269, 1960.

132. Sobue, G, Hashizume, Y, Yasuda, T, et al: Phosphorylated high molecular weight neurofilament protein in lower motor neurons in amyotrophic lateral sclerosis and other neurodegenerative diseases involving ventral horn cells. Acta Neuropathol 79:402–408, 1990.

133. Sobue, G, Matsuoka, Y, Mukai, E, et al: Pathology of myelinated fibers in cervical and lumbar ventral spinal roots in amyotrophic lateral sclerosis. J Neurol Sci 50:413–421, 1981.

134. Sobue, G, Shashi, K, Takahashi, A, et al: Degenerating compartment and functioning compartment of motor neurons in ALS: Possible process of motor neuron loss. Neurology 33:654–657, 1983.

135. Swash, M and Brown, LM: Focal loss of anterior horn cells in the cervical cord in motor neuron disease. Brain 109:939–952, 1986.

136. Swash, M and Fox, KP: The pathology of the muscle spindle: Effect of denervation. J Neurol Sci 22:1–24, 1974.

137. Swash, M, Scholtz, CL, Vowles, G, et al: Selective and asymmetric vulnerability of corticospinal and spinocerebellar tract in motor neuron disease. J Neuro Neurosurg Psychiatry 51:785–789, 1988.

138. Takahashi, H, Oyanagi, K, Ohama, E, et al: Clarke's column in sporadic amyotrophic lateral sclerosis. Acta Neuropathol 84:465–470, 1992.

139. Tomonaga, M, Saito, M, Yoshimura, M, et al: Ultrastructure of the bunina bodies in anterior horn

cells of amyotrophic lateral sclerosis. Acta Neuropathol 42:81–86, 1978.

140. Troost, D, Sillevis Smitt, PAE, De Jon, JMBV, et al: Neurofilament and glial alterations in the cerebral cortex in amyotrophic lateral sclerosis. Acta Neuropathol 84:664–673, 1992.

141. Troost, D, Van Den Oord, JJ, and DeJong, JMBV: Immunohistochemical characterization of the inflammatory infiltrate in amyotrophic lateral sclerosis. Neuropath Applied Neurobiol 16:401–410, 1990.

142. Tsukagoshi, H, Yanagisawa, N, Oguchi, K, et al: Morphometric quantification of the cervical limb motor cells in controls and in amyotrophic lateral sclerosis. J Neurol Sci 41:287–297, 1979.

143. Uebayashi, Y: Epidemiological investigation of motor neuron disease in the Kii Peninsula, Japan and on Guam: The significance of long survival cases. Wakayama Med Rep 23:13–27, 1980.

144. Wakayama, I: Morphometry of spinal motor neurons in amyotrophic lateral sclerosis with special reference to chromatolysis and intracytoplasmic inclusion bodies. Brain Res 585:12–18, 1992.

145. Wilkström, J, Paetau, A, Palo, J, et al: Classic amyotrophic lateral sclerosis with dementia. Arch Neurol 39:681–683, 1982.

146. Williams, C, Kozlowski, MA, Hinton, DR, et al: Degeneration of spinocerebellar neurons in amyotrophic lateral sclerosis. Ann Neurol 27:215–225, 1990.

147. Wohlfart, G: Degeneration and regeneration in the nervous system. World Neurol 2:187–198, 1961.

148. Wohlfart, G and Swank, RL: Pathology of amyotrophic lateral sclerosis. Fiber analysis of the ventral roots and pyramidal tracts of the spinal cord. Arch Neurol Psychiatry 46:783–799, 1941.

149. Wolf, HK, Crain, BJ, and Siddique, T: Degeneration of the substantia nigra in familial amyotrophic lateral sclerosis. Clin Neuropathol 10:291–296, 1991.

150. World Federation of Neurology Research Group on Neuromuscular Diseases Subcommittee on Motor Neuron Disease: El Escorial World Federation of Neurology criteria for the diagnosis of amyotrophic lateral sclerosis. J Neurol Sci 124(suppl): 96–107, 1994.

CHAPTER 12

EXCITO-TOXICITY AND OXIDATIVE DAMAGE IN ALS PATHOGENESIS

EXCITOTOXIC INJURY OF MOTOR
   NEURONS IN ALS
Glutamate: A Potential Excitotoxin
Excitatory Amino Acid Receptors
Potential Causes of Elevated Extracellular
   Glutamate Levels
Mechanisms of Glutamate-Mediated
   Neurotoxicity
Evidence of Excitotoxicity in ALS
Experimental Models of Motor Neuron
   Excitotoxicity
Therapies That Suppress Excitotoxicity
OXIDATIVE NEUROTOXICITY IN ALS
Formation of Reactive Oxygen Species
Superoxide Dismutase (SOD) Protection
   Against Reactive Oxygen Species
SOD1 Gene Mutations in Familial ALS
Therapies That Suppress Oxidative Damage
Relationship Between Oxidative Radical and
   Excitotoxic Processes in ALS

Although the pathogenesis of ALS remains unknown, evidence suggests that excitatory amino acids and free radical–mediated oxidative injury play significant roles in the progressive degeneration and ultimate death of motor neurons in this disease.[41,53,117,223] Irreparable damage to cellular proteins, lipids, organelles, and DNA can result when either of these mechanisms operate individually or jointly.[28] These two processes may contribute to other proposed mechanisms of motor neuron degeneration in ALS, such as abnormal axon transport resulting from defective neurofilament processing (see Chapter 16) and programmed cell death, or apoptosis.[28] This chapter reviews the evidence for these two mechanisms in ALS.

Since Lucas and Newhouse[119] first suggested in 1957 that systemically injected glutamate may have excitotoxic effects on mouse retina, *excitotoxicity* (a term coined 14 years later)[144] has been implicated in the pathogenesis of several human neurologic disorders, including stroke, epilepsy, hypoglycemia, and neurotrauma.[32,128] Accumulating evidence, both clinical and experimental, suggests that glutamate excitotoxicity can also produce chronic neuronal injury in slowly progressive age-related neurodegenerative diseases, such as Huntington's disease and ALS.[32,41,117] The pharmacologic interruption of mechanisms involved in ex-

197

citotoxicity may effectively treat these conditions.

Free radicals, which have also been implicated in causing neuronal injury in various neurodegenerative conditions, such as Parkinson's and Alzheimer's diseases, may play a role in ALS pathogenesis.[11,41] The discovery of mutations in the copper, zinc superoxide dismutase (*SOD1*) gene in a subset of patients with familial ALS (FALS)[166] has significantly bolstered the oxidative damage hypothesis. Although such mutations account for only 1% to 2% of all cases of ALS, the clinical and pathologic similarities of the familial and sporadic forms suggest a common pathogenic mechanism (see Chapters 10 and 11). Therefore, the mechanisms by which the *SOD1* mutation produce motor neuron disease in FALS may provide clues to the cause of sporadic ALS. Development of transgenic mice overexpressing the mutated human *SOD1*, which have behavioral and pathologic features of motor neuron degeneration,[44,45,76,216] has provided a model to examine the mechanisms and potential therapies of the disease.

EXCITOTOXIC INJURY OF MOTOR NEURONS IN ALS

Glutamate: A Potential Excitotoxin

Glutamate and related excitatory amino acids, such as aspartate, are fundamental in excitatory neurotransmission throughout the mammalian CNS, and particularly in motor neurons. Fonnum[61] estimated that approximately 40% of all synapses release excitatory amino acids. Their effects are exerted via excitatory amino acid receptors on both motor and sensory neurons. Overstimulation of excitatory amino acid receptors, however, particularly those allowing intracellular calcium entry, can result in motor neuron death. The influx of excess calcium can trigger a cascade of irreversible intracellular processes leading to neuronal death.[32]

Two factors make glutamate a prime candidate as a cause of motor neuron excitotoxicity in ALS. First, it is the principal excitatory neurotransmitter in the human motor system, including the corticospinal tract,[222] spinal cord interneurons,[142] and corticocortical association pathways.[198] Second, the normal concentration of glutamate is approximately 20,000-fold higher intracellularly ($\approx$10 mmol/L)[111] than it is extracellularly ($\approx$0.6 μmol/L).[21] A tightly regulated energy-dependent system ensures that extracellular glutamate concentrations remain very low to prevent cell injury. Therefore, disruption of this steep concentration gradient would lead to substantial extracellular accumulation of excitatory amino acids. Excitotoxic damage to neurons in intact cortical or hippocampal tissue can occur when the extracellular glutamate concentration increases by as little as 4 to 8 times normal levels (2 to 5 μmol/L).[167]

Excitatory Amino Acid Receptors

Two major classes of excitatory amino acid receptors have been identified: ionotropic receptors, which are ligand-gated ion channels, and metabotropic receptors, which are coupled through G-proteins to second messenger systems.[137] Primarily, ionotropic receptors have been studied in their potential excitotoxic role in neurologic disorders such as stroke, trauma, and ALS.[16,215]

NMDA AND NON-NMDA RECEPTORS

Two main types of ionotropic excitatory amino acid receptors have been identified by examination of their binding characteristics with exogenous agonists, although glutamate binds to all such receptors[212] (Fig. 12–1). The NMDA receptors, so-called because of their preference to bind *N*-methyl-D-aspartate (NMDA), allow calcium and sodium to enter cells when the receptors are activated. Several endogenous compounds, including glutamate, L-aspartate, homocysteate,[51] and quinolinate,[197] can selectively stimulate these receptors. Excitatory transmission mediated by the NMDA receptor has a slow rise time and delay of several hundred milliseconds.[36] Overstimulation of NMDA receptors can result in rapid and fulminant neurotoxicity. Non-NMDA receptors are of two subtypes: AMPA receptors, which prefer to bind α-amino-3-hydroxy-5-methyl-4-isoxazolepropionate (AMPA), and kainate receptors, which preferentially bind kainic acid;

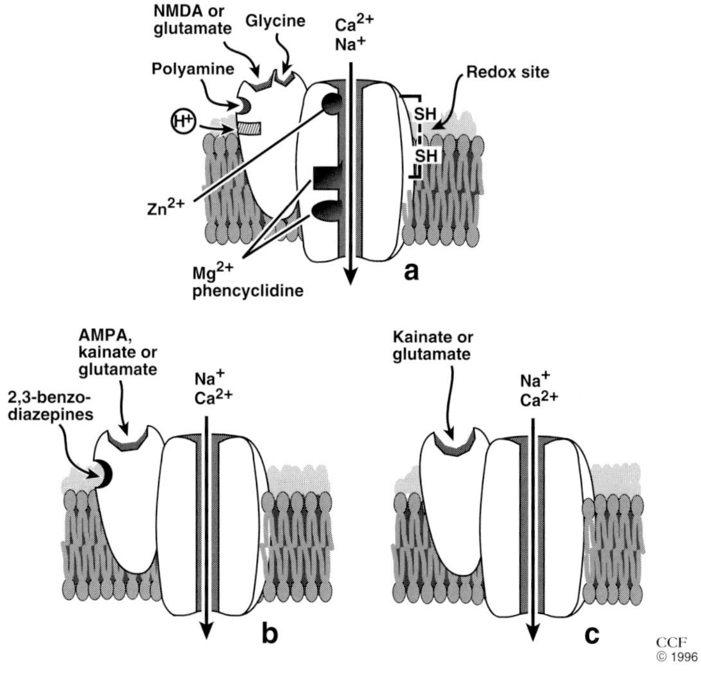

Figure 12–1. The three major types of ionotrophic excitatory amino acid receptor-channel complexes: (a) NMDA, (b) AMPA/kainate, (c) kainate. Common to all types are (1) a binding site for glutamate and a preferred (exogenous) ligand and (2) an ionophore permeable to sodium and calcium (most permeable ion listed first). Modulatory sites (explained in text) are indicated in the NMDA- and AMPA/kainate-receptor subtypes. NMDA, N-methyl-ᴅ-aspartate; AMPA, α-amino-3-hydroxy-5-methyl-4-isoxazolepropionate. (Copyright © 1996 Cleveland Clinic Foundation.)

these are collectively referred to as AMPA/kainate receptors.[133] Although they allow sodium entry predominantly, calcium also enters through the ionophore of the non-NMDA receptor,[90] with the potential to produce a relatively slow neurotoxicity.

The NMDA receptor-channel complex (see Fig. 12–1a) requires glycine for activation and has several modulatory sites that control the degree of cation influx. Those sites in or near the channel that, when occupied, block permeability to calcium and sodium include a voltage-dependent magnesium site[126] and a phencyclidine site where the antagonists ketamine and MK-801 bind.[108] Other modulatory sites are specific for polyamine, hydrogen ions, and zinc. In addition, thiol (sulfhydryl) groups form a redox site (see Fig. 12–1a) that decreases receptor activity when reacting with oxidized nitric oxide (NO^+) to form S-nitrothiol and disulfide bonds.

These characteristics of the NMDA receptor can be exploited pharmacologically to suppress its activity and prevent excitatory amino acid–mediated neuronal damage. Such suppression has been done primarily in experimental models of hypoxia and ischemia.[117] However, these modulatory sites may fail to prevent excess calcium influx when neuron energy production fails.[139] For example, pathologic conditions causing failure of adenosine triphosphate (ATP) production and reduced sodium, potassium–ATPase (Na^+, K^+–ATPase) activity result in partial membrane depolarization and thus removal of the voltage-dependent magnesium block in the ion channel. Such partially open channels would produce slow excitotoxic neuronal death even when extracellular glutamate levels are normal.

The AMPA receptor subtype possesses a modulatory site where benzodiazepines act to desensitize the ionic current to long-term agonist stimulation[224] (see Fig. 12–1b). The 2,3-benzodiazepine antagonist, GYKI 52466, inhibits responses of the AMPA receptor when bound here.[52] The kainate subtype non-NMDA receptor-channel complex, however, does not contain modulatory sites and is more permeable to sodium than to calcium (see Fig. 12–1c).

LOCALIZATION OF AMINO ACID RECEPTORS IN MOTOR NEURONS

Radiolabeled ligand binding studies in normal postmortem human brain and spinal cord tissues using [^{3}H]kainate, [^{3}H]AMPA, or [^{3}H]6-cyano-7-nitroquinoxaline-2,3-dione (CNQX) have revealed a relatively low density of non-NMDA receptors in the ventral horn of the spinal cord.[3,101,183] Radiolabeled NMDA receptors were found in high concentrations in motor neuron regions of the ventral horn.[3,183] Using [^{3}H]MK-801 to label NMDA receptors, Shaw et al.[182] have found higher binding site densities in brainstem nuclei that are affected in ALS compared to nuclei that are spared in this disease. Spinal cord tissue from patients with ALS had fewer radiolabeled NMDA receptors in the ventral horn, consistent with loss of motor neurons.[181]

The differential distribution of NMDA and non-NMDA receptors may explain, at least in part, why only specific motor neuron populations are vulnerable to excitotoxicity. Characterizing the ionotropic receptor types on the basis of genetic sequences may further explain such selective vulnerability. Each ionotropic excitatory amino acid receptor is probably composed of four or five subunits. The subunit composition of the receptor influences its functional characteristics such as ionic permeability of the ion channel.[190]

MOLECULAR CHARACTERIZATION OF THE RECEPTORS

Cloning of the ionotropic excitatory amino acid receptor genes has identified multiple receptor subtypes and revealed the complexity underlying the original pharmacologic classification.[69] So far, at least five NMDA (NMDAR1, NMDAR2A, NMDAR2B, NMDAR2C, and NMDAR2D) and nine non-NMDA receptor subunit genes have been cloned. Of the identified non-NMDA receptor subtypes, at least four prefer AMPA (GluR1, GluR2, GluR3, and GluR4)[107] and five prefer kainate (GluR5, GluR6, GluR7, KA1, and KA2)[137] as the ligand. The gene for one non-NMDA receptor subtype, GluR5, is near the region on chromosome 21[59] that is linked to disease in some patients with familial ALS[184] and had been a candidate gene until the *SOD1* gene mutation was identified.[72]

Alternative splicing (i.e., different transcribed messenger RNAs) of the excitatory amino acid receptor genes results in multiple subunit variants that have diverse functions, pharmacology, and cell specificity.[189] Immunocytochemistry and in situ hybridization have revealed that these receptor subtypes have differing anatomic distributions in the CNS.[18,67,125] Even within AMPA receptor subtypes, motor neurons highly express the GluR3 and GluR4 but not GluR1 and GluR2 subunits; in contrast, dorsal horn sensory neurons predominantly express GluR2 subunits.[67] Presence of the GluR2 subunit in AMPA receptor reduces calcium ion permeability, making the cell less susceptible to excitotoxicity.[90] The relatively low level of GluR2 expression in AMPA receptors of motor neurons[137] and in regions of rat hippocampus vulnerable to ischemia[147] suggests that glutamate receptor subunit distribution may contribute to cellular selective vulnerability by controlling calcium permeability.

Mutations of excitatory amino acid receptor genes or abnormalities in their splicing or editing could perturb normal function and potentially cause neurodegeneration. Examples of animals with genetically altered receptors that result in neurologic disease include the spastic Han-Wistar rat[34] and the myoclonic Poll Hereford calf.[74] Also, global ischemia in rats alters the normal AMPA subunit expression in the hippocampus, resulting in fewer calcium-impermeable GluR2 subunits.[147]

Potential Causes of Elevated Extracellular Glutamate Levels

Extracellular glutamate concentration may increase as a result of several pathologic processes affecting the metabolism of excitatory amino acids. Processes of possible importance in ALS are listed in Table 12–1 and discussed below. Further details on the potential role of excitatory amino acids in the pathogenesis of ALS can be found in several excellent reviews.[6,41,117,134,140,168,179,223]

EXOGENOUS EXCITOTOXINS

That motor neurons degenerate after exposure to various excitotoxins supports the notion that similar environmental toxins could cause sporadic ALS. Neurolathyrism,

Table 12–1. **POSSIBLE CAUSES OF ELEVATED EXTRACELLULAR GLUTAMATE CONCENTRATION IN ALS**

Cause of Increased Glutamate	Mechanism
Increased synthesis	Increased activity of glutamate dehydrogenase or glutaminase
	Decreased activity of glutamine synthetase
Exogenous excitotoxins	Dietary, environmental
Increased release from terminals	Positive feedback of glutamate release
Decreased uptake from synapse	Dysfunction of sodium-dependent glutamate transporter molecules
Failure in ATP production	Loss of the sodium-potassium gradient

Abbreviation: ATP = adenosine triphosphate.

experimental β-*N*-methyl-L-alanine (BMAA) intoxication, and accidental domoic acid intoxication all cause motor neuron degeneration.

Neurolathyrism

Individuals in East Africa and the Indian subcontinent who have ingested flour made from the chickling pea, *Lathyrus sativus*, may develop an acute or insidious spastic paraparesis termed neurolathyrism. It is predominantly an upper motor neuron syndrome, with less than 10% of cases showing lower motor neuron involvement.[35] Neurolathyrism is likely caused by β-*N*-oxalyl-amino-L-alanine (BOAA), a glutamate-like excitotoxin in the chickling pea,[195] although a neurotoxic effect has not been established in humans.[199] BOAA is a specific non-NMDA receptor agonist with particular affinity for the AMPA receptor subtypes.[25] It is excitotoxic to both neurons and astrocytes[26] in mouse spinal cord and cortical explants.[141] Nonhuman primates fed large quantities of BOAA develop corticospinal tract degeneration in the spinal cord.[193,199] Well-nourished macaques fed BOAA develop reversible upper motor neuron signs that resemble those

of the earliest stage of ALS.[194] Pathologic examination has revealed normal-appearing anterior horn cells except for the presence of inclusion bodies.[88]

β-*N*-methyl-L-alanine Intoxication

BMAA is an excitotoxin in the seed of the false sago palm (*Cycas circinalis*), which was processed into flour on Guam and other regions of the Western Pacific until after World War II. It has been implicated as a cause of Western Pacific ALS (see Chapter 3). BMAA stimulates primarily NMDA receptors, but non-NMDA ionotropic receptors and metabotropic receptors are also activated.[39] The initial findings of ALS-like CNS degeneration in macaques fed BMAA[193] was criticized because very large doses (>100 mg/kg per day) were administered compared to the estimated amount ingested by Guamanians (<1 mg/kg per day) after normal processing of the cycad seed, which removes most BMAA.[55] However, subsequent nonhuman primate studies have revealed that nanomolar concentrations of BMAA result in intraneuronal accumulation and abnormalities of mRNA metabolism.[192] Although oral BMAA was not definitely neurotoxic to mice in one study,[149] apoptosis has been found in brain and gut tissue of mice fed cycad seed.[70]

Based on what is known of the acute excitotoxicity resulting from NMDA receptor activation, it is unclear what role BMAA may play in a disease such as ALS because of the disease's long latency period.[55]

Domoic Acid Intoxication

In 1987, an outbreak of toxic encephalopathy in individuals eating mussels contaminated with domoic acid occurred in Canada.[148] Domoic acid is an excitatory amino acid that selectively binds to non-NMDA receptors of the kainate subtype.[221] Acute neurologic deficits ranged from headache, limbic seizures, and short-term memory loss to spastic paraparesis, coma, and death.[205] Postmortem pathologic studies of some patients who were affected acutely revealed substantial neuronal degeneration in the hippocampus and amygdala but not in motor neurons of the brain stem or spinal cord. Survival and initial recovery in some patients was followed by the development of temporal lobe epilepsy caused by the excitotoxicity.[30] No cases of delayed ALS have been reported, however.

INCREASED SYNTHESIS AND RELEASE OF GLUTAMATE

Glutamate synthesis is, in part, regulated by glutamate dehydrogenase, a mitochondrial enzyme found in astroglia.[106] This enzyme catalyzes the interconversion of glutamate and α-ketoglutarate (2-oxoglutarate), which are produced during glucose metabolism[110] (Fig. 12–2). Depending on the cell type, the kinetics of the enzyme-catalyzed reaction are in the direction either of glutamate production or glutamate deamination.[110,153] The main direction of glutamate dehydrogenase activity, however, is probably toward glutamate synthesis.[110] Consequently, whether branched-chain amino acids—which increase glutamate dehydrogenase activity—are beneficial to ALS patients is debatable.[99,158,196,203,206] In addition, reports conflict as to whether the level of glutamate dehydrogenase activity is altered in tissues of patients with ALS. For example, enzyme activity in leukocytes of patients has been found to be normal[156] or decreased[91]; in contrast, glutamate dehydrogenase activity in the descending motor tract regions (lateral and ventral white matter) of the spinal cord was elevated.[122] It is therefore possible that increased glutamate dehydrogenase activity in the ALS spinal cord would result in higher rates of glutamate synthesis.

Glutamate also is produced from interconversion with glutamine. Glutamine is released from astrocytes, shuttled to presynaptic terminals, and converted via glutaminase into glutamate; glutamate released at nerve terminals is taken up by astrocytes and converted back to glutamine through the action of glutamine synthetase[84] (see Fig. 12–2). Overactivity of glutaminase or underactivity of glutamine synthetase (as when ATP production fails) could produce excess glutamate.

Glutamate, released from presynaptic terminals in normal amounts, can stimulate further glutamate release in a positive feedback manner. Although the best example of this is the normal process of long-term potentiation—a cellular model of memory and learning[19]—the reinforcement of glutamate release could initiate excitotoxicity even in the absence of a pathologic state.

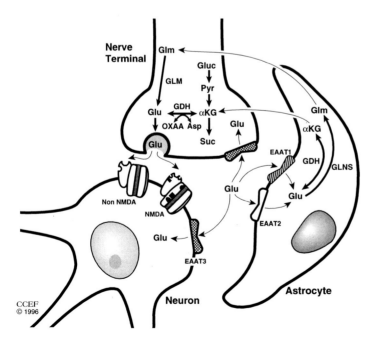

Figure 12–2. Glutamate synthesis, release, and reuptake from the synaptic cleft. Glutamate dehydrogenase (GDH) catalyzes the interconversion of glutamate (Glu) and α-ketoglutarate (αKG) in nerve terminals and astroglia. After release from nerve terminals and interaction with its receptor, glutamate is taken up from the synaptic cleft by astrocytes (via glutamate transporters EAAT1 and EAAT2) and neurons (via EAAT3). Within astrocytes, glutamate is converted into glutamine (Gln) through the action of glutamine synthetase (GLNS), and shuttled to presynaptic terminals where it is converted back into glutamate by glutaminase (GLM). Gluc, Glucose; Pyr, pyruvate; Suc, sucrose; OXAA, oxaloacetate; Asp, aspartate; NMDA, N-methyl-D-aspartate. (Copyright © 1996 Cleveland Clinic Foundation.)

IMPAIRED REMOVAL OF GLUTAMATE TRANSPORTERS

The excitatory activities of glutamate and aspartate are terminated exclusively by their removal from the synaptic cleft by sodium-dependent high-affinity transporters located in neuronal and astrocyte membranes. The three glutamate transporters most fully characterized and cloned[104] are as follows:

- GLAST (new terminology, EAAT1), found predominantly in astrocytes and Bergmann glia of the cerebellum
- GLT1 (EAAT2), which is specific to astrocytes
- EAAC1 (EAAT3), which is localized to neurons (see Fig. 12–2).

Various conditions can compromise glutamate transporter activity. Both arachidonic acid, generated when phospholipase A_2 is activated by abnormally high calcium influx,[210] and free radicals produced through oxidative stress[211] inhibit glutamate transporter function in rat cortical astrocyte cultures. Glutamate transporter function is linked to the sodium gradient and therefore, to Na^+, K^+–ATPase pump activity that maintains the gradient. Because this pump activity depends on ATP, pathologic conditions compromising mitochondrial energy production[11] can indirectly reduce glutamate transporter action. Although unlikely to occur in ALS, a severely reduced sodium gradient can even cause the glutamate transporter to operate in reverse, transporting intracellular glutamate *out* of the cell and increasing its extracellular concentration.[201]

DECREASED ATP PRODUCTION

Mitochondria fail to produce ATP when any process interferes with oxidative phosphorylation. Aging itself is associated with the progressive damage and loss of respiratory enzyme activity because mitochondrial DNA is extremely sensitive to oxidative stress, which increases with age.[11] In addition, mitochondria buffer calcium less efficiently, leading to abnormally high levels of free intracytoplasmic calcium. Such levels could activate harmful enzymatic processes and lead to mitochondrial generation of hydroxyl radicals, as discussed later in this chapter.[56] This process may contribute to the age dependence and delayed onset of neurodegenerative diseases, like ALS (see Chapter 16).

The conversion of glutamate to glutamine in astrocytes is an ATP-dependent process catalyzed by glutamine synthetase. If ATP is not produced, intraglial glutamate would accumulate, overwhelm the glutamate transporters, and thus result in inefficient transport. This, along with reduced Na^+, K^+–ATPase activity that affects the sodium gradient, would increase extracellular glutamate.[177]

Mechanisms of Glutamate-Mediated Neurotoxicity

In vitro studies have identified two phases during which NMDA and non-NMDA receptor overstimulation can injure cells.[31,130] Initially, membrane depolarization allows sodium, chloride, and water through the receptor-associated ion channel to cause acute swelling. Injury at this stage is reversible if receptor stimulation is arrested. If not, subsequent influx of extracellular calcium, along with its release from intracellular stores, elevates cytosolic free calcium to a level that heralds an essentially irreversible phase of calcium-mediated neurotoxicity.

A lesser but significant amount of calcium can also enter through voltage-gated calcium channels, which are activated when membranes are depolarized by ionotropic receptor-mediated cation influx.[200] Of the different channel subtypes, the L-type (long-duration current, large conductance) is most likely to promote glutamate-mediated excitotoxicity because it mediates the most prolonged calcium influx.[115] As discussed in Chapter 13, however, patients with ALS have been found to have IgG antibodies that bind to the L-type channel and appear to enhance calcium influx through the N-type (neuronal) and P-type (Purkinje cell type) voltage-gated calcium channels, causing motor neuron toxicity in vitro.[188]

CALCIUM-MEDIATED NEUROTOXICITY

Although calcium is vital for many cellular processes, intraneuronal excess activates several enzyme systems, including lipases, phospholipases (e.g., phospholipase A_2), proteases, endonucleases, calpains, protein phosphatases, nitric oxide synthase, protein kinase C, calcium/calmodulin–dependent protein kinase II, ornithine decarboxylase, and xanthine oxidase.[32,47,117,208] The uncontrolled activation of these enzymes begins a cascade of harmful processes, including cytoskeletal breakdown, failure to generate ATP, free radical formation, lipid peroxidation, and nucleic acid fragmentation.[128] The neuron-damaging effects of some calcium-activated enzymes are summarized in Table 12–2.

THE PROTECTIVE ROLE OF CALCIUM-BUFFERING PROTEINS

Although the mammalian CNS appears susceptible to glutamate-mediated excitotoxicity, certain safeguards exist. Intraneuronal calcium-binding proteins, such as calbindin-D28K, calretinin, and parvalbumin, are involved in calcium homeostasis and protect against calcium-mediated excitotoxicity.[9,84] Abnormalities of their expression have been found in several human neurodegenerative disorders such as Alzheimer's disease, Parkinson's disease, and Down syndrome.[84] For example, significant reductions (60% to

Table 12–2. ACTIONS AND DAMAGING EFFECTS OF CALCIUM-ACTIVATED ENZYMES

Enzyme	Primary Action	Secondary Action	Damaging Effect
Calcium-calmodulin–dependent protein kinase II	Phosphorylates presynaptic synapsin I	↑Glutamate release[138]	Excitotoxicity
Calpain I and II	Degrade spectrin, microtubules, intermediate filaments, neurofilaments[185]		Cytoskeletal breakdown
	↑Xanthine oxidase	↑Superoxide anion	↑Hydroxyl radicals*
Endonuclease	Fragments DNA[207]		Apoptosis
Nitric oxide synthase	↑Nitric oxide synthesis[68]	↓ATP synthesis	↓Energy
		↓DNA synthesis[87]	↓Transcription
		↑Peroxynitrite	Protein nitration*
	Reacts with superoxide anions	↑Hydroxyl radicals[12]	Lipid peroxidation*
Phospholipase A_2	↑Arachidonic acid[54]	Free radical formation[113]	↑Hydroxyl radicals*
		↑NMDA receptor currents[131]	Excitotoxicity
		↑Glutamate release[63]	Excitotoxicity
		↓Glutamate uptake[10,210]	Excitotoxicity
		↑Protein kinase C synthesis	Excitotoxicity
	↑Platelet-activating factor	↑Glutamate release[17,33]	Excitotoxicity
Phospholipase C	↑Inositol 1,4,5-triphosphate	Releases calcium from intracellular stores	Enzyme activation
	↑Diacylglycerol synthesis	↑Glutamate release[120]	Excitotoxicity
		↑Protein kinase C synthesis	Excitotoxicity
Protein kinase C	↑Synaptic transmission[121]		Excitotoxicity
	↑Duration of calcium influx[37]		Enzyme activation
Xanthine oxidase	Reacts with xanthine	↑Superoxide anions[127]	↑Hydroxyl radicals*

*Oxidative injury arising from initial excitotoxicity.
Abbreviations: ATP = adenosine triphosphate; NMDA = *N*-methyl-D-aspartate.

88%) of calbindin-D28K protein and gene expression have been noted in affected brain regions of patients with Alzheimer's, Parkinson's, or Huntington's diseases, as well as in healthy elderly individuals[94] (see Chapter 16).

Calbindin-D28K and parvalbumin immunoreactivities are markedly lower in motor neurons that degenerate in ALS, including the large cortical Betz cells, motor neurons of the spinal cord, and hypoglossal and vagus motor nuclei. This low reactivity contrasts with the prominent immunoreactivity present in perikarya of the oculomotor nuclei, Onuf's nucleus, most sensory neurons, and cerebellar Purkinje cells, which undergo little or no neurodegeneration.[2,97] This differential distribution of calcium-binding proteins may, in part, explain the selective vulnerability of specific motor neuron populations to excitotoxicity despite the widespread distribution of excitatory amino acid receptors. This aspect of ALS neuropathology was discussed in Chapter 11.

Evidence of Excitotoxicity in ALS

The evidence for excitotoxicity in ALS has been inconsistent.[220] Generally, in patients with classic ALS, glutamate levels are elevated in plasma and cerebrospinal fluid and diminished in postmortem CNS tissue. The contradictory results may be attributed to a heterogeneous patient population or differences in technical handling of blood and cerebrospinal fluid samples.[220]

ELEVATED GLUTAMATE LEVELS IN PLASMA

Plaitakis and Caroscio[156] found that fasting plasma glutamate levels in patients with motor neuron disease were twice normal levels. Patients also experienced higher plasma glutamate and aspartate levels after oral glutamate loading than did normal controls. These findings were interpreted as a generalized defect in the transport or breakdown of excitatory amino acids, which could predispose individuals to neurotoxicity. These findings were confirmed by some investigators[100] but not others,[152] suggesting the influence of technical or other factors (e.g.,

fasting). A follow-up study by Plaitakis et al.[157] of 84 patients with various forms of motor neuron disease revealed elevated plasma glutamate levels in patients with sporadic ALS but no elevation in those with only lower motor neuron dysfunction; the abnormalities were most marked in men.

ELEVATED GLUTAMATE LEVELS IN CEREBROSPINAL FLUID

Cerebrospinal fluid glutamate and aspartate levels in patients with ALS have been reported to be four times higher than in normal individuals.[172,174] In contrast, another study found no significant difference in levels of these excitatory amino acids in the cerebrospinal fluid of patients with ALS compared to control individuals.[152] Differences in the technical handling of the cerebrospinal fluid samples, which can affect glutamate stability and concentration, may explain the discordant results.[172,220]

Levels of N-acetylaspartyl glutamate (NAAG), an excitatory neuropeptide that is metabolized to glutamate,[42] and N-acetylaspartate (NAA), a metabolite of NAAG, have been found to be two to three times higher in the cerebrospinal fluid of patients with ALS than in unaffected individuals.[174] Clinically, minor, although statistically significant, elevations were detected in cerebrospinal fluid levels of serine, threonine, and lysine.[174]

Degeneration of cortical neurons in vitro occurred after exposure to cerebrospinal fluid from patients with ALS but not other neurologic diseases.[40] Prevention of this neurotoxicity with a non-NMDA antagonist (CNQX) but not two NMDA antagonists implicated an excitatory amino acid–like substance (possibly glutamate) acting at the AMPA/kainate receptors.

REDUCED TISSUE LEVELS OF EXCITATORY AMINO ACIDS

Postmortem tissue analyses of patients with sporadic ALS have revealed significant reductions of glutamate in multiple regions of the CNS.[151,152,154,155,209] The decreased glutamate levels, ranging from 55% to 80% of normal, have been detected not only in areas affected in ALS (e.g., spinal cord) but also in unaffected areas.[151,155] For this reason, these changes may reflect not simply a loss of glutamate-containing neurons, but a generalized defect of glutamate metabolism.[153] Statistically significant decreases in concentration have also been noted in NAA (by 40%) and NAAG (by 60%) in the ventral horn of the spinal cord of eight patients with ALS.[174] Similar reductions in glutamate have not been detected in CNS tissue from patients with Guamanian ALS.[150]

GLUTAMATE TRANSPORTER ABNORMALITIES

Rothstein and colleagues[173] first found evidence of a functional defect in the high-affinity sodium-dependent glutamate uptake system in synaptosomes from spinal cord and motor brain regions of patients with ALS. Glutamate transport was 60% to 70% lower than in control individuals, decreased only in brain regions affected by ALS (hippocampus, striatum), and remained normal in patients with other neurodegenerative diseases (Huntington's disease, Alzheimer's disease). Loss of a transporter protein, not just a structural abnormality, was suspected from analyses of the transporter kinetics. Sodium-dependent transporters of other amino acids, like γ-aminobutyric acid and phenylalanine, functioned normally.[173]

The same investigators subsequently identified, by immunoblot analysis, a substantial decrease and even loss of the astrocyte-specific EAAT2 glutamate transporter in the motor cortex and spinal cord in ALS.[175] EAAT2 immunoreactivity was almost nonexistent in most layers of the motor cortex. Little or no significant reduction was detected in two other glutamate transporters.

The role of glutamate transporter abnormalities in the pathogenesis of ALS is unknown. Finding mutations in the glutamate transporter genes in patients with ALS would support a primary role, but so far, no abnormalities have been found in the coding region of the neuronal transporter EAAT3.[129] As discussed above, however, glutamate transporter dysfunction may be a result of other disturbances, such as inadequate ATP[177] or inhibition by oxygen free radicals[211] and arachidonic acid.[210]

Experimental Models of Motor Neuron Excitotoxicity

IN VITRO STUDIES

Whetsell and Schwarcz[213] first showed that chronic administration of low concentrations of quinolinic acid, an NMDA receptor agonist, caused neurodegeneration in organotypic (slice preparation resembling the intact organ) tissue cultures of the rat corticostriatal system. Rothstein and colleagues[170] have used the organotypic postnatal rat spinal cord preparation to study the effects of chronically inhibited glutamate uptake as a model of what may be occurring in some patients with ALS. Blocking the glutamate transporters with competitive inhibitors (e.g., threo-hydroxyaspartate) resulted in elevated extracellular glutamate and slow motor neuron degeneration as revealed by vacuolization and cell loss.[170] The same result was obtained using specific antisense oligonucleotides to EAAT1 and EAAT2, which blocked new synthesis of these two glutamate transporter proteins.[168] This neurotoxicity could be prevented with two non-NMDA antagonists (CNQX and GYKI-52466), which inhibit glutamate synthesis and release, but not by NMDA antagonists.[170]

IN VIVO ANIMAL STUDIES

Only a few in vivo animal studies have examined the neurotoxic effects of increased extracellular excitatory amino acids. Intrathecal administration of kainic acid into mice acutely produced nuclear condensation and cytoplasmic vacuolation, and at several days after injection, progressive neuronal degeneration with axonal dilatation.[91] Neurofilaments were abnormally phosphorylated in the anterior horn cell bodies and proximal dendrites of such animals.[92]

In rats, the chronic intrathecal administration of antisense oligonucleotides to the EAAT1 transporter resulted in degenerated spinal cord motor neurons, paralysis, and muscle denervation.[168] This is the first animal model of defective glutamate uptake that is similar to that found in some patients with ALS.[173]

Therapies That Suppress Excitotoxicity

If neuronal overstimulation by excitatory amino acids contributes to motor neuron degeneration in ALS, interrupting it may retard or even prevent disease progression. The excitotoxic effects of glutamate potentially can be reduced in several ways, including decreasing its synthesis, decreasing its release from nerve terminals, increasing its uptake, blocking the activity of postsynaptic NMDA or non-NMDA receptors, and preventing the secondary intracellular or extracellular events triggered by receptor overstimulation; these latter post-receptor processes will be discussed below. Numerous drugs that interfere with glutamate excitotoxicity have been tested, mostly in vitro and primarily in models of hypoxia or ischemia.[32,128] Such pharmacologic agents have recently been reviewed by Lipton and Rosenberg.[117] Some glutamate-modulating drugs that have been tested or are being tested in ALS clinical trials (Table 12–3) also are discussed.

REDUCTION OF GLUTAMATE SYNTHESIS

Branched-chain amino acids, such as L-leucine, L-isoleucine, and L-valine, are known to increase the activity of glutamate dehydrogenase.[218] This, in turn, is believed to decrease glutamate synthesis by promoting the deamination of glutamate to 2-oxo-glutarate.[58] The first published trial[158] indicated a small transient slowing of ALS progression in 22 patients taking an oral preparation of all three amino acids in a double-blind fashion for a 1-year period. However, four subsequent studies by other groups showed no clinical benefit.[99,196,203,206] In fact, excess mortality in the 24 patients receiving branched-chain amino acids compared to the 13 patients receiving placebo prompted cessation of the Italian ALS Study Group trial.[99] Because glutamate dehydrogenase is believed to act mainly in the direction of glutamate synthesis,[110] as discussed above, stimulating the enzyme with branched-chain amino acids may actually *increase* glutamate synthesis.

INHIBITION OF GLUTAMATE RELEASE

Gabapentin (Neurontin), an anticonvulsant branched-chain amino acid analog, may reduce glutamate synthesis[204] by inhibiting branched-chain amino acid transferase. This enzyme catalyzes the transfer of an amino group from a branched-chain amino acid to α-ketoglutarate to form glutamate.[71] Both gabapentin and riluzole protect motor neurons from glutamate-mediated toxicity in an organotypic rat spinal cord model of neuroprotection.[171] In addition, treating transgenic mice overexpressing mutated human *SOD1* with either of these drugs modestly prolonged survival.[75]

Table 12–3. DRUGS WITH ANTIGLUTAMATE EFFECTS EXAMINED IN ALS

Drug	Mechanism of Action	Potential Use in ALS
Branched-chain amino acid (e.g., leucine)	Reduces glutamate synthesis*	No definite benefit[158,203,206]
Gabapentin (Neurontin)	Reduces glutamate synthesis[204]	ALS clinical trial ongoing; prolonged survival in *SOD1* transgenic mice[75]
Riluzole (Rilutek)[†]	Reduces glutamate release[124]	Prolonged survival in ALS patients[15] and *SOD1* transgenic mice[75]
Lamotrigine	Reduces glutamate release[27]	No benefit[57‡]
Dextromethorphan	Blocks NMDA receptors[62]	No benefit[7,89‡]

*This has been questioned; see text for details.
[†]Approved by the FDA for clinical use.
[‡]See text for further explanation.
Abbreviation: NMDA = *N*-methyl-D-aspartate.

Riluzole (2-amino-6-trifluoromethoxy ben-zothiazole) (Rilutek) is the first drug approved by the Food and Drug Administration (FDA) for treating ALS, although its clinical benefit is limited. It primarily inhibits glutamate release by blocking the voltage-gated sodium channels on presynaptic nerve terminals[85,124] but may also interact with G-proteins and block postsynaptic receptors.[132] Results of the first riluzole trial were criticized,[176] in part because benefit was seen only in patients with bulbar-onset ALS and not limb-onset ALS.[15] At 9 months, 87% (67 of 77) of patients taking riluzole were alive without the need of ventilatory support, compared to 67% (52 of 78) of patients taking placebo. This difference decreased to 49% versus 37%, respectively, at the end of the trial (median, 19 months), but it was still statistically significant. A subsequent multi-center phase 3 trial in Europe and the United States with 959 patients showed a small but statistically significant prolongation of survival (approximately 3 months) without need for ventilatory support in patients taking 100 to 200 mg/d riluzole compared to those taking 50 mg/d riluzole or placebo.[112] The benefit in the larger trial was not restricted to patients with bulbar-onset ALS. There was no statistically significant diminution of the maximal benefit between 12 months and 18 months, when the trial ended. Reportedly, no effect was detected on muscle strength.

Lamotrigine, another inhibitor of glutamate release that blocks voltage-gated sodium channels, is used as an anticonvulsant in Great Britain and Ireland.[27] A small double-blind, placebo-controlled trial showed no significant benefit in patients with ALS after 18 months of taking the drug ($n = 18$) compared to placebo ($n = 21$).[57] Because of its unknown side effects in ALS, however, the dosage tested (100 mg/d) was about half that used to treat refractory seizures. Therefore, the utility of lamotrigine in ALS cannot be excluded and a larger trial with higher dosages (200 to 400 mg/d) may be warranted.

ANTAGONISM OF GLUTAMATE RECEPTORS

Blockers of NMDA receptor activity have been used primarily in clinical trials for stroke (e.g., MK-801), although they are not without side effects that may limit clinical usefulness. Dextromethorphan, a relatively weak NMDA receptor antagonist that blocks the receptor ionophore,[62] has been studied in ALS. Two small studies did not demonstrate efficacy,[7,89] although the relatively short study period (3 months) and the possibility of insufficient blood levels suggest the need for further investigations.

Non-NMDA receptor antagonists such as 1,2,3,4-tetrahydro-6-nitro-2,3-dioxo-benzo[f]-quinoxaline-7-sulfonamide (NBQX), CNQX, and GYKI-52466 prevent excitotoxic neurodegeneration in cultures of rat spinal cord,[170] cerebral cortex,[40] and in animal models of stroke[29] and trauma.[217] Whether these drugs can be tolerated by humans at neuroprotective dosages is not yet known,[117] although clinical trials will probably be conducted soon. Development of clinically usable non-NMDA receptor antagonists is essential, considering they are more effective than NMDA receptor antagonists in preventing glutamate-mediated motor neuron excitotoxicity in vitro.[40,170]

OXIDATIVE NEUROTOXICITY IN ALS

Formation of Reactive Oxygen Species

The human brain and spinal cord derive virtually all their energy from oxidative metabolism in the mitochondrial respiratory chain. During oxidative phosphorylation in mitochondria, oxygen is reduced to water by cytochrome oxidase, and ATP is generated. As high-energy electrons move along the electron transport chain, a small percentage (<5%) normally "leak" onto oxygen to form a free radical,[78] the superoxide anion, $\cdot O_2^-$. A free radical is a molecule that contains one or more unpaired electrons and can exist independently (thus the term "free"); the dot ($\cdot$) denotes the presence of at least one unpaired electron. Such free radicals have been implicated in neurodegenerative diseases, including Alzheimer's disease, Parkinson's disease, and ALS.[78,79,146] Calcium-mediated excitotoxicity can also generate superoxide radicals through activation of xanthine oxidase, and nitric oxide synthase, and the production of arachidonic acid (via phospholipase A_2) (see Table 12–2). Therefore, superoxide anion formation can result from either oxidative or excitoxic processes.

The superoxide anion and other forms of reactive oxygen, like hydrogen peroxide, can damage cells, particularly if present in excess because of increased production or reduced detoxification.

Superoxide Dismutase (SOD) Protection Against Reactive Oxygen Species

Eukaryotic cells possess three types of superoxide dismutase enzyme (SOD) that protect the organism against oxygen free-radical damage.[65] Each SOD is coded by a separate gene and has a distinct distribution; cytosolic copper, zinc superoxide dismutase (SOD1), mitochondrial manganese superoxide dismutase (SOD2), and an extracellular superoxide dismutase (SOD3). SOD1, which has a copper and zinc at the active site, is of particular interest in ALS pathogenesis because *SOD1* gene mutations have been identified in 10% to 20% of patients with autosomally inherited FALS.[166] SOD scavenges the superoxide radical, in the presence of proton (H^+), to form hydrogen peroxide (H_2O_2) and oxygen (Eq. 1). Normally, hydrogen peroxide is then metabolized to water and oxygen by the enzymes glutathione peroxidase (GPx) and catalase (Cat) (Eq. 2).

$$2 \cdot O_2^- + 2H^+ \xrightarrow{\text{SOD}} H_2O_2 + O_2 \quad (1)$$

$$2H_2O_2 \xrightarrow{\text{GPx, Cat}} O_2 + 2H_2O \quad (2)$$

SUPEROXIDE ANION

The superoxide radical is itself relatively unreactive, but it can produce other, more reactive species, including peroxynitrite and hydroxyl radicals. Under normal circumstances, SOD maintains very low levels of the superoxide anion, so such reactive species seldom or never form. However, if enzyme activity is significantly reduced, as has been noted in many patients with FALS who have the *SOD1* gene mutation,[22,50,164] superoxide radicals may accumulate and generate harmful reactive species. Being a radical, the superoxide anion can donate or accept electrons to convert nonradical molecules into radicals; a damaging chain reaction of radical formation can ensue.[82,146]

PEROXYNITRITE

When the superoxide anion reacts with nitric oxide (NO), a highly diffusable radical, peroxynitrite ($ONOO^-$) is formed (Eq. 3).[14] Peroxynitrite is a powerful oxidant that can cause neuronal death.[48,116] It can also react with the copper ion (Cu^{2+}) of *SOD1* (and with other transition metals like manganese and iron) to form the highly reactive and toxic nitronium ion (NOO^+) (Eq. 4).[14] Of note, substantially increased iron levels have been found in the lumbar spinal cord of patients with ALS compared to healthy individuals.[96] The nitronium ion can nitrate the tyrosine residues (H–Tyr) of proteins to form nitrotyrosine (NO_2–Tyr-protein) (Eq. 5).[98]

$$\cdot O_2^- + NO \rightarrow ONOO^- \quad (3)$$

$$ONOO^- + SOD–Cu^{2+} \rightarrow$$
$$SOD–CuO\cdots NOO^+ \quad (4)$$

$$SOD–CuO\cdots NOO^+ + H–Tyr\text{-protein} \rightarrow$$
$$NO_2\text{–Tyr-protein} + SOD–Cu^{2+} + OH^- \quad (5)$$

Beckman and colleagues[13,14] have proposed that this SOD1-dependent protein nitration underlies the pathogenesis of FALS. Several important processes depend on the kinase phosphorylation of intracellular tyrosine targets. Nitration of these tyrosines by peroxynitrite would inactivate them because nitration makes them resistant to phosphorylation.[123] For example, signal transduction of most growth factor receptors (e.g., neurotrophin receptors) involves the phosphorylation of tyrosine residues (see Chapter 15). Kinases may be prevented from normally phosphorylating tyrosine residues on neurofilaments (see Chapter 16). Abnormalities of neurotrophic factor receptors and neurofilament processing have both been implicated in the pathogenesis of ALS (see Chapters 10 and 16).

NITRIC OXIDE

Nitric oxide is a highly diffusable molecule with important functions in the CNS, including acting as a neurotransmitter and vasoregulator.[47] It is produced normally at low levels in macrophages, endothelial cells, and certain neurons by nitric oxide synthase. Nitric oxide synthesis increases during excitotoxicity because nitric oxide synthase is stimulated by calcium influx mediated by activated excitatory amino acid receptors.[48] An abundance of NO would form more peroxynitrite because the superoxide radical highly prefers NO over SOD1.[93] The occurrence of excitotoxicity in certain situations may also require NO (and superoxide anion) as has been shown for hippocampal neurons in culture.[46]

The chemical state of NO, which depends on the availability of electron donors such as ascorbate and cysteine, determines whether or not it is harmful. In its radical state, nitric oxide ($\cdot$NO) damages cells. As a nitrosonium ion (NO^+), it is protective because it binds to a redox modulatory site on the NMDA receptor (see the section on NMDA receptors), decreasing its activity.[116] Drugs resembling nitrosonium, such as nitroglycerin, have been effective in animal models of stroke and may be beneficial in other conditions in which excitotoxicity occurs.[116]

HYDROGEN PEROXIDE

Hydrogen peroxide is a freely diffusable uncharged molecule that is not a radical but can be an intermediate compound in reactions producing highly reactive damaging species. Its rate of production by SOD is limited by the rate of superoxide formation, not by the dismutation of superoxide.[14] Therefore an increase in SOD activity generally does not form more hydrogen peroxide, but a reduction in the activity of glutathione peroxidase or catalase would cause hydrogen peroxide accumulation (see Eq. 2).

In one study of brain tissue from patients with sporadic ALS, the activity of glutathione peroxidase, but not of catalase or SOD, was decreased significantly to approximately 60% of control levels in the motor cortex but not in the cerebellar cortex.[160] The decrease was most marked in those who died from rapidly progressing disease and was less marked in those who died from more slowly progressing disease. These findings contrast with an earlier study that found a marked *increase* in glutathione peroxidase activity in the spinal cord of patients with sporadic motor neuron disease.[96] The cause of the discrepancy is unclear because fairly similar methods were used in both studies.[160]

Hydrogen peroxide becomes reactive when it decomposes to the highly toxic hydroxyl radical ($\cdot$OH) upon gaining an electron from the reduced forms of copper (Cu^+) (Eq. 6), iron (Fe^{2+}) (Eq. 7) or other transition metals.[82] The accompanying hydroxyl ion (OH^-) is relatively harmless, and the transition metal becomes oxidized (loses an electron). These metals have a loosely bound electron in their outer shell and can alternate between different valence states; thus they can either donate or accept a single electron and thereby promote a redox reaction.

$$H_2O_2 + Cu^+ \rightarrow Cu^{2+} + \cdot OH \\ + OH^- \quad (6)$$

$$H_2O_2 + Fe^{2+} \rightarrow Fe^{3+} + \cdot OH \\ + OH^- \quad (7)$$

The formation of hydroxyl radicals further accelerates when the superoxide radical is present because this anion can provide its unpaired electron to again reduce copper (Eq. 8) and iron (Eq. 9).[81]

$$\cdot O_2 + Cu^{2+} \rightarrow Cu^+ + O_2 \quad (8)$$

$$\cdot O_2 + Fe^{3+} \rightarrow Fe^{2+} + O_2 \quad (9)$$

Reduction of hydrogen peroxide by SOD normally occurs at low rates and is not detrimental when the copper ion is in a stable oxidized state (Cu^{2+}) (Eq. 10). Transferrin and ferritin are extracellular metal-binding proteins that normally keep copper and other transition metals in an unreactive state. However, if the copper ion of SOD is in a reduced state (Cu^+), hydrogen peroxide reduction produces harmful hydroxyl radicals ($\cdot$OH) (Eq. 11; also see Eq. 6).

$$SOD-Cu^{2+} + H_2O_2 \rightarrow SOD-Cu^+ \\ + O_2^- + 2H^+ \quad (10)$$

$$SOD–Cu^+ + H_2O_2 \rightarrow SOD–Cu^{2+}$$
$$+ \cdot OH + OH^- \qquad (11)$$

HYDROXYL RADICAL

The hydroxyl radical reacts very rapidly with virtually every molecule in living cells; some of the cellular components damaged by the hydroxyl radical are listed in Table 12–4. The oxidation of polyunsaturated fatty acids (lipid peroxidation) in cell membranes is particularly detrimental. As lipid peroxyl radicals ($\cdot$OO-L) are generated, they themselves react with adjacent membrane fatty acids to generate a chain reaction of continual peroxidation and eventual membrane destruction.[81]

There is evidence of hydroxyl radical damage to the CNS in patients with sporadic ALS. Carbonyl, a marker of oxidative damage to proteins, increases by 85% in the frontal cortex[22] and by 119% in the lumbar spinal cord[180] of patients compared to normal individuals. Also, components of the neuronal cytoskeleton, such as the neurofilaments, could be damaged by hydroxyl radicals in ALS and result in neuronal dysfunction.[1]

SOD1 Gene Mutations in Familial ALS

SOD's beneficial function as a superoxide radical scavenger has been known for over a decade;[66] now functions related to preventing programmed cell death (apoptosis)[73,161] also are being identified. Interest in this enzyme has renewed since Rosen and colleagues[166] discovered dominant mutations in the *SOD1* gene in a proportion of patients with FALS. More than 50 missense mutations have been identified in four of the five exons of *SOD1*, the exception being exon 3, which encodes most of the loop around the metal ions that form the enzyme active site. These mutations were discussed further in Chapter 10. Identification of modifiers of *SOD1* gene expression may explain the clinical variability of ALS in families possessing the same mutation.[5,145] Based on results from numerous patients and studies of transgenic mice overexpressing the mutated human *SOD1* gene, it is now established that the mutated SOD1 enzyme causes motor neuron degeneration, albeit to varying degrees.

ROLE OF MUTATED SOD1 IN MOTOR NEURON DEGENERATION

SOD1 is a dimer of two identical subunits forming a β-barrel structure with the two active sites on opposite sides facing outward.[202] The copper ion, required for enzyme activity, forms the catalytic center that is alternately reduced (Cu^+) and oxidized (Cu^{2+}) by superoxide ions.[178] Most *SOD1* mutations are located in regions coding for the base of the two major loops forming the channel around the active-site copper and at the two ends of the β-barrel.[50] Unlike normal SOD1 in which copper is situated internally, mutated SOD1 may expose the metal ion, making it more accessible to reduction by free radicals.[20,50]

Table 12–4. **CELLULAR MOLECULES DAMAGED BY HYDROXYL RADICALS**

Cellular Component	Type of Damage	Consequence
DNA	Strand breakage Base modification	Apoptosis[80,105]
Protein	Site-specific lesion Fragmentation Cross-linking	Protein inactivation (e.g., glutamine synthetase[136]) Protein degradation
Lipid	Peroxidation of polyunsaturated fatty acids[81]	Loss of membrane potential ↑Permeability to Ca^{2+}, metal ions Formation of toxic aldehydes Loss of membrane integrity

The most frequent mutation is Ala4→Val in exon 1 of the *SOD1* gene. Located in the β-strand region of SOD1, the mutation destabilizes the dimers, decreasing enzyme activity to less than half of normal.[50] The resulting clinical phenotype is one of the most severe, with the average survival after onset being 1.2 years, compared to 2.5 to 3.5 years for all other patients with FALS.[103,165]

Precisely how the *SOD1* mutation results in motor neuron degeneration is unclear. Initially, superoxide radical–induced damage was suspected because SOD1 enzyme activity is decreased by 20% to 50% in most FALS patients with this mutation.[22,50,164] This decrease is attributed to diminished stability of the enzyme dimer, which shortens its half-life by 30% to 75%.[20] Enzyme instability may result in precipitation and formation of toxic cytoplasmic aggregates. At least one *SOD1* mutation, Asp90→Ala, does not diminish SOD1 activity, although development of clinical disease requires homozygosity.[186] No true *SOD1* null mutations have been reported in FALS, although a two-base-pair deletion that produces a truncated SOD1 enzyme has been identified.[159] Therefore, there are no examples of *SOD1*-related FALS in which enzyme activity is completely absent.

Rather than a lack of SOD1 function being responsible for the motor neuron degeneration, the aforementioned features argue for a "gain of function" exerted by the *SOD1* mutation: autosomal-dominant inheritance, lack of decreased SOD1 enzyme activity in at least one type of mutation (Asp90→Ala), and lack of null mutations resulting in total absence of enzyme activity. Furthermore, motor neuron degeneration occurring in transgenic mice overexpressing the mutated, but not the wild-type, human *SOD1*[45,76] suggests that disease results from some novel cytotoxic property of the mutated SOD1 protein. However, inhibition of endogenous SOD1 activity can cause neuronal degeneration in organotypic postnatal spinal cord cultures.[169] In addition, 3-month-old mice deficient in SOD1 had greater neuronal loss after facial nerve axotomy than did animals with normal enzyme levels, although no motor neuron pathology was detected without axotomy.[162] This finding suggests that patients with FALS and diminished SOD1 activity may be less able to compensate for conditions (whatever they may be) that expose motor neurons to physiologic stress.

NOVEL CYTOTOXIC EFFECTS OF MUTATED SOD1

Increased Reactivity with Peroxynitrite

Beckman et al.[13] proposed that the copper ion of the mutated SOD1 has an increased affinity for peroxynitrite, and, as discussed above, forms the highly reactive nitronium ion (see Eq. 4), which subsequently nitrates tyrosine residues in critical proteins (e.g., neurofilaments, tyrosine kinase receptors). The increased affinity may result from a mutation-induced structural change in SOD1, allowing peroxynitrite and other substances greater access to the reactive metal core. In addition to increasing SOD1 affinity for peroxynitrite, the mutation reduces the superoxide scavenging capacity of the enzyme.[13] Crow et al.[43] have demonstrated nitration of neurofilament catalyzed by SOD1 in patients with ALS, supporting the role of peroxynitrite in disease pathogenesis.

Increased Reactivity with Hydrogen Peroxide

Wiedau-Pazos et al.[214] proposed that the mutated SOD1 enzyme can act as a peroxidase, catalysing the reduction of hydrogen peroxide much more rapidly than the wild-type enzyme (see Eq. 10). This reaction becomes harmful when the SOD1 copper ion is in a reduced state (Cu^+), resulting in hydroxyl radical ($\cdot OH$) formation (see Eq. 11). Free radicals can be directly monitored with electron spin resonance spectroscopy by measuring energy changes that occur as unpaired electrons align in an external magnetic field.[102] To facilitate this measurement, the radical is reacted with a "trap" or "spin trap" molecule to produce one or more stable products. (For further explanation of trapping assays, see Reference 82.) In their in vitro experiments, Wiedau-Pazos et al.[214] used this technique to measure the hydroxyl radicals produced by mutated SOD1 containing reduced copper ion. The hydroxyl radicals reacted with the spin trap substrate 5, 5′-dimethyl-1-pyrroline *N*-oxide (DMPO) to form DMPO–OH, a hydroxyl adduct, which was then measured by electron spin resonance spectroscopy (Eq. 12).

$$SOD-Cu^+ + H_2O_2 \rightarrow$$

$$SOD-Cu^{2+} + \cdot OH + OH^- \xrightarrow{\text{DMPO}}$$

$$SOD-Cu^{2+} + DMPO-OH + OH^- \quad (12)$$

Formation of hydroxyl radicals did not occur if the experiments were performed using free copper, metal-free SOD (SOD apoenzyme), or copper chelators (e.g., *d,l*-penicillamine, diethyldithiocarbamate), suggesting that reduced copper was essential for this reaction. Not only does this study[214] support the role of oxidative reactions catalyzed by mutant SOD1 enzyme in the pathogenesis of FALS, but it also reveals the usefulness of copper chelators in inhibiting these reactions.

Proapoptotic Effect

Apoptosis is a means of cell death in which the cell actively participates; it occurs in both physiologic and pathologic processes. Much has been learned of the roles of antiapoptotic (cell death–preventing) and proapoptotic (cell death–inducing) genes in the regulation of neural apoptosis (reviewed in Reference 24). There is no definite evidence of apoptosis in ALS, but detecting it may be difficult because the number of cells dying at any one time is low, as in other chronic neurodegenerative diseases. An immunohistochemical study of 10 patients with sporadic ALS identified DNA fragmentation, an indicator of apoptosis, in spinal cord motor neurons of four to seven patients, depending on the technique used.[219]

In vitro studies have found that wild-type SOD1 is antiapoptotic and abnormal SOD1 (with the Ala4→Val or Gly93→Ala mutation) is proapoptotic. Injecting cultured sympathetic ganglion cells with SOD1 enzyme or an SOD cDNA protected them from apoptosis after deprivation of nerve growth factor.[73] SOD-deficient yeast cells underwent apoptosis when exposed to oxidative stress unless they were injected with SOD1 enzyme, which resulted in survival. However, injection of mutated *SOD1,* even into SOD-containing yeast, enhanced programmed cell death.[161] The same was true for neural cells.[161] Furthermore, a neural cell line expressing mutated forms of human SOD1 underwent apoptosis much more rapidly after serum deprivation than cells expressing the wild-type enzyme.[214] This programmed cell death was suppressed by copper chelators, indicating that hydroxyl radicals may be important in its pathogenesis.

HUMAN *SOD1* MUTATIONS IN TRANSGENIC MICE

Gurney et al.[76] produced the first transgenic mouse model of FALS in which the Ala 4→Val and Gly 93→Ala mutations of the human *SOD1* gene were overexpressed. Motor neuron degeneration was evident in animals with the highest copy number (18) of the Gly 93→Ala mutation. Of note, disease occurred despite normal levels of SOD1 enzyme activity (the mice still possessed their own two alleles). Affected animals began manifesting progressive hind limb weakness by 3 to 4 months of age and became completely paralyzed in two or more limbs by the time of death at approximately 6 months. As in FALS, pathologic changes were essentially limited to motor structures, with progressive motor neuron loss in the brain stem and spinal cord, accumulation of intraneuronal filaments, wallerian degeneration of ventral roots and peripheral nerves, and denervation of muscle.[76] In early stages of the disease, however, motor neuron cell bodies and processes contained varying numbers of vacuoles, which arose from dilations of endoplasmic reticula and mitochondria.[45] Whether these vacuoles represent a significant difference in pathology between the *SOD1* transgenic mouse and FALS or are simply an early phenomenon not evident at later stages of the human disease, when pathologic tissue is usually examined, remains to be clarified.

A transgenic mouse line created by Wong et al.[216] overexpressing a Gly37→Arg *SOD1* mutation had vacuolated mitochondria in axons and dendrites of the lower motor neurons. Higher levels of mutant protein expression in some of the transgenic animals resulted in more extensive pathology involving widespread neuronal populations. In fact, motor neuron degeneration has been reported in the neocortex of transgenic mice expressing an *SOD1* gene mutation that corresponds to one occurring in FALS.[163] Both transgenic mouse experiments support the hypothesis that the *SOD1* mutations produce a dominant gain of function in the mutated SOD1 enzyme.

Transgenic animals in which the wild-type human *SOD1* gene was overexpressed several times above control levels had no clinical signs of motor neuron degeneration,[76,216] although mild vacuolation has been observed in spinal cord motor neurons and motor axons.[45] Other investigators reported retraction and loss of terminal axons at neuromuscular endplates as well as at multiple small terminals in transgenic mice that expressed wild-type SOD1 enzyme at levels as much as 10 times greater than controls.[8] This finding indicates that even the normal enzyme can be neurotoxic when present in high amounts, although the mechanism is unclear. As discussed above, hydrogen peroxide normally should not be overproduced as a result of increased SOD1 enzyme activity.[14] However, the situation may change when the *SOD1* gene is overexpressed in the transgenic mouse, resulting in excessively high levels of mutated SOD1 enzyme. If high levels of hydrogen peroxide are formed and reduced transition metals exist, cytotoxic hydroxyl radicals can be generated.

That oxidative stress contributes to disease in the mutant *SOD1* transgenic mice is also evident by the depletion of α-tocopherol (vitamin E) levels in the brain, rather than the normal age-dependent increase that occurs in unaffected mice.[75] Such depletion is believed to indicate the use of α-tocopherol to scavenge free radicals in tissues.[75]

Therapies That Suppress Oxidative Damage

Because motor neuron degeneration in ALS may, at least in part, be the result of oxidative damage, inhibiting or suppressing its consequences may retard or even arrest disease progression. Several drugs that potentially interrupt oxidative damage have been tested, primarily in vitro or in models of trauma and ischemia; their use in clinical trials has been limited.[117] Only a few of these drugs have been or are being tested for the treatment of ALS (Table 12–5).

ANTIOXIDANTS

Vitamin E (α-tocopherol) is one of the body's most important lipophilic antioxidants, which diffuses into cell membranes and protects polyunsaturated fatty acids against lipid peroxide–mediated damage.[4] HO–tocopherol donates a hydrogen atom (with its single electron) to a lipid peroxide radical ($\cdot$OO–L) to form a lipid hydroperoxide (HOO–L) and a vitamin E radical ($\cdot$O–tocopherol) (Eq. 13). This reaction occurs faster than the lipid peroxide radical

Table 12–5. ANTIOXIDANT DRUGS TESTED IN ALS

Drug	Mechanism of Action	Potential Use in ALS
α-Tocopherol (vitamin E)	Reduces lipid peroxidation[4]	Delayed onset of disease in *SOD1* transgenic mice[75]; no benefit in ALS[60]
SOD	Increases dismutation of superoxide radicals[66]	Reduced motor deficit in wobbler mouse model of ALS (subcutaneous injection of lecithinized SOD)[95]; stabilization on muscle testing in one patient with late-stage FALS[187] (intracerebroventricular infusion of bovine SOD)
N-acetylcysteine	Scavenges free radicals	Randomized, double-blind, placebo-controlled trial showed no improvement at 12 months in survival or ALS progression;[118] open study of large daily subcutaneous injections for 6 months showed "modest" clinical improvement[49]
Metal chelator (e.g., *d,l*-penicillamine)	Inactivates reduced transition metals	Reduced free-radical formation by mutant *SOD1* enzyme in vitro[214]; no benefits in ALS

Abbreviations: FALS = familial ALS; SOD = superoxide dismutase.

can react with adjacent fatty acid chains or membrane proteins. The lipid hydroperoxides are then eliminated by glutathione peroxidase. Part, but not all, of the relatively unreactive vitamin E radical is regenerated by vitamin C (ascorbate) as reduced tocopherol (Eq. 14). In this way, vitamins E and C may act as an antioxidant team.[146]

$$HO\text{--}tocopherol + \cdot OO\text{--}L \rightarrow$$
$$O\text{--}tocopherol + HOO\text{--}L \qquad (13)$$

$$\cdot O\text{--}tocopherol + ascorbate \rightarrow$$
$$semihydroascorbate +$$
$$HO\text{--}tocopherol \qquad (14)$$

Previous trials of vitamin E to treat ALS revealed no detectable benefit, although studies usually involved small numbers of patients treated for relatively short periods (for review see Reference 60). However, the delay of disease onset when transgenic mice overexpressing mutant *SOD1* were given α-tocopherol[75] suggests that antioxidants may benefit patients with FALS caused by *SOD1* mutations. Presymptomatic treatment may be needed because vitamin E only delayed disease onset and did not prolong survival (in contrast to drugs that inhibit glutamate-mediated neurotoxicity).

Vitamin C (L-ascorbate) generally is an excellent antioxidant[64] that is highly concentrated in the CNS; active transport mechanisms can raise the L-ascorbate levels in the cerebrospinal fluid to 10 times that in plasma and to an even higher level in cells.[191] However, vitamin C and other flavonoids can stimulate production of hydroxyl radicals in the abnormal presence of transition metals (e.g., catalytic iron, Fe^{3+}).[79,114] Therefore, caution is required when selecting antioxidant flavonoid therapies to treat ALS. Because mutations in the SOD1 enzyme of patients with FALS may make the internal copper more accessible,[20,50] administration of vitamin C may actually be detrimental.

FREE RADICAL SCAVENGERS

Superoxide scavengers, such as exogenously administered SOD, may be useful in preventing ALS progression, especially if diminished enzyme activity is important in pathogenesis. Because SOD poorly penetrates into the CNS, delivery of the enzyme may be difficult. Lecithinized SOD given subcutaneously to wobbler mice (a model of motor neuron disease) significantly retarded disease progression.[95] Also, muscle strength stabilized in a patient with advanced FALS who received intrathecal SOD.[187]

N-acetylcysteine is a free radical scavenger and precursor of glutathione, an important intracellular antioxidant. A recent randomized, double-blind, placebo-controlled trial of N-acetylcysteine in 110 patients with ALS resulted in a decrease in mortality of 29% at the 1-year endpoint in patients taking the drug who had spinal-onset ALS, but not in those with bulbar-onset ALS; this difference was not statistically significant, however.[118] An earlier open study with large daily subcutaneous injection (up to 100 mL) of 5% N-acetylcysteine in ALS patients for 6 months showed modest improvement,[49] although another study failed to demonstrate any benefit.[109]

METAL CHELATORS

Chelating agents prevent reactive iron or other transition metals from participating in reactions producing hydroxyl radicals and lipid peroxidation. The prototype, desferrioxamine, prevents most iron-dependent radical reactions and has successfully decreased oxidative damage in animal models of human disease.[77] Because desferrioxamine and most antioxidants do not cross the blood-brain barrier, alternative chelating agents with antioxidant activity have been developed, including a group of 21-aminosteroids that include tirilazad mesylate (U74006F).[23]

Mutations of SOD1 destabilize the folded enzyme[20] and likely expose the normally shielded active-site copper, so that if it is reduced (Cu^+), it can react with hydrogen peroxide to produce damaging hydroxyl radicals (see Eq. 11). The metal chelators d,l-penicillamine and ethylenediaminetetraacetic acid (EDTA) can minimize the production of free radicals by the mutant SOD1 enzyme in vitro.[214] Administering penicillamine to ALS patients (more to increase heavy metal excretion) did not reveal any clinical benefit.[38] This finding may, in part, be owing to poor penetration of chelating agents into the CNS.

Relationship Between Oxidative Radical and Excitotoxic Processes in ALS

Two of the neurodegenerative mechanisms hypothesized to be involved in ALS—glutamate-mediated excitotoxicity and oxidative damage—probably interact, and even potentiate each other's effects, at various steps along a final common pathway to cell death.[41,117] Figure 12–3 illustrates how the effects of excitotoxicity and oxidative damage are interrelated to perpetuate cellular injury.[113,135,143,211]

The co-occurrence of these processes is likely in *SOD1*-related FALS. For example, motor neuron degeneration in transgenic mice overexpressing the mutated human *SOD1* gene responded differently to treatment suppressing oxidative damage or excitotoxicity: vitamin E delayed the onset of disease, whereas riluzole or gabapentin extended survival. This difference suggests that mutant SOD1 enzyme, at least in the mouse model, produces oxidative damage initially and slow or weak excitotoxicity subsequently.[75]

Another example of such interacting excitotoxic and oxidative effects in ALS involves cysteine, an amino acid required for the synthesis of the free radical scavenger glutathione. Cysteine is transported into neurons and glia, and glutamate is transported out. If extracellular glutamate is elevated, this cotransport stops, and cysteine influx is terminated. As a result, less glutathione is synthesized and free radical–induced damage is more likely.[135] Elevation of plasma cysteine levels in patients with ALS provides evidence for this process.[83]

Combination therapy using drugs with different mechanisms of action (e.g., inhibitors of glutamate toxicity and antioxidants) may provide the greatest therapeutic benefit in ALS. For example, cotreatment of wobbler mice with brain-derived neurotrophic factor and ciliary neurotrophic factor resulted in a greater-than-additive benefit compared to either factor used alone (see Chapter 15). Future treatment of ALS will probably involve

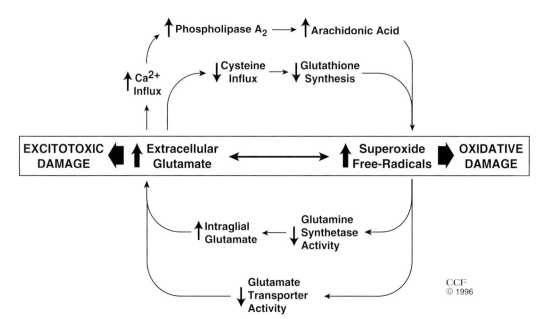

Figure 12–3. Interrelationship of glutamate-mediated excitotoxicity and oxidative damage leading to cellular injury and death. The effects of increased extracellular glutamate, such as increased calcium (Ca^{2+}) influx and decreased cysteine influx, cause increased superoxide free-radical formation which decreases activities of glutamine synthetase and glutamate transporters to again increase extracellular glutamate. Based on information from references 113, 135, 143, 211. (Copyright © 1996 Cleveland Clinic Foundation.)

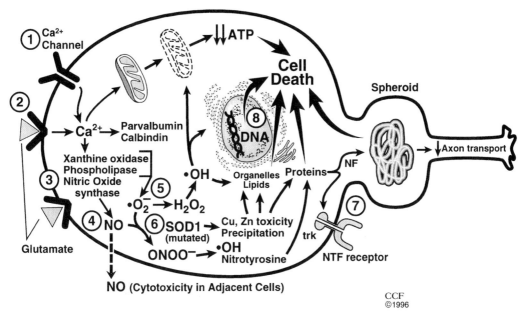

Figure 12–4. Potential mechanisms of motor neuron degeneration in ALS and possible sites of therapeutic intervention: (1) Calcium channel antagonists; (2) glutamate receptor antagonists; (3) nitric oxide synthase inhibitors; (4) nitric oxide scavengers; (5) free-radical scavengers; (6) exogenous SOD enzyme; (7) neurotrophic factors; (8) antiapoptotics. NO, nitric oxide; $\cdot O_2^-$, superoxide anion; $ONOO^-$, peroxynitrite; SOD1, copper, zinc-superoxide dismutase; H_2O_2, hydrogen peroxide; $\cdot OH$, hydroxyl radical; ATP, adenosine triphosphate; DNA, deoxyribonucleic acid; trk, tyrosine kinase receptor; NF, neurofilament; NTF, neurotrophic factor. (Copyright © 1996 Cleveland Clinic Foundation.)

coadministering inhibitors of excitotoxicity and oxidative damage, along with neurotrophic factors to block mechanisms of motor neuron degeneration and enhance recovery and sprouting of already damaged neurons. Figure 12–4 summarizes the various mechanisms proposed to cause motor neuron degeneration in ALS and the sites of action of potential treatments.

SUMMARY

Evidence is accumulating that excitotoxicity and free radical–mediated oxidative injury are important in ALS pathogenesis. They may also contribute to other mechanisms of motor neuron degeneration, including axon transport abnormalities and programmed cell death (apoptosis).

Glutamate and related excitatory amino acids are fundamental in motor transmission. Overstimulation of excitatory amino acid receptors can result in excess intracel-

lular calcium entry and a cascade of processes leading to neuronal death. Of the two classes of excitatory amino acid receptors identified, ionotropic receptors have been implicated in excitotoxicity in ALS. Named for their preferential binding of either NMDA or AMPA and kainate, stimulation of either receptor subtype by endogenous glutamate causes intracellular sodium and calcium influx. This influx is regulated by modulatory sites that can be pharmacologically manipulated to suppress receptor activity and prevent neuronal damage. Features of these ionotropic receptors that may in part make certain motor neuron populations vulnerable to excitotoxicity and degeneration in ALS include their differential distribution in the CNS, differences in ionic permeability, and several receptor genes coding for subunit variants with diverse functions, pharmacology, and anatomic distribution.

Pathologic processes can increase the extracellular glutamate concentration, including exposure to exogenous excitotoxins, increased synthesis and release of glutamate, impaired removal of glutamate transporters, and ATP deficiency. The excitatory amino acid–mediated cation influx through NMDA and AMPA/kainate receptors also activates voltage-gated calcium channels to allow additional calcium influx. Excessive calcium influx activates several enzyme systems that induce cytoskeletal breakdown, free radical formation, and lipid peroxidation, among other events. Intraneuronal calcium-binding proteins protect against calcium-mediated excitotoxicity; motor neurons that degenerate in ALS are relatively deficient in these proteins.

Evidence for excitotoxicity in patients with ALS includes elevated glutamate plasma levels, elevated glutamate and NAAG cerebrospinal fluid levels, presence of a non-NMDA-like substance in cerebrospinal fluid, and diminished tissue glutamate levels. Certain exogenous excitotoxins can result in motor neuron degeneration, such as BOAA, which has been implicated in neurolathyrism, and BMAA, which has been implicated in Western Pacific ALS. Glutamate-uptake transporters, particularly the astrocyte-specific EAAT2, are reduced in ALS motor cortex and spinal cord. Several in vivo and in vitro experiments to increase extracellular excitatory amino acid concentration resulted in motor neuron degeneration.

Therapies suppressing excitotoxicity, and therefore reducing motor neuron degeneration, have been tested. Branched-chain amino acids have been ineffective in most clinical trials. Gabapentin and riluzole have prevented glutamate-mediated excitotoxicity in spinal cord explants and extended survival in transgenic mice that overexpress the mutated human *SOD1* gene. Further, riluzole, which inhibits glutamate release, extended survival in ALS patients by approximately 3 months and is the first drug approved by the FDA for treatment of ALS. Lamotrigine, another inhibitor of glutamate release, may prove useful. Antagonists of non-NMDA receptors but not of NMDA receptors effectively prevented motor neuron degeneration in tissue culture.

Oxidative neurotoxicity, the second possible cause of ALS, begins when reactive oxygen species, such as superoxide ions, are generated during oxidative phosphorylation and calcium-mediated neurotoxicity. Superoxide anions are potentially cytotoxic, and SOD converts them to hydrogen peroxide, which is metabolized to water and oxygen by glutathione peroxidase and catalase. *SOD1* is mutated in 10% to 20% of patients with autosomal-dominant FALS. The abnormal *SOD1* may allow accumulation of superoxide anions and production of reactive species, such as peroxynitrite and hydroxyl radicals. Peroxynitrite, which is formed when the superoxide anion reacts with nitric oxide, can interact with the SOD1 copper ion to form the harmful nitronium ion; the nitronium ion nitrates the tyrosine residues of proteins. Increased nitric oxide generation, occurring when nitric oxide synthase is stimulated by excitatory amino acid–mediated calcium influx, generates more peroxynitrite. Hydrogen peroxide can accumulate if glutathione peroxidase or catalase activity decreases, as occurs in the motor cortex of patients with sporadic ALS. Hydrogen peroxide can produce hydroxyl radicals when it gains an electron from reduced transition metals, such as copper (in mutated SOD1). Although hydroxyl radical production is accelerated when the superoxide radical further reduces the transition metal, it is inhibited by metal chelators. Hydroxyl radical–mediated damage has been detected in the CNS of patients with sporadic ALS. Apoptosis of motor neurons, which may occur in ALS, is induced by mutated SOD1; this can be suppressed in a neural cell line by copper chelators.

More than 50 missense mutations have been discovered in the *SOD1* gene in patients with autosomal-dominant FALS. The most frequent mutation (Ala4→Val) destabilizes the SOD1 dimer, markedly reduces enzyme activity, and produces a severe clinical phenotype. It is unclear how SOD1 mutations result in motor neuron degeneration, but it is probably not simply a result of diminished enzyme activity. Evidence for a "gain of function" exerted by the mutation includes autosomal-dominant inheritance, lack of decreased SOD1 enzyme activity in at least one mutation, lack of null mutations, and progressive motor neuron degeneration in transgenic mice overexpressing the mutated (but not wild-type) human *SOD1* gene.

Therapies suppressing oxidative damage may benefit patients with ALS. Antioxidants inhibit lipid peroxidation and include the lipid-soluble vitamin E and vitamin C, which may act as an antioxidant team. Vitamin E delays disease onset but not survival in transgenic mice overexpressing mutant *SOD1*. The superoxide scavenger SOD may also be beneficial, although delivery into the CNS would be problematic. The free-radical scavenger *N*-acetylcysteine was of some benefit in patients with spinal-onset ALS. Metal chelators, such as desferrioxamine and *d,l*-penicillamine, may prevent hydroxyl radical formation by inactivating reduced transition metals, although trials in ALS have been disappointing.

Glutamate-mediated excitotoxicity and oxidative damage probably occur concurrently in ALS, particularly in *SOD1*-related FALS. Motor neuron degeneration in transgenic mice overexpressing the mutated human *SOD1* gene was reduced by drugs suppressing oxidative damage and excitotoxicity. This effect suggests that therapies that combine drugs with different mechanisms of action may most effectively treat ALS.

REFERENCES

1. Al-Chalabi, A, Powell, JF, and Leigh, PN: Neurofilaments, free radicals, excitotoxins and amyotrophic lateral sclerosis. Muscle Nerve 18:540–545, 1995.
2. Alexianu, ME, Ho, B-K, Mohamed, AH, et al: The role of calcium-binding proteins in selective motor neuron vulnerability in amyotrophic lateral sclerosis. Ann Neurol 36:846–858, 1994.
3. Allaoua, H, Chaudieu, I, Kreiger, C, et al: Alterations in spinal cord excitatory amino acid receptors in amyotrophic lateral sclerosis patients. Brain Res 579:169–172, 1992.
4. Ames, BN, Shigenaga, MK, and Hagen, TM: Oxidants, antioxidants and the degenerative diseases of aging. Proc Nat Acad Sci USA 90:7915–7922, 1993.
5. Aoki, M, Abe, K, Houi, K, et al: Variance of age at onset in a Japanese family with amyotrophic lateral sclerosis associated with a novel Cu/Zn superoxide dismutase mutation. Ann Neurol 37:676–679, 1995.
6. Appel, SH: Excitotoxic neuronal cell death in amyotrophic lateral sclerosis. Trends Neurosci 16:3–5, 1993.
7. Asmark, H, Aquilonius, SM, Gillberg, PG, et al: A pilot trial of dextromethorphan in amyotrophic lateral sclerosis. J Neurol Neurosurg Psychiatry 56:197–200, 1993.
8. Avraham, KB, Sugarman, H, Rotshenker, S, et al: Down's syndrome: Morphological remodeling and increased complexity in the neuromuscular junction of transgenic Cu,Zn-superoxide dismutase mice. J Neurocytol 20:208–215, 1991.
9. Baimbridge, KG, Celio, MR, and Rogers, JH: Calcium-binding proteins in the nervous system. Trends Neurosci 15:303–308, 1992.
10. Barbour, B, Szatkowski, M, Ingledew, N, et al: Arachidonic acid induces a prolonged inhibition of glutamate uptake into glial cells. Nature 342:918–920, 1989.
11. Beal, MF: Aging, energy, and oxidative stress in neurodegenerative diseases. Ann Neurol 38:357–366, 1995.
12. Beckman, JS, Beckman, TW, Chen, J, et al: Apparent hydroxyl radical production by peroxynitrite: Implications for endothelial injury from nitric oxide and superoxide. Proc Nat Acad Sci USA 87:1620–1624, 1990.
13. Beckman, JS, Carson, M, Smith, CD, et al: ALS, SOD and peroxynitrite [letter]. Nature 364:584, 1993.
14. Beckman, JS, Chen, J, Crow, JP, et al: Reactions of nitric oxide, superoxide and peroxynitrite with superoxide dismutase in neurodegeneration. Prog Brain Res 103:371–380, 1994.
15. Bensimon, G, Lacomblez, L, Meininger, V, et al: A controlled trial of riluzole in amyotrophic lateral sclerosis. N Engl J Med 330:585–591, 1994.
16. Bettler, B and Mulle, C: Review: Neurotransmitter receptors. II. AMPA and kainate receptors. Neuropharmacology 34:123–139, 1995.
17. Bito, H, Nakamura, M, Honda, Z, et al: Platelet-activating factor (PAF) receptor in rat brain: PAF mobilizes intracellular Ca^{2+} in hippocampal neurons. Neuron 9:285–294, 1992.
18. Blackstone, CD, Levey, AI, Martin, LJ, et al: Immunological detection of glutamate receptor subtypes in human central nervous system. Ann Neurol 31:680–683, 1992.
19. Bliss, TVP and Collingridge, GL: A synaptic model of memory: Long-term potentiation in the hippocampus. Nature 361:31–39, 1993.
20. Borchelt, DR, Lee, MK, Slunt, HS, et al: Superoxide dismutase 1 with mutations linked to familial amyotrophic sclerosis possesses significant activity. Proc Nat Acad Sci USA 91:8292–8296, 1994.
21. Bouvier, M, Szatkowski, M, Amato, A, et al: The glial cell glutamate uptake carrier countertransports pH-changing anions. Nature 360:471–474, 1992.
22. Bowling, AC, Schulz, JB, Brown, RH Jr, et al: Superoxide dismutase activity, oxidative damage, and mitochondrial energy metabolism in familial and sporadic amyotrophic lateral sclerosis. J Neurochem 61:2322–2325, 1993.
23. Braughler, JM, Pregenzer, JF, Chase, RL, et al: Novel 21-amino steroids as potent inhibitors of iron-dependent lipid peroxidation. J Biol Chem 262:10438–10440, 1987.
24. Bredesen, DE: Neural apoptosis. Ann Neurol 38:839–851, 1995.
25. Bridges, RJ, Kadri, MM, Monaghan, DT, et al: Inhibition of [^{3}H]AMPA binding by the excitotoxin beta-N-oxalyl-L-alpha,beta-diaminopropionic acid. Eur J Pharmacol 145:357–359, 1988.
26. Bridges, RJ, Hatalski, C, Shim, SN, et al: Gliotoxic properties of *Lathyrus* excitotoxin β-N-oxalyl-L-α,β-

diamino-propionic acid (β-L-ODAP). Brain Res 561:262–268, 1991.

27. Brodie, MJ: Drug profiles: Lamotrigine. Lancet 339:1397–1400, 1992.

28. Brown, RH, Jr: Amyotrophic lateral sclerosis: Recent insights from genetics and transgenic mice. Cell 80:687–692, 1995.

29. Buchan, AM, Li, H, Cho, S, et al: Blockade of the AMPA receptor prevents CA1 hippocampal injury following severe but transient forebrain ischemia in adult rats. Neurosci Lett 132:255–258, 1991.

30. Cendes, F, Andermann, F, Carpenter, S, et al: Temporal lobe epilepsy caused by domoic acid intoxication: Evidence for glutamate receptor-mediated excitotoxicity in humans. Ann Neurol 37:123–126, 1995.

31. Choi, DW: Ionic dependence of glutamate neurotoxicity in cortical cell culture. J Neurosci 7:369–379, 1987.

32. Choi, DW: Glutamate neurotoxicity and diseases of the nervous system. Neuron 1:623–634, 1988.

33. Clark, GD, Happel, LT, Zorumski, CF, et al: Enhancement of hippocampal excitatory synaptic transmission by platelet-activating factor. Neuron 9:1211–1216, 1992.

34. Cohen, RW, Fisher, RS, Duong, T, et al: Altered excitatory amino acid function and morphology of the cerebellum of the spastic Han-Wistar rat. Mol Brain Res 11:27–36, 1991.

35. Cohn, DF and Streifler, M: Human neurolathyrism, a follow-up study of 200 patients. Arch Schweiz Archiv Neurol Neurochir Psychiatry 128:151–156, 1981.

36. Collingridge, GL and Lester, AJ: Excitatory amino acid receptors in the vertebrate central nervous system. Pharmacol Rev 40:143–210, 1989.

37. Connor, JA, Wadman, WJ, Hockberger, PE, et al: Sustained dendritic gradients of Ca^{2+} induced by excitatory amino acids in CA1 hippocampal neurons. Science 240:649–653, 1988.

38. Conradi, S, Ronnevi, LO, Nise, G, et al: Long-term penicillamine treatment in amyotrophic lateral sclerosis with parallel determination of lead in blood, plasma and urine. Acta Neurol Scand 65:203–211, 1982.

39. Copani, A, Canonico, PL, Catania, MV, et al: Interaction between β-N-methylamino-L-alanine and excitatory amino acids in brain slices and neuronal cultures. Brain Res 558:76–86, 1991.

40. Couratier, P, Hugon, J, Sindou, P, et al: Cell culture evidence for neuronal degeneration in amyotrophic lateral sclerosis being linked to glutamate AMPA/kainate receptors. Lancet 341:265–268, 1993.

41. Coyle, JT and Puttfarcken, P: Oxidative stress, glutamate, and neurodegenerative disorders. Science 262:689–694, 1993.

42. Coyle, JT, Robinson, MB, Blakely, RD, et al: The neurobiology of N-acetyl-aspartyl glutamate. In Barnard, EA, and Costa, E (eds): Allosteric Modulation of Amino Acid Receptors: Therapeutic Implications. Raven Press, New York, 1989, pp 319–333.

43. Crow, JP and Beckman, JS, personal communication, August 1996.

44. Dal Canto, MC and Gurney, ME: Development of central nervous system pathology in a murine transgenic model of human amyotrophic lateral sclerosis. Am J Pathol 145:1271–1279, 1994.

45. Dal Canto, MC and Gurney, ME: Neuropathological changes in two lines of mice carrying a transgene for mutant human Cu, Zn SOD, and in mice overexpressing wild type human SOD: A model of familial amyotrophic lateral sclerosis (FALS). Brain Res 676:25–40, 1995.

46. Dawson, VL, Dawson, TM, Bartley, DA, et al: Mechanisms of nitric oxide: Mediated neurotoxicity in primary brain cultures. J Neurosci 13:2651–2661, 1993.

47. Dawson, TM, Dawson, VL, and Snyder, SH: A novel neuronal messenger molecule in brain: The free radical, nitric oxide. Ann Neurol 32:297–311, 1992.

48. Dawson, VL, Dawson, TM, London, ED, et al: Nitric oxide mediates glutamate neurotoxicity in primary cortical cultures. Proc Nat Acad Sci USA 88:6368–6371, 1991.

49. de Jong, JMBV, Den Hartog Jager, WA, Posthumus Meyjes, FE, et al: N-acetylcysteine and N-acetylmethionine treatment of amyotrophic lateral sclerosis (ALS) and of rapidly progressive motor neuron disease (MND). In Tsubaki, T and Yase Y (eds): Amyotrophic Lateral Sclerosis. Elsevier, Amsterdam, 1988, pp 313–318.

50. Deng, H-X, Hentati, A, Tainer, JA, et al: Amyotrophic lateral sclerosis and structural defects in Cu, Zn superoxide dismutase. Science 261:1047–1051, 1993.

51. Do, KQ, Herrling, PL, Streit, P, et al: In vitro release and electrophysiological effects in situ of homocysteic acid, an endogenous N-methyl-(D)-aspartic acid agonist, in the mammalian striatum. J Neurosci 6:2226–2234, 1986.

52. Donevan, SD and Rogawski, MA: GYKI 52466, a 2,3-benzodiazepine, is a highly selective, noncompetitive antagonist of AMPA/kainate receptor responses. Neuron 10:51–59, 1993.

53. Dugan, LL and Choi, DW: Excitotoxicity, free radicals, and cell membrane changes. Ann Neurol 35:S17–S21, 1994.

54. Dumuis, A, Sebben, M, Haynes, L, et al: NMDA receptors activate the arachidonic acid cascade system in striatal neurons. Nature 336:68–70, 1988.

55. Duncan, MW, Steele, JC, Kopin, IJ, et al: 2-amino-3-(methylamino)-propanoic acid (BMAA) in cycad flour: An unlikely cause of amyotrophic lateral sclerosis and parkinsonism-dementia of Guam. Neurology 40:767–772, 1990.

56. Dykens, JA: Isolated cerebral and cerebellar mitochondria produce free radicals when exposed to elevated Ca^{2+} and Na^{+}: Implications for neurodegeneration. J Neurochem 63:584–591, 1994.

57. Eisen, A, Stewart, H, Schulzer, M, et al: Anti-glutamate therapy in amyotrophic lateral sclerosis: A trial using lamotrigine. J Can Sci Neurol 20:297–301, 1993.

58. Erecinska, M and Nelson, D: Activation of glutamate dehydrogenase by leucine and its non-metabolisable analogue in rat brain synaptosomes. J Neurochem 54:1335–1343, 1990.

59. Eubanks, JH, Puranam, RS, Kleckner, NW, et al: The gene encoding the glutamate receptor sub-

unit GluR5 is located on human chromosome 21q21.1-22 in the vicinity of the gene for familial amyotrophic lateral sclerosis. Proc Nat Acad Sci USA 90:178–182, 1993.

60. Festoff, BW and Crigger, NJ: Therapeutic trials in amyotrophic lateral sclerosis: A review. In Mulder, DW (ed): The Diagnosis and Treatment of Amyotrophic Lateral Sclerosis. Houghton Mifflin, Boston, 1980, pp 337–370.

61. Fonnum, F: Glutamate: A neurotransmitter in mammalian brain. J Neurochem 42:1–11, 1984.

62. Foster, AC: Channel blocking drugs for the NMDA receptor. In Meldrum, BS (ed): Excitatory Amino Acid Antagonists. Blackwell, Oxford, 1991, pp 164–179.

63. Freeman, EJ, Terrian, DM, and Dorman, RV: Presynaptic facilitation of glutamate release from isolated hippocampal mossy fiber nerve endings by arachidonic acid. Neurochem Res 15:743–750, 1990.

64. Frei, B, England, L, and Ames, BN: Ascorbate is an outstanding antioxidant in human blood plasma. Proc Nat Acad Sci USA 86:6377–6381, 1989.

65. Fridovich, I: The biology of oxygen radicals. Science 209:875–877, 1978.

66. Fridovich, I: Biological effects of the superoxide radical. Arch Biochem Biophys 247:1–11, 1986.

67. Furuyama, T, Kiyama, H, Sato, K, et al: Region-specific expression of subunits of ionotropic glutamate receptors (AMPA-type, KA-type and NMDA receptors) in the rat spinal cord with special reference to nociception. Mol Brain Res 18:141–151, 1993.

68. Garthwaite, J, Charles, SL, and Chess-Williams, R: Endothelium-derived relaxing factor release on activation of NMDA receptors suggests role as intercellular messenger in the brain. Nature 336:385–388, 1988.

69. Gasic, GP and Hollmann, M: Molecular neurobiology of glutamate receptors. Annu Rev Physiol 54:1335–1343, 1992.

70. Gobe, GC: Apoptosis in brain and gut tissue of mice fed a seed preparation of the cycad *Lepidozami peroffskyana*. Biochem Biophys Res Comm 205:327–333, 1994.

71. Goldlust, A, Su, T-Z, Welty, DF, et al: Effects of the anticonvulsant drug gabapentin on the enzymes in the metabolic pathways of glutamate and GABA. Epilepsy Res 22:1–11, 1995.

72. Gregor, P, Reeves, RH, Jabs, EW, et al: Chromosomal localization of glutamate receptor genes: Relationship to familial amyotrophic lateral sclerosis and other neurological disorders of mice and humans. Proc Nat Acad Sci USA 90:3052–3057, 1993.

73. Greenlund, LJS, Deckwerth, TL, and Johnson, EM, Jr: Superoxide dismutase delays neuronal apoptosis: A role for reactive oxygen species in programmed neuronal death. Neuron 14:303–315, 1995.

74. Gundlach, AL: Disorder of the inhibitory glycine receptor: inherited myoclonus in Poll Hereford calves. FASEB J 4:2761–2766, 1990.

75. Gurney, ME, Cutting, FB, Zhai, P, et al: Benefit of vitamin E, riluzole, and gabapentin in a transgenic model of familial amyotrophic lateral sclerosis. Ann Neurol 39:147–157, 1996.

76. Gurney, ME, Pu, H, Chiu, AY, et al: Motor neuron degeneration in mice that express a human Cu, Zn superoxide dismutase mutation. Science 264:1772–1775, 1994.

77. Halliwell, B: Protection against tissue damage in vivo by desferrioxamine. What is its mechanism of action: Free Radic Biol Med 7:645–651, 1989.

78. Halliwell, B: Reactive oxygen species and the central nervous system. In Packer, L, Prilipko, L, and Christen, Y (eds): Free Radicals in the Brain: Aging, Neurological and Mental Disorders. Springer-Verlag, New York, 1992, pp 21–40.

79. Halliwell, B: Oxygen radicals as key mediators in neurological disease: Fact or fiction? Ann Neurol 32:S10–S15, 1992.

80. Halliwell, B and Aruoma, OI: DNA damage by oxygen-derived species. Its mechanism and measurement in mammalian systems. FEBS Lett 281:9–19, 1991.

81. Halliwell, B and Gutteridge, JMC: Role of free radicals and catalytic metal ions in human disease: An overview. Methods Enzymol 186:1–85, 1990.

82. Halliwell, B, Gutteridge, JMC, and Cross, CE: Free radicals, antioxidants, and human disease: Where are we now? J Lab Clin Med 119:598–620, 1992.

83. Heafield, MT, Fearn, S, Steventon, GB, et al: Plasma cysteine and sulphate levels in patients with motor neurone, Parkinson's and Alzheimer's disease. Neurosci Lett 110:216–220, 1990.

84. Heizmann, CW and Braun, K: Changes in Ca^{2+}-binding proteins in human neurodegenerative disorders. Trends Neurosci 15:259–264, 1992.

85. Herbert, T, Drapeau, P, Pradier, L, et al: Block of the rat brain IIA sodium channel alpha subunit by the neuroprotective drug riluzole. Mol Pharmacol 45:1055–1060, 1994.

86. Hertz, L: Functional interactions between neurons and astrocytes I. Turnover and metabolism of putative amino acid transmitters. Prog Neurobiol 13:277–323, 1979.

87. Hibbs, JB Jr, Taintor, RR, Vavrin, Z, et al: Nitric oxide: A cytotoxic activated macrophage effector molecule. Biochem Biophys Res Commun 157:87–94, 1988.

88. Hirano, A, Llena, JF, Streifler, M, et al: Anterior horn cell changes in a case of neurolathyrism. Acta Neuropathol 35:277–283, 1976.

89. Hollander, D, Pradas, J, Kaplan, R, et al: High-dose dextromethorphan in amyotrophic lateral sclerosis: Phase I safety and pharmacokinetic studies. Ann Neurol 36:920–924, 1994.

90. Hollman, M, Hartley, M, and Heinemann, S: Ca^{2+} permeability of KA-AMPA–gated glutamate receptor channels depends on subunit composition. Science 252:851–853, 1991.

91. Hugon, J, Tabaraud, F, Rigaud, M, et al: Glutamate dehydrogenase and aspartate aminotransferase in leukocytes of patients with motor neuron disease. Neurology 39:956–958, 1989.

92. Hugon, J and Vallat, JM: Abnormal distribution of phosphorylated neurofilaments in neuronal degeneration induced by kainic acid. Neurosci Lett 119:45–48, 1990.

93. Huie, RE and Padmaja, S: The reaction rate of nitric oxide with superoxide. Free Rad Res Commun 18:195–199, 1993.

94. Iacopino, AM and Christakos, S: Specific reduction of calcium-binding protein (28-kilodalton calbindin-D) gene expression in aging and neurodegenerative diseases. Proc Nat Acad Sci USA 87:4078–4082, 1990.

95. Ikeda, K, Kinoshita, M, Iwasaki, Y, et al: Lecithinized superoxide dismutase retards wobbler mouse motor neuron disease. Neuromusc Disord 5:383–390, 1995.

96. Ince, PG, Shaw, PJ, Candy, JM, et al: Iron, selenium and glutathione peroxidase activity are elevated in sporadic motor neuron disease. Neurosci Lett 182:87–90, 1994.

97. Ince, P, Stout, N, Shaw, P, et al: Parvalbumin and calbindin D-28k in the human motor system and in motor neuron disease. Neuropathol Appl Neurobiol 19:291–299, 1993.

98. Ischiropoulos, H, Zhu, L, Chen, J, et al: Peroxynitrite-mediated tyrosine nitration catalyzed by superoxide dismutase. Arch Biochem Biophys 298:431–437, 1992.

99. The Italian ALS Study Group: Branched-chain amino acids and amyotrophic lateral sclerosis: A treatment failure? Neurology 43:2466–2470, 1993.

100. Iwasaki, Y, Ikeda, K, and Kinoshita, M: Plasma amino acid levels in patients with amyotrophic lateral sclerosis. J Neurol Sci 107:219–222, 1992.

101. Jansen, KLR, Faull, RLM, Dragunow, M, et al: Autoradiographic localisation of NMDA, quisqualate and kainic acid receptors in human spinal cord. Neurosci Lett 108:53–57, 1990.

102. Janzen, EG: Spin trapping and associated vocabulary. Free Radical Res Commun 10:63–68, 1990.

103. Juneja, T, Dave, S, Pericak-Vance, M, et al: Prognosis in familial ALS: Progression and survival in patients with E100G and A4V mutations in Cu, Zn superoxide dismutase. Neurology, 1997, in press.

104. Kanai, Y, Smith, CP, and Hediger, MA: A new family of neurotransmitter transporters: The high affinity glutamate transporters. FASEB J 8:1450–1459, 1994.

105. Kane, DJ, Sarafian, TA, Anton, R, et al: Bcl-2 inhibition of neural death: Decreased generation of reactive oxygen species. Science 262:1274–1277, 1993.

106. Kaneko, T, Akiyama, H, and Mizuno, N: Immunohistochemical demonstration of glutamate dehydrogenase in astrocytes. Neurosci Lett 77:171–175, 1987.

107. Keinanen, K, Wisden, W, Sommer, B, et al: A family of AMPA-selective glutamate receptors. Science 249:556–560, 1990.

108. Kemp, JA, Foster, AC, and Wong, EHF: Noncompetitive antagonists of excitatory amino acid receptors. Trends Neurosci 10:294–298, 1987.

109. Kuther, G and Struppler, A: Therapieversuch der amyotrophischen lateralsklerose mit N-acetylcystein. Fortschr Myol 8:51–57, 1986.

110. Kvamme, E: Deaminases and amidases. In Lajtha, A (ed): Handbook of Neurochemistry, Vol 4, ed 2. Plenum Press, New York, 1983, pp 85–105.

111. Kvamme, E, Schousboe, A, Herz, L, et al: Developmental change of endogenous glutamate and gamma-glutamyl transferase in cultured cerebral cortical interneurons and cerebellar granule cells, and in mouse cerebral cortex and cerebellum in vivo. Neurochem Res 10:993–1008, 1985.

112. Lacomblez, L, Bensimon, G, Guillet, P, et al: Riluzole: A double-blind randomised placebo-controlled dose-range study in amyotrophic lateral sclerosis (ALS). [abstract] Electroenceph Clin Neurophysiol 97:S68, 1995.

113. Lafon-Cazal, M, Pietri, S, Culcasi, M, et al: NMDA-dependent superoxide production and neurotoxicity. Nature 364:535–537, 1993.

114. Laughton, MJ, Halliwell, B, Evans, PJ, et al: Antioxidant and pro-oxidant actions of the plant phenolics quercetin, gossypol and myricetin. Effects on lipid peroxidation, hydroxyl radical generation and bleomycin-dependent damage to DNA. Biochem Pharmacol 38:2859–2865, 1989.

115. Lipton, SA: Calcium channel antagonists in the prevention of neurotoxicity. Adv Pharmacol 22:271–297, 1991.

116. Lipton, SA, Choi, Y-B, Pan, Z-H, et al: A redox-based mechanism for the neuroprotective and neurodestructive effects of nitric oxide and related nitroso- compounds. Nature 364:626–632, 1993.

117. Lipton, SA and Rosenberg, PA: Excitatory amino acids as a final common pathway for neurologic disorders. N Engl J Med 330:613–622, 1994.

118. Louwerse, ES, Weverling, GJ, Bossuyt, PMM, et al: Randomized, double-blind, controlled trial of acetylcysteine in amyotrophic lateral sclerosis. Arch Neurol 52:559–564, 1995.

119. Lucas, DR and Newhouse, JP: The toxic effect of sodium L-glutamate on the inner layers of the retina. Arch Ophthalmol 58:193–201, 1957.

120. Lynch, MA and Bliss, TV: Long-term potentiation of synaptic transmission in the hippocampus of the rat; effect of calmodulin and oleoyl-acetyl-glycerol on release of [^{3}H]glutamate. Neurosci Lett 65:171–176, 1986.

121. Malenka, RC, Kauer, JA, Perkel, DJ, et al: The impact of postsynaptic calcium on synaptic transmission—Its role in long-term potentiation. Trends Neurosci 12:444–450, 1989.

122. Malessa, S, Leigh, PN, Bertel, O, et al: Amyotrophic lateral sclerosis: Glutamate dehydrogenase and transmitter amino acids in the spinal cord. J Neurol Neurosurg Psychiatry 54:984–988, 1991.

123. Martin, BL, Wu, D, Jakes, S, et al: Chemical influences on the specificity of tyrosine phosphorylation. J Biol Chem 265:7108–7111, 1990.

124. Martin, D, Thompson, MA, and Nadler, JV: The neuroprotective agent riluzole inhibits release of glutamate and aspartate from slices of hippocampal area CA1. Eur J Pharmacol 250:473–476, 1993.

125. Martin, LJ, Blackstone, CD, Levey, AI, et al: AMPA glutamate receptor subunits are differentially distributed in rat brain. Neuroscience 53:327–358, 1993.

126. Mayer, ML, Westbrook, GL, and Guthrie, PB: Voltage-dependent block by Mg^{2+} of NMDA responses in spinal cord neurones. Nature 309:261–263, 1984.

127. McCord, JM: Oxygen-derived free radicals in postischemic tissue injury. N Engl J Med 312:159–163, 1985.

128. Meldrum, B and Garthwaite, J: Excitatory amino

acid neurotoxicity and neurodegenerative disease. Trends Pharmacol Sci 11:379–387, 1990.

129. Meyer, T, Lenk, U, Kuther, G, et al: Studies of the coding region of the neuronal glutamate transporter gene in amyotrophic lateral sclerosis. Ann Neurol 37:817–819, 1995.

130. Miller, RJ, Murphy, SN, and Glaum, SR: Neuronal Ca^{2+} channels and their regulation by excitatory amino acids. Ann NY Acad Sci 568:149–158, 1989.

131. Miller, B, Sarantis, M, Traynelis, SF, et al: Potentiation of NMDA receptor currents by arachidonic acid. Nature 355:722–725, 1992.

132. Mizoule, J, Meldrum, B, Mazadier, M, et al: 2-amino-6-trifluoromethoxy benzothiazole, a possible antagonist of excitatory amino acid neurotransmission—I. Anticonvulsant properties. Neuropharmacology 24:767–773, 1985.

133. Monaghan, DT, Bridges, RJ, and Cotman, CW: The excitatory amino acid receptors: Their classes, pharmacology and distinct properties in the function of the central nervous system. Annu Rev Pharmacol Toxicol 29:365–402, 1989.

134. Munsat, TL and Hollander, D: Excitotoxins and amyotrophic lateral sclerosis. Therapie 45:277–279, 1990.

135. Murphy, TH, Miyamoto, M, Sastre, A, et al: Glutamate toxicity in a neuronal cell line involves inhibition of cystine transport leading to oxidative stress. Neuron 2:1547–1558, 1989.

136. Nakamura, K and Stadtman, ER: Oxidative inactivation of glutamine synthetase subunits. Proc Nat Acad Sci USA 81:2011–2015, 1984.

137. Nakanishi, S: Molecular diversity of glutamate receptors and implications for brain function. Science 258:597–603, 1992.

138. Nichols, RA, Sihra, TS, Czernik, AJ, et al: Calcium/calmodulin-dependent protein kinase II increases glutamate and noradrenaline release from synaptosomes. Nature 343:647–651, 1990.

139. Novelli, A, Reilly, JA, Lysko, PG, et al: Glutamate becomes neurotoxic via the N-methyl-D-aspartate receptor when intracellular energy levels are reduced. Brain Res 451:205–212, 1988.

140. Nunn, PB: Toxicology of Motor Systems. In Leigh, PN and Swash, M (eds): Motor Neuron Disease: Biology and Management. Springer-Verlag, New York, 1995, pp 201–218.

141. Nunn, PB, Seelig, M, and Spencer, PS: Stereospecific acute neuronotoxicity of uncommon plant amino acids linked to human motor system diseases. Brain Res 561:262–268, 1987.

142. O'Brien, RJ and Fischbach, GD: Modulation of embryonic chick motor neuron glutamate sensitivity by interneurones and agonists. J Neurosci 6:3290–3296, 1986.

143. Oliver, CN, Starke-Reed, PE, Stadtman, ER, et al: Oxidative damage to brain proteins, loss of glutamine synthetase activity, and production of free radicals during ischemia/reperfusion-induced injury to gerbil brain. Proc Nat Acad Sci USA 87:5144–5147, 1990.

144. Olney, JW and Sharpe, LG: Brain lesions in infant rhesus monkey treated with monosodium glutamate. Science 166:386–388, 1969.

145. Orrell, RW, King, AW, Hilton, DA, et al: Familial amyotrophic lateral sclerosis with a point mutation of SOD-1: Intrafamilial heterogeneity of disease duration associated with neurofibrillary tangles. J Neurol Neurosurg Psychiatry 59:266–270, 1995.

146. Patterson, D, Warner, HR, Fox, LM, et al: Superoxide dismutase, oxygen radical metabolism, and amyotrophic lateral sclerosis. Molec Genet Med 4:79–119, 1994.

147. Pellegrini-Giampietro, DE, Zukin, RS, Bennett, MVL, et al: Switch in glutamate receptor subunit gene expression in CA1 subfield of hippocampus following global ischemia in rats. [published erratum appears in Proc Nat Acad Sci USA 90:780, 1993]. Proc Nat Acad Sci USA 89:10499–10503, 1992.

148. Perl, TM, Bedard, L, Kosatsky, T, et al: An outbreak of toxic encephalopathy caused by eating mussels contaminated with domoic acid. N Engl J Med 322:1775–1780, 1990.

149. Perry, TL, Bergeron, C, Biro, AJ, et al: β-N-Methylamino-L-alanine: Chronic oral administration is not toxic to mice. J Neurol Sci 94:173–180, 1989.

150. Perry, TL, Bergeron, C, Steele, JC, et al: Brain amino acid contents are dissimilar in sporadic and Guamanian amyotrophic lateral sclerosis. J Neurol Sci 99:3–8, 1990.

151. Perry, TL, Hansen, S, and Jones, K: Brain glutamate deficiency in amyotrophic lateral sclerosis. Neurology 37:1845–1848, 1987.

152. Perry, TL, Krieger, C, Hansen, S, et al: Amyotrophic lateral sclerosis: Amino acid levels in plasma and CSF. Ann Neurol 28:12–17, 1990.

153. Plaitakis, A: Glutamate dysfunction and selective motor neuron degeneration in amyotrophic lateral sclerosis: A hypothesis. Ann Neurol 28:3–8, 1990.

154. Plaitakis, A and Constantakakis, E: Altered metabolism of excitatory amino acids, N-acetyl-aspartate and N-acetyl-aspartyl-glutamate in amyotrophic lateral sclerosis. Brain Res 30:381–386, 1993.

155. Plaitakis, A, Constantakakis, E, and Smith, J: The neuro-excitotoxic amino acids glutamate and aspartate are altered in the spinal cord and brain in amyotrophic lateral sclerosis. Ann Neurol 24:446–449, 1988.

156. Plaitakis, A and Caroscio, JT: Abnormal glutamate metabolism in amyotrophic lateral sclerosis. Ann Neurol 22:575–579, 1987.

157. Plaitakis, A, Mandeli, J, Fesdjian, C, et al: Dysregulation of glutamate metabolism in ALS: Correlation with gender and disease type. Neurology 41:392–393, 1991.

158. Plaitakis, A, Mandeli, J, Smith, J, et al: Pilot trial of branched-chain amino acids in amyotrophic lateral sclerosis. Lancet 1:1015–1018, 1988.

159. Pramatarova, A, Goto, J, Nanba, E, et al: A two base pair deletion in the SOD1 gene causes familial amyotrophic lateral sclerosis. Hum Mol Genet 3:2061–2062, 1994.

160. Przedborski, S, Donaldson, D, Jakowec, M, et al: Brain superoxide dismutase, catalase, and glutathione peroxidase activities in amyotrophic lateral sclerosis. Ann Neurol 39:158–165, 1996.

161. Rabizadeh, S, Gralla, EB, Borchelt, DR, et al: Mutations associated with amyotrophic lateral sclerosis convert superoxide dismutase from an anti-

apoptotic gene to a proapoptotic gene: Studies in yeast and neural cells. Proc Nat Acad Sci USA 92:3024–3028, 1995.

162. Reaume, AG, Elliott, JL, Hoffman, EK, et al: Motor neurons in Cu/Zn superoxide dismutase-deficient mice develop normally but exhibit enhanced cell death after axonal injury. Nature Genet 13:43–47, 1996.

163. Ripps, ME, Huntley, GW, Hof, PR, et al: Transgenic mice expressing an altered murine superoxide dismutase gene provide an animal model of amyotrophic lateral sclerosis. Proc Nat Acad Sci USA 92:689–693, 1995.

164. Robberecht, W, Sapp, P, Viaene, MK, et al: Cu/Zn superoxide dismutase activity in familial and sporadic amyotrophic lateral sclerosis. J Neurochem 62:384–387, 1994.

165. Rosen, DR, Bowling, AC, Patterson, D, et al: A frequent Ala 4 to Val superoxide dismutase-1 mutation is associated with a rapidly progressive familial amyotrophic lateral sclerosis. Hum Mol Genet 3:981–987, 1994.

166. Rosen, DR, Siddique, T, Patterson, D, et al: Mutations in Cu/Zn superoxide dismutase are associated with familial amyotrophic lateral sclerosis. Nature 362:59–62, 1993.

167. Rosenberg, PA, Amin, S, and Leitner, M: Glutamate uptake disguises neurotoxic potency of glutamate agonists in cerebral cortex in dissociated cell culture. J Neurosci 12:56–61, 1992.

168. Rothstein, JD: Excitotoxic mechanisms in the pathogenesis of amyotrophic lateral sclerosis. In Serratrice, G and Munsat, T (eds): Pathogenesis and Therapy of Amyotrophic Lateral Sclerosis. Adv Neurol, vol 68. Lippincott-Raven, Philadelphia, 1995, pp 7–20.

169. Rothstein, JD, Bristol, LA, Hosler, B, et al: Chronic inhibition of superoxide dismutase produces apoptotic death of spinal neurons. Proc Nat Acad Sci 91:4155–4159, 1994.

170. Rothstein, JD, Jin, L, Dykes-Hoberg, M, et al: Chronic inhibition of glutamate uptake produces a model of slow neurotoxicity. Proc Nat Acad Sci USA 90:6591–6595, 1993.

171. Rothstein, JD and Kuncl, R: Neuroprotective strategies in a model of chronic glutamate-mediated motor neuron toxicity. J Neurochem 65:643–651, 1995.

172. Rothstein, JD, Kuncl, R, Chaudhry, V, et al: Excitatory amino acids in amyotrophic lateral sclerosis: An update. Ann Neurol 30:224–225, 1991.

173. Rothstein, JD, Martin, LJ, and Kuncl, RW: Decreased glutamate transport by the brain and spinal cord in amyotrophic lateral sclerosis. N Engl J Med 326:1464–1468, 1992.

174. Rothstein, JD, Tsai, G, Kuncl, RW, et al: Abnormal excitatory amino acid metabolism in amyotrophic lateral sclerosis. Ann Neurol 28:18–25, 1990.

175. Rothstein, JD, Van Kammen, M, Levey, AI, et al: Selective loss of glial glutamate transporter GLT-1 in amyotrophic lateral sclerosis. Ann Neurol 38:73–84, 1995.

176. Rowland, LP: Riluzole for the treatment of amyotrophic lateral sclerosis—Too soon to tell? N Engl J Med 330:636–637, 1994.

177. Schousboe, A: Transport and metabolism of glutamate and GABA in neurons and glial cells. Int Rev Neurobiol 22:1–45, 1981.

178. Scozzafava, A and Viezzoli, MS: The role of the active site amino acid residues on the catalytic activity on CuZnSod. Mol Chem Neuropathol 19:193–204, 1993.

179. Shaw, PJ: Excitotoxicity and motor neuron disease: A review of the evidence. J Neurol Sci 124(suppl):6–13, 1994.

180. Shaw, PJ, Ince, PG, Falkous, G, et al: Oxidative damage to protein in sporadic motor neuron disease spinal cord. Ann Neurol 38:691–695, 1995.

181. Shaw, PJ, Ince, PG, Johnson, M, et al: N-methyl-D-aspartate (NMDA) receptors in the spinal cord and motor cortex in motor neuron disease: A quantitative autoradiographic study using [^{3}H]MK-801. Brain Res 637:297–302, 1994.

182. Shaw, PJ, Ince, PG, Johnson, M, et al: The quantitative autoradiographic distribution of [^{3}H]MK-801 binding sites in the normal human brainstem in relation to motor neuron disease. Brain Res 572:276–280, 1992.

183. Shaw, PJ, Ince, PG, Johnson, M, et al: An autoradiographic study of glutamate receptor subtypes in the normal human motor system. In Rose, FC (ed): New Evidence in MND/ALS Research. Smith-Gordon, London, 1991, pp 237–249.

184. Siddique, T, Figlewicz, DA, Pericak-Vance, MA, et al: Linkage of a gene causing familial amyotrophic lateral sclerosis to chromosome 21 and evidence of genetic-locus heterogeneity. N Engl J Med 324:1381–1384, 1991.

185. Siman, R and Noszek, JC: Excitatory amino acids activate calpain I and induce structural protein breakdown in vivo. Neuron 1:279–287, 1988.

186. Själander, A, Beckman, G, Deng, H-X, et al: The D90A mutation results in a polymorphism of Cu, Zn superoxide dismutase that is prevalent in northern Sweden and Finland. Hum Mol Genet 4:1105–1108, 1995.

187. Smith, RA, Balis, FM, Ott, KH, et al: Pharmacokinetics and tolerability of ventricularly administered superoxide dismutase in monkeys and preliminary clinical observations in familial ALS. J Neurol Sci 129(suppl):13–18, 1995.

188. Smith, RG, Alexianu, ME, Crawford, G, et al: Cytotoxicity of immunoglobulins from amyotrophic lateral sclerosis patients on a hybrid motoneuron cell line. Proc Nat Acad Sci USA 91:3393–3397, 1994.

189. Sommer, B, Kohler, M, Sprengel, R, et al: RNA editing in brain controls a determinant of ion flow in glutamate-gated channels. Cell 67:11–19, 1991.

190. Sommer, B and Seeburg, PH: Glutamate receptor channels: Novel properties and new clones. Trends Pharmacol Sci 13:291–296, 1992.

191. Spector, R and Eells, J: Deoxynucleotide and vitamin transport into the central nervous system. Fed Proc 43:196–200, 1984.

192. Spencer, PS, Allen, CN, Kisby, CE, et al: Lathyrism and Western Pacific amyotrophic lateral sclerosis: Etiology of short- and long-latency motor system disorders. Adv Neurol 56:287–299, 1991.

193. Spencer, PS, Nun, PB, Hugon, J, et al: Guam amyotrophic lateral sclerosis-parkinsonism-dementia

linked to a plant exicitant neurotoxin. Science 237:517–522, 1987.

194. Spencer, PS, Roy, DN, Ludolph, A, et al: Primate model of lathyrism: A human pyramidal disorder. In Nappe, F (ed): Neurodegenerative Disorders: The Role Played by Endotoxins and Xenobiotics. Raven Press, New York, 1988, pp 231–238.

195. Spencer, PS, Roy, DN, Ludolph, A, et al: Lathyrism: Evidence for role of the neuroexcitatory amino-acid BOAA. Lancet 2:1066–1067, 1986.

196. Steiner, TJ, for Scientific Pan-European Collaboration in ALS: Multinational trial of branched-chain amino acids in amyotrophic lateral sclerosis. [abstract]. Muscle Nerve 1(suppl):S166, 1994.

197. Stone, TW and Connick, JH: Quinolinic acid and other kynurenines in the central nervous system. Neuroscience 15:597–617, 1985.

198. Storm-Mathison, J and Otterson, OP: Localisation of excitatory amino acid transmitters. In Lodge, D (ed): Excitatory Amino Acids in Health and Disease. John Wiley, Chichester, 1988, pp 107–143.

199. Streifler, M, Cohn, DF, Hirano, A, et al: The central nervous system in a case of neurolathyrism. Neurology 27:1176–1178, 1977.

200. Sucher, NJ, Lei, SZ, and Lipton, SA: Calcium channel antagonists attenuate NMDA-receptor mediated neurotoxicity of retinal ganglion cells in culture. Brain Res 551:297–302, 1991.

201. Szatkowski, M, Barbour, B, and Attwell, D: Nonvesicular release of glutamate from glial cells by reversed electrogenic glutamate uptake. Nature 348:443–446, 1990.

202. Tainer, JA, Getzoff, ED, Beem, KM, et al: Determination and analysis of the 2-A structure of copper, zinc superoxide dismutase. J Mol Biol 160:181–217, 1982.

203. Tandan, R, Bromberg, MB, Forshew, D, et al: A controlled trial with amino acid therapy in amyotrophic lateral sclerosis: I. Clinical, functional, and isometric torque data. Neurology 47:1220–1226, 1996.

204. Taylor, CP: Emerging perspectives on the mechanism of action of gabapentin. Neurology 44(suppl 5):S10–S16, 1994.

205. Teitelbaum, JS, Zatorre, RJ, Carpenter, S, et al: Neurotoxic sequelae of domoic acid intoxication due to the ingestion of contaminated mussels. N Engl J Med 322:1781–1787, 1990.

206. Testa, D, Caraceni, T, and Fetoni, V: Branched-chain amino acids in the treatment of amyotrophic lateral sclerosis. J Neurol 236:445–447, 1989.

207. Tomei, LD and Cope, OF (eds): Apoptosis: The Molecular Basis of Cell Death. Cold Spring Harbor Laboratory Press, Plainview, NY, 1991.

208. Trout, JJ, Koenig, H, Goldstone, AD, et al: N-Methyl-D-aspartate receptor excitotoxicity involves activation of polyamine synthesis: Protection by α-difluoromethylornithine. J Neurochem 60:352–355, 1993.

209. Tsai, GC, Stauch-Slusher, B, Sim, L, et al: Reductions in acidic amino acids and N-acetylaspartyl-

glutamate in amyotrophic lateral sclerosis CNS. Brain Res 556:151–156, 1991.

210. Volterra, A, Trotti, D, Cassutti, P, et al: High sensitivity of glutamate uptake to extracellular free arachidonic acid levels in rat cortical synaptosomes and astrocytes. J Neurochem 59:600–606, 1992.

211. Volterra, A, Trotti, D, Tromba, C, et al: Glutamate uptake inhibition by oxygen free radicals in rat cortical astrocytes. J Neurosci 14:2924–2932, 1994.

212. Watkins, JC and Olverman, HJ: Agonists and antagonists for excitatory amino acid receptors. Trends Neurosci 10:265–272, 1987.

213. Whetsell, WO, Jr and Schwarcz, R: Prolonged exposure to submicromolar concentrations of quinolinic acid causes excitotoxic damage in organotypic cultures of rat corticostriatal system. Neurosci Lett 97:271–275, 1989.

214. Wiedau-Pazos, M, Goto, JJ, Rabizadeh, S, et al: Altered reactivity of superoxide dismutase in familial amyotrophic lateral sclerosis. Science 271:515–518, 1996.

215. Wisden, W and Seeburg, PH: Mammalian ionotropic glutamate receptors. Curr Opin Neurobiol 3:291–298, 1993.

216. Wong, PC, Pardo, CA, Borchelt, DR, et al: An adverse property of a familial ALS-linked *SOD1* mutation causes motor neuron disease characterized by vacuolar degeneration of mitochondria. Neuron 14:1105–1116, 1995.

217. Wrathall, JR, Teng, YD, Choiniere, D, et al: Evidence that local non-NMDA receptors contribute to functional deficits in contusive spinal cord injury. Brain Res 586:140–143, 1992.

218. Yielding, KL and Tomkins, GM: An effect of L-leucine and other essential amino acids on the structure and activity of glutamate dehydrogenase. Proc Nat Acad Sci USA 47:983, 1961.

219. Yoshiyama, Y, Yamada, T, Asanuma, K, et al: Apoptosis related antigen, Le(Y) and nick-end labeling are positive in spinal cord motor neurons in amyotrophic lateral sclerosis. Acta Neuropathol 88: 207–211, 1994.

220. Young, AB: What's the excitement about excitatory amino acids in amyotrophic lateral sclerosis? [editorial]. Ann Neurol 28:9–11, 1990.

221. Young, AB and Fagg, GE: Excitatory amino acids in the brain: Membrane binding and receptor autoradiographic approaches. Trends Pharmacol Sci 11:126–133, 1990.

222. Young, AB, Penney, JB, Dauth, GW, et al: Glutamate or aspartate as a possible neurotransmitter of the cerebral cortico-fugal fibres in the monkey. Neurology 33:1513–1516, 1983.

223. Zeman, S, Lloyd, C, Meldrum, B, et al: Excitatory amino acids, free radicals and the pathogenesis of motor neuron disease. Neuropathol Appl Neurobiol 20:219–231, 1994.

224. Zorumski, CF, Yamada, KA, Price, MT, et al: A benzodiazepine recognition site associated with the non-NMDA glutamate receptor. Neuron 10:61–67, 1993.

CHAPTER 13

THE IMMUNE HYPOTHESIS

At first glance, the suggestion that ALS might be immunologic or autoimmune in nature strikes most clinicians as unlikely. From a clinical standpoint, there are no consistent features of systemic illness, such as rash, arthritis, or other major organ disturbance so often seen in the well-established autoimmune diseases. The usual laboratory markers of autoimmune disease such as elevated erythrocyte sedimentation rate, the presence of antinuclear antibodies or rheumatoid factor, or the features of an inflammatory cerebrospinal fluid (CSF) are conspicuously absent.[10] Except for occasional paraproteinemic abnormalities (see below), levels of immunoglobulins G (IgG), A (IgA), and M (IgM) are normal.[77] Total B-cell and T-cell numbers and T-cell immunoregulatory subsets also appear to be normal in ALS.[7] Biopsy studies of accessible tissue such as peripheral nerve and muscle have shown only the expected nerve fiber loss and denervation atrophy. There has been no indication of inflammation (with the exception of nonspecific mononuclear infiltrates in muscle biopsy specimens of longstanding cases), and, with some notable exceptions, postmortem studies of brain and spinal cord have not disclosed evidence for an inflammatory autoimmune condition.

Appel and colleagues,[1] however, found an increased incidence of thyroid disease in ALS patients compared with controls, and a greater number of ALS patients (compared to controls) with a family history of possible autoimmune diseases. Also noted was increased expression of Ia antigen on T cells in ALS patients compared to controls, suggesting immune activation.[1] Because of the possibility that ALS is an unconventional autoimmune disorder,[20] clinicians have attempted a multiplicity of immunosuppressive and immunomodulatory therapies. Regrettably, none of these therapeutic interventions, to be described later in this chapter, has been successful.

Despite the clinical view that ALS is unlikely to be immune-mediated, a considerable literature has developed on the immune hypothesis (Table 13–1). In this chapter, we review early studies that generated the hy-

Table 13–1. **SELECTED LITERATURE CONCERNING THE IMMUNE HYPOTHESIS**

Study	Finding
1973, *Wolfgram and Myers*[83] In vitro cultures of anterior horn cells with ALS sera	Serum factor(s) toxic to anterior horn cells
1976, *Oldstone et al.*[48] Studies of glomerular basement membrane in ALS	Immune complex deposition in rapidly progressive ALS
1982, *Rowland et al.*[59] Clinical-pathologic correlation in patient presenting with progressive muscular atrophy syndrome	Motor neuron syndrome associated with monoclonal (immunoglobin M) gammopathy
1986, *Shy et al.*[67] Study of paraproteins and ALS	4.8% of motor neuron disease patients had paraprotein (vs. 1% controls)
1986, *Freddo et al.*[29] Clinical-immunologic study in patient with lower motor neuron syndrome and immunoglobulin M gammopathy	1gM bound to gangliosides (asialo-GM1, GM1, and GD1B); M-proteins might cause motor neuron degeneration in some patients
1990, *Troost et al.*[81] Neuropathology of ALS spinal cord	Infiltration of lymphocytes; predominance of suppressor-cytotoxic T cells; T-cell immune responses occur in ALS
1990, *Englehardt et al.*[26] Experimental autoimmune gray matter disease in guinea pigs	Acute motor neuron syndrome; immunoglobulin G localized to motor endplate
1992, *Smith et al.*[71] The effect of ALS and control sera on voltage-gated calcium channels	Sera from ALS patients showed greater calcium channel binding of immunoglobin G than controls (but effect not specific; seen in Lambert-Eaton myasthenic syndrome and Guillain-Barré syndrome)
1994, *Drachman et al.*[21] Total lymph node irradiation in ALS	No beneficial effect despite virtually complete immunosuppression
1996, *Arsac et al.*[5a] Immunoassay of anti-calcium channel specificity in ALS sera	Failure to detect antibodies against neuronal calcium channels in ALS serum

pothesis, subsequent studies that maintained an interest in it, and finally, current work that suggests a role for specific calcium channel autoantibodies in the pathogenesis of ALS.

EFFECTS OF ALS SERUM FACTORS ON MOTOR NEURONS

In 1973, Wolfgram and Myers[83] reported that sera from patients with ALS were toxic to monolayer cultures of anterior horn motor neurons of 3-day-old mice grown in tissue culture. The effect was specific to ALS sera and was not found in sera from disease controls, including patients with Werdnig-Hoffmann disease and polio. Motor neurons were selectively vulnerable; cells in the culture other than neurons remained intact. Almost a decade later, the presence of a nondialyzable, highly specific, heat-labile antineuronal agent in the sera of most ALS patients was confirmed.[56] These findings suggested the presence of a neuronal cytotoxic protein in ALS sera and led to the notion that a circulating immunoglobulin might be involved in causing the disease.

There are many difficulties, however, in interpreting results of culture systems that study morphologic reactions of spinal tissue to sera. These difficulties include inherent problems with standardizing and comparing experiments involving heterogeneous culture techniques, the variability in species chosen for the studies, the different developmental stages of the tissue source, and the potential for contamination of neuronal cultures by supporting cells.[10] Indeed, other investigations failed to reproduce the first culture system results.[34,42] Additional studies on the effects of ALS sera on cultured chick ciliary ganglion neurons[80] and ALS CSF on rat motor neurons[6] also found no neurotoxic effect. Ronnevi and colleagues,[57] however, have shown that ALS immunoglobulins, particularly the IgA and IgG fractions, are toxic to red blood cells. These findings support the possibility of an immunologic abnormality that could adversely affect the lower motor neuron, whose distal portion, the motor endplate, lies outside the blood-brain barrier and might therefore be susceptible to such cytotoxic antibodies.

To test the hypothesis that a serum factor might help cause ALS, either serum or fractionated IgG from ALS patients obtained by plasmapheresis was injected intraperitoneally into mice for 3 months.[16] The absence of any ill effects argued against an immune pathogenesis. In another experiment, enhanced binding of serum immunoglobulins from patients with ALS to rat spinal cord cells compared with control sera was found,[17] raising the possibility of an immune response in ALS, but the primacy of an immunologic reaction in the pathogenesis of ALS could not be demonstrated. In a third study, ALS serum diminished the level of neurofilament protein expressed in cultured chick spinal neurons, but no toxic action in immunoglobulin fractions was found, nor was there evidence of antibodies against the neuronal surface membrane or against serum-borne or muscle-borne trophic factors.[18] Last, using immunoblotting techniques, antineural antibodies were found in ALS sera;[9] the target antigens appeared to be neurofilament proteins. The significance of the antibodies was uncertain, but their low titer argued against a central role in ALS pathogenesis. However, in one ALS patient,[46] in whom postmortem examination revealed accumulations of IgA monoclonal antibody in surviving motor

neurons, the antibody had inhibited phosphorylation of high-molecular-weight neurofilament protein. This observation suggested the possibility that disruption of kinase-mediated phosphorylation may be a mechanism of cell death in ALS.

In 1984, the observation was made that antibodies associated with ALS could mediate their toxicity not by damaging motor neurons per se but by inhibiting sprouting of neurites and subsequent reinnervation of previously denervated skeletal muscle.[32] Further work showed that the antibody inhibiting sprouting is directed against a soluble factor elaborated by target muscle cells, a 56-kd protein designated *neuroleukin*. It is likely, however, that antibodies to neuroleukin in ALS are an epiphenomenon secondary to massive denervation rather than a primary cause of the disease.[10] Of interest, serum from a patient with ALS associated with an IgG kappa paraproteinemia did not inhibit experimentally induced sprouting of motor nerve terminals.[19]

IMMUNE COMPLEX DEPOSITION IN ALS PATIENTS

In 1976, Oldstone and colleagues[48] reported that 10 of 25 samples of ALS sera bound significantly greater quantities of radiolabeled complement component Clq than 15 samples from healthy controls. These investigators also found moderate amounts of both IgG and complement component C3 of granular appearance along the glomerular basement membrane and mesangia in a pattern characteristic of immune complex deposition, in 9 of 33 patients with ALS. Of these 9 patients, 8 had a rapidly progressive neurologic course, in contrast to slowly progressive or stable disease in patients without glomerular deposition. Abnormal deposits of complement and immunoglobulins have also been found in the jejunal lamina propria of ALS patients.[11] Because immune complexes are an important feature of autoimmune disease, these findings support the autoimmune hypothesis. There has been little additional support, however, for the notion that ALS is an immune complex disease. Although these complexes are occasionally found in ALS patients, they are probably of secondary origin and do not reflect a generalized immunologic reaction.[49]

PARAPROTEIN ABNORMALITIES IN ALS PATIENTS

In 1982, Rowland and colleagues[59] described a patient with a progressive lower motor neuron syndrome with clinical features resembling progressive spinal muscular atrophy. Laboratory features were unusual for ALS, however, in that nerve conduction velocities were less than 70% of normal, CSF protein was elevated (132 mg/dL), and the patient had a monoclonal IgM gammopathy. Postmortem examination revealed that the total number of motor neurons was essentially normal, although there was central chromatolysis of anterior horn cells. The brunt of the pathology was found in the ventral nerve roots. The condition resembled motor neuron disease clinically, but was best characterized as a predominantly proximal motor demyelinating radiculoneuropathy. This intriguing observation—that motor neuropathy associated with monoclonal gammopathy could clinically simulate motor neuron disease or neuronopathy—led Rowland and colleagues[62] on a long and fruitful quest to understand the relationship of paraproteins to motor neuron and motor nerve disorders.

Among the questions that generated research in this area, three are especially germane to the immune hypothesis of ALS: What is the frequency of monoclonal gammopathy in patients with ALS? Among patients with apparent ALS, is there a subset with a treatable neuropathic (not neuronal) disorder caused by autoantibody? Might the study of autoantibody-associated motor disorders provide clues to the pathogenesis of ALS per se? Studies in the last decade by several groups of investigators have begun to answer these questions (Table 13–2).

First, 4.8% of motor neuron disease patients had paraproteinemia, compared with only 1% of age-matched controls.[67] Using a more sensitive method of immunofixation electrophoresis, 9.8% of patients with motor

Table 13–2. **PARAPROTEINS AND MOTOR NEURON DISEASE**

- Paraproteinemia—almost 10% of patients with motor neuron disease
- The protein (often immunoglobulin M) reacts with neural antigens (glycoconjugates)
- Glycoconjugates (ganglioside antigens) are located in spinal motor neuron membrane, motor axon, and motor nerve terminal
- Antiganglioside antibodies:
  - High titer and frequent: lower motor neuron syndromes, multifocal motor neuropathy
  - High titer, infrequent: ALS
  - Found in immune disorders without major motor neuron involvement
  - May reflect ongoing humoral immune process
  - Probably not primary pathophysiologic factor

neuron disease were found to have paraproteins.[41,84] Most patients had ALS or ALS with probable upper motor neuron signs, and one patient had a pure lower motor neuron disorder. This disproportionately frequent association of paraproteinemia and motor neuron disease implicated the immune system in the pathogenesis of ALS.[60] Second, a subset of patients with lower motor neuron syndromes resembling ALS have improved with immunosuppressive treatment.[50] The motor disorder in these cases, multifocal motor neuropathy, is often accompanied by antibodies directed against neural antigens (see below), sometimes in the context of a paraproteinemia. Third, whether these antibodies are pathogenetic in lower motor neuron syndromes is relevant to our understanding of ALS. Indeed, the literature on the antibody–motor neuron disorder association is now large, and much of it is based on the discovery that in some patients with monoclonal gammopathy, the M protein (IgM) has antibody activity against specific neural antigens.

Antibody Activity Against Glycoconjugates

In 1986, Freddo and colleagues[29] studied a patient with a progressive lower motor neuron disease associated with an IgM gammopathy (M-protein). They seized the op-

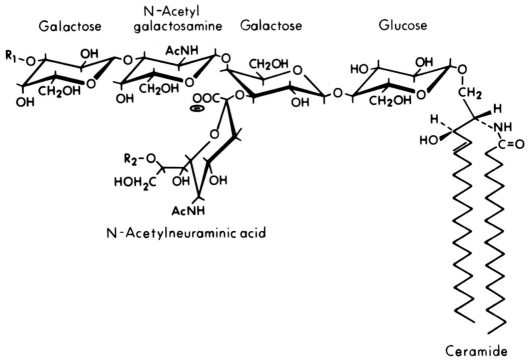

Galactose   N-Acetyl galactosamine   Galactose   Glucose

N-Acetylneuraminic acid

Ceramide

Figure 13–1. Structure of the gangliosides GM1, GD1B, and GD1A. GM1, $R_1 = R_2 = H$; GD1B, $R_1 = H$, $R_2 = NeuAc$; GD1A, $R_1 = NeuAc$, $R_2 = H$. NeuAc, *N*-acetylneuraminic acid. The zig-zag lines of ceramide (hydrophobic unit anchors the molecule to the membrane) represent hydrocarbon chains. (From Ledeen, R: Gangliosides of the neuron. Trends in Neurosciences, p 169, April 1985.)

portunity to identify the antigens to which the M-protein bound. Immunostains for serum IgM identified two sialic-acid-containing glycospingolipids or gangliosides, designated GM1 and GD1B (Fig. 13–1). The IgM M-protein also bound to asialo-GM1, indicating reactivity to the galactosyl (β 1-3) *N*-acetylgalactosaminyl moiety shared by GM1, GD1B, and asialo-GM1 (Fig. 13–2). The IgM binding to the two gangliosides was detectable by enzyme-linked immunosorbent assay (ELISA) at serum dilutions of greater than 1:10,000. Further work on the specificities of monoclonal IgM and on the neural structures that serve as targets for the antibodies was reported by Latov and colleagues.[39] In two additional patients with lower motor neuron disorders and IgM lamb-

GM1:   Gal(β1-3) GalNAc(β1-4) Gal(β1-4) Glc-Cer
                                              |(α 2-3)
                                              NeuAc

ASIALO-GM1:   Gal(β1-3) GalNAc(β1-4) Gal(β1-4) Glc-Cer

GD1B: Gal(β1-3) GalNAc(β1-4) Gal(β1-4) Glc-Cer
                                           |(α 2-3)
                                           NeuAc
                                           |(α 2-8)
                                           NeuAc

Figure 13–2. Structure of the cross-reactive glycolipids GM1, asialo GM1, and GD1B. NeuAc = *N*-acetylneuraminic acid; cer = ceramide. (From Latov, H: Antibodies to glycoconjugates in neurologic disease. Clinical Aspects of Autoimmunity 4:18–29, 1990, with permission.)

da monoclonal proteins, the IgM antibodies had unique specificity for gangliosides GM1 and GD1B. On immunofluorescence microscopy, the antibodies were noted to be bound to central and peripheral nerve tissue and to motor endplates of the neuromuscular junction. These interesting results prompted the question of whether the M-proteins were pathogenic.[39] Supporting an important pathogenetic role for the antibodies in these lower motor neuron syndromes is the observation of IgM binding of patient serum to neural tissues and the clinical improvement in several patients with immunotherapy as the serum IgM concentration was reduced.[39,69] Of note, increased antiganglioside antibody titers were also detected in the absence of monoclonal gammopathy.[68]

Pathogenic Role for Autoantibodies

To explore the mechanisms underlying antibody activity, antibody localization needed to be characterized more precisely. Ganglioside epitopes are widely distributed in the CNS peripheral nervous system, although they are frequently shielded and not available for antibody binding.[40] Possible sites for an antibody to exert its deleterious effects include the motor neuron cell body, nerve terminal, and motor axon.[78]

BINDING TO THE MOTOR NEURON CELL BODY

Human IgM anti-Gal(β1-3)GalNAc (from patients with motor neuron disease) binds to bovine spinal motor neurons;[79] the specific targets appear to be both glycoproteins and glycolipids.[44] In other experiments, anti-GM1 antibodies also bound to bovine spinal motor neuron membrane, the target antigen being GM1 itself.[12] Perhaps of most interest has been the observation that IgM M-proteins (immunoreactive with GM1 and GD1B) from patients with motor neuron disease bound to and damaged human spinal cord motor neurons cocultured with human myotubes.[33] Antibodies against motor neuron membrane could be detrimental in various ways, such as by damaging the cell surface by complement fixation, by interfering with adhesion to neighboring cells or to components of the extracellular matrix, or by disrupting vital trophic or metabolic interactions with other cells or circulating factors.[40]

BINDING TO THE NEUROMUSCULAR JUNCTION

The binding of IgM M-protein with known antibody activity against GM1, GD1B, and asialo-GM1 to the mammalian neuromuscular junction has also been reported.[66,78] Antibodies binding to the external surface of axon terminal membranes might be internalized and carried via retrograde transport to the neuronal cell body where they could interfere with neuronal function.[66]

BINDING TO THE MOTOR AXON

IgM anti-GM1 binds to the nodes of Ranvier as shown by Santoro and colleagues[64] with serum obtained from a patient with the rare combination of ALS *and* motor neuropathy (multifocal motor neuropathy with conduction block). Anti-GM1 antibodies binding to nodal and paranodal regions might cause motor fiber conduction disturbances by inducing demyelination through complement activation or by interfering with sodium channels.[65] Studies of the mouse phrenic nerve–diaphragm preparation have found that anti-GM1 antibodies in sera from patients with multifocal neuropathy can block nerve conduction at distal motor nerves, which is consistent with a direct or indirect effect on sodium channel function.[55] Further work on the influence of antiganglioside antibodies on potassium and sodium currents in isolated rat myelinated nerve fibers showed that the antibodies themselves can uncover potassium channels in the paranodal region, whereas in the presence of complement, the antibodies probably form antigen-antibody complexes and thereby block sodium channels.[75]

Clinical Spectrum

The spectrum of neurologic disease associated with antiganglioside antibodies is broad and includes lower motor neuron disease, sensorimotor neuropathy, and multifocal motor neuropathy.[63] Antibodies are frequently present in high titers in multifocal motor neuropathy and lower motor neuron syndromes (with primarily distal involvement). On the other hand, in ALS, only occasional patients (5% to 15%) have high anti-GM1 titers.[52] In sera from ALS patients, low-titer polyclonal IgM antibodies to GM1 or GD1A ganglioside (see Fig. 13–1), or both, are present in 78% of patients. On further analysis, selective reactivity to GD1A ganglioside is common when upper motor neuron signs are prominent, and reactivity to GM1 is common when lower motor neuron signs predominate.[51] Casting doubt on a pathologic role for these antibodies in ALS is their presence in immune disorders without motor neuron involvement, such as multiple sclerosis, idiopathic demyelinating neuropathy, and lupus erythematosus.[22] Most investigators now believe that the presence of anti-ganglioside antibodies reflects an ongoing humoral immune process in many patients with ALS, but their role in motor neuron destruction is still unresolved.[40,51]

NEUROPATHOLOGIC FINDINGS SUGGEST IMMUNE MECHANISMS

Conventional wisdom has held that ALS is characterized by motor neuron loss and astroglial proliferation, with either no or only minimal inflammation in the form of mild perivascular cuffing in the brain and spinal cord. This traditional view of ALS is based on classic histologic techniques in which tissues are first fixed in formalin and then embedded in paraffin. Such techniques would, however, destroy many surface antigens, making important functional proteins undetectable by immunohistochemistry and preventing the identification of pathophysiologically significant cells.[35] Therefore, in the late 1980s, a number of investigators applied newer immunohistochemical techniques that revealed findings suggestive of an immune pathogenesis (Table 13–3).

Cellular Infiltrates

Inflammatory cell infiltrates were identified in CNS tissue from ALS patients more

Table 13–3. NEUROPATHOLOGY OF ALS: POSSIBLE CLUES TO IMMUNE PATHOGENESIS

- Inflammatory infiltrates in spinal cord
- Suppressor-cytotoxic T cells outnumber helper-inducer T cells
- Major histocompatibility complex-II expression in macrophages
- Immunoglobulin G localization in spinal motor neurons

commonly than originally suspected. Spinal cords from eight patients with sporadic ALS were analyzed in which infiltration of lymphocytes was found on routine histologic examination and from which frozen tissue was available.[81] Leukocyte common antigen–positive cells were identified as T lymphocytes, macrophages, and dendritic cells. Suppressor-cytotoxic T cells outnumbered helper-inducer T cells. The results suggested that T-cell–mediated immune responses occur in the spinal cords of some ALS patients.

The presence of lymphocytic infiltrates in ALS-affected spinal cords was confirmed by others.[27] T-helper cells were found close to areas of corticospinal tract degeneration, whereas T-helper and T-suppressor cytotoxic cells were present in the ventral horns. There was no immunohistochemical evidence of B cells. No association was noted between the presence of lymphocytic infiltrates and the clinical course of ALS.

Lampson and colleagues[38] were unable to detect major histocompatibility complex (MHC) expression by motor neurons, which argues against an ongoing MHC-restricted T-cell response directed at affected cells. However, in affected areas they did find MHC II–positive antigen-laden phagocytes and occasional T cells, suggesting a potential for cellular immune activity, and they proposed that the phagocytes themselves may cause secondary tissue damage that exacerbates the original insult. The authors speculated that vessel-associated phagocytes might be a source of antigen to peripheral lymphoid tissue, stimulating production of autoantibodies. Kawamata and colleagues[35] used several immunologic markers in an extensive autopsy study of 13 human brains and spinal cords of ALS patients, confirming earlier findings of immune-effector changes consistent with autoimmunity; these findings were, however, also compatible with reactive changes secondary to neuronal degeneration.

Immunoglobulin Deposition

The presence of immunoglobulin within motor neurons in experimental autoimmune motor neuron disease (see below) prompted studies of IgG reactivity in the spinal cord and motor cortex of patients with ALS.[25] A population of spinal motor neurons from 13 of 15 patients with ALS exhibited patchy or coarse granular cytoplasmic localization of IgG. The reactivity for IgG was more intense in patients at an earlier stage of disease or with relatively preserved motor neuron morphologic patterns. No control spinal cords exhibited the same intensity or patchy distribution of endogenous IgG staining. In ALS, spinal cord astrocytes were also stained, but less intensely and specifically than motor neurons. IgG was also found in a number of pyramidal cells in the motor cortices of 6 of 11 patients with ALS but not in the brains of control subjects. (Astrocytic staining for IgG was also seen in the motor cortex of brains of both patients with ALS and controls.) IgG in motor neurons may have reached the cell body by retrograde transport after being taken up at presynaptic terminals outside the blood-brain barrier. The IgG noted in upper motor neurons might have originated from IgG in destroyed lower motor neurons, or it might have entered the CNS at sites where blood-brain barrier function is altered.

EXPERIMENTAL AUTOIMMUNE ALS

In the first immune-mediated animal model, guinea pigs were immunized with motor neurons from swine spinal cords and had a delayed, progressive chronic course similar histologically to human spinal muscular atrophy.[23]

In a subsequent animal model, designated "experimental allergic motor neuron disease" (EAMND), guinea pigs were inoculated with bovine motor neurons.[24] Selective and slow destruction of lower motor neurons resulted in clinical weakness after 4 months of inoculations. This period was associated with continuously high levels of anti–motor neuron IgG in the blood. Only lower motor neurons were lost, whereas all other parts of the CNS and peripheral nervous system were unaffected. No inflammatory foci were noted in parenchyma or meninges of the CNS. Immunohistochemical studies documented the presence of IgG in spinal cord motor neurons and at the motor endplates of immunized animals. However, motor neuron–inoculated animals that did not develop clinical and pathologic evidence of motor unit destruction still had the same IgG localization as symptomatic animals. IgG at the neuromuscular junction may have been taken up at the axon terminal and carried by retrograde transport to the cell body.

A third model, experimental autoimmune gray matter disease (EAGMD), was produced by immunizing guinea pigs with bovine spinal cord ventral horn homogenate.[26] This syndrome occurs much more acutely than EAMND and involves lower and upper motor neurons. Denervation is present, as indicated by electromyography and histologic tissue analysis. Pathologic examination reveals loss of motor neurons and scattered inflammatory foci, mostly localized to the spinal cord. Immunohistochemical techniques reveal IgG at the motor endplate and around the external membrane and within the cytoplasm of motor neurons. Of interest, cyclophosphamide prevented or attenuated motor neuron destruction when administered before or immediately after inoculation of gray matter.[74]

IgG at the external membrane of motor neurons in EAGMD might have arisen from passage of the anti–motor neuronal IgG through a defect in the blood-brain barrier at the site of multiple inflammatory foci.[26] The brisk focal inflammatory cell infiltrates in the CNS during the early stages suggest the importance of cellular immunity as a contributing factor, whereas the deposition of immunoglobulin and the C3 component of complement point to the potential importance of humoral immune mechanisms.

THE ROLE OF ANTIBODIES TO CALCIUM CHANNELS IN ALS

In the immune-mediated models of motor neuron disease, IgG is bound to the neuromuscular junction and is detectable there by immunoblot techniques before the onset of significant weakness.[26] Accordingly, studies were done to determine whether IgG at the endplate is associated with abnormal physiology of the neuromuscular junction, which in turn might reflect early immune-mediated dysfunction of motor neurons.[30] The frequency of miniature endplate potentials in the experimental models was significantly higher than in controls. This increased frequency was proportional to the level of serum IgG (it was greater earlier in the course of the disease when titers are highest, and decreased later, when titers are lowest). Serum from experimental models or from patients with sporadic ALS passively transferred to mice resulted in a similar increase in frequency of miniature endplate potentials reflecting increased acetylcholine release.[3]

Effect on L-Type Calcium Channels

According to classic concepts of neuromuscular transmission, acetylcholine release at the neuromuscular junction requires increased presynaptic cytosolic calcium. Thus ALS IgG might be expected to facilitate calcium channel opening in the motor axon terminal. Therefore the effects on calcium channels of IgG from patients with ALS was studied.[14,15] Paradoxically, ALS IgG was found to reduce peak calcium currents through L-type calcium channels in individual mammalian muscle fibers. Mean channel open time was reduced, suggesting that ALS IgG can interact directly with L-type calcium channels to alter their activity. To identify the antibody-channel interaction biochemically, an enzyme-linked immunoabsorbent assay (ELISA) was used to detect the reaction of serum IgG with purified complexes of L-type voltage-gated calcium channels (VGCCs) from rabbit skeletal muscle.[71] With this assay, 75% of sera from ALS patients showed significantly higher calcium channel binding of IgGs than sera from controls. Serum reactivity by ELISA correlated with the rate of disease progression. The presence of these reactive antibodies was not specific, however, because they were found in two-thirds of patients with Lambert-Eaton myasthenic syn-

drome and in one-fifth of patients with Guillain-Barré syndrome. Additional studies have shown that the ALS IgG binds the calcium ionophore-forming α1 subunit of the VGCC and does not bind other VGCC subunits;[37] in contrast, VGCC-binding IgG from patients with Lambert-Eaton myasthenic syndrome reacts with α1 and β subunits. These findings suggest that anti-VGCC antibodies have a pathogenic role, although it is also possible they might reflect secondary immune responses to constituents released from damaged cells.[31] It has also been suggested that raised proteolytic activity in ALS IgG preparations may be partly responsible for some of the effects described for ALS IgG.[45a]

Effect on N- and P-Type Calcium Channels

The paradoxic finding that IgG antibodies *inhibit* the function of L-type VGCCs and yet *increase* acetylcholine release[60,71] suggests that antibodies to calcium channels in ALS may have different results when interacting with other subtypes of VGCCs located in motor nerve terminals, such as N- or P-type channels.[4] Adding ALS IgG to purified P-type VGCC protein enhances inward calcium current,[43] and ALS IgGs are cytotoxic in a motor neuron–neuroblastoma hybrid cell line, a cytotoxicity dependent on calcium and mediated by normal N- and P-type VGCCs.[72] Further studies with this hybrid cell line[73] showed that ALS IgG-mediated toxicity could be prevented by a thousand-fold reduction of extracellular calcium concentration with ethylenediamine tetraacetic acid, by preincubating IgG with purified intact L-type VGCC or with VGCC α1 subunit, and by preincubating cells with inhibitors of N- and P-type VGCCs. In this cell system, cell death was apoptotic and could be prevented by previous incubation with the protein synthesis inhibitor cycloheximide but not by inhibitors of glutamate receptors.

Effect on Morphology of Nerve Terminals

Repeated passive transfer of IgG from sporadic ALS patients to mice led to some instances of axonal degeneration and denervated motor endplates.[82] Immunoglobulin fractions from patients with ALS injected into mice increased vesicle density in presynaptic boutons and increased the calcium content of motor axon terminals.[28] In parallel with these passive transfer studies of IgG to mice, motor nerve terminals from sporadic ALS patients contain significantly increased calcium, increased mitochondrial volume, and increased numbers of synaptic vesicles compared with control groups.[70]

Thus ALS IgG–containing antibodies to calcium channels seem able to passively transfer functional and structural alterations of motor axon terminals in vitro and in vivo,[5] but it is not clear that these immunoglobulins play a role in the loss of motor neurons in ALS.

Indeed, other investigations have raised doubts about the existence of antibodies to calcium channels in ALS sera.[82a] In one study, using a sensitive radioimmunoassay, only one of 26 ALS sera gave a weakly positive result for binding to either N-type or P-type calcium channels.[21a] By contrast, 44% of Lambert-Eaton sera were positive in the N-type assay and 95% were positive in the P-type assay. In a second study,[5a] using immunoprecipitation assays and ELISA with purified N-type calcium channels from rat brain to detect anti-neuronal calcium channel antibodies, immunoreactivity was not consistently detected in sera from patients with ALS.

IMMUNOTHERAPY OF ALS

Some motor neuron syndromes respond to immunosuppressive treatments. These include multifocal motor neuropathy with conduction block, with or without antiganglioside antibodies;[13,76] distal lower motor neuron syndromes with anti-GM1 antibodies but without conduction block;[53] and some patients with both ALS and lymphoproliferative disease.[61] As pointed out by Rowland,[61] these potentially treatable patients account for no more than 5% to 10% of all clinically diagnosed cases of motor neuron disease (in our experience, perhaps closer to 5%). Other patients with ALS have not responded to treatment with a wide array of immunosuppressive or immunomodulatory agents including azathioprine, cyclophosphamide, cyclosporine, plasmapheresis, and human immune globu-

Table 13–4. **IMMUNOTHERAPY OF ALS: METHODS FOUND INEFFECTIVE**

- Intrathecal corticosteroid (and vitamin B_{12})[54]
- Plasmapheresis[45,47]
- Plasmapheresis and azathioprine[36]
- Cyclophosphamide (intravenous) and corticosteroid[8,76]
- Cyclosporine[2]
- Total lymph node irradiation[21]
- Intravenous gammaglobulin[13]

lin (Table 13–4). Drachman and colleagues[21] found no beneficial effect of total lymph node irradiation, despite virtually complete immunosuppression. The authors noted continued antiganglioside antibody production in some patients, however, which suggests incomplete immunosuppression and thus does not exclude a pathogenic role of these antibodies in ALS. Attributing a lack of benefit to powerful immunosuppression does not entirely disprove the immune theory of ALS. It is conceivable, albeit unlikely, that an immune mechanism acts early in the course of the illness to induce motor neuron loss and irreversible injury that cannot be ameliorated with immunotherapies in the later stages of ALS.[4,21]

SUMMARY

In the past two decades, a number of intriguing observations have kindled interest in an immune theory of ALS. Perhaps the first was the detection in ALS patients of serum factors toxic to motor neurons in culture, followed by the identification of immune complexes in the kidney and small bowel of ALS patients. Although these findings were not consistently noted, subsequent observations continued to support the idea of an immune process in ALS and to suggest mechanisms whereby motor neurons could be damaged. These observations included the presence of monoclonal gammopathy, specifically antiganglioside antibodies in some patients with ALS, as well as the detection of immunoglobulin binding to motor nerve terminals in immunologically produced animal models and in patients with ALS. Although it is unlikely that antiganglioside antibodies cause ALS, they are perhaps manifestations of an ongoing humoral immune process in ALS patients. The immunoglobulin found in antigenically induced animal models reacts with calcium channels and could theoretically lead to an excess of intracellular calcium and eventually to neuronal demise. A major stumbling block to accepting immune mechanisms as important in ALS pathogenesis, however, is the uniform lack of response of the disease to any immunologic treatment, even one that achieves virtually complete immunosuppression.

REFERENCES

1. Appel, SH, Appel, VS, Stewart, SS, et al: Amyotrophic lateral sclerosis. Associated clinical disorders and immunological evaluations. Arch Neurol 43:234–238, 1986.
2. Appel, SH, Stewart, SS, Appel, V, et al: A double-blind study of cyclosporine in amyotrophic lateral sclerosis. Arch Neurol 43:234–238, 1988.
3. Appel, SH, Engelhardt, JI, Garcia, J, et al: Immunoglobulins from animal models of motor neuron disease and from human amyotrophic lateral sclerosis patients passively transfers physiologic abnormalities to the neuromuscular junction. Proc Nat Acad Sci (USA) 88:647–651, 1991.
4. Appel, SH, Smith, RG, Engelhardt, JI, et al: Evidence for autoimmunity in amyotrophic lateral sclerosis. J Neuro Sci 118:169–174, 1993.
5. Appel, SH, Smith, G, Alexianu, MF, et al: Autoimmunity as an etiological factor in sporadic Amyotrophic Lateral Sclerosis. In Serratrice, G and Munsat, TL (eds): Pathogenesis and Therapy of Amyotrophic Lateral Sclerosis. Vol 68, Adv Neurol, Lippincott-Raven Press, Philadelphia, 1995, pp 47–57.
5a. Arsac, C, Raymond, C, Martin-Mourot, N, et al. Immunoassays fail to detect antibodies against neuronal calcium channels in amyotrophic lateral sclerosis serum. Ann Neurol 40:695–700, 1996.
6. Askanas, V, Marangos, PJ, and Engel, WK. CSF from amyotrophic lateral sclerosis patients applied to motor neurons in culture fails to alter neuron-specific enolase. Neurology 31:1196–1197, 1981.
7. Bartfeld, H, Dham, C, Donnenfeld, H, et al: Immunological profile of amyotrophic lateral sclerosis patients and their cell-mediated immune responses to viral and CNS antigens. Clin Exp Immunol 48:137–146, 1982.
8. Brown, RH, Hauser, SL, Harrington, H, et al: Failure of immunosuppression with a 10- to 14-day course of high-dose intravenous cyclophosphamide to alter the progression of amyotrophic lateral sclerosis. Arch Neurol 43:383–384, 1986.
9. Brown, RH, Johnson, D, Ogonowski, M, et al: Antineural antibodies in the serum of patients with amyotrophic lateral sclerosis. Neurology 37:152–155, 1987.
10. Cashman, NR and Antel, JP: Amyotrophic lateral sclerosis: An immunologic perspective. Immunol Allergy Clin North Am 8:331–342, 1988.
11. Cook, AW, Pertschuk, LP, and Gupta, JK: Jejunal viral antigens in multiple sclerosis and amyotrophic lateral sclerosis. Lancet 19:434, 1977.
12. Corbo, M, Quattrini, A, Lugaresi, A, et al: Patterns of reactivity of human anti-GM1 antibodies with spinal cord and motor neurons. Ann Neurol 32:487–493, 1992.
13. Dalakas, MC, Stein, DP, Otero, C, et al: Effect of high-dose intravenous immunoglobulin on amyotrophic lateral sclerosis and multifocal motor neuropathy. Arch Neurol 51:861–864, 1994.
14. Delbono, O, Garcia, J, Appel, SH, et al: IgG from amyotrophic lateral sclerosis affects tubular calcium channels of skeletal muscle. Am J Physiol 260: C1347–C1351, 1991.
15. Delbono, O, Garcia, J, Appel, SH, et al: Calcium current and charge movement of mammalian muscle: Action of amyotrophic lateral sclerosis immunoglobulin. J Physiol 444:723–742, 1991.
16. Denys, EH, Jackson, JE, Aguilar, MJ, et al: Passive transfer experiments in amyotrophic lateral sclerosis. Arch Neurol 41:161–163, 1984.
17. Digby, J, Harrison, R, Jehanli, A, et al: Cultured rat spinal cord neurons: Interaction with motor neuron disease immunoglobulins. Muscle Nerve 8:595–605, 1985.
18. Doherty, P, Dickson, JG, Flanigan, TP, et al: Effects of amyotrophic lateral sclerosis serum on cultured chick spinal neurons. Neurology 36:1330–1334, 1986.
19. Donaghy, M and Duchen, LW: Sera from patients with motor neuron disease and associated paraproteinemia fail to inhibit experimentally induced sprouting of motor nerve terminals. J Neurol Neurosurg Psychiatry 49:817–819, 1986.
20. Drachman, DB and Kuncl, RW: Amyotrophic lateral sclerosis: An unconventional autoimmune disease? Ann Neurol 26:269–274, 1992.
21. Drachman, DB, Chaudhry, V, Cornblath, D, et al: Trial of immunosuppression in amyotrophic lateral sclerosis using total lymphoid irradiation. Ann Neurol 35:142–150, 1994.
21a. Drachman, DB, Fishman, PS, Rothstein, JD, et al. Amyotrophic lateral sclerosis. An autoimmune disease? In Serratice, G and Munsat, TL (eds): Pathogenesis and Therapy of Amyotrophic Lateral Sclerosis. Vol. 68, Adv Neurol, Lippincott-Raven Press, Philadelphia, 1995, pp. 59–65.
22. Endo, T, Scott, DD, Stewart, SS, et al: Antibodies to glycosphingolipids in patients with multiple sclerosis and SLE. J Immunol 132:1793–1797, 1984.
23. Engelhardt, J and Joo, F: An immune-mediated guinea pig model for lower motor neuron disease. J Neuroimmunol 12:279–290, 1986.
24. Engelhardt, JI, Appel, SH, and Killian, JM: Experimental autoimmune motoneuron disease. Ann Neurol 26:368–376, 1989.
25. Engelhardt, JI and Appel, SH: IgG reactivity in the spinal cord and motor cortex in amyotrophic lateral sclerosis. Arch Neurol 47:1210–1216, 1990.
26. Engelhardt, JI, Appel, SH, and Killian, JM: Motor neuron destruction in guinea pigs immunized with bovine spinal cord ventral horn homogenate: Experimental autoimmune gray matter disease. J Neuroimmunol 27:21–31, 1990.
27. Engelhardt, JI, Tajti, J, and Appel, SH: Lymphocyt-

ic infiltrates in the spinal cord in amyotrophic lateral sclerosis. Arch Neurol 50:30–36, 1993.

28. Engelhardt, JI, Siklos, L, Kouves, L, et al: Antibodies to calcium channels from ALS patients passively transferred to mice selectively increase intracellular calcium and induce ultrastructural changes in motoneurons. Synapse 20:185–199, 1995.

29. Freddo, L, Yu, RK, Latov, N, et al: Gangliosides GM1 and DG1b are antigens for IgM-protein in a patient with motor neuron disease. Neurology 36:454–458, 1986.

30. Garcia, J, Engelhardt, JI, Appel, SH, et al: Increased MEPP frequency as an early sign of experimental immune-mediated motoneuron disease. Ann Neurol 28:329–334, 1990.

31. Greenberg, DA: Calcium channels and neuromuscular disease. Ann Neurol 35:131–132, 1994.

32. Gurney, ME, Belton, AC, Cashman, N, et al: Inhibition of terminal axon sprouting by serum from patients with amyotrophic lateral sclerosis. N Engl J Med 311:933–939, 1984.

33. Heiman-Patterson, T, Krupa, T, Thompson, P, et al: Anti-GM1/GD1B M-proteins damage human spinal cord neurons co-cultured with muscle. J Neurol Sci 120:38–45, 1993.

34. Horwich, MS, Engel, WK, and Chauvin, PB: Amyotrophic lateral sclerosis sera applied to cultured human spinal cord neurons. Arch Neurol 30:332–333, 1974.

35. Kawamata, T, Akiyama, H, Yamada, T, et al: Immunologic reactions in amyotrophic lateral sclerosis brain and spinal cord tissue. Am J Pathol 140:691–707, 1992.

36. Kelemen, J, Hedlund, W, Orlin, JB, et al: Plasmapheresis with immunosuppression in amyotrophic lateral sclerosis. Arch Neurol 40:752–753, 1983.

37. Kimura, F, Smith, RG, Delbono, O, et al: Amyotrophic lateral sclerosis patient antibodies label Ca^{2+} channel alpha1 subunit. Ann Neurol 35:164–171, 1994.

38. Lampson, LA, Kushner, PD, and Sobel, RA: Major histocompatibility complex antigen expression in the affected tissues in amyotrophic lateral sclerosis. Ann Neurol 28:365–372, 1990.

39. Latov, N, Hays, AP, Donofrio, PD, et al: Monoclonal IgM with unique specificity to gangliosides GM1 and GD1B and to lacto-N-tetraose associated with human motor neuron disease. Neurology 38:763–768, 1988.

40. Latov, N: Antibodies to glycoconjugates in neurologic disease. Clin Aspects Autoimmun 4:18–29, 1990.

41. Lavrnic, D, Vidakovic, A, Miletic, V, et al: Motor neuron disease and monoclonal gammopathy. Eur Neurol 35:104–107, 1995.

42. Liveson, J, Frey, H, and Bornstein, MB: The effect of serum from ALS patients on organotypic nerve and muscle tissue cultures. Acta Neuropathol 32:127–131, 1975.

43. Llinas, R, Sugimori, M, Cherksey, BD, et al: IgG from amyotrophic lateral sclerosis patients increases current through P-type calcium channels in mammalian cerebellar Purkinje cells and in isolated channel protein in lipid bilayer. Proc Nat Acad Sci (USA) 90:11743–11747, 1993.

44. Lugaresi, A, Corbo, M, Thomas, FP, et al: Identification of glycoconjugates which are targets for anti-Gal(β1-3)GalNAc autoantibodies in spinal motor neurons. J Neuroimmunol 34:69–76, 1991.

45. Norris, FH, Denys, EH, and Mielke, CH: Plasmapheresis in amyotrophic lateral sclerosis. Muscle Nerve 1:342 (A), 1978.

45a. Nyormoi, O. Proteolytic activity in amyotrophic lateral sclerosis IgG preparations. Ann Neurol 40:701–706, 1996.

46. Ogino, Y, Hisanaga, S, Lee, G, et al: IgA monoclonal antibody of an ALS patient that recognizes NFH and a 65-kD neuronal protein that inhibits phosphorylation of NFH by cdc2 kinase in vitro. Neurol 45:221 (Abstract), 1995.

47. Olarte, MR, Schoenfeldt, RB, McKiernan, G, et al: Plasmapheresis in amyotrophic lateral sclerosis. Ann Neurol 8:644–645, 1980.

48. Oldstone, MBA, Wilson, CB, Perrin, LH, et al: Evidence for immune complex formation in patients with amyotrophic lateral sclerosis. Lancet 2:169–172, 1976.

49. Palo, J, Rissanen, A, Jokinenn, E, et al: Kidney and skin biopsy in amyotrophic lateral sclerosis. Lancet 1:1270, 1978.

50. Pestronk, A, Adams, RN, Clawson, L, et al: Serum antibodies to GM1 ganglioside in amyotrophic lateral sclerosis. Neurology 38:1457–1461, 1988.

51. Pestronk, A, Adams, RN, Cornblath, D, et al: Patterns of serum IgM antibodies to GM1 and GD1a gangliosides in amyotrophic lateral sclerosis. Ann Neurol 25:98–102, 1989.

52. Pestronk, A: Invited review: Motor neuropathies, motor neuron disorders, and antiglycolipid antibodies. Muscle Nerve 14:927–936, 1991.

53. Pestronk, A, Lopate, G, Kornberg, AJ, et al: Distal lower motor neuron syndromes with high titer serum IgM anti-GM1 antibodies: Improvement following immunotherapy with monthly plasma exchange and intravenous cyclophosphamide. Ann Neurol 36:285, 1994.

54. Pieper, SJL and Fields, WS: Failure of ALS to respond to intrathecal steroid and vitamin B12. Arch Neurol 19:522–526, 1957.

55. Roberts, M, Willison, HJ, Vincent, A, et al: Multifocal motor neuropathy human sera block distal motor nerve conduction in mice. Ann Neurol 38:111–118, 1995.

56. Roisen, FJ, Bartfeld, H, Donnenfeld, H, et al: Neuron specific in vitro cytotoxicity of sera from patients with amyotrophic lateral sclerosis. Muscle Nerve 5:48–53, 1982.

57. Ronnevi, L-O, Conradi, S, Karlsson, E, et al: Nature and properties of cytotoxic plasma activity in amyotrophic lateral sclerosis. Muscle Nerve 10:734–743, 1987.

58. Rothstein, JD, Martin, LJ, and Kuncl, RW: Decreased glutamate transport by the brain and spinal cord in amyotrophic lateral sclerosis. N Engl J Med 326:1464–1468, 1992.

59. Rowland, LP, Defendini, R, Sherman, W, et al: Macroglobulinemia with peripheral neuropathy simulating motor neuron disease. Ann Neurol 11:532–536, 1982.

60. Rowland, LP: Amyotrophic lateral sclerosis and autoimmunity. N Engl J Med 327:1752–1753, 1992.

61. Rowland, LP: Amyotrophic lateral sclerosis: Theories and therapies. Ann Neurol 35:129–130, 1994.

62. Rowland, LP. Amyotrophic lateral sclerosis with paraproteins and antibodies. In Serratice, G and Munsat, TL (eds): Pathogenesis and Therapy of Amyotrophic Lateral Sclerosis. Vol. 68, Adv Neurol, Lippincott-Raven Press, Philadelphia, 1995, pp. 93–105.

63. Sadiq, SA, Thomas, FP, Kilidireas, K, et al: The spectrum of neurologic disease associated with anti-GM1 antibodies. Neurology 40:1067–1072, 1990.

64. Santoro, M, Thomas, FP, Fink, ME, et al: IgM deposits at nodes of Ranvier in a patient with amyotrophic lateral sclerosis, anti-GM1 antibodies, and multifocal motor conduction block. Ann Neurol 28:373–377, 1990.

65. Santoro, M, Uncini, A, Corbo, M, et al: Experimental conduction block induced by serum from a patient with anti-GM1 antibodies. Ann Neurol 32:487–493, 1992.

66. Schluep, M and Steck, AJ: Immunostaining of motor nerve terminals by IgM M protein with activity against gangliosides GM1 and GD1B from a patient with motor neuron disease. Neurology 38:1890–1892, 1988.

67. Shy, ME, Rowland, LP, Smith, T, et al: Motor neuron disease and plasma cell dyscrasia. Neurology 36:1429–1436, 1986.

68. Shy, ME, Evans, VA, Lublin, FD, et al: Antibodies to GM1 and GD1B in patients with motor neuron disease without plasma cell dyscrasia. Ann Neurol 25:511–513, 1989.

69. Shy, ME, Heiman-Patterson, T, Parry, GJ, et al: Lower motor neuron disease in a patient with autoantibodies against Gal(B1-3)GalNAc in gangliosides GM1 and GD1B: Improvement following immunotherapy. Neurology 40:842–844, 1990.

70. Siklos, L, Engelhardt, J, Harati, Y, et al: Ultrastructural evidence for altered calcium in motor nerve terminals in amyotrophic lateral sclerosis. Ann Neurol 39:203–216, 1996.

71. Smith, RG, Hamilton, S, Hoffmann, F, et al: Serum antibodies to L-type calcium channels in patients with amyotrophic lateral sclerosis. N Engl J Med 327:1721–1728, 1992.

72. Smith, RG, Alexianu, ME, Crawford, G, et al: Cytotoxicity of immunoglobulins from amyotrophic lateral sclerosis patients on a hybrid motor neuron cell line. Proc Nat Acad Sci (USA) 91:3393–3397, 1994.

73. Smith, RG and Appel, SH: Molecular approaches to amyotrophic lateral sclerosis. Annu Rev Med 46:133–145, 1995.

74. Tajti, J, Stefani, E, and Appel, SH: Cyclophosphamide alters the clinical and pathological expression of experimental autoimmune gray matter disease. J Neuroimmunol 34:143–151, 1991.

75. Takigawa, T, Yasuda, H, Kikkawa, R, et al: Antibodies against GM1 ganglioside affect K and Na currents in isolated rat myelinated nerve fibers. Ann Neurol 37:436–442, 1995.

76. Tan, E, Lynn, J, Amato, AA, et al: Immunosuppressive treatment in motor neuron syndromes. Attempts to distinguish a treatable disorder. Arch Neurol 51:194–200, 1994.

77. Tarolato, BF, Licandro, AC, and Saia, A: Motor neuron disease: An immunological study. Eur Neurol 13:433, 1975.

78. Thomas, FP, Adapon, PH, Goldberg, GP, et al: Localization of neural epitopes that bind to IgM monoclonal autoantibodies (M-proteins) from two patients with motor neuron disease. J Neuroimmunol 21:31–39, 1989.

79. Thomas, FP, Thomas, JE, Sadiq, SA, et al: Human monoclonal IgM anti-Gal(B1-3)GalNAc autoantibodies bind to the surface of bovine spinal motoneurons. J Neuropathol Exp Neurol 49:89–95, 1990.

80. Touzeau, G and Kato, AC: Effects of amyotrophic lateral sclerosis sera on cultured cholinergic neurons. Neurology 33:317–322, 1983.

81. Troost, D, Van Den Oord, JJ, and Vianney DeJong, JMB: Immunohistochemical characterization of the inflammatory infiltrate in amyotrophic lateral sclerosis. Neuropathol Applied Neurobiol 16:401–410, 1990.

82. Uchitel, OD, Scornik, F, Protti, DA, et al: Long-term neuromuscular dysfunction produced by passive transfer of amyotrophic lateral sclerosis immunoglobulins. Neurology 42:2175–2180, 1992.

82a. Vincent, A, and Drachman, DB. Amyotrophic lateral sclerosis and antibodies to voltage-gated calcium channels—New doubts. Ann Neurol 40:691–692, 1996.

83. Wolfgram, F and Myers, L: Amyotrophic lateral sclerosis: Effect of serum on anterior horn cells in tissue culture. Science 179:579–580, 1973.

84. Younger, DS, Rowland, LP, Latov, N, et al: Motor neuron disease and amyotrophic lateral sclerosis: Relation of high CSF protein content to paraproteinemia and clinical syndromes. Neurology 40:595–599, 1990.

CHAPTER 14

HYPOTHESES FOR VIRAL AND OTHER TRANSMISSIBLE AGENTS IN ALS

A viral hypothesis of ALS evolved in parallel with our understanding of the role of poliovirus in the pathogenesis of acute and chronic disorders of motor neurons. In 1875, poliomyelitis was already known to cause both acute paralytic illness and chronic progressive weakness and muscular atrophy.[5] In 1906, a new pathogen, poliovirus, was found to cause acute poliomyelitis.[31] Zilkha[69] in 1962 and Poskanzer et al.[46] in 1969 suggested a close association between ALS and a history of paralytic polio. Mulder and col-

leagues[41] pointed out that acute poliomyelitis may, many years later, give rise to a syndrome resembling ALS that they called a "forme fruste ALS."

In the past several decades, increasing knowledge of poliovirus and other neurotropic viruses has continued to renew the hypothesis that ALS may be caused by one of these viruses.[36] However, extensive investigations have demonstrated no solid evidence for such a hypothesis. Jolicoeur[22] pointed out that:

1) absence of viral particles in the diseased tissues does not indicate absence of viral infection. Several viruses, including retroviruses, can infect cells and remain in a latent form, expressing only part of their genome, thus preventing the formation of virus particles;
2) the absence of an inflammatory reaction seen in ALS lesions can no longer be used to indicate lack of viral infection. The Creutzfeldt-Jakob and kuru transmissible agent and the neurovirulent murine retroviruses induce neurologic diseases in the absence of inflammatory reactions in the affected lesions and even in the absence of a general immune response; and
3) failure to transmit ALS to primates or other mammals does not disprove that viruses are involved, but rather, only that the result is negative. Viral infection might be present, but infectious particles might be absent; or the range of hosts the virus can infect might be highly restricted.

239

Therefore, a viral theory remains a viable hypothesis for the cause of ALS. This chapter reviews clinical manifestations of poliovirus, other neurotropic viruses, and prion agents, and potential causal relationships with ALS. Results of limited therapeutic trials attempted to date are also reviewed briefly.

POLIOVIRUS

Acute Poliomyelitis

Acute poliomyelitis had been endemic for hundreds of years until the mid-19th century, when it became epidemic, creating a major health problem in many parts of the world. Poliovirus is extremely infectious, but only a small fraction of those infected become demonstrably ill. In most patients, the initial infection causes only minor symptoms and resembles a nonspecific febrile illness. These symptoms are manifestations of the prodromal (first) stage of acute poliomyelitis. Patients may proceed to the second stage, in which poliovirus invades the CNS. The second stage is designated as nonparalytic or preparalytic poliomyelitis and is characterized clinically by severe flulike symptoms and acute meningoencephalitis. Symptoms abate in several days unless the infection advances to the third stage—paralytic poliomyelitis, which develops with incredible rapidity. It begins with focal weakness and may advance to widespread and complete paralysis within hours. Patients who survive acute paralytic poliomyelitis invariably recover with various degrees of residual weakness. With the advent of poliovirus vaccine, acute poliomyelitis from poliovirus infection has nearly disappeared, whereas acute poliomyelitis provoked by poliovirus vaccine has been reported, particularly associated with any intramuscular injections given after polio vaccination.[58] Acute poliomyelitis has no resemblance to ALS, but its remote effects are similar to some features of ALS.

Postpolio Progressive Muscular Atrophy

After many years of clinical stability following recovery from acute poliomyelitis, some patients may develop slowly progressive muscle weakness and atrophy, called *postpolio progressive muscular atrophy* (PPMA), which superficially resembles ALS.[7,25,41] Other clinical manifestations, such as muscle and joint pains and multiple musculoskeletal and orthopedic problems, are often called postpolio syndrome and represent an inclusive clinical complex seen in many patients with remote polio infection. Table 14–1 summarizes similarities and differences between PPMA and ALS; clinical features of PPMA are discussed in Chapter 6. Perhaps the most

Table 14–1. SIMILARITIES AND DIFFFERENCES BETWEEN ALS AND PROGRESSIVE POSTPOLIOMYELITIS MUSCULAR ATROPHY

Characteristics	ALS	PPMA
Clinical Features		
UMN involvement	100%	8.3%*
LMN involvement	100%	100%
Rate of progression	Rapid	Very slow
Electromyographic Findings		
Fibrillations	Widespread, abundant	Limited
Chronic MUPs	Mild to moderate	Prominent
Cerebrospinal Fluid Findings		
Routine tests	Normal	Normal
Oligoclonal bands	Absent	Often present
Muscle Histology		
Denervation	Active (small groups)	Active (fascicular)
Reinnervation	Limited	Extensive
Chronic inflammation	Absent	May be present
Spinal Cord Pathology		
Neuronal loss	Present	Present
Chronic inflammation	Rare	Frequent
Ubiquitin inclusions	Present	Absent

*According to Jubelt and Drucker (1993), the percentage of UMN signs is very similar in both patients with acute paralytic poliomyelitis and those with PPMA.

Abbreviations: LMN = lower motor neuron; MUP = motor unit potential; PPMA = progressive postpoliomyelitis muscular atrophy; UMN = upper motor neuron.

compelling and prognostically significant clinical feature that distinguishes PPMA from ALS is the slow progression of PPMA.[7,8] Pathologically, chronic lymphocytic infiltration in the spinal cord and occasionally in skeletal muscles is evident in PPMA. Ubiquitin-positive intracytoplasmic inclusions are not present in the anterior horn cells in PPMA, but they are consistently found in ALS.[21] In contrast to ALS, the incidence of PPMA is not well established, but ranges from 0%[18] to 64%.[67] Although PPMA appears to be well defined,[8,41] such an unusually wide disparity in occurrence raises the concern that the identity of PPMA may be more ambiguous than we have suspected.

History of Prior Paralytic Poliomyelitis in ALS Patients

Since the initial reports suggesting frequent prior polio infection in patients with ALS,[46,69] subsequent studies of patients with ALS have shown a surprisingly low frequency (Table 14–2). In fact, unequivocal cases of ALS occurring in those with prior acute paralytic poliomyelitis are rare.[1,50] Investigators have even speculated as to whether prior polio infection may protect against the development of ALS. Recent epidemiologic studies do not support a close relationship between ALS and prior poliomyelitis. Moriwaka et al.[39] surveyed this relationship in Japan and found no significant correlation between ALS and poliomyelitis. The incidence of ALS has not declined in a population in Scotland who have been vaccinated against polio, suggesting that preventing paralytic poliomyelitis does not reduce the frequency of ALS.[59] In fact, the rates of hospital

Table 14–2. **HISTORY OF ACUTE POLIOMYELITIS IN ALS**

Investigator	Acute Poliomyelitis/ALS
Zilkha[69] (1962)	11/37 (30.0%)
Poskanzer[46] (1969)	5/196 (5.2%)
Codd et al.[5a] (1985)	0/316 (0%)
Norris et al.[42a] (1993)	10/710 (1.4%)
Moriwaka et al.[39] (1993)	1/220 (0.5%)

discharge and mortality resulting from ALS are increasing in this particular population.

Evidence of Poliovirus Infection in ALS

Laboratory studies have not produced convincing evidence of ongoing, active poliovirus infection in patients with ALS. Poliovirus has not been identified by culturing or by immunofluorescence staining of various tissues from ALS patients at necropsy.[6,45,62] An RNA in situ hybridization assay has shown that picornaviruses may persist in the human nervous system in normal individuals as well as in ALS patients.[28] The specificity of such findings remains to be resolved.[33,57] Barfeld et al.[2] found a significantly increased in vitro, cell-mediated immune response to poliovirus in tissues obtained from ALS patients at autopsy. This increase suggests that specific sensitization to poliovirus takes place and that a resulting autoimmune process may be involved in ALS.

Failure to identify poliovirus, however, does not exclude the possibility that a defective poliovirus is involved in the pathogenesis of ALS.[61] It is most puzzling and instructive to know that the results of virologic and immunologic studies in PPMA, presumably a certain indicator of a remote polio infection, are at best equivocal in identifying evidence of prior poliovirus infection. Sharief et al.[53] found poliovirus antibodies and poliovirus-sensitized cells in the cerebrospinal fluid of PPMA patients. Other investigators, however, found no such evidence.[29,51] Studies with polymerase chain reaction to look for poliovirus RNA in skeletal muscles have been negative.[34] More recent investigations with polymerase chain reaction have revealed the presence of a poliovirus RNA fragment in cerebrospinal fluid samples obtained from several patients with PPMA (Marinos Dalakas, MD HIN, personal communication, 1995). This finding suggests that poliovirus and similar viruses, such as coxsackievirus or a defective poliovirus (all of which may share the same RNA sequence), may persist in patients with PPMA. Further studies in PPMA are important in understanding the disease mechanisms involved with PPMA and ALS.

Experimental Poliomyelitis

A persistent poliomyelitis infection occurs when the virus is directly inoculated into mouse brain.[35] Despite documented infection of brain homogenates on viral cultures in these animals, serum-neutralizing antibodies to poliovirus are not detected, and poliovirus RNA is detected in only half the animals. Another model is produced by direct intracerebral inoculation of diluted poliomyelitis virus after immunosuppression with cyclophosphamide.[26] These models require direct virus inoculation to the brain and always show persistent lymphocytic infiltration when the disease develops. If persistent poliomyelitis infection can cause an ALS-like syndrome (i.e., progressive motor neuron degeneration, weakness, and muscle atrophy), experimental techniques have not successfully reproduced it in an animal model.

RNA AND DNA VIRUSES

Jubelt[24] and Jubelt and Drucker[25] reviewed ALS-like syndrome and motor neuron disease caused by viral infections. The viruses included RNA viruses, such as coxsackievirus, Vilyuisk encephalitis, Russian spring-summer encephalitis, Schu virus, and mumps virus, and DNA viruses, including adenovirus and herpesviruses (see review by Salazar-Gruesco and Roos[52]). Extensive studies investigating antibodies against these viruses in patients with ALS have been uniformly negative.[27] Hudson and Rice[20] hypothesized that the Guamanian ALS-parkinsonism-dementia complex may be caused by persistent infection by encephalitis lethargica virus because of clinical and pathologic similarities between the two conditions. This presumably already-extinct virus is most likely to closely resemble the DNA adenovirus, which is well known to cause persistent infections and has a high mutation frequency. Mulder[40] believes that muscle atrophy in patients with ALS on Guam differs from that found in patients with encephalitis lethargica. Furthermore, this hypothesis cannot explain why the disease has been confined to the Mariana Islands, whereas encephalitis lethargica was distributed worldwide in the early part of this century.

RETROVIRUSES

Retroviruses are a heterogeneous group of RNA viruses that are classified in a distinct taxonomic group because they share a pattern of replication. Upon entering the cell, these viruses synthesize a DNA copy of their genome (the provirus), which then integrates into the host's cellular DNA. After integration, cellular enzymes synthesize virus-specific mRNA transcripts that are translated into proteins. The viral proteins package the viral genomic RNA, and the viral particles exit the cell by budding through the cellular membrane. Retrovirus replication usually, although not always, has no cytotoxic effects on the infected cell.[32] Interest in the biology of retroviruses has markedly intensified in recent years after the discovery that some are pathogenic to humans.

Human Immunodeficiency Virus

Human immunodeficiency virus (HIV) infection causes a wide range of neurologic disorders involving the CNS and peripheral nervous system.[9,56] Only three anecdotal case reports of ALS-like motor neuron disease occurring in patients with known HIV infection have been published.[17,25] Autopsy studies were performed in two patients; a myeloradiculoneuropathy existed in both, but one patient also had a myopathy without motor neuron loss,[60] whereas the other had motor neuron loss and reactive gliosis.[54] A few additional reported cases clinically resemble motor neuron disease, but most likely are instances of motor axonal polyradiculoneuropathy; cerebrospinal fluid protein level is modestly increased in these patients.[16,19] The disease course is an important feature in these cases: the course was not progressive, but in some patients, weakness appeared to improve slowly with or without steroids or intravenous immunoglobulin treatment. The patient reported by Verma et al.[60] (see above) also had scattered chronic lymphocytic infiltration in a muscle biopsy specimen, again a feature not seen in ALS.

We treated a 35-year-old man, known to be HIV seropositive and previously treated with zidovudine, who developed progressive weakness (Medical Research Council [MRC] scale range 4), predominantly in the lower extremities, and nonpathologic hyperreflexia. Weakness progressed to the point that he could walk only with a cane. On electromyographic (EMG) studies, the needle electrode examination showed widespread acute and chronic denervation predominantly in the lower extremities. We found no evidence of a demyelinating neuropathy. The cerebrospinal fluid study was normal, and a muscle biopsy specimen showed neurogenic atrophy with occasional degenerating muscle fibers and mild lymphocytic infiltration. Initially, we suspected ALS. Over several months, however, his muscle strength improved. A repeated EMG study also showed no evidence of acute denervation. Therefore, one must include ALS-like syndromes among the many neurologic complications of HIV infection. It is generally agreed that no previously reported cases established a causal relationship between HIV and motor neuron disease per se.

Human T-Lymphotrophic Virus Type 1

In 1985, a high prevalence of antibodies against human T-lymphotrophic virus type 1 (HTLV-1) was noted in the Caribbean region.[14] Subsequently, HTLV-1, the first human exogenous retrovirus, was determined to cause tropical spastic paraparesis (TSP) in the Pan-Caribbean areas. About the same time, cases of endogenous myelopathy in southern Japan were found to be caused by HTLV-1; this myelopathy was termed HTLV-1-associated myelopathy (HAM).[44] Since then, the condition caused by this retrovirus has been called TSP/HAM. HTLV-1 infection causes leukomyelitis, which is clinically characterized by spastic paraparesis, urinary frequency, urinary incontinence, and sensory impairment.[3,44,55] Although the predominant clinical picture is that of a pure upper motor neuron syndrome, EMG study shows reduced compound motor action potentials, a delayed F-wave response, and giant motor unit potentials, suggesting that lower motor neurons or their axons are clearly involved, perhaps chronically.[3] In fact, motor neuron disease indistinguishable from ALS has been reported in a patient who had typical TSP/

HAM.[30] The autopsy showed widespread neuronal degeneration, including pyramidal tract and anterior horn cell lesions, in addition to a prominent lymphocytic infiltration throughout the spinal cord. Therefore, HTLV-1 infection may cause an ALS-like syndrome.

Murine Retroviruses

Gardner et al.[13] originally discovered a murine disease that produced both hindlimb paralysis and lymphoma or leukemia and was caused by infection with a murine retrovirus, type-C RNA leukemia virus. Subsequently, several murine retroviruses have been identified, and the genome responsible for the neurotropic infection, leukemia, and disease virulence has been identified.[22] Only neonatal mice are susceptible to this retrovirus; older mice are immune. In neonatal mice inoculated with the virus, hindlimb paralysis develops in 4 weeks, and a marked spongy degeneration develops in endothelial and glial cells but not in neurons. Virion budding is found in the granular and agranular endoplasmic reticulum. No signs of inflammation exist. Neuronal degeneration appears to be indirect and not the result of neuronal infection (the viral infection perhaps blocks neurotrophic receptor sites). This model provides an extremely intriguing paradigm for the investigation of retrovirus infection, immune response, and the mechanism of viral neurotropism.[22,23] However, this model differs from ALS because of its distinctive pathology.

Retrovirus in ALS

Recently, Younger and associates[68] have suggested that the occurrence of lymphoma in patients with ALS may be more than coincidental and suspect that either an immunologically mediated process in the course of lymphoma or a retrovirus like HTLV-1 might be involved in the pathogenesis of ALS. Engel[11] also endorsed a viral hypothesis and offered the term *human ALS virus* (HAV) for such a virus. If ALS should be a viral disease, the story of HTLV-1 infection may provide an interesting model. HTLV-1 infection probably occurs throughout the world but is rare; areas of endemic infection include Africa, the Pan-Caribbean, South America, and Japan. The latency period after the initial HTLV-1 infection can be several decades. ALS may behave similarly to TSP/HAM, occurring after many years' latency in an endemic pattern, as is seen in Guam, the Kii peninsula of Japan, and New Guinea. However, the inflammatory reaction occurring in the spinal cord of patients with TSP/HAM is generally absent in ALS. On the other hand, some retrovirus infections cause no inflammation.

With intriguing theories, searches of HTLV-1/2 proviral genomes have been continued. Dekaban et al.[10] did not find proviral genome at autopsy in the brains of five patients with ALS. On the other hand, HTLV genome and its highly conserved genomic regions were found in some sera obtained from ALS patients but not from controls by using polymerase chain reaction techniques.[4] Other retroviruses have also been investigated in ALS. In fact, Westarp and colleagues[63] found that patients with sporadic ALS are seropositive for human foamy retrovirus and visna virus. These viral epitopes appear to share motor neuron receptor polypeptides, perhaps interfering with neuronotrophic signaling.[65] Further studies clearly are necessary.[22,23]

PRIONS

Prusiner[47] introduced the term *prions* to distinguish the proteinaceous infectious particles that cause scrapie, Creutzfeldt-Jakob disease, Gerstmann-Sträussler-Scheinker syndrome, and kuru from viroids and viruses. According to Prusiner,[48] prions cause transmissible and genetic neurodegenerative diseases, including scrapie and bovine spongiform encephalopathy in agricultural animals, and Creutzfeldt-Jakob disease, Gerstmann-Sträussler-Scheinker syndrome, thalamic dementia, and fatal familial insomnia syndrome in humans. Infectious prion particles are composed largely, if not entirely, of an abnormal isoform of the prion protein, the gene for which is encoded on a chromosome. A posttranslational process, as yet unidentified, converts the cellular prion pro-

tein into an abnormal isoform. Point mutations in the prion protein genes of animals and humans are genetically linked to neurodegeneration.[48]

An extensive study of ALS transmission to primates has been performed, but transmission was unsuccessful, indicating that ALS is unlikely to be a well-established prion disease.[15] Nevertheless, in one study, arginase activity increased in the cerebrospinal fluid of patients with ALS, suggesting a possible relationship to prions in ALS, because in scrapie-infected mice a markedly increased arginase activity coincides with the appearance of intracellular multilayer membranes, but its activity falls when status spongiosus develops.[49] Thus, a similar elevation of arginase activity in ALS may suggest an underlying process that may involve prion infection. To date, however, no evidence shows that prions cause ALS. Furthermore, ALS histopathology is distinct from that in prion-induced disease (see Chapters 6 and 11). We are, however, only at the beginning of our understanding of novel genetic and transmissible prion-related neurodegenerative disorders: "lessons learned from prion diseases may give insight into the etiologies, as well as the pathogenic mechanisms, of such common CNS degenerative disorders as Alzheimer's disease, ALS, and Parkinson's disease."[48]

THERAPEUTIC TRIALS

Despite unsuccessful attempts to find evidence of viral infection in ALS, antiviral treatment has been tested.[37] Table 14–3 summarizes antiviral treatment trials that have been performed. Only a small number of antiviral agents have been available. None has shown clinical benefits although exploratory clinical trials with α- and β-interferon have been done.

SUMMARY

A viral hypothesis of ALS has evolved in parallel with our understanding of the role of poliovirus in the pathogenesis of acute and chronic disorders of motor neurons. In this chapter, we reviewed the clinical manifestations of acute paralytic poliomyelitis and

Table 14–3. SUMMARY OF TRIALS OF ANTIVIRAL TREATMENT FOR ALS

Agents	Mechanisms	Study Design	Results	Reference
Amantadine	Antiviral, prophylaxis of influenza-A	Controlled	Negative	38, 42
Levamisole	Immunostimulatory	Controlled	Negative	43
α-Interferon	Antiviral, immunomodulation	Exploratory, open trials	Negative	12, 57
Zidovudine	Antiretroviral	Open trials	Negative	64
β-Interferon	Antiviral, immunomodulation	Exploratory, open trials	—*	66

*Intrathecal administration with no clinical therapeutic assessment available.

PPMA, which may develop many years after recovery from acute poliomyelitis. Although PPMA superficially resembles ALS, the clinical, EMG, histopathologic, and epidemiologic features of PPMA are quite different from those of ALS. True ALS occurring in those with prior acute paralytic poliomyelitis is unusually rare, suggesting that poliovirus might even protect against developing ALS. Extensive investigation to find evidence of prior poliovirus infection in ALS has been negative, and the studies in PPMA are at best equivocal.

Other candidate viruses include HIV and HTLV-1. HIV can involve lower motor neurons and multiple spinal motor roots and thus may mimic motor neuron disease, whereas HTLV-1 can cause progressive myelopathy characterized by spastic paraparesis and, rarely, by lower motor neuron signs. Based on the observation that human retroviruses can produce motor neuron disease–like manifestations and the existence of murine retrovirus motor neuron disease, the possibility that ALS is caused by an as yet unidentified retrovirus cannot be excluded. The novel transmissible agents, prions, have emerged as an increasingly important causative factor in neurodegenerative disorders, but their role, if any, in ALS remains to be determined. The results of previous and current therapeutic trials with antiviral agents so far have been negative.

REFERENCES

1. Armon, C, Daube, JR, Windebank, AJ, et al: How frequently does classic amyotrophic lateral sclerosis develop in survivors of poliomyelitis? Neurology 40:172–174, 1990.
2. Barfeld, H, Dham, C, Donnenfeld, H, et al: Immunological profile of amyotrophic lateral sclerosis patients and their cell-mediated immune responses to viral and CNS antigen. Clin Exp Immunol 48:137–146, 1982.
3. Bhagavati, S, Ehrlich, G, Kula, RW, et al: Detection of human T-cell lymphoma/leukemia virus type I DNA and antigen in spinal fluid and blood of patients with chronic progressive myelopathy. N Engl J Med 318:1141–1147, 1988.
4. Caputo, D, Westarp, ME, Mancuso, R, et al: HTLV antibodies and DNA sequences in sporadic amyotrophic lateral sclerosis. Neurology 45(suppl 4): A221, 1995.
5. Cornil, V and Lépine, R: Sur un cas de paralysie générale spinale antérieure subaiguë, suivi d'autopsie. Gaz Med Paris 4:127–129, 1875.
5a. Codd, MB, Mulder, DW, Kurland, LT, et al: Poliomyelitis in Rochester, Minnesota, 1935–1995. In Halstead, LS and Weicher, DO (eds): Late Effects of Poliomyelitis. Miami: Symposia Foundation, 1985, pp. 121–134.
6. Cremer, NE, Oshiro, LS, Norris, FH, et al: Cultures of tissues from patients with amyotrophic lateral sclerosis. Arch Neurol 29:331–333, 1973.
7. Cwik, VA and Mitsumoto, H: Postpoliomyelitis syndrome. In Smith, RA (ed): Handbook of Amyotrophic Lateral Sclerosis. Marcel Dekker, New York, 1992, pp 77–91.
8. Dalakas, MC, Elder, G, Hallett, M, et al: A long-term follow-up study of patients with post-poliomyelitis neuromuscular symptoms. N Engl J Med 314:959–963, 1986.
9. Dalakas, MC and Pezeshkpour, GH: Neuromuscular diseases associated with human immunodeficiency virus infection. Ann Neurol 23(suppl): S38–S48, 1988.
10. Dekaban, GA, Hudson, AJ, and Rice, GPA: Absence of HTLV-I and HTLV-II proviral genome in the brains of patients with multiple sclerosis and amyotrophic lateral sclerosis. Can J Neurol Sci 19:458–461, 1992.
11. Engel, WK: Does a retrovirus cause amyotrophic lateral sclerosis? Ann Neurol 30:431–433, 1991.
12. Färkkilä, M, Iivanainen, M, and Roine, R: Neurotoxic and other side effects of high-dose interferon in amyotrophic lateral sclerosis. Acta Neurol Scan 69:42–46, 1984.
13. Gardner, MB, Henderson, BE, Officer, JE, et al: A spontaneous lower motor neuron disease apparently caused by indigenous type-C RNA virus in wild mice. J Nat Cancer Inst 51:1243–1254, 1973.
14. Gessain, A and Gout, O: Chronic myelopathy asso-

ciated with human T-lymphotropic virus type I (HTLV-I). Ann Intern Med 117:933–946, 1992.

15. Gibbs, CJ Jr and Gajdusek, DC: An update on long term in vivo and in vitro studies designed to identify a virus as the cause of amyotrophic lateral sclerosis, parkinsonism, dementia, and Parkinson's disease. In Rowland, LP (ed): Human Motor Neuron Diseases. Raven Press, New York, 1982, pp 343–351.

16. Goldstein, JM, Azizi, SA, Booss, J, et al: Human immunodeficiency virus-associated motor axonal polyradiculoneuropathy. Arch Neurol 50:1316–1319, 1993.

17. Hoffman, PM, Festoff, BW, Giron, LT, et al: Isolation of LAV-HTLV-III from a patient with amyotrophic lateral sclerosis. N Engl J Med 313:324–325, 1985.

18. Howard, RS, Wiles, CM, and Spencer, GT: The late sequelae of poliomyelitis. Q J Med 66:219–232, 1988.

19. Huang, PP, Chin, R, Son, S, et al: Lower motor neuron dysfunction associated with human immunodeficiency virus infection. Arch Neurol 50:1328–1330, 1993.

20. Hudson, AJ and Rice, GPA: Similarities of Guamanian ALS/PD to postencephalitic Parkinsonism/ALS: Possible viral cause. Can J Neurol Sci 17:427–433, 1990.

21. Ito, H and Hirano, A: Comparative study of spinal cord ubiquitin expression in post-poliomyelitis and sporadic amyotrophic lateral sclerosis. Acta Neuropathol (Berl) 87:425–429, 1994.

22. Jolicoeur, P: Retrovirus-induced lower motor neuron disease in mice: A model for amyotrophic lateral sclerosis and human spongiform neurological disease. In Hudson, AJ (ed): Amyotrophic Lateral Sclerosis. University Toronto Press, Toronto, 1990, pp 53–75.

23. Jolicoeur, P: Neuronal loss in a lower motor neuron disease induced by a murine retrovirus. Can J Neurol Sci 18:411–413, 1991.

24. Jubelt, B: Viruses and motor neuron diseases. Adv Neurol 56:463–472, 1991.

25. Jubelt, B and Drucker, J: Post-polio syndrome: An update. Semin Neurol 13:283–289, 1993.

26. Jubelt, B and Meagher, JB: Poliovirus infection of cyclophosphamide-treated mice results in persistence and late paralysis: I. Clinical, pathologic, and immunologic studies. Neurology 34:486–493, 1984.

27. Kascsak, RJ, Carp, RI, Vilcek, JT, et al: Virological studies in amyotrophic lateral sclerosis. Muscle Nerve 5:93–101, 1982.

28. Kohne, DE, Gibbs, CJ, White, L, et al: Virus detection by nucleic acid hybridization: Examination of normal and ALS tissue for the presence of poliovirus. J Gen Virol 56:223–233, 1981.

29. Kurent, JE, Brooks, BR, Madden, DL, et al: CSF viral antibodies. Evaluation in amyotrophic lateral sclerosis and late-onset postpoliomyelitis progressive muscular atrophy. Arch Neurol 36:269–273, 1979.

30. Kuroda, Y and Sugihara, H: Autopsy report of HTLV-I-associated myelopathy presenting with ALS-like manifestations. J Neurol Sci 106:199–205, 1991.

31. Landsteiner, K and Popper, E: Übertragung der Poliomyelitis acuta auf Affen. Z Immun Forsch 2:377–390, 1909.

32. Lazo, PA and Tsichlis, PN: Biology and pathogenesis of retroviruses. Semin Oncol 17:269–294, 1990.

33. McClure, MA and Perrault, J: Poliovirus genome RNA hybridizes specifically to higher eukaryotic rRNAs. Nucleic Acids Res 13:6797–6816, 1985.

34. Melchers, W, de Visser, M, Jongen, P, et al: The postpolio syndrome: No evidence for poliovirus persistence. Ann Neurol 32:728–732, 1992.

35. Miller, JR: Prolonged intracerebral infection with poliovirus in asymptomatic mice. Ann Neurol 9:590–596, 1981.

36. Mitsumoto, H, Hanson, MR, and Chad, DA: Amyotrophic lateral sclerosis: Recent advances in pathogenesis and therapeutic trails. Arch Neurol 45:189–202, 1988.

37. Mitsumoto, H: New therapeutic approaches: Rationale and results. In Leigh, PN and Swash, M (eds): Motor Neuron Disease. Biology and Management. Springer-Verlag, London, 1995, pp 419–441.

38. Mora, JS, Munsat, TL, Kao, K-P, et al: Intrathecal administration of natural human interferon alpha in amyotrophic lateral sclerosis. Neurology 36:1137–1140, 1986.

39. Moriwaka, F, Okumura, H, Tashiro, K, et al: The ALS Study Group: Motor neuron disease and past poliomyelitis. J Neurol 240:13–16, 1993.

40. Mulder, DW: The etiology of amyotrophic lateral sclerosis: What do the clinical patterns tell us? Neurol Forum 4:2–5, 1993.

41. Mulder, DW, Rosenbaum, RA, and Layton, DD: Late progression of poliomyelitis or forme fruste amyotrophic lateral sclerosis? Mayo Clin Proc 47:756–761, 1972.

42. Norris, FH, Calanchini, PR, Fallat, RJ, et al: The administration of guanidine in amyotrophic lateral sclerosis. Neurology 24:721–728, 1974.

42a. Norris, FW, Shepherd, R, Denys, E, et al: Onset, natural history and outcome in idiopathic adult motor neuron disease. J Neurol Sci 118:48–55, 1993.

43. Olarte, MR and Shaffer, SQ: Levamisole is ineffective in the treatment of amyotrophic lateral sclerosis. Neurology 35:1063–1066, 1985.

44. Osame, M, Matsumoto, M, Usuku, K, et al: Chronic progressive myelopathy associated with elevated antibodies to human T-lymphotropic virus type 1 and adult T-cell leukemia-like cells. Ann Neurol 21:117–122, 1987.

45. Oshiro, LS, Cremer, NE, Norris, FH, et al: Viruslike particles in muscle from a patient with amyotrophic lateral sclerosis. Neurology 26:57–60, 1976.

46. Poskanzer, DC, Cantor, HM, and Kaplan, GS: The frequency of preceding poliomyelitis in amyotrophic lateral sclerosis. In Norris, FH and Kurland, LT (eds): Motor Neuron Diseases. Grune & Stratton, New York, 1969, pp 286–290.

47. Prusiner, SB: Novel proteinaceous infectious particles cause scrapie. Science 216:136–144, 1982.

48. Prusiner, SB: Molecular biology of prion diseases. Science 252:1515–1522, 1991.

49. Roikhel, VM, Fokina, GI, Khokhlov, AI, et al: Al-

terations of arginase activity in scrapi-infected mice and in amyotrophic lateral sclerosis. Acta Virol 34:545–553, 1990.

50. Roos, R, Viola, MV, Wollmann, R, et al: Amyotrophic lateral sclerosis with antecedent poliomyelitis. Arch Neurol 37:312–313, 1980.

51. Salazar-Grueso, EF, Grimaldi, LM, Roos, RP, et al: Isoelectric focusing studies of serum and cerebrospinal fluid in patients with antecedent poliomyelitis. Ann Neurol 26:709–713, 1989.

52. Salazar-Grueso, EF and Roos, RP: Viruses and amyotrophic lateral sclerosis. In Smith, RA (ed): Handbook of Amyotrophic Lateral Sclerosis. Marcel Dekker, New York, 1992, pp 453–477.

53. Sharief, MK, Hentges, R, and Ciardi, M: Intrathecal immune response in patients with the post-polio syndrome. N Engl J Med 325:749–755, 1991.

54. Sher, J, Wrzolek, M, and Shmuter, Z: Motor neuron disease associated with AIDS. J Neuropathol Exp Neurol 47:303, 1988.

55. Shibasaki, H, Endo, C, Kuroda, Y, et al: Clinical picture of HTLV-I associated myelopathy. J Neurol Sci 87:15–24, 1988.

56. Simpson, DM and Tagliati, M: Neurologic manifestations of HIV infection. Ann Intern Med 121:769–785, 1994.

57. Smith, RA and Norris, FH, Jr: Treatment of amyotrophic lateral sclerosis with interferon. In Smith, RA (ed): Interferon Treatment of Neurologic Disorders. Marcel Dekker, New York, 1988, pp 265–275.

58. Strebel, PM, Ion-Nedelcu, N, Baughman, A, et al: Intramuscular injections within 30 days of immunization with oral poliovirus vaccine—A risk factor for vaccine-associated paralytic poliomyelitis. N Engl J Med 332:500–506, 1995.

59. Swingler, RJ, Fraser, H, and Warlow, CP: Motor neuron disease and polio in Scotland. J Neurol Neurosurg Psychiatry 55:1116–1120, 1992.

60. Verma, RK, Ziegler, DK, and Kepes, JJ: HIV-related neuromuscular syndrome simulating motor neuron disease. Neurology 40:544–546, 1990.

61. Viola, MV, Lararus, M, Antel, J, et al: Nucleic acid probes in the study of amyotrophic lateral sclerosis. In Rowland, LP (ed): Human Motor Neuron Disease. Raven Press, New York, 1982, pp 312–327.

62. Weiner, LP, Stohlman, SA, and Davis, RL: Attempts to demonstrate virus in amyotrophic lateral sclerosis. Neurology 30:1319–1322, 1980.

63. Westarp, ME, Bartmann, P, Hoff-Jorgensen, R, et al: Amyotrophic lateral sclerosis—Indications of increased antiretroviral seroreactivity without obvious epidemiology [German]. Nervenarzi 64:384–389, 1993.

64. Westarp, ME, Bartmann, P, Rossler, J, et al: Antiretroviral therapy in sporadic adult amyotrophic lateral sclerosis. Neuroreport 4:819–822, 1993.

65. Westarp, ME, Westphal, KP, Clausen, J, et al: Retroviral interference with neuronotrophic signaling in human motor neuron disease? Clin Phys Biochem 10:1–7, 1993.

66. Westarp, ME, Westphal, KP, Kolde, G, et al: Dermal, serological and CSF changes in amyotrophic lateral sclerosis with and without intrathecal beta treatment. Int J Clin Pharmacol Ther Toxicol 30:81–93, 1992.

67. Windebank, AJ, Litchy, WJ, Daube, JR, et al: Late effects of paralytic poliomyelitis in Olmsted County, Minnesota. Neurology 41:501–507, 1991.

68. Younger, DS, Rowland, LP, Latov, N, et al: Lymphoma, motor neuron diseases, and amyotrophic lateral sclerosis. Ann Neurol 29:78–86, 1991.

69. Zilkha, KJ: Discussion on motor neuron disease. Proc R Soc Med 55:1028–1029, 1962.

CHAPTER 15

NEUROTROPHIC FACTORS FOR MOTOR NEURONS

After 90 years of small, incremental advances, the study of neurotrophic factors has become one of the most rapidly evolving and expanding fields in neuroscience today. Ramòn y Cajal[131] introduced the terms *neurotropism* and *neurotrophism* at the turn of this century in his extensive studies of neuronal development and axonal regeneration. Gowers[54] presented a more clinical concept, *abiotrophy,* or lack of vital nutrition, explaining that "neurons depend for vitality on the cell from which the fibers proceed," and suggested that abiotrophy may cause various neurodegenerative disorders.

During the first part of this century, neuronal tissue was transplanted or ablated in extensive experiments in amphibian and chick embryos. These investigations clearly suggested that the survival of developing vertebrate neurons was determined by the fields they innervated.[91,122] A series of the experiments showing that the mouse sarcoma-180 cells secreted a growth-stimulating substance (see a review by Levi-Montalcini[91]) led Levi-Montalcini and Hamburger[92] to discover nerve growth factor (NGF) in 1951. After its discovery, NGF remained the only well-characterized trophic substance for more than 30 years.[91,98] In the late 1970s and early 1980s, many laboratories began to discover trophic agents that were similar to NGF but had specific actions on other types of neurons.[4]

In 1982, Barde and colleagues[15] undertook the painstaking task of isolating a

12.3-kda basic protein called brain-derived neurotrophic factor (BDNF).[90] The relatively slow progress in characterizing novel factors undoubtedly was related to the low abundance of such neurotrophic molecules. In the initial purification of BDNF, for example, only 1 μg of BDNF was obtained from 1.5 kg of porcine brain.[98] Once BDNF was purified, sequenced, and cloned, however, recombinant biotechnology revolutionized access to such rare endogenous proteins and changed research in neurotrophic factors. This progress has led to the recent discovery of several classes of novel neurotrophic factors with biologic specificities that are different from NGF.[87,146,154] In this chapter, we review the neurobiology of neurotrophic factors, characteristics of each neurotrophic factor, their clinical relevance, and the results of recent ALS clinical trials of neurotrophic factors.

NEUROTROPHIC FACTOR NEUROBIOLOGY

Definition of the Neurotrophic Factor

Neurotrophic agents enhance neuronal survival, maintenance, and differentiation but also can increase neurite growth and neurotransmitter production. Prepared on the basis of extensive analysis of NGF, criteria to define "target-derived" neurotrophic factors have been proposed (Table 15–1).[14] As knowledge accumulates, however, exactly what defines a neurotrophic factor changes,

Table 15–1. **SUGGESTED CRITERIA TO DEFINE TARGET-DERIVED NEUROTROPHIC FACTORS**

- Must keep vertebrate neurons alive that would die if the factor were absent
- Must be present in the biologically active form and synthesized in the target tissue of the very neurons that need them for survival
- Must be present in the target tissue in very small amounts and limit the survival of specific neurons
- Must affect the development or maintenance of neurons in vivo

Source: Based on Barde, Y-A: What, if anything, is a neurotrophic factor? Trends Neurosci 11:343–346, 1988.

Table 15–2. **NEUROTROPHIC FACTORS AND RELATED PROTEINS**

Neurotrophin Family
Nerve growth factor
Brain-derived neurotrophic factor*
Neurotrophin 3*
Neurotrophin 4/5*
Neurotrophin 6†

Hemopoietic Cytokine Family
Ciliary neurotrophic factor*
Leukemia inhibitory factor*
Interleukin 6
Oncostatin-M
Cardiotrophin 1*

Other Trophic Factors
Fibroblast growth factor family*
Insulin-like growth factor I*
Glial cell line–derived neurotrophic factor*

*Motor neuron survival-promoting effects are shown.
†A new neurotrophin reported by Götz et al.[53]

so these criteria may be, at best, tentative. The complexity of the individual neurotrophic factors is evident even in their names. For instance, the names of individual factors, such as NGF, ciliary neurotrophic factor (CNTF), BDNF, or fibroblast growth factor (FGF), do not reflect their function, because the names generally are based on how the neurotrophic factor was discovered. Table 15–2 lists the currently known neurotrophic factors.

Mode of Action

Neurotrophic factors were originally described as being target-derived; that is, neurons derive trophic support by means of retrograde transport from the "target" cells they innervate. However, the sources of such neurotrophic support are far more complicated than previously suspected,[88] and retrograde transport appears to be only one of several mechanisms. Figure 15–1 depicts several such mechanisms. Many neurons likely depend on anterograde trophic support, the lack of which may lead to anterograde degeneration. Neurotransmitters may exert such trophic influences on target cells.[120] Nerve-sheathing cells, such as Schwann cells, astrocytes, and oligodendroglia, are now

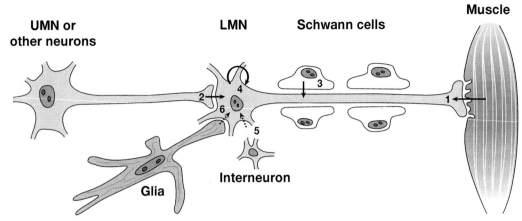

Figure 15–1. Six different mechanisms of trophic support. 1. Traditional target-derived, retrograde mechanism. 2. Anterograde mechanism. 3. Schwann cell to axon. 4. Autocrine loop. 5. Paracrine influence. 6. Neuroglial cell influence.

considered sources of neurotrophic factors. In the event of a nerve lesion, neurotrophic factor production is up-regulated, and regenerating axons receive this trophic message.[30,31,36,87,111] Some neurons not only synthesize neurotrophic factors but also express their cognate receptors, which allow them to respond to their own factors.[1,88] This type of neurotrophic action is called an *autocrine loop*. Such examples are found in motor and sensory neurons that express both a member of the FGF family and the FGF receptor. Several types of neurons both secrete BDNF and express the BDNF receptor, TrkB. Autocrine trophic factors may function to keep neurons alive until the target cell is established, or to maintain survival in the adult once mature contact with the target has been established. Secreted neurotrophic factors also may support adjacent neurons. The survival of cerebellar granular cells, for example, appears to depend on Purkinje cells, which may mediate local action of endogenous trophic substances on granular cells, an effect called *paracrine secretion*.[137] Glial cells synthesize neurotrophic factors that may mediate indirect trophic actions on nearby neurons and cause glial cell proliferation.

Not all neurotrophic proteins may be secreted from cells. For example, CNTF and FGF lack the N-terminal signal sequence required for cellular secretion.[155] These neurotrophic proteins may be secreted by different mechanisms, or they may not be released

from the cell until it is damaged.[155] Such a mechanism may function as a lesion factor.[32]

Overlapping and Pleiotropic Actions and Specificity

The actions of neurotrophic factors on even a single neuron are diverse. A single neurotrophic factor can cause neuronal cell proliferation, differentiation, maintenance, repair, and regeneration.[91,97,146] A single neurotrophic factor can also influence diverse neuron types. For example, BDNF has trophic influences on dorsal root ganglion cells, motor neurons, basal forebrain cholinergic neurons, neurons in the substantia nigra, retinal ganglion cells, and auditory and vestibular neurons. In many cases, classic neurotrophic factors also affect certain nonneuronal cells in different tissues. NGF influences some hemopoietic immune cells[162] and neuronal precursor cells. BDNF, neurotrophin-3 (NT-3), FGF, CNTF, and leukemia-inhibitory factor (LIF) enhance proliferation of neuronal precursor cells. CNTF stimulates glial cell proliferation. Thus, neurotrophic factors have pleiotropic actions.

Different neurotrophic factors have overlapping, yet distinctive, patterns of activity. Dorsal root ganglion cells as a whole respond to many neurotrophic factors. On the other hand, it is suspected that the functions of individual neurotrophic factors are distinct to specific subpopulations of dorsal root ganglion cells. Such overlap is also found in motor neurons that respond to several different neurotrophic factors. Different neurotrophic factors share receptor subunits. For example, at least four distinct neurotrophins share three different receptors, and CNTF shares its receptor complex with members of the hemopoietic cytokines, such as interleukin-6 (IL-6), LIF, and oncostatin-M (OSM).[76,77]

Neurotrophic factors thus must have exceedingly complex overlapping functions. However, a high degree of specificity is achieved by the interaction of different determinants.[88] The access of a particular neuronal type to a specific neurotrophic factor depends on the distinct anatomic location of the neuron, temporal factors, expression of specific receptors, and activation of appropriate intracellular signaling cascades.

NEUROTROPHIC FACTORS THAT AFFECT MOTOR NEURONS

Three features of neurotrophic factors have a major role in the biology of motor (and sensory) neurons: (1) specific survival-promoting activities of the factor in motor neurons in vitro and in vivo;[97,146,155] (2) in vivo accumulation of these factors in motor neurons by receptor-mediated uptake and retrograde axonal transport; and (3) altered expression of these factors in distal nerve segments after nerve injury.[30] Table 15–3 summarizes the biologic characteristics of factors that exert neurotrophic effects on motor neurons. NGF, the prototypic neurotrophic factor, has no discernible neurotrophic effects on motor neurons.[116,122] As of yet, no single molecule has shown a unique specificity for motor neurons.

Furthermore, it has been a surprise to find that if neurotrophic factors (such as BDNF and NT-3) that promote the survival of motor neurons in vitro and in vivo are congenitally absent, the number of motor neurons is not appreciably different from that in normal animals. Null mutation ("knockout") mice, in which both alleles of a specific gene coding for a given neurotrophic factor are disrupted, have no motor neuron loss except for CNTF and glial cell line–derived neurotrophic factor (GDNF) knockout mice.[145] In the CNTF knockout mice, a modest loss of motor neurons, approximately 20% in controls, occurs only in adults, along with a mild loss of muscle strength.[109] In humans, spontaneous null mutation of the CNTF gene oc-

Table 15–3. CHARACTERISTICS OF NEUROTROPHIC FACTORS ASSOCIATED WITH MOTOR NEURONS

| | SURVIVAL-PROMOTING EFFECTS | | | | FACTOR SYNTHESIS | | RECEPTOR PRESENCE | | |
Factors	In Vitro Culture	Naturally Occurring Developmental Death	Facial Axotomy	Sciatic Axotomy	Motor Neuron	Muscle*	Motor Neuron	Muscle	Retrograde Transport
CNTF	Yes	Yes	Yes	Yes	?	No	Yes	Yes	Yes
LIF	Yes	?	?	?	No	Yes	Yes	?	Yes
BDNF	Yes	Yes	Yes	Yes	Yes	Yes	Yes	Yes	Yes
NT-3	Yes	No	Yes (modest)	Yes	Yes	Yes	Yes	Yes	Yes
NT-4/5	Yes	Yes	Yes	Yes	?	Yes	Yes	?	?
bFGF	No	?	?	No	Yes	?	?	?	?
IGF-I	Yes	Yes	Yes	Yes	Yes	Yes	Yes	Yes	No†
GDNF	Yes	Yes	Yes	Yes	?	Yes	Yes	?	Yes

*Peripheral nerves, particularly Schwann cells, probably function as the target organs that synthesize neurotrophic factors, such as CNTF, NGF, LIF, BDNF, and interleukin 6.

†A retrograde signal transduction system may be present.

Abbreviations: BDNF = brain-derived neurotrophic factor; bFGF = basic fibroblast growth factor; CNTF = ciliary neurotrophic factor; GDNF = glial cell line–derived neurotrophic factor; IGF-I = insulin-like growth factor I; LIF = leukemia inhibitory factor; NT-3 = neurotrophin 3; and NT-4/5 = neurotrophin 4/5.

curs in 2.6% of apparently healthy people, suggesting that the lack of CNTF in humans apparently has very little clinical significance.[153] A recent study of mice lacking a CNTF receptor α gene, however, showed a profound motor neuron deficit at birth,[35] implying that the CNTF receptor is crucial for motor neuron development as long as CNTF and other yet-to-be-discovered trophic factors provide signal transduction through this receptor. These findings suggest that the development and growth of motor neurons is apparently maintained by overlapping, possibly redundant motor neuron survival factors.[26,44,79,84,101] GDNF knockout mice which have only recently been produced showed a variable degree of motor neuron loss (none to 30%), depending on the type of motor neurons.[134]

The Hemopoietic Cytokine Family

CILIARY NEUROTROPHIC FACTORS

CNTF was first described as an agent that supports the survival of embryonic chick ciliary ganglion neurons.[4,104] After recombinant CNTF became available, further characterization was possible.[96,107,151] The CNTF molecule is a weakly acidic protein comprised of 200 amino acids. Messenger RNA coding for CNTF is most evident in the brain, spinal cord, and sciatic nerves.[105,160] CNTF is expressed in large quantities, particularly in Schwann cells[142,160] and glial cells,[75] but it is not expressed at detectable levels in skeletal muscle. Two excellent reviews are available on CNTF.[76,139]

Biologic Effects of CNTF

The biologic actions of CNTF have been extensively investigated, and CNTF was initially considered to be the most potent motor neuron neurotrophic factor.[13] In tissue culture studies, only a minute amount of CNTF prolongs survival of motor neurons,[13,138] In in ovo studies, CNTF markedly reduces natural neuronal cell death occurring during development, specifically in spinal motor neurons.[124] When applied to the distal stump of a transected rat neonatal facial nerve, CNTF can rescue 80% of facial motor

neurons that normally degenerate after axotomy.[141] It also prevents postnatal sexually dimorphic motor neuron death that occurs in the spinal bulbocavernosus nucleus of female animals and thus prevents bulbocavernosus muscle degeneration.[47] Although under certain conditions CNTF may induce natural cell death in cultured sympathetic neurons,[82] this effect has not been reported in cultures of developing motor neurons.[56] The effects of CNTF are found in not only developing but also mature animals. Systemically injected CNTF markedly reduces the degree of muscle atrophy after axotomy.[61] CNTF also induces sprouting of motor neuron neurites in adult mouse gluteus muscle when injected subcutaneously over it.[55]

CNTF is unusual in that high levels are found in the cytoplasm of Schwann cells.[49,75,160] The CNTF protein is rapidly depleted from Schwann cells after axotomy and is restored when axon repair begins.[49,143] This behavior contrasts with that of other target-derived neurotrophic factors, whose expression in the distal nerve increases after axotomy. That abundant levels of CNTF are maintained in Schwann cells suggests that CNTF plays a dual role: It maintains differentiated axons, and it functions as a lesion factor that is rapidly released on axotomy to signal injury. Such injury-induced regulation of CNTF occurs not only in the peripheral nerves but also in the brain.[75]

The CNTF Receptor

Although CNTF does not cross the blood-brain barrier, it is transported to spinal cord motor neurons by retrograde axonal transport.[31] Furthermore, it is suspected that binding of CNTF to its receptor induces signal transduction in neurons directly at the axon terminals.[22,73,76,77] The CNTF receptor complex is a heterotrimeric structure consisting of a CNTF receptor α component (CNTFR α), gp-130, and leukemia inhibitory factor receptor β (LIFR β). The CNTFR α component is a CNTF-binding protein that lacks a transmembrane domain but is linked to the plasma membrane by a glycophosphatidylinositol linkage. The gp-130 component is an IL-6 β-subunit (Fig. 15–2). After ligand binding to the receptor α subunit, the two transmembrane β components undergo heterodimerization, which activates tyrosine

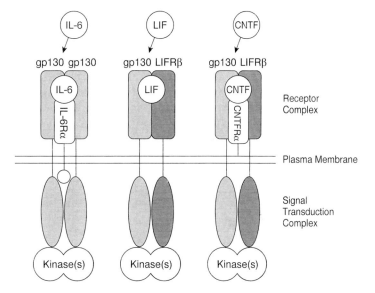

Figure 15–2. The heterotrimeric structure of the ciliary neurotrophic factor (CNTF) receptor, composed of CNTF receptor α (CNTFR α), gp-130 (an interleukin-6 β subunit), and leukemia inhibitory factor receptor β (LIFR β). After binding to the receptor α subunit, the transmembrane β components undergo heterodimerization to activate tyrosine kinase to induce signal transduction. (Adapted from Davis, S and Yancopoulos, G: The molecular biology of the CNTF receptor. Cur Biol 3:22, 1993, with permission).

kinase to induce signal transduction (tyrosine phosphorylation).

Recent studies have uncovered the mechanisms by which CNTF signal transduction occurs. CNTF and other members of the CNTF cytokine family use the Jak-Tyk kinases in their signal transduction after heterodimerization of the β-receptor components.[150] Apparently, different cells express the distinctive Jak-Tyk phosphorylation cascade, providing cell-specific reaction patterns in different cell lines.[150] Jak-Tyk kinases are linked to a CNTF-signaling protein called p91 (a 91-kda protein), and to p91-related proteins. Tyrosine-phosphorylated p91 translocates to the nucleus, where p91 and p91-related proteins bind to a DNA sequence found in the promoters of genes responsive to CNTF.[17] CNTF also activates the immediate-early gene *tis-11* through the CNTF receptor-mediated signaling pathway.[74] Interestingly, one of the DNA sequences resembling the CNTF response element is the superoxide dismutase 1 (*SOD1*) promoter, suggesting that CNTF may enhance the expression of *SOD1*, which is implicated in certain cases of familial ALS.[17] Furthermore, CNTF may trigger signal transduction associated with other neurotrophic factors: When CNTF prevents neuronal degeneration, low-affinity NGF receptor expression is up-regulated.[56]

That components of the CNTF receptor complex are common to LIF and IL-6 receptors suggests that the action of CNTF might be similar to that of a hemopoietic cytokine.[83,126] Thus, CNTF is considered to be a distant member of the hemopoietic cytokines, such as LIF, IL-6, OSM, and granulocyte colony-stimulating factor. However, CNTF is highly specific to the nervous system, because CNTFR α is only expressed at high levels in the brain, spinal cord (including motor neurons), sympathetic ganglia, skeletal muscles, and hepatic cells, thus limiting its physiologic actions to these tissues.[33,38,73,148]

The CNTFR α component that is anchored to the cell membrane may be released from the cell surface, as occurs in other receptors that have a structure similar to CNTFR α.[32,73,78] In fact, IL-6 receptor α is released from the cell surface and activates the biologic effects of IL-6. When skeletal muscle is acutely denervated by motor nerve axotomy, CNTFR α is released from the muscle surface. Released CNTFR α is a soluble protein that reacts with CNTF to form a CNTF-CNTFR α complex. This complex is believed to affect hemopoietic cells expressing both gp-130 and LIFR β, such as macrophages, monocytes, and perhaps fibroblasts (all LIF-responsive cells).[32] Substantial amounts of soluble CNTFR α are found in human cerebrospinal fluid, suggesting a role for soluble CNTFR in the CNS.

Effects of CNTF in Natural Motor Neuron Disease Models

The effects of CNTF have been tested in three different natural motor neuron disease models. Characteristics of each model are discussed in Chapter 17. In the primary motor neuronopathy (pmn) model, CNTF is delivered by intraperitoneally injected mouse tumor D3 cells that have a CNTF genomic DNA construct.[141] The predictable mortality (most affected animals die by 6 to 7 weeks of age), the number of motor neurons in the facial nucleus, the number of phrenic nerve myelinated fibers, and a behavioral test (ability to hang onto a metal bar) are used to measure the effects of CNTF. CNTF treatment markedly delayed mortality, lessened motor dysfunction, and rescued 65% of motor neurons in the degenerating facial nucleus, and significantly increased phrenic nerve fibers.[142]

The second animal model is the progressive motor neuron degeneration (mnd) mouse. The speed of gait and stride length are analyzed. CNTF administration slowed gait abnormalities in this disease model.[60]

The third animal model is the wobbler mouse. CNTF treatment in wobbler mice was analyzed by using several quantitative and semiquantitative measurement techniques, which are described in Chapter 17. Subcutaneous CNTF injections 3 times per week for 4 weeks retarded deterioration of grip strength, running speed, muscle physiology, and other semiquantitative measures of motor function.[114] Denervation-induced muscle atrophy also significantly decreased in wobbler mice treated with CNTF. Electron microscopic examination of the wobbler mouse spinal cord, however, showed no differences in vacuolar degeneration between CNTF-treated mice and controls. This finding suggests that CNTF does not inhibit the process underlying vacuolar degeneration, a pathognomonic finding in the wobbler mouse, but rather delays motor neuron disease progression.[71]

CNTF treatment in all these animal models reduced motor dysfunction, and in the wobbler and pmn models, such effects were substantiated by morphologic evidence. These results in animal models encouraged clinical trials in patients with ALS, but the results were disappointing. Preliminary studies with CNTF treatment in transgenic mice with the human *SOD1* mutation, an animal model of human familial ALS (see Chapter 17), showed no benefit (Ronald M. Lindsay, PhD, Regeneron Pharmaceuticals, personal communication, 1996).

LEUKEMIA INHIBITORY FACTOR

LIF, formerly called cholinergic differentiation factor, is a pleiotropic cytokine with widespread actions, including the stimulation of hepatic acute phase responses, bone resorption, lipid metabolism, megakaryocyte proliferation, myoblast proliferation, and neuronal differentiation.[66] In the CNS, LIF is identified only by highly sensitive polymerase chain reaction techniques, indicating that it is present in very low amounts.[127] In peripheral nerves, Schwann cells are a main source of LIF; released LIF may attract LIF receptor-expressing monocytes and macrophages.[30] These cells may participate in the degradation of degenerating axons and myelin during axonal regeneration. Based on the composite structure of functional LIF and CNTF receptors, it is likely that CNTF-responsive cells will also respond to LIF.[30]

As shown in Table 15–3, LIF has survival-promoting effects in motor neurons in tissue culture.[106] LIF is readily detectable in the distal peripheral nerves and in Schwann cells.[163] It is retrogradely transported to the motor neuron cell body in increasing amounts after axotomy.[30] Although the effects of LIF on natural neuronal death and axotomy are not known, LIF may be a neurotrophic factor for motor neurons.

CARDIOTROPHIN-1

Recently, a novel cytokine, cardiotrophin-1 (CT-1) has been cloned.[127] It induces cardiac myocyte hypertrophy in tissue culture and is a potent pleiotropic cytokine.[23] The amino acid sequence of CT-1 is somewhat similar to that of IL-6, CNTF, LIF, and OSM, and CT-1 shares a common signaling subunit, gp-130, with these cytokines. In neuronal cells, CT-1 induces a cholinergic change in rat sympathetic neurons and promotes the survival of rat dopaminergic and chick ciliary neurons.[127] Prolonged motor neuron survival effects have been observed in tissue culture studies.[129]

The Neurotrophin Family

The prototypic neurotrophic factor, NGF, has no trophic effects on motor neurons in vitro or in vivo.[122] As discussed above, for many years NGF was the only fully characterized neurotrophic factor. However, soon after BDNF was purified, sequenced, and cloned,[90] molecular cloning techniques led to the discovery of NT-3 and NT-4/5 (NT-4 or NT-5), the two other members of what is now known as the *neurotrophin family*.[57,67,72,103] The neurotrophins have at least 50% amino acid sequence homology with each other; each has survival-promoting effects on a specific subpopulation of dorsal root ganglion cells; and each factor is widely distributed in the CNS and peripheral nervous system.[97,163]

The neurotrophins appear to use a dual set of receptors: (1) high-affinity receptors of Trk (pronounced "truck"), a family of receptor tyrosine kinases, which are similar to those used by traditional mitogenic growth factors, FGF[77]; (2) the common low-affinity neurotrophin receptor (LNR), which is expressed in many neurons where Trk receptors are present. The high-affinity Trk receptors are almost exclusively expressed in postmitotic neurons. Ligand-induced dimerization of Trk receptors mediates signaling in responsive neurons.[52,77] There are three different Trk receptors: Trk A, Trk B, and Trk C (Fig. 15–3). Trk A receptor responds primar-

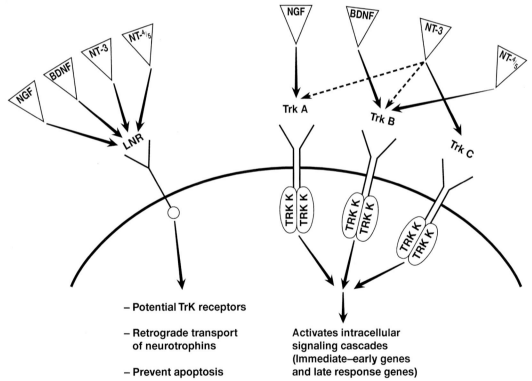

- Potential TrK receptors

- Retrograde transport
  of neurotrophins

- Prevent apoptosis

Activates intracellular
signaling cascades
(Immediate–early genes
and late response genes)

Figure 15–3. Schematic diagram illustrating the high-affinity tyrosine kinase (Trk) receptors, Trk A, Trk B, and Trk C. mRNA for Trk B and Trk C, but not Trk A, are found in developing and adult spinal cord motor neurons. Ligand-induced autophosphorylation and dimerization of the Trk receptors activate cascades of signaling events. The low-affinity neurotrophin receptor (LNR) is in all cells with expressed Trk receptors and responds to all the neurotrophins. This receptor appears to potentiate Trk receptor function and also to have independent neurobiological function. (Adapted from Neuroscience 5, Ip, NP and Yancopoulos, GD: Receptors and signaling pathways of ciliary neurotrophic factor and the neurotrophins, p 250, 1993; with kind permission from Elsevier Science Ltd, The Boulevard, Langford Lane, Kidlington OX5 1GB, UK.)

ily to NGF, and Trk C responds only to NT-3; in comparison, Trk B in vitro responds to BDNF, NT-4/5, and to a lesser extent, NT-3.[147,149] A recent study also indicates that Trk A responds to NT-3.[24] When a ligand activates its Trk receptor, tyrosine kinase activity stimulates the small guanosine triphosphate–binding protein, *ras*. Activated *ras* triggers a cascade of phosphorylation events that ultimately activate immediate-early genes and late-response genes to initiate neural growth and differentiation.[51]

In contrast to high-affinity Trk receptors, the function of LNR remains relatively unclear. A series of recent studies has suggested several important functions of the low-affinity receptor. LNR is a potentially universal potentiator for each Trk, displaying a marked ability to interact functionally with each Trk receptor to potentiate autocrine loops as well as responses to limited amounts of exogenously provided neurotrophins.[59] However, it is unclear whether this receptor acts as a ligand reservoir or as a ligand clearance molecule to control the overall ligand activity. Alternatively, it is unknown whether LNR activates signaling on its own or somehow regulates the Trk signaling capabilities. Another study has suggested that LNR may control apoptosis because unbound LNR induces neural cell death.[130] Further studies suggest that LNR mediates the retrograde axonal transport of neurotrophins, specifically BDNF and NT-4/5, but not NGF.[29]

BRAIN-DERIVED NEUROTROPHIC FACTOR

BDNF is another potent neurotrophic factor for motor neurons (see the review by Lindsay[97]). It is expressed in spinal motor neurons and skeletal muscles, and its Trk B receptor is expressed in adult motor neurons. BDNF may be important as a target-derived neurotrophic factor for motor neurons.[97,155] Levels of BDNF are low in intact peripheral nerves, but after a crush or transection nerve injury, BDNF messenger RNA production increases in muscle tissue and the distal nerve stump, suggesting that BDNF may participate in regeneration.[87,111] BDNF is transported retrogradely from its target field—in the sciatic nerve model, from tran-

sected sciatic nerve to motor neurons and dorsal root sensory neurons.[37,166]

BDNF has potent survival-promoting effects for developing motor neurons in the in ovo,[125] in vitro,[62] and in vivo facial nerve models,[87,140] and as seen in sciatic nerve axotomy studies (see Table 15–3).[94,165,166] It also enhances choline acetyltransferase activity in cultured motor neurons[161] and the activity and maturation of developing neuromuscular synapses in vitro.[102,158] Although the survival-promoting effects of BDNF are seen in motor neurons derived from the spinal cord, BDNF appears to potentiate necrosis in cultured motor neurons derived from cerebral cortex.[86]

The above studies were performed in developing or neonatal animals, and the duration of BDNF treatment was brief, at most several days. Treatment given in a similar setting for a longer period, approximately 3 weeks, does not appear to rescue motor neurons after sciatic nerve axotomy but does rescue sensory neurons.[42] These results raise the possibility that the effects of BDNF in developing motor neurons are transient. However, studies in wobbler mice suggest that this idea is not correct. BDNF treatment beginning at 3 to 4 weeks of age and lasting for 4 weeks slows the disease process in wobbler mice when measurement techniques are used that are identical to those used in CNTF preclinical studies:[70] grip strength and muscle physiology tests showed significant differences between the vehicle and BDNF-treated groups. Slowing of denervation atrophy explains why BDNF-treated mice perform better than vehicle-treated mice. Furthermore, BDNF treatment reduces motor axon loss at the cervical ventral roots.[70] Preliminary studies with BDNF treatment in transgenic mice with the human *SOD1* mutation, however, found no beneficial effects (Ronald M. Lindsay, PhD, Regeneron Pharmaceuticals, personal communication, 1996). Why neither BDNF nor CNTF was beneficial in these transgenic mice requires further clarification.

In adult animals, nerve transection causes the loss of choline acetyltransferase activity in motor neurons and re-expression of the LNR.[48] BDNF treatment after sciatic nerve transection significantly reduces the loss of choline acetyltransferase activity and increases LNR re-expression, suggesting that

BDNF exerts its neurotrophic effects also on adult motor neurons.[48] In adult rats, retrograde cell death induced by ventral root avulsion is prevented by BDNF when given through a subcutaneous pump delivery system. BDNF appears to block nitric oxide synthase expression, which is activated after ventral root avulsion.[119] Therefore, BDNF has some of the most promising therapeutic implications of the motor neuron trophic factors.

NEUROTROPHIN 3

The effect of NT-3 on developing motor neurons are somewhat similar to those of BDNF in in vitro studies,[62,161] in the facial axotomy models,[140] and in sciatic nerve axotomy models.[94] NT-3 is synthesized in Schwann cells and muscles.[41] As with BDNF, NT-3 is transported retrogradely from axotomized nerve to motor and sensory neurons.[37,166] The NT-3 receptor, Trk C, is expressed in motor neurons.[110] Like BDNF, NT-3 promotes the maturation of developing neuromuscular synapses.[102,158]

NT-3 may be unique in that it affects upper motor neurons.[135] NT-3 and, to a lesser degree, NGF (but not BDNF) enhances sprouting of corticospinal tract fibers in response to traumatic axotomy in adult rats, suggesting that at least NT-3 has neurotrophic effects on upper motor neurons. However, regenerated axons do not elongate unless anti–myelin-associated neurite growth-inhibitory proteins are applied to the lesion.[135] These findings support the idea that NT-3 is similar to BDNF in acting as a neurotrophic factor for motor neurons but may also influence upper motor neurons. However, further studies are clearly needed to define the significance of NT-3 in motor neurons.

NEUROTROPHIN 4/5

The effects of NT-4/5 on motor neurons are broadly similar to those of BDNF. In cultured motor neurons, NT-4/5 promotes motor neuron survival[62] and enhances choline acetyltransferase activity.[161] In ovo studies, NT-4/5 reduced naturally occurring cell death, although less so than BDNF.[125] In sciatic nerve transection studies, NT-4/5 treatment rescues only 20% to 30% of motor neurons.[94] Neurotrophic effects of NT-4/5 also occur in adult animals. As seen with BDNF, NT-4/5 treatment attenuates the loss of choline acetyltransferase activity and increases re-expression of the LNR after axotomy.[48] A recent study showed that NT-4/5 is derived from muscle, particularly from type I muscle fibers, and that its synthesis increases with muscle activity.[50] Furthermore, NT-4/5 markedly enhances sprouting of intramuscular terminal axons. Unlike other neurotrophins, such as BDNF and NT-3, which increase after denervation, synthesis of NT-4/5 appears to depend on muscle activity: intact motor neuron innervation is required. Muscle NT-4/5 production is proportional to the intensity of electrical stimulation, suggesting that exercise training may increase nerve sprouting. This raises an intriguing question of whether certain exercise training may benefit patients with ALS.

The Fibroblast Growth Factor Family

FGFs comprise a family of at least nine different proteins that are structurally related as revealed by the 30% to 50% homology of their amino acid sequences. Among them, acidic and basic FGF (aFGF and bFGF) have been of particular interest in neurobiology, because they exist in the adult CNS and support nerve fiber outgrowth and survival of a variety of neurons in vitro.[40] Acidic FGF is present in astrocytes and in a specific group of hippocampal neurons, whereas bFGF is found in other selected sets of neurons, such as the basal forebrain cholinergic neurons, substantia nigra neurons, and motor neurons.

Survival-promoting effects of bFGF on in vitro cultured motor neurons have been extensively studied.[13,62,106] In vivo sciatic nerve axotomy studies failed to reveal that bFGF affects degenerating neurons (see Table 15–3).[94,123] In the adult nervous system, large quantities of aFGF and bFGF are stored in neuron cell bodies. When motor neurons are injured, bFGF is believed to be released to initiate repair that is possibly autocrine in nature. At the same time, injured astrocytes release bFGF, which stimulates astrocyte mitogenesis and perhaps indirectly stimulates motor neuron survival. Basic FGF may be involved only in the initial stages of the repair process, with other neurotrophic factors involved at subsequent stages.[41]

Recent studies have suggested that FGF-5 is a motor neuron trophic factor. It is found in embryonic and adult skeletal muscles and has a hydrophobic N-terminal, as is typical of secreted proteins.[68] FGF-5 may be a target-derived neurotrophic factor, but further studies are required to determine this.

Other Trophic Factors

INSULIN-LIKE GROWTH FACTOR I

Insulin-like growth factors (IGF), peptides structurally related to the insulin precursor (proinsulin), are found in a wide variety of tissues and the circulation. Their key function is thought to be mediation of growth hormone activity. Two genes encode IGF-I and IGF-II; IGF-I is expressed postnatally, whereas IGF-II is expressed abundantly in fetal tissues. Recent studies have shown that IGF-I, independent of growth hormone levels, has growth-promoting actions.[46] Transgenic mice overexpressing IGF-I have increased brain growth and enhanced myelination.[21] In contrast, IGF-I knockout mice have markedly reduced body weight, muscle immaturity, and white matter defects, and most (95%) die during gestation.[159]

IGF-I is expressed in many cells, including motor neurons, glial cells, and skeletal muscles. The IGF-I receptor has an intracellular tyrosine kinase domain, probably sharing its signaling pathways with other neurotrophic factors (see the review by Lewis[93]). The receptor also is expressed in glial cells, motor neurons, and skeletal muscles. The neurotrophic effects of IGF-I have been found in many experimental settings. It has modest survival-promoting effects in cultured motor neurons, attenuates natural cell death,[118] and reduces motor neuron death in neonatal rats after transection of facial[69] and sciatic nerves.[94] One study found that IGF-I enhanced regeneration but not survival of cultured sensory neurons.[45] This study was performed with insulin in the tissue culture medium, however, resulting in minimal survival-promoting effects.[13] A more recent study using insulin-free culture medium showed a markedly enhanced survival-promoting effect.[27]

IGF-I expression is rapidly up-regulated when skeletal muscles are paralyzed by botulinum toxin or denervated.[78] Intramuscular terminal nerve sprouting is triggered by IGF-I administration. This sprouting can be blocked by simultaneous injection of IGF-I receptor protein, suggesting that IGF-I can specifically induce nerve sprouting.[20] In addition, in developing animals, growth-associated protein (GAP) 43 expression is down-regulated in motor neurons during normal elimination of extraneuromuscular synapses.[19] Administration of IGF-I prevents the GAP-43 down-regulation to maintain its production.[19] Furthermore, GAP-43 up-regulation is believed to coincide with increased nerve sprouting in adult animals.[20] Although IGF-I is not retrogradely transported along the motor neurons, signal transduction of IGF-I probably occurs via a retrograde pathway, conveying the second messenger protein G_i from the axon terminal to the neuron cell body.[28,65]

IGF-I may also have direct myotrophic effects.[47] When overexpressed in muscle fibers isolated from neural influence in tissue culture, IGF-I stimulates myofiber differentiation and hypertrophy.[25] This myotrophic effect appears to be sustained by autocrine or paracrine mechanisms, or possibly both, which are stimulated by overexpressed IGF-I in muscle fibers.

Recombinant human IGF-I has been tested in wobbler mice.[58] Daily treatment with IGF-I at 1 mg/kg for 6 weeks significantly increased body weight, grip strength, and muscle fiber diameter compared to control treatment. Motor neuron loss still occurred. The effects of IGF-I also were tested in transgenic mice with the human *SOD1* mutation, but no benefit occurred in this motor neuron disease (Jeffry Vaught, PhD, Cephalon Inc., personal communication, 1996).

GLIAL CELL LINE–DERIVED NEUROTROPHIC FACTOR

GDNF is a distant member of the transforming growth factor β gene superfamily and was originally found to have potent trophic effects on dopaminergic neurons[95] and motor neurons.[63] It is expressed in limb buds, Schwann cells, and cultured embryonic myotubes. It is retrogradely transported to motor neuron perikarya.[167] All these findings suggest that GDNF is a target-derived neurotrophic factor for motor neurons. The structure of GDNF differs from that of the hemopoietic cytokines such as CNTF or LIF, and the neurotrophin family, suggesting that the GDNF receptor is distinct from those of other identified neurotrophic factors. In fact, very recent studies have shown that the GDNF receptor is involved in two components: the one is a nontransmembrane component, called GDNFR α, which resembles CNTFR α in relation to the cell membrane, and the other is a transmembrane component called c-Ret, which is one of the oncogenes and widely distributed among many cells, including renal epithelial cells and enteric neurons.[108,156] GDNF knockout mice are born with no kidneys and markedly deficient enteric neurons. Motor neurons are also deficient, ranging from none to 40% depending on the type of motor neurons.[134]

Impressive survival-promoting effects have been seen in motor neuron tissue culture models,[63,121] in an in ovo model in which GDNF prevents natural neuronal death,[121] and in a facial nerve axotomy model[63,167] (see Table 15–3). In the adult rat, GDNF markedly attenuates the decrease in choline acetyltransferase activity that occurs in motor neurons after nerve transection.[167] Preliminary studies with GDNF in transgenic mice with human mutated *SOD1*, showed no beneficial effects (Qiao Yan, PhD, Amgen Inc., personal communication, 1996). GDNF treatment in pmn mice, administered by means of a polymer capsule containing hamster kidney cells transfected with human GDNF gene, neither prevented motor axon degeneration nor prolonged survival of affected animals, although GDNF slowed motor neuron loss.[133] However, in wobbler motor neuron disease, GDNF has remarkable beneficial effects. Using assessment techniques that are routinely used in one of our laboratories, subcutaneously injected GDNF was tested in the wobbler mouse model. GDNF significantly reduced the rate of motor dysfunction and rescued more than 50% of choline acetyltransferase immunoreactive anterior horn cells and 20% of motor axons at the ventral roots (H. Mitsumoto, unpublished observation, 1996). This result was in contrast to the recent study in pmn mice.

The differences in response to GDNF treatment among the animal models may be derived from different disease processes. All the experimental data suggest that GDNF is one of the most promising neurotrophic factors for the treatment of ALS as well as Parkinson's disease.

COTREATMENT WITH NEUROTROPHIC FACTORS

The combined use of neurotrophic factors may have important therapeutic implications in the future treatment of ALS.[115a] Combination treatment with diverse therapeutic agents has been widely practiced in patients with advanced cancers, resistant infectious diseases, and many other difficult medical diseases.

Cotreatment in Tissue Culture Studies

Motor neuron survival in vitro is enhanced by neurotrophic factors used in combination. In a study with IGF-I, CNTF, and bFGF, any combination was more beneficial than a single factor, but CNTF with bFGF was most effective.[13] Using insulin-free culture medium, the combination of IGF-I and CNTF produced markedly synergistic effects in vitro.[27] However, when up-regulation of choline acetyltransferase activity was measured, the effect of CNTF and LIF together was no better than that of either factor alone, suggesting that combining neurotrophic factors of the same family may not provide superior benefit as compared to combining different classes of neurotrophic factors.[106] In this respect, a combination of CNTF and BDNF or CNTF and NT-4/5 showed remarkable synergy in increasing choline acetyltransferase activity in cultured motor neurons.[161] Other combinations (CNTF and NT-3 or NT-3 and NT-4/5) showed the same additive effects.[161]

Cotreatment in Normal Laboratory Animal Studies

Axonal sprouting at the motor endplate in mouse skeletal muscle is stimulated by CNTF but not bFGF; combining both factors produces markedly synergistic effects.[55] In the sciatic nerve axotomy model, a combination of BDNF and GDNF has a synergistic effect on survival.[157] Recent studies in *Xenopus* nerve-muscle cultures showed that CNTF and BDNF exerted synergistic effects in synaptic development and function.[152]

Cotreatment in Motor Neuron Disease Models

Whereas CNTF or BDNF treatment slows disease progression in wobbler mice,[70,114] CNTF and BNDF cotreatment arrests clinical progression (as determined by semiquantitative paw position and walking pattern abnormalities).[115] Although some animals lose grip strength, in others it actually increases above the baseline with combination treatment, so that the mean effect is one of no deterioration. The effect on running speed was slightly more than additive with CNTF and BDNF cotreatment. Histometric analyses of muscle histology and ventral root motor myelinated fibers also showed that the protection from denervation and motor axon loss distinctly improved more with cotreatment than with single-factor treatment.[70,71] The results of CNTF and BDNF cotreatment suggest that the effect is synergistic compared to that attained with either CNTF or BDNF alone (Fig. 15–4).

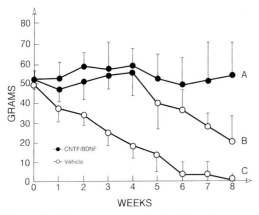

Figure 15–4. Mean grip strength of wobbler mice treated with ciliary neurotrophic factor (CNTF) and brain-derived neurotrophic factor (BDNF) (CNTF/BDNF 8 weeks, line A), CNTF/BDNF (4 weeks) followed by vehicle (4 weeks) (line B), or vehicle only (8 weeks) (line C). Vertical bars indicate standard deviations.

A recent preliminary study indicated that long-term CNTF and BDNF cotreatment (8 weeks in contrast to the previously discussed 4-week studies; see also Chapter 17) can sustain grip strength and running speed as long as the cotreatment is continued, indicating that the synergy of these two factors is not transient. However, in this study more cotreated wobbler mice than vehicle-treated animals died at the later stages of the treatment period because of presumed toxic effects.[85]

NEUROTROPHIC FACTOR DEFICIT IN ALS

Appel[11] proposed in 1981 that neurodegenerative disorders, such as ALS, Parkinson's disease, and Alzheimer's disease, may result from a lack of specific trophic hormone in target neurons. Such a hypothesis is not easily tested. Survival-promoting effects on cultured motor neurons of extracts from skeletal muscles, autopsied spinal cord, or sera obtained from patients with ALS do not differ from those from controls.[39] The low-affinity NGF receptor found in ventral root and peripheral nerve Schwann cells is not different between ALS patients and controls.[81] The re-expression of high- and low-affinity NGF receptors is not increased in the motor neurons of autopsied spinal cord from patients with ALS.[2,12,81] Immunoreactive IGF-I, aFGF, and bFGF are all present in motor neurons and axons in ALS spinal cord at autopsy. IGF-I immunoreactivity is present in glial cells and Schwann cells, and aFGF immunoreactivity is found in oligodendroglia. IGF-I and aFGF, but not bFGF, are expressed in muscles. Control and ALS tissue do not differ, indicating that a deficit of these neurotrophic factors is unlikely in ALS etiology.[80]

When IGF-I binding and IGF-I receptors are studied in spinal cord tissue from patients with ALS, IGF-I binding is not different from healthy controls, but IGF-receptor immunoreactivity significantly increases in the cervical and sacral spinal cord from patients with ALS.[3] Although an IGF-I deficiency is unlikely to cause ALS, increased levels of IGF-I receptor expression in ALS suggests that a regenerative and repair process, such as increased terminal sprouting, does increase in motor neurons in ALS.[3] Serum IGF-I levels in patients with ALS are the same as those of controls.[18] Clinical trials with recombinant human growth hormone in patients with ALS found higher levels of serum IGF-I levels in patients treated with growth hormone but showed no clinical benefits, suggesting that the elevation of serum IGF-I levels itself may not achieve clinical benefits in ALS patients.[144]

Recently, Anand and colleagues[10] may have found the first evidence of a neurotrophic factor abnormality in ALS. In autopsy brain and spinal cord from patients with ALS and matched healthy controls, CNTF was markedly decreased in the ventral horn in the ALS spinal cord but not in the motor cortex. In contrast, NGF levels were decreased in ALS motor cortex and increased in the lateral column of the spinal cord. These intriguing findings cannot be readily explained. Recently Yamamoto and colleagues[164] measured GDNF messenger RNA in the spinal cord and skeletal muscles in ALS. Increased levels of GDNF messenger RNA were found in the spinal cord (where pathology was severe), whereas the level was reduced in the muscles. An explanation is not apparent at this point. The pathogenic significance of various neurotrophic factors in patients with ALS requires further investigation.

CLINICAL TRIALS WITH NEUROTROPHIC FACTORS

Molecular biotechnology has made recombinant human neurotrophic factors available in large quantities, and thus it is now possible to test the therapeutic potential of pharmacologic doses of neurotrophic proteins in ALS and other neurologic disorders. At the early stages of clinical application of neurotrophic factors, undoubtedly unforeseen problems will have to be overcome.[132] Research in neurotrophic factors has been moving rapidly from the laboratory to clinical trials.[99,100]

Ciliary Neurotrophic Factor

The clinical effects of CNTF have been investigated by two independent research teams.[6,113] In the phase I and II studies, the ALS CNTF Treatment Study (ACTS) group[7] found that doses of 30 μg/kg recombinant human CNTF increased plasma CNTF levels above the concentrations that maximally potentiate motor neuron survival in vivo. This study showed that subcutaneous injection of CNTF produced a prolonged terminal disposition phase, the so-called β phase, which has more practical importance for clinical effects than the rapid-clearance α phase, because drug levels are sustained in the serum.[9,22,38] The dosage was associated with activation of the acute-phase response, suggesting that CNTF produces biologic systemic responses.[8] The phase III studies involved 730 patients who were randomly assigned to one of three groups (30 μg/kg, 15 μg/kg, and placebo) and received subcutaneous injections 3 times a week.[6] The specifics of these clinical trials, including primary and secondary outcomes, are summarized in Chapter 20, Table 20–13.

Neither the slopes of megascore (see Chapter 20) of maximal voluntary isometric muscle contraction (MVIC) (the primary outcome) (Fig. 15–5) nor those of most secondary outcomes differed in any treatment groups. Patients in the CNTF-treated groups rapidly lost strength over the first 2 to 3 months and then at a much slower rate (see Fig. 15–5A). Body weight loss was significant in CNTF-treated patients, with an abrupt reduction in the first 2 months of the study (Fig. 15–5B). Commonly reported adverse events included cough, asthenia, nausea, anorexia, stomatitis, injection site reactions, and fever. Among these adverse effects, the mechanisms of intractable cough and dose-related frequency of stomatitis remain unclear. Other side effects were most likely caused by a systemic cytokine reaction induced by CNTF.[38,43,64,136] Despite these side effects, however, survival was similar among all treatment groups. On the other hand, the dropout rate was higher in the high-dose patient group (26%) than in the low-dose and placebo groups (both approximately 10%). Anti-CNTF antibodies, which were associated with an increased capacity for neutralizing CNTF in an in vitro test system, were detected in more than 60% of patients receiving the factor. Antibody production coincided with a lessening in frequency and severity of CNTF side effects, suggesting that the anti-

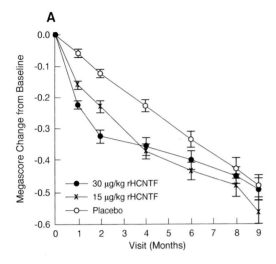

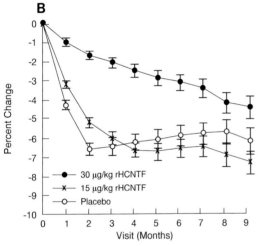

Figure 15–5. Change from baseline in megascore of maximal voluntary isometric contraction (MVIC) (Plate A) and percent change from baseline in body weight (Plate B) in the ALS ciliary neurotrophic factor treatment studies (ACTS). Muscle strength deteriorated rapidly in CNTF-treated patients, more prominently in patients with the higher dose than those with the lower dose (Plate A). Weight reduction was also marked in patients treated with CNTF, although the weight reduction slowly recovered (Plate B). Vertical lines represent mean ± standard errors. (Modified from Neurology Vol. 46, pages 1247 and 1248, 1996, by permission of Little, Brown and Company, Inc.).

bodies may have played a role not only in reducing adverse effects but also in the therapeutic effects of CNTF.[6]

Another study used smaller dosages of CNTF (0.5, 2, and 5 μg/kg) and a daily injection schedule.[113] The study characteristics are summarized in Chapter 20, Table

20–13. The dosages were determined based on findings in preliminary studies.[112] The primary outcomes, including the MVIC megascore, changed from entry to the end of the study; the mean of arm, combined leg and forced vital capacity (FVC) scores, as well as the secondary outcomes, such as arm megascore, leg megascore, FVC, and sickness index profile (see Chapter 20), showed no benefit in any CNTF-treated groups. The overall frequency of adverse events was less than that found in the ACTS CNTF study, and the quality of adverse events was similar between the two. The dropout rate was highest (27%) among the highest-dose group. The death rate did not differ during the study period among the groups, but it increased 1 month after the end of the study in patients who received the highest CNTF dose. The reasons for such results are unclear, but they may be the result of cumulative toxic effects of CNTF or withdrawal effects.

Systemic injection may be a difficult method to use because of unexpected adverse reactions. Two other approaches to deliver CNTF into the CNS have been tested. Because CNTF does not cross the blood-brain barrier and systemic injection causes cytokine reactions, direct infusion into the intrathecal space using an intrathecal pump has been explored in a small number of patients. Some patients developed modest cytokine-related adverse effects (Dr J. Cedarbaum, personal communication, 1995). Another approach is to deliver CNTF using hamster kidney cells transfected with the human CNTF gene in a special capsule attached to a tether and implanted directly into the intrathecal space. Preliminary results of the phase I studies with this encapsulated transfected cell therapy have been reported.[5] Controlling the CSF concentration of CNTF may be difficult with this technique. However, these new approaches have a great potential for delivering neurotrophic factors in patients with ALS.

Insulin-Like Growth Factor I

Phase III studies with IGF-I have been performed in the United States and Europe. The characteristics of the American study are summarized in Chapter 20, Table 20–13. The patients were randomized into three dosage groups (0.05 mg/kg, 0.1 mg/kg, placebo) and received daily subcutaneous drug injections for 9 months. The IGF-I was generally well tolerated and caused no major adverse events. Injection-site reaction was the most common adverse reaction. The Appel ALS score (see Chapter 20) declined at a rate of 4.2 points per month in patients with placebo, 3.7 points per month with the low dose, and 3.3 points per month with high dose. The psychologic domain of the sickness impact profile quality of life assessment (see Chapter 20) also showed significantly better results in patients treated with IGF-I.[89,117] The results from the European studies were not robust but were supportive of the American studies (Discussed by Robert Miller, MD, American Academy of Neurology, San Francisco, April 1996). In June 1996, the Food and Drug Administration approved IGF-I as a treatment investigational new drug (IND; or "early access" IND) to test IGF-I.

Brain-Derived Neurotrophic Factor

Randomized, placebo-controlled, double-blind-dose-escalating phase I and phase II clinical trials with BDNF have been completed. These studies involved 283 patients (six doses were tested among 224 patients treated with BDNF; 59 received placebo).[16] BDNF was generally well tolerated; BDNF-treated patients experienced minor gastrointestinal symptoms and injection-site reactions more frequently than placebo patients. At the completion of the 6-month study, loss of respiratory function as measured by the percent predicted forced vital capacity significantly slowed in BDNF-treated patients, compared with those receiving placebo. Similarly, BDNF-treated patients experienced a slower decline in walking speed than did placebo patients. The BDNF-treated patients also showed a trend toward improved survival after 9 months of therapy.[16] Based on these encouraging results, phase III studies involving more than 1,000 patients in 38 centers in North America were started in August 1995 and completed in September 1996. Despite the earlier promising results, the phase III study turned out to be negative.

SUMMARY

Only recently have the full importance and clinical potential of neurotrophic factors begun to be realized. At least 12 neurotrophic factors and related proteins are now well characterized. Neurotrophic factors are typically target derived and transported to the neuronal cell body by retrograde axonal transport, although other mechanisms also exist. Although neurotrophic factors have extensive overlap and redundancy in their distribution and activity, they are believed to achieve high specificity through a precise combination of factors, such as the temporal and neuroanatomic distribution of neurotrophic factors and their receptors, alteration of receptor characteristics, and diverse intracellular signaling pathways.

Several neurotrophic factors support motor neuron survival, but no single factor is absolutely essential. In most cases, mice genetically engineered to develop without a certain factor (null mutation) have normal motor neurons, again suggesting that the trophic factor support overlaps extensively. Ciliary neurotrophic factor was one of the first molecules identified that promoted motor neuron survival in tissue cultures, embryonic motor neurons, axotomy models, and animal models of motor neuron disease. This factor is a hemopoietic cytokine. Therefore, overlapping actions between ciliary neurotrophic factor and related cytokine, such as leukemia inhibitory factor and interleukin 6, may trigger cytokine reactions.

Except nerve growth factor, all members of the neurotrophin family promote motor neuron survival. BDNF has been extensively studied for its motor neuron trophic effects. NT-3 and NT-4/5 have similar survival-promoting effects, but NT-3 appears to be unique in enhancing axonal regeneration of upper motor neurons, and NT-4/5 depends on muscle activity for its expression. Therefore, these neurotrophins, some of which share the same receptor, may exert different effects on different motor neurons.

Three factors of the FGF family influence motor neurons. IGF-I has also motor neuron survival-promoting effects. This factor may promote axonal regeneration and exerts direct trophic effects on skeletal muscles.

GDNF appears to strongly promote motor neuron survival.

Neurotrophic factor cotreatment, particularly when the factors belong to different families, produces additive or synergistic effects in cultured motor neurons and in animal models of motor neuron disease. Studies of such combinations may have important therapeutic implications.

Ciliary neurotrophic factor is the only factor that has been found to be abnormal in the ventral horn of ALS spinal cords. Whether such findings indicate that abnormal neurotrophic factors are closely associated with the ALS disease process or whether other neurotrophic factors may cause ALS remain unanswered. Regardless, neurotrophic factor research in ALS has moved rapidly from the laboratory to clinical trials. Ciliary neurotrophic factor was the first factor clinically investigated in patients with ALS. Unfortunately, two independent clinical trials, one using lower dosages and the other using higher dosages, showed no clinical benefits, primarily because of adverse reactions. Clinical trials with IGF-I have been promising, and this factor now has the treatment IND status. Phase I and II clinical trials with BDNF also showed promise in slowing the deterioration of pulmonary function. The results of the phase III clinical trial with BDNF become available in the spring of 1997.

REFERENCES

1. Acheson, A, Conover, JC, Fandi, JP, et al: A BDNF autocrine loop in adult sensory neurons prevents cell death. Nature 374:450–453, 1995.
2. Adem, A, Ekblom, J, and Gillberg, PG: Growth factor receptors in amyotrophic lateral sclerosis. Mol Neurobiol 9:225–231, 1994.
3. Adem, A, Ekblom, J, Gillberg, PG, et al: Insulin-like growth factor-I receptors in human spinal cord: Changes in amyotrophic lateral sclerosis. J Neural Transm Gen Sect 97:73–84, 1994.
4. Adler, R, Landa, KB, Manthorpe, M, et al: Cholinergic neuronotrophic factors: Intraocular distribution of trophic activity for ciliary neurons. Science 204:1434–1436, 1979.
5. Aebischer, P, Déglon, N, Heyd, B, et al: A gene therapy approach for the treatment of amyotrophic lateral sclerosis. Soc Neurosci Abstr 21:1563, 1995.
6. ALS CNTF Treatment Study (ACTS) Study Group: A double-blind placebo-controlled clinical trial of subcutaneous recombinant human ciliary neuro-trophic factor (rHCNTF) in amyotrophic lateral sclerosis. Neurology 46:1244–1249, 1996.
7. ALS CNTF Treatment Study Group: Recombinant human ciliary neurotrophic factor (rHCNTF) in amyotrophic lateral sclerosis (ALS) patients: Phase I-II safety, tolerability, and pharmacokinetic studies [abstract]. Neurology 43:A416, 1993.
8. ALS CNTF Treatment Study (ACTS) Phase I-II Study Group: The pharmacokinetics of subcutaneously administered recombinant human ciliary neurotrophic factor (rHCNTF) in patients with amyotrophic lateral sclerosis: Relationship to parameters of the acute phase response. Clin Neuropharmacol 18:500–514, 1995.
9. ALS CNTF Treatment Study (ACTS) Phase I-II Study Group: A phase I study of recombinant human ciliary neurotrophic factor (rHCNTF) in patients with amyotrophic lateral sclerosis. Clin Neuropharmacol 18:515–532, 1995.
10. Anand, P, Parrett, A, Martin, J, et al: Regional changes in ciliary neurotrophic factor and nerve growth factor levels in the post mortem spinal cord and cerebral cortex from patients with motor disease. Nature Med 1:168–178, 1995.
11. Appel, SH: A unifying hypothesis for the cause of amyotrophic lateral sclerosis, parkinsonism, and Alzheimer disease. Ann Neurol 10:499–505, 1981.
12. Aquilonius, S-M, Askmark, H, Ebendal, T, et al: No re-expression of high-affinity nerve growth factor binding sites in spinal motor neurons in amyotrophic lateral sclerosis. Eur Neurol 32:216–218, 1992.
13. Arakawa, Y, Sendtner, M, and Thoenen, H: Survival effect of ciliary neurotrophic factor (CNTF) on chick embryonic motoneurons in culture: Comparison with other neurotrophic factors and cytokines. J Neurosci 10:3507–3515, 1990.
14. Barde, Y-A: What, if anything, is a neurotrophic factor? Trends Neurosci 11:343–346, 1988.
15. Barde, Y-A, Edgar, D, and Thoenen, H: Purification of a new neurotrophic factor from mammalian brain. EMBO J 1:549–553, 1982.
16. BDNF Study Group: Recombinant methionyl human brain-derived neurotrophic factor (r-met HuBDNF) in the treatment of patients with amyotrophic lateral sclerosis. Ann Neurol (in press).
17. Bonni, A, Frank, DA, Schindler, C, et al: Characterization of a pathway for ciliary neurotrophic factor signaling to the nucleus. Science 262:1575–1579, 1993.
18. Braunstein, GD and Reviczky, AL: Serum insulin-like growth factor-I levels in amyotrophic lateral sclerosis. J Neurol Neurosurg Psychiatry 50:792–794, 1987.
19. Caroni, P and Becker, M: The downregulation of growth-associated proteins in motoneurons at the onset of synapse elimination is controlled by muscle activity and IGF-I. J Neurosci 12:3849–3861, 1992.
20. Caroni, P, Schneider, C, Kiefer, MC, et al: Role of muscle insulin-like growth factors in nerve sprouting: Suppression of terminal sprouting in paralyzed muscle by IGF-binding protein 4. J Cell Biol 125:893–902, 1994.
21. Carson, MJ, Behringer, RR, Brinster, RL, et al: Insulin-like growth factor-I increases brain growth

and central nervous system myelination in transgenic mice. Neuron 10:729–740, 1993.

22. Cedarbaum, JM, DiStefano, PS, Lakings, DB, et al: Pharmacokinetics and pharmacodynamics of rHCNTF in rodents. Ann Neurol 39:552–553, 1996.

23. Cheng, G, Pennica, D, and Patterson, PH: Cardiotrophin-1 induces the same neuropeptides in sympathetic neurons as the neuropoietic cytokines [abstract]. Soc Neurosci Abstr 21:1544, 1995.

24. Clary, DO and Reichardt, LF: An alternative spliced form of the nerve growth factor receptor Trk A confers an enhanced response to neurotrophin 3. Proc Nat Acad Sci USA 91:11133–11137, 1994.

25. Coleman, ME, DeMayo, F, Yin, KC, et al: Myogenic vector expression of insulin-like growth factor I stimulates muscle cell differentiation and myofiber hypertrophy in transgenic mice. J Biol Chem 270:12109–12116, 1995.

26. Conover, JC, Erickson, JT, Katz, DM, et al: Neuronal deficits, not involving motor neurons, in mice lacking BDNF and/or NT4. Nature 375:235–238, 1995.

27. Costa, APD, Wang, S, Prevette, DM, et al: Insulin attenuates the survival effects of IGF-I on chick motoneurons in vitro [abstract]. Soc Neurosci Abstr 21:1548, 1995.

28. Crouch, MF and Hendry, IA: Growth factor second messenger systems: Oncogenes and the heterotrimeric GTP-binding protein connection. Med Res Rev 13:105–123, 1993.

29. Curtis, R, Adryan, KM, Stark, JL, et al: Differential role of the low affinity neurotrophic receptor (p75) in retrograde axonal transport of the neurotrophins. Neuron 14:1201–1211, 1995.

30. Curtis, R, Scherer, SS, Somogyi, R, et al: Retrograde axonal transport of LIF is increased by peripheral nerve injury: Correlation with increased LIF expression in distal nerve. Neuron 12:191–204, 1994.

31. Curtis, R, Adryan, KM, Zhu, Y, et al: Retrograde axonal transport of ciliary neurotrophic factor is increased by peripheral nerve injury. Nature 365:253–255, 1993.

32. Davis, S, Aldrich, TH, Ip, NY, et al: Released form of CNTF receptor α component as a soluble mediator of CNTF responses. Science 259:1736–1739, 1993.

33. Davis, S, Aldrich, TH, Valenzuela, DM, et al: The receptor for ciliary neurotrophic factors. Science 253:59–63, 1991.

34. Davis, S and Yancopoulos, G: The molecular biology of the CNTF receptor. Cur Biol 3:20–24, 1993.

35. DeChira, TM, Vejsada, R, Poueymirou, WT, et al: Mice lacking the CNTF receptor, unlike mice lacking CNTF, exhibit profound motor neuron deficits at birth. Cell 83:313–322, 1995.

36. Diamond, J, Foerster, A, Holmes, A, et al: Sensory nerves in adult rats regenerate and restore sensory function to the skin independently of endogenous NGF. J Neurosci 12:1467–1476, 1992.

37. DiStefano, PS, Friedman, B, Radziejewski, C, et al: The neurotrophins, BDNF, NT-3, and NGF display distinct patterns of retrograde axonal transport in peripheral and central neurons. Neuron 8:983–993, 1992.

38. Dittrick, F, Thoenen, H, and Sendtner, M: Ciliary

39. Ebendal, T, Askmark, H, and Aquilonius, S-M: Screening for neurotrophic disturbances in amyotrophic lateral sclerosis. Acta Neurol Scand 79:188–193, 1989.

40. Eckenstein, FP, Andersson, C, Kuzis, K, et al: Distribution of acidic and basic fibroblast growth factors in the mature, injured, and developing rat nervous system. Prog Brain Res 103:55–64, 1994.

41. Ernfors, P, Merlio, JP, and Perssön, H: Cells expressing mRNA for neurotrophins and their receptors during embryonic rat development. Eur J Neurosci 4:1140–1158, 1992.

42. Ericksson, NP, Lindsay, RM, and Aldskogius, H: BDNF and NT-3 rescue sensory but not motoneurones following axotomy in the neonate. NeuroReport 5:1445–1448, 1994.

43. Fantuzzi, G, Benigni, F, Sironi, M, et al: Ciliary neurotrophic factor (CNTF) induces serum amyloid A, hypoglycaemia and anorexia, and potentiates IL-1 induced corticosterone and IL-6 production in mice. Cytokine 7:150–156, 1995.

44. Fariñas, I, Jones, KR, Backus, C, et al: Severe sensory and sympathetic deficits in mice lacking neurotrophin-3. Nature 369:658–661, 1994.

45. Fernyhough, P, Willars, GB, Lindsay, RM, et al: Insulin and insulin-like growth factor I enhance regeneration in cultured adult rat sensory neurons. Brain Res 607:117–124, 1993.

46. Florini, JR, Ewton, DZ, and Magri, KA. Hormones, growth factors, and myogenic differentiation. Annu Rev Physiol 53:201–216, 1991.

47. Forger, NG, Roberts, SL, Wong, V, et al: Ciliary neurotrophic factor maintains motor neurons and their target muscles in developing rats. J Neurosci 13:4720–4726, 1993.

48. Friedman, B, Kleinfeld, D, Ip, NY, et al: BDNF and NT-4/5 exert neurotrophic influences on injured adult spinal motor neurons. J Neurosci 15:1044–1056, 1995.

49. Friedman, B, Scherer, SS, Rudge, JS, et al: Regulation of ciliary neurotrophic factor expression in myelin-related Schwann cells in vivo. Neuron 9:295–305, 1992.

50. Funakoshi, H, Belluardo, N, Arenas, E, et al: Muscle-derived neurotrophin-4 as an activity-dependent trophic signal for adult motor neurons. Science 268:1495–1499, 1995.

51. Ginty, DD, Bonni, A, and Greenberg, ME: Nerve growth factor activates a Ras-dependent protein kinase that stimulates c-fos transcription via phosphorylation of CREB. Cell 77:713–725, 1994.

52. Glass, DJ and Yancopoulos, GD: The neurotrophins and their receptors. Trends Cell Biol 3:262–268, 1993.

53. Götz, R, Köster, R, Winkler, C, et al: Neurotrophin-6 is a new member of the nerve growth factor family. Nature 372:266–269, 1994.

54. Gowers, WR: A lecture on abiotrophy. Lancet 1:1003–1007, 1902.

55. Gurney, ME, Yamamoto, H, and Kwon, Y: Induction of motor neuron sprouting in vivo by ciliary neurotrophic factor and basic fibroblast growth factor. J Neurosci 12:3241–3247, 1992.

56. Hagg, T, Quon, D, Higaki, J, et al: Ciliary neurotrophic factor prevents neuronal degeneration and promotes low-affinity NGF receptor expression in the adult rat CNS. Neuron 8:145–158, 1992.

57. Hallböök, F, Ibáñez, CF, and Persson, H: Evolutionary studies of the nerve growth factor family reveal a novel member abundantly expressed in *Xenopus* ovary. Neuron 6:845–858, 1991.

58. Hantai, D, Akaaboune, M, Lagord, C, et al: Beneficial effects of insulin-like growth factor-I on wobbler mouse motoneuron disease. J Neurol Sci 129:122–126, 1995.

59. Hantzopoulos, PA, Suri, C, Glass, DJ, et al: The low affinity NGF receptor can collaborate with each of the Trks to potentiate functional responses to the neurotrophins. Neuron 13:187–201, 1994.

60. Helgren, ME, Friedman, B, Kennedy, M, et al: Ciliary neurotrophic factor (CNTF) delays motor impairments in the Mnd mouse, a genetic model for motor neuron disease [abstract]. Soc Neurosci Abstr 18:618, 1992.

61. Helgren, ME, Squinto, SP, Davis, HL, et al: Trophic effect of ciliary neurotrophic factor on denervated skeletal muscle. Cell 76:1–20, 1994.

62. Henderson, CE, Camu, W, Mettling, C, et al: Neurotrophins promote motor neuron survival and are present in embryonic limb bud. Nature 363:266–270, 1993.

63. Henderson, CE, Phillips, HS, Pollock, RA, et al: GDNF: A potent survival factor for motoneurons present in peripheral nerve and muscle. Science 266:1062–1063, 1994.

64. Henderson, JT, Seniuk, NA, Richardson, PM, et al: Systemic administration of ciliary neurotrophic factor induced cachexia in rodents. J Clinical Invest 93:2632–2638, 1994.

65. Hendry, IA and Crouch, MF: Retrograde axonal transport of the GTP-binding protein-G_{ia}: A potential neurotrophic intra-axonal messenger. Neurosci Lett 133:29–32, 1991.

66. Hilton, DJ and Gough, NM: Leukemia inhibitory factor: A biological perspective. J Cell Biochem 46:21–26, 1991.

67. Hohn, A, Leibrock, J, Bailey, K, et al: Identification and characterization of a novel member of the nerve growth factor/brain-derived neurotrophic factor family. Nature 344:339–341, 1990.

68. Hughes, RA, Sendtner, M, Goldfarb, M, et al: Evidence that fibroblast growth factor 5 is a major muscle-derived survival factor for cultured spinal motoneurons. Neuron 10:369–377, 1993.

69. Hughes, RA, Sendtner, M, and Thoenen, H: Members of several gene families influence survival of rat motoneurons *in vitro* and *in vivo*. J Neurosci Res 36:663–671, 1993.

70. Ikeda, K, Klinkosz, B, Greene, T, et al: Effects of brain-derived neurotrophic factor (BDNF) on motor dysfunction in wobbler mouse motor neuron disease. Ann Neurol 37:505–511, 1995.

71. Ikeda, K, Wong, V, Holmlund, TH, et al: Histometric effects of ciliary neurotrophic factor in wobbler mouse motor neuron disease. Ann Neurol 37:47–54, 1995.

72. Ip, NY, Ibanez, CF, Nye, SH, et al: Mammalian neurotrophin-4: Structure, chromosomal localization, tissue distribution, and receptor specificity. Proc Nat Acad Sci 89:3060–3064, 1992.

73. Ip, NY, McClain, J, Barrezueta, NX, et al: The alpha component of the CNTF receptor is required for signaling and defines potential CNTF targets in the adult and during development. Neuron 10:89–102, 1993.

74. Ip, NY, Nye, SH, Boulton, TG, et al: CNTF and LIF act on neuronal cells via shared signaling pathways that involve the IL-6 signal transducing receptor component gp 130. Cell 69:1121–1132, 1992.

75. Ip, NY, Wiegand, SJ, Morse, J, et al: Injury-induced regulation of ciliary neurotrophic factor mRNA in the adult rat brain. Eur J Neurosci 5:25–33, 1993.

76. Ip, NY and Yancopoulos, GD: Ciliary neurotrophic factor and its receptor complex. Prog Growth Factor Res 4:139–155, 1992.

77. Ip, NY and Yancopoulos, GD: Receptors and signaling pathways of ciliary neurotrophic factor and the neurotrophins. Neuroscience 5:249–257, 1993.

78. Ishii, DN, Glazner, GW, and Whalen, LR: Regulation of peripheral nerve regeneration by insulin-like growth factor. Ann NY Acad Sci 692:172–183, 1993.

79. Jones, KR, Fariñas, I, Backus, C, et al: Targeted disruption of the BDNF gene perturbs brain and sensory neuron development but not motor neuron development. Cell 76:989–999, 1994.

80. Kerkhoff, H, Hassan, SM, Troost, D, et al: Insulin-like and fibroblast growth factors in spinal cords, nerve roots and skeletal muscle of human controls and patients with amyotrophic lateral sclerosis. Acta Neuropathol 87:411–421, 1994.

81. Kerkhoff, H, Jennekens, FGI, Troost, D, et al: Nerve growth factor receptor immunostaining in the spinal cord and peripheral nerves in amyotrophic lateral sclerosis. Acta Neuropathol 81:649–656, 1991.

82. Kessler, JA, Ludlan, WH, Freidin, MM, et al: Cytokine-induced programmed death of cultured sympathetic neurons. Neuron 11:1123–1132, 1993.

83. Kishimoto, T, Akira, S, and Taga, T: Interleukin-6 and its receptor: A paradigm for cytokines. Science 258:593–596, 1992.

84. Klein, R, Smeyne, RJ, Wurst, W, et al: Targeted disruption of trkB neurotrophin receptor gene results in nervous system lesions and neonatal death. Cell 75:113–122, 1993.

85. Klinkosz, B, Mitsumoto, H, Cedarbaum, JM, et al: The effects of prolonged co-administration of CNTF and BDNF in wobbler mice [abstract]. Soc Neurosci Abstr 21:1005, 1995.

86. Koh, JY, Gwag, BJ, Lobner, D, et al: Potentiated necrosis of cultured cortical neurons by neurotrophins. Science 268:573–575, 1995.

87. Koliatsos, VE, Clatterbuck, RE, Winslow, JW, et al: Evidence that brain-derived neurotrophic factor is a trophic factor for motor neurons in vivo. Neuron 10:359–367, 1993.

88. Korsching, S: The neurotrophic factor concept: A reexamination. J Neurosci 13:2739–2748, 1993.

89. Lange, DJ: Clinical trials in patients with amyotrophic lateral sclerosis: Experience and myotrophin. In Armon, C and Rowland, LP (co-directors): Critical Issues in ALS Trials: Update, Consensus and Controversy (CME Course 171). American Academy of Neurology, Minneapolis, 1995, pp 27–28.

90. Leibrock, J, Lottspeich, F, Hohn, A, et al: Molecu-

lar cloning and expression of brain-derived neurotrophic factor. Nature 341:149–152, 1989.

91. Levi-Montalcini, R: The nerve growth factor 35 years later. Science 237:1154–1162, 1987.

92. Levi-Montalcini, R and Hamburger, V: Selective growth stimulating effects of sarcoma on the sensory and sympathetic system of the chick embryo. J Exp Zool 116:321–362, 1951.

93. Lewis, ME, Neff, NT, Contreras, PC, et al: Insulin-like growth factor-I: Potential for treatment of motor neuronal disorders. Exp Neurol 124:73–88, 1993.

94. Li, L, Oppenheim, RW, Lei, M, et al: Neurotrophic agents prevent motoneuron death following sciatic nerve section in the neonatal mouse. J Neurobiol 25:759–766, 1994.

95. Lin, LFH, Doherty, DH, Lile, JD, et al: GDNF: A glial cell line-derived neurotrophic factor for midbrain dopaminergic neurons. Science 260:1130–1132, 1993.

96. Lin, LFH, Mismer, D, Lile, JD, et al: Purification, cloning and expression of ciliary neurotrophic factors (CNTF). Science 246:47–56, 1989.

97. Lindsay, RM: Brain-derived neurotrophic factor: An NGF-related neurotrophin. In Loughlin, SE and Fallon, JH (eds): Neurotrophic Factors. Academic Press, San Diego, 1993, pp 257–284.

98. Lindsay, RM: The role of neurotrophic growth factors in development, maintenance, and regeneration of sensory neurons. In Parnavelas, JG, Stern, CD, and Stirling, RV (eds): The Making of the Nervous System. Oxford University Press, Oxford, 1988, pp 148–165.

99. Lindsay, RM, Wiegand, SJ, Altar, CA, et al: Neurotrophic factors: From molecule to man. Trends Neurosci 17:182–190, 1994.

100. Lindsay, RM: Neuron saving schemes. Nature 373:289–290, 1995.

101. Liu, X, Ernfors, P, Wu, H, et al: Sensory but not motor neuron deficits in mice lacking NT4 and BDNF. Nature 375:238–241, 1995.

102. Lohof, AM, Ip, NY, and Poo, M: Potentiation of developing neuromuscular synapses by the neurotrophins NT-3 and BDNF. Nature 363:350–353, 1993.

103. Maisonpierre, PC, Belluscio, L, Squinto, S, et al: Neurotrophin-3: A neurotrophic factor related to NGF and BDNF. Science 247:1446–1451, 1990.

104. Manthorpe, M, Skaper, S, Adler, R, et al: Cholinergic neurotrophic factors: Fractionation properties of an extract from selected chick embryonic eye tissues. J Neurochem 34:69–75, 1980.

105. Manthorpe, M, Skaper, S, Williams, L, et al: Purification of adult rat sciatic nerve ciliary neurotrophic factor. Brain Res 367:282–286, 1986.

106. Martinou, J-C, Martinou, I, and Kato, AC: Cholinergic differentiation factor (CDF/LIF) promotes survival of isolated rat embryonic motoneurons in vitro. Neuron 8:737–744, 1992.

107. Masiakowski, P, Liu, H, Radziejewski, C, et al: Recombinant human and rat ciliary neurotrophic factors. J Neurochem 57:1003–1012, 1991.

108. Massagué, J: Crossing receptor boundaries. Nature 382:29–30, 1996.

109. Masu, Y, Wolf, E, Holtmann, B, et al: Disruption of the CNTF gene results in motor neuron degeneration. Nature 365:27–32, 1993.

110. Merlio, JP, Ernfors, P, Jaber, M, et al: Molecular cloning of rat trkC and identification of cells expressing mRNAs for members of the trk family in the rat central nervous system. Neuroscience 51:513–532, 1992.

111. Meyer, M, Matsuoka, I, Wetmore, C, et al: Enhanced synthesis of brain-derived neurotrophic factor in the lesioned peripheral nerve: Different mechanisms are responsible for the regulation of BDNF and NGF mRNA. J Cell Biol 119:45–54, 1992.

112. Miller, RB, Bryan, WW, Munsat, TL, et al: Safety, tolerability and pharmacokinetics of recombinant human ciliary neurotrophic factor (rhCNTF) in patients with amyotrophic lateral sclerosis (ALS) [abstract]. Ann Neurol 34:241, 1993.

113. Miller, RG, Petajan, J, Bryan, WW, et al: A placebo-controlled trial of recombinant human ciliary neurotrophic factor (rhCNTF) in amyotrophic lateral sclerosis. Ann Neurol 39:256–260, 1996.

114. Mitsumoto, H, Ikeda, K, Holmlund, TH, et al: The effects of ciliary neurotrophic factor on motor dysfunction in wobbler mouse motor neuron disease. Ann Neurol 36:142–148, 1994.

115. Mitsumoto, H, Ikeda, K, Klinkosz, B, et al: Arrest of motor neuron disease in wobbler mice co-treated with CNTF and BDNF. Science 265:1107–1110, 1994.

115a. Mitsumoto, H and Olney, RK: Drug combination treatment in patients with ALS: Current status and future directions. Neurology 47 (Suppl. 2): s103–s107, 1996.

116. Miyata, Y, Kashihara, Y, Homma, S, et al: Effects of nerve growth factor on the survival and synaptic function of Ia sensory neurons axotomized in neonatal rats. J Neurosci 6:2012–2018, 1986.

117. Murphy, MF, Flice, K, Gavel, M, et al: A double-blind, placebo-controlled study of myotrophin (CEP-151) in the treatment of amyotrophic lateral sclerosis. Ann Neurol 38:335, 1995.

118. Neff, NT, Prevette, D, Houenou, LJ, et al: Insulin-like growth factors: Putative muscle-derived trophic agents that promote motoneuron survival. J Neurobiol 24:1578–1588, 1993.

119. Novikov, L, Novikova, L, and Kellerth, J-O: Brain-derived neurotrophic factor promotes survival and blocks nitric oxide synthase expression in adult rat spinal motoneurons after ventral root avulsion. Neurosci Lett 200:45–48, 1995.

120. Oppenheim, RW: Cell death during development of the nervous system. Ann Rev Neurosci 14:453–501, 1991.

121. Oppenheim, RW, Houenou, LJ, Johnson, JE, et al: Developing motor neurons rescued from programmed and axotomy-induced cell death by GDNF. Nature 373:344–346, 1995.

122. Oppenheim, RW, Maderdrut, JL, and Wells, DJ: Cell death of motoneurons in the chick embryo spinal cord. Reduction of naturally occurring cell death in the thoracolumbar column of Terni by nerve growth factor. J Comp Neurol 210:174–189, 1982.

123. Oppenheim, RW, Prevette, D, and Fuller, F: The lack of effect of basic and acidic fibroblast growth factors on the naturally occurring death of neurons in the chick embryo. J Neurosci 12:2726–2734, 1992.

124. Oppenheim, RW, Prevette, D, Qin-Wei, Y, et al: Control of embryonic motoneuron survival in vivo by ciliary neurotrophic factor (CNTF). Science 251:1616–1618, 1991.

125. Oppenheim, RW, Qin-Wei, Y, Prevette, D, et al: Brain-derived neurotrophic factor rescues developing avian motoneurons from cell death. Nature 360:755–757, 1992.

126. Patterson, PH: The emerging neuropoietic cytokine family: First CDF/LIF, CNTF and IL-6; next ONC, MGF, GCSF? Cur Opin Neurobiol 2:94–97, 1992.

127. Patterson, PH and Fann, MJ: Further studies of the distribution of CDF/LIF mRNA. Ciba Found Symp 167:125–135, 1992.

128. Pennica, D, King, KL, Shaw, KJ, et al: Expression cloning of cardiotrophin 1, a cytokine that induces cardiac myocyte hypertrophy. Proc Nat Acad Sci 92:1142–1146, 1995.

129. Pennica, D, Arce, V, Swanson, TA, et al: Cardiotrophin-1, a cytokine present in embryonic muscle, supports long term survival of spinal motoneurons. Neuron 17:63–74, 1996.

130. Rabizadeh, S, Oh, J, Zhong, L, et al: Induction of apoptosis by the low-affinity NGF receptor. Science 261:345–348, 1993.

131. Ramòn y Cajal, S: Degeneration and Regeneration of the Nervous System, Vol 1. Hafner, New York, 1928.

132. Rowland, LP: Amyotrophic lateral sclerosis: Theories and therapies. Ann Neurol 35:129–130, 1994.

133. Sagot, Y, Tan, SA, Hammang, JP, et al: GDNF slows loss of motoneurons but not axonal degeneration or premature death of pmn/pmn mice. J Neurosci 16:2335–2341, 1996.

134. Sánchez, M, Silos-Santiago, I, Frisén, J, et al: Renal agenesis and the absence of enteric neurons in mice lacking GDNF. Nature 382:70–73, 1996.

135. Schnell, L, Schneider, R, Kolbeck, R, et al: Neurotrophin-3 enhances sprouting of corticospinal tract during development and after adult spinal cord lesion. Nature 367:170–173, 1994.

136. Schooltink, H, Stoyan, T, Roeb, E, et al: Ciliary neurotrophic factor induces acute-phase protein expression in hepatocytes. FEBS Lett 314:280–284, 1992.

137. Segal, RA, Takahashi, H, and McKay, RDG: Changes in neurotrophin responsiveness during the development of cerebellar granule neurons. Neuron 9:1041–1052, 1992.

138. Sendtner, M, Arakawa, Y, Stöckli, KA, et al: Effect of ciliary neurotrophic factor (CNTF) on motoneuron survival. J Cell Sci 15:103–109, 1991.

139. Sendtner, M, Carroll, P, Holtmann, B, et al: Ciliary neurotrophic factor. J Neurobiol 25:1436–1453, 1994.

140. Sendtner, M, Holtmann, B, Kolbeck, H, et al: Brain-derived neurotrophic factor prevents the death of motoneurons in newborn rats after nerve section. Nature 360:757–759, 1992.

141. Sendtner, M, Kreutzberg, GW, and Thoenen, H: Ciliary neurotrophic factor prevents the degeneration of motor neurons after axotomy. Nature 345:440–441, 1990.

142. Sendtner, M, Schmalbruch, H, Stöckli, KA, et al: Ciliary neurotrophic factor prevents degeneration of motor neurons in mouse mutant progressive motor neuronopathy. Nature 358:502–504, 1992.

143. Sendtner, M, Stöckli, KA, and Thoenen, H: Synthesis and localization of ciliary neurotrophic factor in the sciatic nerve of the adult rat after lesion and during regeneration. J Cell Biol 118:139–148, 1992.

144. Smith, RA, Melmed, S, Sherman, B, et al: Recombinant growth hormone treatment of amyotrophic lateral sclerosis. Muscle Nerve 16:624–633, 1993.

145. Snider, WD: Functions of the neurotrophins during nervous system development: What the knockouts are teaching us. Cell 77:627–638, 1994.

146. Snider, WD, Johnson, EM, Jr: Neurotrophic molecules. Ann Neurol 26:489–506, 1989.

147. Soppet, D, Escandon, E, Maragos, J, et al: The neurotrophic factors, brain-derived neurotrophic factor, and neurotrophin-3 are ligands for the trkB tyrosine kinase receptor. Cell 65:895–903, 1991.

148. Squinto, SP, Aldrich, TH, Lindsay, RM, et al: Identification of functional receptors for ciliary neurotrophic factor on neuronal cell lines and primary neurons. Neuron 5:757–766, 1990.

149. Squinto, SP, Stitt, TN, Aldrich, TH, et al: TrkB encodes a functional receptor for brain-derived neurotrophic factor and neurotrophin-3 but not nerve growth factor. Cell 65:885–893, 1991.

150. Stahl, N, Boulton, TG, Farruggella, T, et al: Association and activation of Jak-Tyk kinases by CNTF-LIF-OSM-IL-6 β receptor components. Science 263:92–94, 1994.

151. Stöckli, KA, Lottspeich, F, Sendtner, M, et al: Molecular cloning, expression, and regional distribution of rat ciliary neurotrophic factor. Nature 342:920–923, 1989.

152. Stoop, R and Poo, M: Synaptic modulation by neurotrophic factors: Differential and synergistic effects of brain-derived neurotrophic factor and ciliary neurotrophic factor. J Neurosci 16:3256–3264, 1996.

153. Takahashi, R, Yokoji, H, Misawa, H, et al: A null mutation in the human CNTF gene is not causally related to neurological diseases. Nature Genet 7:79–84, 1994.

154. Thoenen, H: The changing scene of neurotrophic factors. Trends Neurosci 14:165–170, 1991.

155. Thoenen, H, Hughes, RA, and Sendtner, M: Trophic support of motoneurons: Physiological, pathophysiological, and therapeutic implications. Exp Neurol 124:47–55, 1993.

156. Treanor, JJS, Goodman, L, de Sauvage, F, et al: Characterization of a multicomponent receptor for GDNF. Nature 382:80–83, 1996.

157. Vejsada, R, Lindsay, RM, and Kato, AC: Additive rescue effects of GDNF and BDNF axotomized sciatic motoneurons in newborn rats [abstract]. Soc Neurosci Abstr 21:1536, 1995.

158. Wang, T, Zie, K, and Lu, B: Neurotrophins promote maturation of developing neuromuscular synapses. J Neurosci 15:4796–4805, 1995.

159. Warburton, C and Braxton-Powell, L: Mouse models of IGF-I deficiency generated by gene targeting. Receptor 5:35–41, 1995.

160. Williams, L, Manthorpe, M, Barbin, G, et al: High ciliary neuronotrophic specific activity in rat peripheral nerve. Int J Dev Neurosci 2:177–180, 1984.

161. Wong, V, Arriaga, R, Ip, NY, et al: The neurotrophins BDNF, NT-3 and NT-4/5, but not NGF, up-regulate the cholinergic phenotype of developing motor neurons. Eur J Neurosci 5:466–474, 1993.

162. Yaar, M, Grossman, K, Eller, M, et al: Evidence for nerve growth factor-mediated paracrine effects in human epidermis. J Cell Biol 115:821–828, 1991.

163. Yamamori, T: Localization of cholinergic differentiation factor/leukemia inhibitory factor mRNA in the rat brain and peripheral tissues. Proc Nat Acad Sci 88:7298–7302, 1991.

164. Yamamoto, M, Sobue, G, Yamamoto, K, et al: Expression of glial cell line-derived growth factor mRNA in the spinal cord and muscle in amyotrophic lateral sclerosis. Neurosci Lett 204:117–120, 1996.

165. Yan, Q, Elliott, JL, Matheon, C, et al: Influence of neurotrophins on mammalian motoneurons in vivo. J Neurobiol 4:1555–1577, 1993.

166. Yan, Q, Elliott, J, and Snider, WD: Brain-derived neurotrophic factor rescues spinal motor neurons from axotomy-induced cell death. Nature 360:753–755, 1992.

167. Yan, Q, Matheson, C, and Lopez, OT: *In vivo* neurotrophic effects of GDNF on neonatal and adult facial motor neurons. Nature 373:341–343, 1995.

CHAPTER 16

OTHER HYPOTHESES OF ALS PATHOGENESIS

Motor neurons are large, complex cells with axons sometimes longer than a meter that extend into the periphery. Because protein synthesis is restricted to cell bodies, there are special metabolic demands on the neuron to maintain the integrity of distal axons;[12] accordingly, the motor neuron is vulnerable, perhaps more so than other cells, to a wide variety of insults. Because multiple endogenous and exogenous factors can injure the neuron, neuronal degeneration in an individual patient with ALS may result from a set of predisposing factors and a trigger, possibly environmental, that initiates a cascade leading to a progressive loss of motor neu-

rons.[96b] In previous chapters, we have explored several different mechanisms that can lead to motor neuron death, including oxidative damage and excitotoxicity (see Chapter 12) and loss of neurotrophic influence (see Chapter 15). In this chapter, we consider a variety of additional factors that may play a role in the pathogenesis of ALS, including androgen receptor disturbances, systemic neoplasms, disturbances in trace metal metabolism, abnormalities in neurofilaments, and aging.

THE ANDROGEN/ANDROGEN RECEPTOR HYPOTHESIS

In 1980, Weiner[106] proposed the androgen hypothesis to explain a number of features of ALS. Clinical features pointing to a possible role for androgens include the preponderance of male to female patients (in a ratio of 1.5 to 2.5:1), and an incidence of ALS equal in men and postmenopausal women with an average age of onset between 56 and 58 years.[18] Weiner pointed to work that revealed sparse androgen receptors in the ocular nuclei, dorsal motor nucleus of the vagus nerve, and sensory nerve nuclei[96]—all structures spared in ALS. In contrast, spinal motor neurons and motor nuclei of cranial nerves V, VII, and XII, as well as the nucleus ambiguous, had androgen receptors. Hence, the presence of androgen receptors appeared to coincide generally with neurons damaged in ALS. Weiner hypothesized that various insults—toxins, viruses, trauma, and an accelerated aging process—damage normal nerves and muscles hundreds of times in a lifetime but with the trophic stimulation of androgen on their androgen receptors, neurons can repair their axons. According to this hypothesis, the decline in androgen levels with age (in men), combined with a defect or loss of androgen receptors, has a permissive effect on motor neuron degeneration.[106]

The androgen receptor hypothesis of ALS received little notice until about a decade ago when attention turned to unraveling the molecular genetics of bulbospinal neuronopathy (BSN), first described by Kennedy and colleagues.[59] Understanding this condition is relevant to the study of ALS because some of its clinical features, most importantly amyotrophy and fasciculations of bulbar and spinal innervated musculature, are shared with ALS (see Chapter 6). Like ALS, the disease is progressive, although it tends to evolve much more slowly. In contrast to ALS, however, there are no upper motor neuron features. The observation that patients with BSN have signs of androgen insensitivity, such as gynecomastia, testicular atrophy, and reduced fertility, rekindled interest in the androgen hypothesis.

In 1986, the gene for BSN was mapped to the proximal arm of the X chromosome,[33] and subsequently the human androgen receptor was cloned and mapped to the same region; hence, it became a candidate gene

for this disease.[34] Subsequent work disclosed that a trinucleotide repeat $(CAG)_n$ in the first exon of the androgen receptor gene was without exception expanded in BSN patients. Normally, the cytosine-adenine-guanine (CAG) repeat encodes a tract of 11 to 34 glutamines in the androgen receptor protein (Fig. 16–1). In BSN, the polyglutamine tract, located in a large amino-terminal regulatory domain separate from the DNA and hormone binding sites, lengthens to 40 to 62 amino acids.[62] The molecular mechanism whereby the trinucleotide expansion leads to motor neuron degeneration is not yet clear, but it does not cause a simple loss of activity of the receptor; rather, it creates a novel gain of function toxic to motor neurons.[15] It is thought that the gene product in BSN is a regulatory protein or transcription factor whose function is disturbed when the polyglutamine tract is expanded, leading to aberrant transcriptional regulation of target genes and ultimately motor neuron death; alternatively, it may lead to the formation of a novel protein complex that is toxic to neurons and unrelated to transcription.

Although in BSN the plasma testosterone level decreases and the estrogen level variably increases, resulting in an abnormality in the estrogen to androgen ratio,[43,51] no evidence of an abnormality in the hypothalamic-pituitary axis or in the interaction of testosterone with its receptors has been found in sporadic ALS.[54,72] Weekly intramuscular injections of testosterone have not had a definite ameliorating effect on the progression of ALS.[54] When combined with the findings that no patient with ALS has been found to

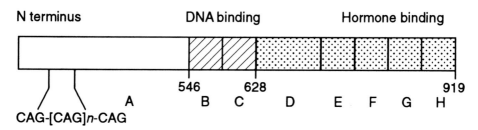

Figure 16–1. Schematic diagram of the human androgen receptor. The androgen receptor, like other steroid hormone receptors, is comprised of an N-terminus domain, a DNA-binding domain, and a hormone-binding domain. Capital letters designate the exons of the receptor, and numbers indicate amino acid position. The CAG-trinucleotide repeat begins at position 58, in the N-terminus domain. (From Brooks, BP and Fischbeck, KH: Spinal and bulbar muscular atrophy: A trinucleotide-repeat expansion neurodegenerative disease. Trends Neurosci 18:460, 1995.)

have an increase in $(CAG)_n$ repeats,[31,36] it is not likely that androgen receptor abnormalities are relevant to the pathogenesis of ALS.

THE PARANEOPLASTIC SYNDROME HYPOTHESIS

A paraneoplastic neurologic disorder is one that occurs in association with cancer but is not a direct result of a primary or metastatic tumor in the nervous system.[93] Potential mechanisms of nervous system damage in the paraneoplastic syndromes are varied and include poor nutrition, metabolic derangement, vascular occlusion, and infection, but an immunopathogenesis is now considered most likely.[89] A possible cause-and-effect relationship between neoplasia and ALS was proposed by Norris and Engel,[80] who found the frequency of cancer in their series of 130 ALS patients to be 10% compared to 1.6% in a concurrently observed group of 312 stroke patients. A number of epidemiologic surveys from around the world, however, have not confirmed an increased presence of cancer in patients dying of ALS.[4,89] Nonetheless, because neurologic paraneoplastic syndromes are extremely rare and ALS is relatively common, it remains possible that neoplasia and ALS could be etiologically linked in a very small number of patients, a number too small to be identified in statistical data.[94]

There are three clinical situations in which a cause-and-effect relationship is regarded to exist between ALS or an ALS-like syndrome and neoplasia (Table 16–1). First, when patients with ALS substantially improve or stabilize with treatment of the underlying cancer, the ALS is considered paraneoplastic. Such occurrences are rare, with

Table 16–1. **ALS AS PARANEOPLASTIC SYNDROME**

- ALS or ALS-like syndrome resolves or stabilizes with treatment or removal of neoplasm
- ALS-like syndrome as a part of an encephalomyelitis with antineuronal antibodies (anti-Hu antibodies)
- Lower motor neuron syndrome (rarely ALS per se) in setting of lymphoma

only eight patients reported in almost 30 years.[13,17,29,39,75,80,84,86] For example, a 74-year-old man has been described with a lower motor neuron syndrome characterized by atrophy of both thighs; fasciculations in arm, calf, and thigh muscles; pelvic girdle weakness; and essentially normal reflexes without Babinski signs.[29] An electromyographic (EMG) study showed chronic denervation and reinnervation. Removal of a renal cell carcinoma by right radical nephrectomy was followed by improved strength and resolution of EMG abnormalities. Patients have also been described with a combination of lower and upper motor neuron findings. A 53-year-old man experienced wasting of small muscles of the hands; fasciculations of the arms, forearms, and thighs; increased tone, and hyperactive reflexes.[13] After lobectomy for an adenocarcinoma, he returned to work, and at examination 11 months after presentation, his muscle strength was normal, although occasional fasciculations were seen. The tumor recurred 7 months later but the patient had no signs of neurologic deterioration; postmortem examination showed a reduced anterior horn cell density at cervical and lumbar spinal levels.

An ALS-like syndrome probably has a paraneoplastic origin when the neurologic syndrome is tightly associated with the presence of a serum autoantibody. In this instance, patients with cancer develop neurologic signs referable to various parts of the nervous system, and postmortem examination reveals inflammation in the brain, brain stem, spinal cord, dorsal root ganglia, and nerve roots. The neurologic signs have been termed *encephalomyelitis associated with carcinoma*,[44] and *paraneoplastic sensory neuronopathy*.[45] Further studies indicate that this paraneoplastic neurologic syndrome can be associated with virtually any type of tumor, but in more than 75% of patients, the underlying tumor is a small-cell lung cancer.[45] With few exceptions, patients with small-cell lung carcinoma and paraneoplastic encephalomyelitis or a sensory neuronopathy have antineuronal antibodies (designated anti-Hu) in serum and cerebrospinal fluid (CSF).[27] Anti-Hu reacts with a protein antigen or antigens of molecular weight 35 to 40 kd expressed in the neuronal nuclei and to a lesser extent in the cytoplasm of neurons and small-cell lung cancer cells. Autopsy studies of such patients disclose antibody deposits in the tumor and in areas of the nervous system with corresponding neurologic symptoms, suggesting that the antibody has a role in disease pathogenesis.

Only one patient has been described with isolated lower motor neuron disease in the presence of a small-cell cancer of the lung in association with high titers of anti-Hu antibody in serum and CSF.[104b] In most patients with paraneoplastic encephalomyelitis, motor neuron signs are accompanied by abnormal findings referable to other areas of the nervous system. Thus, ALS per se is not generally a part of paraneoplastic encephalomyelitis, although motor weakness is occasionally the first neurologic symptom, and motor neuron dysfunction is prominent in about 20% of patients with the anti-Hu antibody.[27] In general, symptoms begin with loss of strength proximally that affects the lower or upper extremities or both, sometimes in an asymmetric pattern mimicking ALS. Weakness, atrophy, and fasciculations of the distal muscles are common; tendon reflexes may decrease or increase, and some patients have pathologic reflexes. Rarely, the patient presents with a floppy-head syndrome.

A third circumstance in which there appears to be a paraneoplastic relationship between ALS and neoplasia is found in rare patients with lymphoma who develop a pure lower motor neuron syndrome that is designated as motor neuronopathy.[97] It is subacute, progressive, painless, and often asymmetric, with the legs more affected than the arms. These clinical features may occur at any time during the course of lymphoma but most often occur when the tumor is in remission or after radiation therapy to the mantle and para-aortic regions. The neurologic syndrome tends to stabilize or improve over months to years and is rarely severely debilitating. Pathologically, there is loss of neurons in the anterior horn and Clarke's column, as well as demyelination of anterior roots and posterior columns. This syndrome was originally described in two patients with Hodgkin's lymphoma but has also been reported in non-Hodgkin's lymphoma.[95] The cause of this syndrome is not certain, but infection of the anterior horn cells has been proposed, particularly in view of the fact that patients with lymphoma are at risk for immunosuppression and opportunistic viral infection.

In a small number of patients with lymphoma or Hodgkin's disease, a motor neuron disorder occurs with signs of both upper and lower motor neuron dysfunction that qualify such patients for the diagnosis of ALS. It is not clear whether this disorder is the same as the disorder described above, but almost half the patients with lymphoma and ALS have a paraproteinemia, two thirds have elevated CSF protein levels, and a third have oligoclonal bands in the CSF. The relationship between the lymphoma and ALS is not clear, but a retroviral infection has been proposed. The paraproteinemia suggests that an immunologic disorder may have a role in ALS pathogenesis.[111]

THE NEUROTOXIC METALS HYPOTHESIS

The Role of Lead and Mercury

Epidemiologic studies have raised the possibility that metals may be involved in the pathogenesis of ALS[57] (Table 16–2). Since the observations of Wilson,[107] there has been an interest in the relationship of lead to the pathogenesis of ALS. A number of investigators have pointed out that lead may cause a clinical syndrome and pathologic changes similar to those of ALS.[8,50,67] Lead poisoning may cause ALS-like clinical features (see Chapter 6) that are helped by chelating agents.[76] In a systematic survey of heavy metal exposure in ALS, there was evidence of lead exposure before onset of disease in 24 out of 31 patients.[26] Lead or other heavy metal exposure was a significant antecedent event more frequently in patients with ALS than in controls.[90] Increased levels of lead have also been found in nerve, muscle, and the spinal cord of patients who died of ALS,[87] with the spinal cord lead levels correlating with disease duration.[61] A variety of analytic procedures have revealed increased lead in the CSF of patients with ALS.[22] When lead is added to plasma, erythrocytes from patients with ALS have an increased lead uptake and are more fragile to mechanical stimuli than

Table 16–2. **METALS THAT MAY BE INVOLVED IN ALS PATHOGENESIS**

Metal	Findings and Comments
Lead and mercury	• Increased in spinal cord in sporadic ALS*
	• May cause a reversible ALS-like syndrome
	• Probably not involved in typical sporadic ALS
Aluminum	• Interferes with neurofilament transport
	• Increased in brain and spinal cord in Guamanian Western Pacific ALS*
	• May play a pathogenic role in Western Pacific ALS
Calcium	• Increased in spinal cord in Guamanian Western Pacific ALS*
	• Important mediator of neuron damage
Silicon	• Increased in brain and spinal cord in Guamanian Western Pacific ALS*
Iron	• Increased in spinal cord in sporadic ALS*
	• Ferrous state may facilitate free radical formation
Manganese	• Increased in brain and spinal cord in sporadic ALS*
Selenium	• Increased in spinal cord in sporadic ALS*

*In some studies, however, not significantly different compared with normal tissue.[57]

normal control erythrocytes.[91] The increased plasma lead level found in ALS patients may be a result of the leakage of lead from hemolyzed erythrocytes;[91] a generalized membrane defect was hypothesized to cause such erythrocyte fragility in ALS.[92]

These interesting clinical, pathologic, epidemiologic, and biochemical observations implicating lead in the pathogenesis of ALS have been tempered, however, by the inability to confirm abnormal lead concentrations in blood, CSF, erythrocytes, and plasma from patients with ALS.[101] There was also no significant difference in lead content of muscles between ALS patients and controls.[21] Also, lead deposition in ALS might be a secondary phenomenon, resulting from alterations of the blood-brain or blood-nerve barrier.[69] ALS clinical trials with chelating agents such as penicillamine have been unsuccessful,[23,48] although long-term urinary excretion of lead was achieved.[23]

The possibility of mercury toxicity in ALS has also raised interest. Progressive muscle atrophy developed in two young men who worked with mercury oxide and had high urinary mercury levels.[3] Withdrawal from the exposure was followed by resolution of signs and symptoms and a fall of urinary mercury levels to acceptable levels. A progressive muscular atrophy syndrome developed in a 54-year-old man who had been salvaging mercury from thermometers and showed increased urinary mercury levels.[1] Symptoms and signs resolved when exposure ended. Thus, reversible ALS-like disorders may be caused by mercury toxicity. In other reports, mercury exposure is suspected as a causative factor in patients with an ALS-like clinical picture except that adequate chelating therapy has no ameliorating effect,[16,56] and in one case, postmortem examination showed anterior horn cell changes consistent with ALS per se.[16] The inference is that in these latter cases, mercury exposure is incidental to the development of ALS.

The Role of Metals in Western Pacific ALS

Further interest in the mineral hypothesis was kindled by the environmental and epidemiologic studies of neurodegenerative disorders (including ALS) among three genetically and geographically distinct populations in the Western Pacific region (see Chapter 3).[109,110] Although the incidence of ALS in these regions has decreased markedly, levels of metals in the environment appear to have a role, possibly acting in combination with another factor (e.g., excitotoxin).[102] In these regions, which include Guamanian villages, areas of the Kii peninsula of Japan, and the southern coastal plain of West New Guinea, drinking water and garden soil show comparatively high levels of aluminum and manganese and unusually low levels of calcium and magnesium.[110] Scanning electron microscopy with energy-dispersive x-ray spectrometry analysis of the elemental content of hippocampal neurons in Guamanian Chamorran natives with ALS showed prominent accumulations of aluminum in the nuclear region and perikaryal cytoplasm.[85] In another study, calcium and aluminum were found in neurons in patients with Guamanian ALS.[37] Further investigations using a computer-driven electron β-x-ray microprobe with wavelength-dispersive spectrometry detected silicon in the cell bodies and dendritic processes of hippocampal neurons bearing neurofibrillary tangles in patients with ALS[38]; the distribution of silicon was similar to that of calcium and aluminum. The colocalization of silicon, calcium, and aluminum suggests that these elements are involved in the pathogenesis of Western Pacific ALS. These mineral deposits are stable, immobile, and are thought to be aluminosilicates and calcium hydroxyapatites.[110] It has been proposed that silicon and aluminum could each interfere with slow axonal transport.[38] Various in vivo and in vitro studies have established that aluminum disrupts the neuronal cytoskeleton,[103] leading to the accumulation of neurofilaments in motor neurons (see below)—one of the ultrastructural hallmarks of ALS (see Chapter 10).

Proponents of a role for abnormal mineral metabolism in the pathogenesis of Western Pacific ALS propose that deposition of minerals in the CNS of patients may have occurred during a period of secondary hyperparathyroidism provoked by deficiencies of calcium and magnesium endemic to the high-incidence foci.[109] Because detailed metabolic studies of calcium and vitamin D metabolism in Chamorrans did not disclose significant abnormalities, accumulation and deposition of metals in the CNS must have occurred long before onset of symptoms; any detectable abnormalities of calcium and vitamin D metabolism would have normalized by symptom onset.[109] Although subsequent adequate calcium and magnesium intake might have corrected secondary hyperparathyroidism acquired early in life, disappearance of hydroxyapatite deposits in neurons or reversal of neuronal damage would not be expected.

Manganese has also been implicated in the pathogenesis of Guamanian ALS because it was found in increased amounts in water, soil, cattle hair, and plants in Guam.[110] In a group of seven autopsied cases with sporadic ALS, anterior horn cervical spinal cord manganese concentrations were significantly higher compared to six control subjects.[77] Of note, the elevation of manganese levels in the ALS subjects was more prominent in the anterior horn and lateral columns than in the posterior columns. It was speculated that local disturbances of manganese metabolism in the spinal cord may have contributed to neurologic degenerative changes.[77] A 37-year-old man with manganese poisoning has been described who developed ALS with severe bulbar symptoms.[105]

The Role of Metals in Sporadic ALS

The possibility that disturbed calcium metabolism might play a role in the pathogenesis of sporadic ALS is suggested by clinical similarities between ALS and neuromuscular syndromes of primary and secondary hyperparathyroidism,[83] by more frequent skeletal abnormalities and fractures in patients with ALS,[68] and by the observation that the spinal cord calcium content, in the form of calcium hydroxyapatite, is greater in patients compared to controls.[53] The calcium content of erythrocytes from patients with ALS is normal,[30] but the calcium level in muscle is low although calmodulin levels are normal.[74] In contrast, peripheral blood lymphocytes from patients with sporadic ALS were found to have higher levels of resting free cytosolic calcium with respect to control lymphocytes.[26a] Additionally, in human autopsy studies, immunoreactive calbindin-D28K and parvalbumin are absent in those motor neurons lost early in ALS, including the cortical, lower cranial, and spinal motor neurons; those neurons damaged infrequently (ocular motor neurons and Onuf's nucleus) expressed markedly higher levels.[2] In view of the importance of increased intracellular calcium as a mediator of cell death (by activating calcium-dependent proteases and phospholipases and triggering hydroxyl radical release from mitochondria[47a]), mechanisms controlling intraneuronal calcium homeostasis may influence the selective vulnerability seen in ALS, irrespective of the disease-triggering mechanism.

Although aluminum is found in excess in Guamanian ALS, a recent study of aluminum concentration in the spinal cord of patients with sporadic ALS using laser microprobe mass spectroscopy did not detect any increase of this metal in motor neurons, neuropil, or capillaries.[58] In contrast, iron and calcium increased 1.5- to 2-fold in the nucleus and cytoplasm of ALS neurons, but not in capillaries and neuropil. Increased iron and transferrin levels have been found in regenerating motor neurons after axotomy,[40] an experimental finding that may be relevant at some point during the course of ALS. Although the presence of intraneuronal iron in sporadic ALS may be a normal physiologic response, in its ferrous state it may make motor neurons more susceptible to degeneration by facilitating the production of hydroxyl free radicals from hydrogen peroxide generated by copper-zinc superoxide dismutase (SOD1) (see Chapter 12). Also implicating metal toxicity in ALS is the observation that the iron-binding protein lactotransferrin, which also transports aluminum, is strongly immunoreactive with Betz cells, the cells that are severely affected in ALS.[65] It is hypothesized that these cells take up lactotransferrin at an elevated rate, resulting in accumulation of potentially damaging iron and aluminum.[65]

In addition to iron, significant elevations of selenium have been found in the lumbar spinal cord from patients with sporadic ALS.[52] Also elevated was glutathione peroxidase, which is a selenoprotein enzyme that in concert with SOD1 provides a coupled detoxifying system that catalyzes the reduc-

tion of superoxide radicals via hydrogen peroxide and hydroxyl radicals to water (see Chapters 11 and 12). One might speculate that glutathione peroxidase elevation may be a response to oxidative stress occurring in sporadic ALS. Of note, earlier studies raised the possibility that selenium could be implicated in the pathogenesis of ALS. Four cases of ALS were described in a region with high selenium content in the soil and where selenium intoxication of farm animals occurred.[60] However, an additional epidemiologic study[7] and findings that patients with ALS excrete normal levels of selenium[81] have failed to support a role for this element.

THE NEUROFILAMENT HYPOTHESIS

Neurofilament Structure and Function

Neurofilaments are neuron-specific, metabolically stable, cytoskeletal elements whose normal production and transport to the nerve terminal are critical to the health and integrity of the motor neuron.[11] They play key roles in bidirectional axonal transport of organelles and substances vital to the integrity of the motor neuron and its lengthy axon. Neurofilaments, 10 nm in diameter and many microns long, are composed of individual proteins of molecular mass 200 kd (the neurofilament heavy [NF-H] subunit), 160 kd (neurofilament medium [NF-M]), and 68 kd (neurofilament light [NF-L]).[11] Each subunit is regulated during production and coded by a separate gene; the three proteins rapidly self-assemble into a larger triplet protein after translation. This larger structure consists of a core filament, NF-L, from which the carboxy-terminal portions of NF-M and NF-H subunits project. The serine residues of the NF-M and NF-H carboxy-terminal side arms are highly phosphorylated, with up to 50 phosphates per NF-H subunit;[63] therefore they are designated as multiphosphorylation sites. Phosphorylation of NF-M and NF-H may control the dynamics of cytoskeletal interactions by altering the sidearm conformation, charge, or both; an increase in the overall level of phosphorylation is associated with a reduced rate of neurofilament transport.[66] Once phosphorylated, the neurofilament is transported distally via the slow axonal transport system[47] and, together with microtubules, is a major determinant of myelinated axon diameter. The neurofilaments are rapidly degraded by calcium-activated proteases when they reach the nerve terminal.

Neurofilament Abnormalities in ALS

We can trace the development of the neurofilament hypothesis in ALS (Table 16–3) from observations made by Carpenter,[19] who noted focal enlargements of axons in cells in the anterior horn of the spinal cord and in the somatic motor nuclei of the brain stem. These large argentophilic spheroids (axonal swellings) are now widely accepted as highly characteristic pathologic findings in the spinal cords of patients with ALS. The clinical course of the disease correlates with this pathologic feature, with a tendency for the enlargements to be seen in the more rapidly progressive cases of 10 months or less.[19] The swellings are similar to structures produced in experimental models of toxicity with iminodipropionitrile (IDPN) and aluminum, and

Table 16–3. EVIDENCE FOR NEURO-FILAMENT INVOLVEMENT IN ALS

- Neurofilament accumulation (axonal spheroids) in perikarya and proximal axons in ALS
- Neurofilament accumulations and abnormal slow axon transport in experimental toxic neuropathies and some animal motor neuron diseases
- Increased phosphorylation of neurofilaments in ALS
- Neurofilament accumulations, similar to those in ALS, in transgenic mice overexpressing normal wild-type genes for NF-L or NF-H proteins, or a mutant NF-L gene
- NF-H gene deletions in a few cases of sporadic ALS*
- Neurofilament accumulations in transgenic mice expressing *SOD1* mutations and in familial ALS caused by certan *SOD1* mutations

*These deletions were not found in a subsequent study.[104a]
Abbreviations: NF-H = neurofilament-heavy, NF-L = neurofilament-light, *SOD1* = superoxide dismutase 1.

to neurofilamentous abnormalities in spontaneously occurring motor neuron disorders in animals (see below). Subsequent studies found that 10-nm neurofilaments were seen not only in patients with a short course but also in most patients with longer duration illness.[46]

The mechanism underlying neurofilament swelling and whether these swellings provide a clue to the pathogenesis of ALS potentially are issues of great importance in understanding ALS. Experimental toxic neuropathies produced by β, β'-IDPN[41] or aluminum[104] and motor diseases of animals[24] have neurofilamentous swellings and abnormal slow axonal transport. (In ALS, however, only fast axonal transport has been studied.[10,14,79,96a]) Phosphorylation of neurofilaments is also altered in ALS. In normal neurons, nonphosphorylated neurofilaments are found in the soma and proximal axon, whereas phosphorylated neurofilaments are located in distal axons and terminals.[100] In ALS, however, most focal collections of neurofilaments in anterior horn cell perikarya are phosphorylated.[70,78] It is likely that neurofilaments are prematurely phosphorylated in ALS, but whether this is the result or the cause of altered neurofilament transport from the perikaryon to the proximal axon is not clear.[70] When the SMI31 antibody, which reacts with the multiphosphorylation sites on the carboxy-terminal extension of NF-M and NF-H, is microinjected into spinal cord motor neurons in culture, antibody-decorated neurofilaments accumulate in proximal axonal segments and cause them to swell.[28] SMI31 preserves the phosphorylated conformation of the neurofilament side arms and possibly prevents dephosphorylation, thereby preventing effective transport. This finding, therefore, supports a role for phosphorylation of neurofilament side arms in controlling neurofilament transport and demonstrates that direct interference with the multiphosphorylation sites of neurofilament proteins can cause axonal swellings. Furthermore, the lack of effect when SMI31 was injected into dorsal root ganglia neurons suggested that the neurofilament network of motor neurons is inherently susceptible to disruption, which may help explain the selective vulnerability of motor neurons in ALS.[28]

Animal Models of Neurofilament Overexpression

To further explore the possible role of neurofilaments in ALS, overexpression of neurofilament protein in transgenic mice has been examined. Transgenic mice overexpressing the human NF-H gene twofold to fourfold developed progressive neurologic defects and abnormal neurofilamentous swellings in the perikarya and proximal axons of spinal motor neurons reminiscent of those found in motor neurons of patients with ALS.[25] An increased amount of NF-H was postulated to cause extra NF-H crossbridges that would in turn impose additional drag on neurofilament transport, reduce intracellular transport of newly synthesized neurofilaments, and lead to the piling up of newly synthesized neurofilaments.

To clarify the mechanism of neurodegeneration of NF-H transgenic mice, intracellular transport of axonal proteins was studied.[20] In motor axons, the transport rates of neurofilament proteins as well as those of tubulin and actin decreased remarkably. Electron microscopy confirmed the accumulation of filamentous structures and depletion of mitochondria and endoplasmic reticulum in atrophied axons. Examination of the L5 ventral roots from NF-H transgenics 2 years old revealed massive degeneration of large axons derived from spinal motor neurons, providing direct evidence that neurofilament abnormalities can contribute to motor neuron degeneration. It is likely that the neurofilament accumulation in these transgenic animals interfered with transport of the intracellular components necessary for axonal integrity and therefore contributed to motor neuron degeneration. A similar mechanism may be involved in the pathogenesis of human ALS.[55] The high level of neurofilament protein synthesis may account for the observation that large motor neurons in ALS are selectively vulnerable to disturbances in neurofilament production.[20]

In transgenic mice expressing four times the normal mouse NF-L level,[108] motor neurons of the ventral horn showed early onset of massive accumulations of neurofilaments, swollen perikarya, and eccentrically localized nuclei, which were accompanied by more frequent axonal degeneration, proximal axon swelling, and severe skeletal muscle atrophy. The pathology in mice that overexpress NF-L appears similar to that in the early stages of ALS and suggests that neurofilament overaccumulation may cause motor neuron dysfunction before widespread neuronal loss. Thus, primary alterations in neurofilament production may lead to structural changes as occur in ALS, that is, axonal breakdown and loss. The axonal swellings could be a result of disturbed axon transport, either from an increase in the amount of neurofilaments synthesized or from changes in their structure and organization because of a proportionately high NF-L concentration. Another pathologic feature in these mice was the accumulation of phosphorylated NF-H in the soma of motor neurons. The relatively minor loss of axons despite the marked neurofilament accumulation suggests that the neuron has a substantial "tolerance" for such increases. Such tolerance implies that filament-induced degeneration would be a slow process and therefore consistent with the gradual progression of a disorder like ALS.

The overexpression in transgenic mice of a mutant disrupting NF-L assembly[64] led to massive, selective degeneration of spinal motor neurons accompanied by abnormal accumulations of neurofilaments and severe neurogenic muscle atrophy. Sensory neurons showed only modest degenerative changes. The pathologic changes in mice expressing this mutant neurofilament resemble those found in mice overexpressing human NF-H except for earlier onset and faster progression.[55] These findings demonstrate that aberrant accumulation of mutated neurofilament may play a causal role in selective motor neuron death.

Pathogenic Role for Neurofilaments in ALS

These transgenic mouse studies clearly implicate neurofilament accumulation in the pathogenesis of motor neuron degeneration. Neurofilament accumulation in human ALS may result from a decrease in slow axonal transport of this key element of the motor neuron cytoskeleton.[35] This notion is supported by pathologic findings in human

ALS and animal models of ALS in which organelles, in addition to neurofilaments, accumulate in perikarya and proximal axons, pointing to a transport defect that affects both neurofilaments and other organelles.[24,46,96a] It is also known that there is a retardation in slow axonal transport of cytoskeletal elements during aging,[71] a risk factor for ALS. In ALS, defective neurofilament transport could result from a variety of lesions, including an intrinsic alteration of neurofilament structure, so that filaments can no longer be adequately transported.[108] In fact, cases are described in which abnormal filament structure and organization exist, including paracrystalline arrays, beaded filaments, and various types of focal accumulations of neurofilaments.[46] Motor neurons might be selectively targeted in diseases like ALS because they are naturally rich in neurofilaments and therefore most susceptible to defects triggering overaccumulation.[108] The striking similarities in pathologies of human motor neuron disease and transgenic mice expressing the NF-L mutation suggest that mutations in neurofilament subunits may be responsible for, or at least contribute to, a proportion of ALS cases.[64] The more severe neurofilament mutations could underlie the occasional ALS case that has an early onset and rapid progression, whereas mutations with more subtle effects on neurofilament assembly and organization could cause a later onset and possibly more slowly progressive disease, as in some instances of sporadic and familial ALS.

In this regard, a pathogenic role for neurofilaments in the development of ALS is suggested by novel mutations in the C-terminal region of the NF-H subunit in 5 patients with ALS that were not found in 306 normal controls.[32] The mutations may have affected the cross-bridging properties of NF-H and perhaps contributed to the development of neurofilamentous swellings in ALS. Of interest, four of five of the patients with ALS had the same three base-pair deletion—AAG codon for lysine. The deleted lysine residue is part of a consensus sequence that serves as a substrate for a neurofilament kinase called *cdk5* kinase.[99] Such a mutation may have led to the gradual development of aberrant neurofilamentous accumulations and hence be in keeping with the usual later onset of ALS. Al-

though the NF-H mutation alone may predispose a patient to ALS, the development of neuronal degeneration per se is likely to require additional environmental or genetic factors unique to each individual. For example, a patient with a C-terminal region NF-H mutation[32] was exposed to long-lived toxins (hydrazine and morpholene), which may have accelerated the onset of the disease. The possible importance of mutations in NF-H led to the hypothesis that a defect on chromosome 22 band q12 may be involved in the pathogenesis of ALS.[73] In addition to NF-H, this region encodes the P2 blood group phenotype (significantly more prevalent in ALS patients than normal controls)[88] and leukemia inhibitory factor (a ciliary neurotrophic factor–related cytokine that prevents motor neuron death in vivo and in vitro[49]).

Further studies, however, by Vechio and colleagues[104a] seeking to confirm and extend the earlier work on NF-H gene deletions[32] failed to find mutations as primary causes of ALS. These investigators examined almost all of the coding domains of all three neurofilament subunits in DNAs from 100 familial as well as 75 sporadic ALS patients. Nonetheless, it is likely that aberrant accumulations of axonal neurofilaments contribute to progression of disease in ALS.[104a] There is evidence that disturbances in neurofilament structure and transport may be affected by oxidative stress (see Chapter 12) (Fig. 16–2). For example, neurofilament accumulation occurs in motor neurons of some familial ALS cases induced by mutations in *SOD1*,[94a] and aberrant neurofilament swellings are found in degenerating motor neurons of transgenic mice expressing a mutant form of human *SOD1*.[42] There is also evidence from immunohistochemical studies of familial and sporadic ALS of nitration of tyrosine residues in NF-L by peroxynitrite[19a] that would inhibit NF phosphorylation and thereby disturb subsequent assembly and transport of NF subunits. Neurofilaments, the most abundant structural proteins in large myelinated axons, are an obvious target for cumulative oxidative damage because they require 1 to 2 years to travel the length of a 1-m sciatic nerve.[64] Downregulation of neurofilament expression in patients with ALS has been suggested as a potential means to retard disease progression.[55]

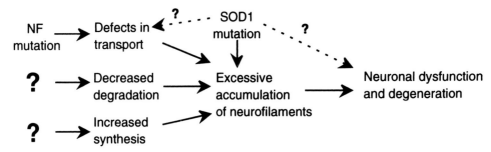

Figure 16–2. Schematic model for involvement of neurofilaments in motor neuron disease. (From Lee, MK, Marszalek, JR, and Cleveland, DW: A mutant neurofilament subunit causes massive, selective motor neuron death: Implications for the pathogenesis of human motor neuron disease. Neuron 13:984, 1994, with permission of Cell Press.)

THE AGING HYPOTHESIS

Aging is undoubtedly an important risk factor for a variety of neurodegenerative diseases, including ALS (see Chapter 3). Evidence is growing that the mitochondria are central in the process of motor neuronal damage in ALS.[5] With increasing age, mitochondrial function progressively declines as a result of mitochondrial DNA deletions, point mutations, and oxidative damage. Disturbed mitochondrial function is expressed by a decline in oxidative phosphorylation and ultimately by a reduction in ATP production. This defect in energy metabolism may lead to neuronal depolarization, followed by a relief of the magnesium block of the N-methyl-D-aspartate receptor, persistent receptor activation by ambient glutamate levels, and a resulting influx of calcium.[82] Increased intracellular calcium increases the activity of potentially damaging proteases, phospholipases, and endonucleases, and activates nitric oxide synthase, thereby enhancing the formation of nitric oxide. In buffering the large calcium load, the mitochondria generate the superoxide free radical that reacts with nitric oxide to increase formation of peroxynitrite, which may be a key mediator of oxidative damage in motor neurons.[6] Indeed, protein carbonyl groups, a marker of oxidative damage, are found in greater amounts in sporadic ALS frontal cortex compared to control normal values,[9] and in ALS spinal cord[98] compared to normal and neurologic disease controls.

SUMMARY

The androgen receptor hypothesis was proposed to explain the selective vulnerability of particular motor neurons in ALS. Disordered androgen receptor function is probably critically important in the pathogenesis of bulbospinal neuronopathy but in the contemporary view is unlikely to play a role in ALS. In most ALS patients, motor neuron degeneration and neoplasia are not related, but in a very small subset of patients, ALS or an ALS-like condition is paraneoplastic and probably immune-mediated. (As discussed in Chapter 13, the immune hypothesis of ALS has been difficult to establish despite some suggestive experimental studies.)

Various metals have also been implicated in ALS pathogenesis. Patients with Western Pacific ALS have aluminum deposits in the CNS that are likely to play a role in this disease, perhaps by interfering with neurofilament function. Rarely, lead or mercury exposure has caused an ALS-like syndrome. In most cases of sporadic ALS, however, all three metals, as well as selenium and manganese, have a marginal role at most. Iron may be involved in generating hydroxyl radicals, which may mediate oxidative damage in motor neurons. Calcium may also be important in the pathogenesis of ALS, and the lack of calcium-binding proteins in certain subsets of motor neurons may enhance their vulnerability to calcium-mediated injury.

It has long been known from ALS autopsy specimens that neurofilaments accumulate prominently in motor neurons and proximal axons. Much attention has recently been focused on the structure and transport of neurofilaments because clinical and pathologic features of ALS can be produced in transgenic mice overexpressing various neurofilament protein subunits. In humans, impaired transport of neurofilaments may be involved in ALS pathogenesis. Defective transport could result from a neurofilament gene mutation or an acquired lesion of the neurofilament subunit proteins.

The increased risk of ALS apparent with aging may stem from declining mitochondrial function with age. A defect in energy metabolism could lead to a metabolic cascade that ultimately generates free radicals that damage macromolecules critical to the motor neuron's survival and thereby trigger ALS.

REFERENCES

1. Adams, CR, Ziegler, DK, and Lin, JT: Mercury intoxication simulating amyotrophic lateral sclerosis. JAMA 250:642–643, 1983.
2. Alexianu, ME, Bao-Kuang, H, Mohamed, H, et al: The role of calcium-binding proteins in selective motoneuron vulnerability in amyotrophic lateral sclerosis. Ann Neurol 36:846–858, 1994.
3. Barber, TE: Inorganic mercury intoxication reminiscent of amyotrophic lateral sclerosis. J Occup Med 20:667–669, 1978.
4. Barron, KD and Rodichok, LD: Cancer and disorders of motor neurons. In Rowland, LP (ed): Human Motor Neuron Diseases. Raven Press, New York, 1982, pp 267–272.
5. Beal, MF: Aging, energy, and oxidative stress in neurodegenerative diseases. Ann Neurol 38:357–366, 1995.
6. Beckman, JS and Crow, JP: Pathological implications of nitric oxide, superoxide and peroxynitrite formation. Biochem Soc Trans 21:330–334, 1993.
7. Bharucha, NE, Schoenberg, BS, Raven, RH, et al: Geographic distribution of motor neuron disease and correlation with possible etiologic factors. Neurology 33:911–915, 1983.
8. Boothby, JA, deJesus, PV, and Rowland, LP: Reversible forms of motor neuron disease: Lead "neuritis." Arch Neurol 31:18–23, 1974.
9. Bowling, AC, Schultz, JB, Brown, RH Jr, et al: Superoxide dismutase activity, oxidative damage, and mitochondrial energy metabolism in familial and sporadic amyotrophic lateral sclerosis. J Neurochem 61:2322–2325, 1993.
10. Bradley, WG, Good, P, Rasool, CG, et al: Morphometric and biochemical studies of peripheral nerves in amyotrophic lateral sclerosis. Ann Neurol 14:267–277, 1983.
11. Brady, ST: Motor neurons and neurofilaments in sickness and health. Cell 73:1–3, 1993.
12. Brady, ST: Interfering with the runners. [letter] Nature 375:12–13, 1995.
13. Brain, L, Croft, PB, and Wilkinson, M. Motor neuron disease as a manifestation of neoplasm. Brain 88:479–500, 1965.
14. Breuer, AC, Lynn, MP, Atkinson, MB, et al: Fast axonal transport in amyotrophic lateral sclerosis: An intra-axonal organelle traffic analysis. Neurology 37:738–748, 1987.
15. Brooks, BP and Fischbeck, KH: Spinal and bulbar muscular atrophy: A trinucleotide-repeat expansion neurodegenerative disease. Trends Neurosci 18:459–461, 1995.
16. Brown, IA: Chronic mercurialism—A case of the clinical syndrome of amyotrophic lateral sclerosis. Arch Neurol Psychiatry 72:674–681, 1954.
17. Buchanan, DS and Malamud, N: Motor neuron disease with renal cell carcinoma and postoperative neurologic remission. Neurology 23:891–894, 1973.
18. Caroscio, JT, Mulvihill, MN, Sterling, R, et al: Amyotrophic lateral sclerosis. Its natural history. Neurol Clin 5:1–8, 1987.
19. Carpenter, S: Proximal axonal enlargement in motor neuron disease. Neurology 18:841–851, 1968.
19a. Chou, SM, Wang, HS, Taniguchi, A: Role of SOD-1 and nitric oxide/cyclic GMP cascade on neurofilament aggregation in ALS/NMD. J Neurol Sci 139(suppl.):16–26, 1996.
20. Collard, J-F, Cote, F, and Julien, J-P: Defective axonal transport in a transgenic mouse model of amyotrophic lateral sclerosis. Nature 375:61–64, 1995.
21. Conradi, S, Ronnevi, LO, and Vesterberg, O: Lead concentration in skeletal muscle in amyotrophic lateral sclerosis patients and control subjects. J Neurol Neurosurg Psychiatry 41:1001–1004, 1978.
22. Conradi, S, Ronnevi, L-O, Nise, G, et al: Abnormal distribution of lead in amyotrophic lateral sclerosis: Reestimation of lead in the cerebrospinal fluid. J Neurol Sci 48:413–418, 1980.
23. Conradi, S, Ronnevi, L-O, Nise, G, et al: Long time penicillamine treatment in amyotrophic lateral sclerosis with parallel determination of lead in blood, plasma and urine. Acta Neurol Scand 65:203–211, 1982.
24. Cork, LC, Troncoso, JC, Klavano, GG, et al: Neurofilamentous abnormalities in motor neurons in spontaneously occurring animal disorders. J Neuropathol Exp Neurol 47:420–431, 1988.
25. Cote, F, Collard, J-F, and Julien, J-P: Progressing neuronopathy in transgenic mice expressing the human neurofilament heavy gene: A mouse model of amyotrophic lateral sclerosis. Cell 73:35–46, 1993.
26. Currier, RD and Haerer, AF: Amyotrophic lateral sclerosis and metallic toxins. Arch Environ Health 17:712–719, 1968.
26a. Curti, D, Malaspina, A, Facchetti, G, et al: Amyotrophic lateral sclerosis: Oxidative energy metabolism and calcium homeostasis in peripheral blood lymphocytes. Neurology 47:1060–1064, 1996.
27. Dalmau, J, Graus, F, Rosenblum, MK, et al: Anti-

Hu-associated paraneoplastic encephalomyelitis/sensory neuronopathy. A clinical study of 71 patients. Medicine 71:59–72, 1992.

28. Durham, HD: An antibody against hyperphosphorylated neurofilament proteins collapses the neurofilament network in motor neurons but not in dorsal root ganglion cells. J Neuropathol Exp Neurol 51:287–297, 1992.

29. Evans, BK, Fagan, C, Arnold, T, et al: Paraneoplastic motor neuron disease and renal cell carcinoma: Improvement after nephrectomy. Neurology 40:960–962, 1990.

30. Felmus, MT, Rasool, CG, and Bradley, WG: Calcium content of RBCs from patients with amyotrophic lateral sclerosis. Arch Neurol 39:454, 1982.

31. Ferlini, A, Patrosso, MC, Guidetti, D, et al: Androgen receptor gene (CAG)n repeat analysis in the differential diagnosis between Kennedy disease and other motorneuron disorders. Am J Med Gen 55:105–111, 1995.

32. Figlewicz, DA, Krizus, A, Martinoli, MG, et al: Variants of the heavy neurofilament subunit are associated with the development of amyotrophic lateral sclerosis. Hum Mol Genet 3:1757–1761, 1994.

33. Fischbeck, KH, Ionasescu, V, Ritter, AW, et al: Localization of the gene for X-linked spinal muscular atrophy. Neurology 36:1595–1598, 1986.

34. Fischbeck, KH, Souders, D, and La Spada, AR: A candidate gene for X-linked spinal muscular atrophy. Adv Neurol 56:209–214, 1991.

35. Gajdusek, DC: Hypothesis: Interference with axonal transport of neurofilament as a common pathogenetic mechanism in certain diseases of the central nervous system. N Engl J Med 312:714–719, 1985.

36. Garafalo, O, Figlewicz, DA, Leigh, PN, et al: Androgen receptor gene polymorphism in amyotrophic lateral sclerosis. Neuromusc Disorder 3:195–199, 1993.

37. Garruto, RM, Swyt, C, Fiori, CE, et al: Intraneuronal deposition of calcium and aluminum in amyotrophic lateral sclerosis of Guam. [letter] Lancet 2:1353, 1985.

38. Garruto, RM, Swyt, C, Yanigahara, R, et al: Intraneuronal co-localization of silicon with calcium and aluminum in amyotrophic lateral sclerosis and parkinsonism with dementia of Guam. N Engl J Med 315:711, 1986.

39. Gerling, GM and Woolsey, RM: Paraneoplastic motor neurone disease. Case reports. Modern Med 64:503–506, 1967.

40. Graebner, MB, Raivich, G, and Kreutzberg, GW: Increase of transferrin receptors and iron uptake in regenerating motor neurons. J Neurosci Res 23:342–345, 1989.

41. Griffin, JW, Hoffman, PN, Clark, AW, et al: Slow axonal transport of neurofilament proteins: Impairment by β, β′-iminodipropionitrile administration. Science 202:633–635, 1978.

42. Gurney, ME, Pu, H, Chiu, AY, et al: Motor neuron degeneration in mice that express a human Cu, Zn superoxide dismutase mutation. Science 264:1772–1775, 1994.

43. Hausmanowa-Petrusewicz, I, Borkowska, J, and Janczewski, Z: X-linked adult form of spinal muscular atrophy. J Neurol 229:175–178, 1983.

44. Henson, RA, Hoffman, HL, and Urich, H: Encephalomyelitis with carcinoma. Brain 88:449–464, 1965.

45. Henson, RA, and Urich, H: Encephalomyelitis with carcinoma. In Henson, RA and Urich, H (eds): Cancer and the Nervous System. Blackwell Scientific, Oxford, 1982, pp 314–345.

46. Hirano, A, Donnenfield, H, Sasaki, S, et al: Fine structural observations of neurofilamentous changes in amyotrophic lateral sclerosis. J Neuropathol Exp Neurol 43:461–470, 1984.

47. Hoffman, PN and Lasek, RJ: The slow component of axonal transport. Identification of the major structural polypeptides of the axon and their generality among mammalian neurons. J Cell Biol 66:351–366, 1975.

47a. Hosler, BA, and Brown, RH: Copper/zinc superoxide dismutase mutations and free radical damage in amyotrophic lateral sclerosis. Adv Neurol 68:41–46, 1995.

48. House, AO, Abbott, RJ, Davidson, DLW, et al: Response to penicillamine of lead concentrations in CSF and blood in patients with motor neuron disease. Br Med J 2:1684, 1978.

49. Hughes, RA, Sendtner, M, and Thoenen, H: Members of several gene families influence survival of rat motor neurons in vitro and in vivo. J Neurosci Res 36:663–671, 1993.

50. Hylsop, GH and Kraus, WM: The pathology of motor paralysis by lead. Arch Neurol Psychiatry 10:444–455, 1923.

51. Imai, H, Beppu, H, Uono, M, et al: Endocrinological investigation in patients with progressive proximal spinal and bulbar muscular atrophy of late onset (Kennedy-Alter-Sung type). Clin Neurol 20:704–712, 1980.

52. Ince, PG, Shaw, PJ, Candy, JM, et al: Iron, selenium and glutathione peroxidase activity are elevated in sporadic motor neuron disease. Neurosci Lett 182:87–90, 1994.

53. Iwata, S: Structural analysis of metal coprecipitated calcification products in the central nervous system with particular reference to ALS. Neurol Med Chir (Tokyo) 13:103–107, 1980.

54. Jones, TM, Yu, R, and Antel, JP: Response of patients with amyotrophic lateral sclerosis to testosterone therapy. Arch Neurol 39:721–722, 1982.

55. Julien, J-P: A role for neurofilaments in the pathogenesis of amyotrophic lateral sclerosis. Biochem Cell Biol 73:593–597, 1995.

56. Kantarjian, AD: A syndrome clinically resembling amyotrophic lateral sclerosis following chronic mercurialism. Neurology 11:639–644, 1961.

57. Kasarskis, EJ: Neurotoxicology: Heavy metals. In Smith, RA (ed): Handbook of Amyotrophic Lateral Sclerosis. Marcel Dekker, New York, pp 559–573, 1992.

58. Kasarskis, EJ, Tandon, L, Lovell, MA, et al: Aluminum, calcium, and iron in the spinal cord of patients with sporadic amyotrophic lateral sclerosis using laser microprobe mass spectroscopy: A preliminary study. J Neurol Sci 130:203–208, 1995.

59. Kennedy, WB, Alter, M, and Sung, JG: Report of an X-linked form of spinal muscular atrophy. Neurology 18:671–680, 1968.

60. Kilness, AW and Hochberg, FH. Amyotrophic lat-

eral sclerosis in a high selenium environment. JAMA 237:2843–2844, 1977.

61. Kurlander, HM and Patten, BM: Metals in spinal cord tissue of patients dying of motor neuron disease. Ann Neurol 6:21–24, 1979.

62. La Spada, AR, Paulson, HL, and Fischbeck, KH: Trinucleotide repeat expansion in neurological disease. Ann Neurol 36:814–822, 1994.

63. Lee, M-YV, Otvos, L, Carden, MJ, et al: Identification of the major multiphosphorylation site in mammalian neurofilaments. Proc Natl Acad Sci U S A 85:1998–2002, 1988.

64. Lee, MK, Marszalek, JR, and Cleveland, DW: A mutant neurofilament subunit causes massive, selective motor neuron death: Implications for the pathogenesis of human motor neuron disease. Neuron 13:975–988, 1994.

65. Leveugle, B, Spik, G, Perl, DP, et al: The iron-binding protein lactotransferrin is present in pathological lesions in a variety of neurodegenerative disorders: A comparative immunohistochemical analysis. Brain Res 650:320–331, 1994.

66. Lewis, SE and Nixon, RA: Multiple phosphorylation variants of the high molecular mass subunit neurofilaments in axons of retinal cell neurons: Characterization and evidence for their differential association with stationary and moving neurofilaments. J Cell Biol 107:2689–2701, 1988.

67. Livesley, B and Sissons, CE: Chronic lead intoxication mimicking motor neurone disease. Br Med J 4:387–388, 1968.

68. Mallette, L, Patten, B, Cook, J, et al: Calcium metabolism in amyotrophic lateral sclerosis. Diseases of Nervous System 38:457–461, 1977.

69. Mandybur, TI and Cooper, GP: Increased spinal cord lead content in amyotrophic lateral sclerosis—possibly a secondary phenomenon. Med Hypotheses 5:1313–1315, 1979.

70. Manetto, V, Sternberger, NH, Perry, G, et al: Phosphorylation of neurofilaments is altered in amyotrophic lateral sclerosis. J Neuropathol Exp Neurol 47:642–653, 1988.

71. McQuarrie, IG, Brady, ST, and Lasek, RJ: Retardation in the slow axonal transport of cytoskeletal elements during maturation and aging. Neurobiol Aging 10:359–365, 1989.

72. Melmed, S and Braunstein, GD: Endocrine function in amyotrophic lateral sclerosis. A review. Neurol Clin 5:33–42, 1987.

73. Meyer, MA and Potter, NT: Sporadic ALS and chromosome 22: Evidence for a possible neurofilament gene defect. Muscle Nerve 18:536–539, 1995.

74. Mishra, SK and Kumar, S: Muscle calcium, calmodulin levels in amyotrophic lateral sclerosis. [abstract] Neurology 35(suppl 1):73, 1985.

75. Mitchell, DM and Olczak, SA: Remission of a syndrome indistinguishable from motor neurone disease after resection of bronchial carcinoma. [abstract] Br Med J 2:176, 1979.

76. Mitchell, JD: Heavy metals and trace elements in amyotrophic lateral sclerosis. Neurol Clin 5:43–60, 1987.

77. Miyata, S, Nakamura, S, Nagata, H, et al: Increased manganese level in spinal cords of amyotrophic lateral sclerosis determined by radiochemical neuron activation analysis. J Neurol Sci 61:283–293, 1983.

78. Munoz, DG, Greene, C, Perl, DP, et al: Accumulation of phosphorylated neurofilaments in anterior horn motorneurons of amyotrophic lateral sclerosis patients. J Neuropathol Exp Neurol 47:9–18, 1988.

79. Norris, FH: Moving axon particles of intercostal nerve terminals in benign and malignant ALS. In Tsubaki, T and Toyokura, Y. (eds): Amyotrophic Lateral Sclerosis. University Park Press, Baltimore, 1979, pp 375–385.

80. Norris, FH and Engel, WK: Carcinomatous amyotrophic lateral sclerosis. In Brain, L and Norris, FH (eds): The Remote Effects of Cancer on the Nervous System. Grune & Stratton, New York, 1995, pp 24–41.

81. Norris, FH and U, KS. Amyotrophic lateral sclerosis and low urinary selenium levels. [letter] JAMA 239:404, 1978.

82. Novelli, A, Reilly, JA, Lysko, PG, et al: Glutamate becomes neurotoxic via the N-methyl-D-aspartate receptor when intracellular energy levels are reduced. Brain Res 451:205–212, 1988.

83. Patten, BM, Bilezekian, JP, Maillette, LE, et al: Neuromuscular disease in primary hyperparathyroidism. Ann Intern Med 80:182–193, 1974.

84. Peacock, A, Dawkins, K, and Rushworth, G: Motor neurone disease associated with bronchial carcinoma? Br Med J 2:499–500, 1979.

85. Perl, DP, Gajdusek, DC, Garruto, RM, et al: Intraneuronal aluminum accumulation in amyotrophic lateral sclerosis and parkinsonism-dementia on Guam. Science 217:1053–1055, 1982.

86. Peters, HA and Clatanoff, DV: Spinal atrophy secondary to macroglobulinemia. Neurology 18:101–108, 1968.

87. Petkau, A, Sawatzky, A, Hillier, CR, et al: Lead content of neuromuscular tissue in amyotrophic lateral sclerosis—Case report and other considerations. British Journel Industrial Medicine 31:275–287, 1974.

88. Plato, CC, Rucknagel, DL, and Kurland, LT. Blood group investigations on the Carolinians and Chamorros of Saipan. Am J Phys Anthropol 24:147–154, 1966.

89. Posner, JB: Neurologic Complications of Cancer. FA Davis, Philadelphia, 1995.

90. Roelofs-Iverson, RA, Mulder, DW, Elveback, LR, et al: ALS and heavy metals: A pilot case-control study. Neurology 34:393–395, 1984.

91. Ronnevi, L-O, Conradi, S, and Nise, G: Further studies on the erythrocyte uptake of lead in vitro in amyotrophic lateral sclerosis (ALS) patients and controls. Abnormal erythrocyte fragility in ALS. J Neurol Sci 57:143–156, 1982.

92. Ronnevi, L-O and Conradi, S: Increased fragility of erythrocytes from amyotrophioc lateral sclerosis (ALS) patients provoked by mechanical stress. Acta Neurol Scand 69:20–26, 1984.

93. Rosenfeld, MR and Dalmau, J: Paraneoplastic syndromes and progressive motor dysfunction. Semin Neurol 13:291–298, 1993.

94. Rosenfeld, MR and Posner, JB: Paraneoplastic motor neuron disease. Adv Neurol 56:445–459, 1991.

94a. Rouleau, GA, Clark, AW, Rooke, K, et al: SOD1 mutation is associated with accumulation of neurofilaments in amyotrophic lateral sclerosis. Ann Neurol 39:128–131, 1996.

95. Rowland, LP and Schneck, SA: Neuromuscular disorders associated with malignant neoplastic disease. J Chronic Dis 16:777–795, 1963.

96. Sar, M and Stumpf, WE: Androgen concentration in motor neurons of cranial nerves and spinal cord. Science 197:77–79, 1977.

96a. Sasaki, S and Iwata, M: Impairment of fast axonal transport in the proximal axons of anterior horn neurons in amyotrophic lateral sclerosis. Neurology 47:535–540, 1996.

96b. Serratrice, GT and Munsat, TL: Overview of the pathogenesis and therapy of amyotrophic lateral sclerosis. Adv Neurol 68:1–5, 1995.

97. Schold, SC, Cho, E-S, Somasundaram, M, et al: Subacute motor neuronopathy: A remote effect of lymphoma. Ann Neurol 5:271–287, 1979.

98. Shaw, PJ, Ince, PG, Falkous, G, et al: Oxidative damage to protein in sporadic motor neuron disease spinal cord. Ann Neurol 38:691–695, 1995.

99. Shetty, KT, Link, WT, and Pant, HC: cdc-2 like kinase from rat spinal cord specifically phosphorylates KSPXK motifs in neurofilament proteins: Isolation and characterization. Proc Natl Acad Sci U S A 90:6844–6848, 1993.

100. Sternberger, LA and Sternberger, NH: Monoclonal antibodies distinguish phosphorylated and nonphosphorylated forms of neurofilaments in situ. Proc Natl Acad Sci U S A 80:6126–6130, 1983.

101. Stober, T, Stelte, W, and Kunze, K: Lead concentration in blood, plasma, erythrocytes, and cerebrospinal fluid in amyotrophic lateral sclerosis. J Neurol Sci 61:21–26, 1983.

102. Stone, R. Guam: Deadly disease dying out. Science 261:424–426, 1993.

103. Strong, MJ and Garruto, RM: Experimental paradigms of motor neuron degeneration. In Woodruff, ML and Nonneman, AL (eds): Toxin-induced models of neurological disorders. Plenum Press, New York, 1994, pp 39–88.

104. Troncoso, JC, Price, DL, Griffen, JW, et al: Neurofibrillary axonal pathology in aluminum intoxication. Ann Neurol 12:278–283, 1982.

104a. Vechio, JD, Bruijn, LI, Zuoshang, X, Brown, RH, and Cleveland, DW: Sequence variants in human neurofilament proteins: Absence of linkage to familial amyotrophic lateral sclerosis. Ann Neurol 40:603–610, 1996.

104b. Verma, A, Berger, JR, Snodgrass, S, and Petito, C: Motor neuron disease: A paraneoplastic process associated with anti-Hu antibody and small-cell lung carcinoma. Ann Neurol 40:112–116, 1996.

105. Voss, H: Cited by Yanagihara, R: Heavy metals and essential minerals in motor neuron disease. Adv Neurol 36:233–247, 1982.

106. Weiner, LP: Possible role of androgen receptors in amyotrophic lateral sclerosis. A hypothesis. Arch Neurol 37:129–131, 1980.

107. Wilson, SAK: The amyotrophy of chronic lead poisoning—Amyotrophic lateral sclerosis of toxic origin. Rev Neurol Psychiatry 5:441–455, 1907.

108. Xu, Z, Cork, L, Griffin, JW, et al: Increased expression of neurofilament subunit NF-L produces morphological alterations that resemble the pathology of human motor neuron disease. Cell 73:23–33, 1993.

109. Yanagihara, R, Garruto, RM, Gajdusek, C, et al: Calcium and vitamin D metabolism in Guamanian Chamorros with amyotrophic lateral sclerosis and parkinsonism-dementia. Ann Neurol 15:42–48, 1984.

110. Yase, Y: The pathogenesis of amyotrophic lateral sclerosis. Lancet 2:292–296, 1972.

111. Younger, DS, Rowland, LP, Latov, N, et al: Lymphoma, motor neuron diseases, and amyotrophic lateral sclerosis. Ann Neurol 29:78–86, 1991.

CHAPTER 17

ANIMAL MODELS OF ALS

The investigation of how to solve the mystery of ALS has been difficult, and thus its pathogenesis and cause remain enigmatic. In any difficult human disease, the studying of appropriate animal models is a standard approach to expanding the knowledge of the disease. ALS is no exception. Animal models have several advantages: The disease can be studied at any stage, any organ can be investigated, the disease can be studied serially, radioisotope use or surgical manipulation is possible, and the effects of new biologic agents can be easily analyzed. Nevertheless, a potential disadvantage is that motor neuron disease (MND) in animal models may not be a true counterpart to ALS in the human.

The search for an animal model of ALS first was begun in naturally occurring MNDs, which were often incidentally discovered.[23] ALS investigators have been searching for clues in animal diseases that resemble ALS to solve arising questions. At the same time, several attractive hypotheses were proposed about the cause of ALS. In order to test such hypotheses, healthy laboratory animals have been used to induce experimentally a disease or a process that resembles ALS.[92,100] Animal models offer an invaluable opportunity to investigate the neurobiology of motor neuron degeneration.

Table 17–1 summarizes the different experimental animal models. In this chapter, we discuss animal models that have been frequently or extensively studied and those that have been recently developed.[79,84] For each model, we specifically discuss which features represent ALS and which do not. Advantages and disadvantages of each model in the investigation of ALS are reviewed. We also briefly review the techniques and results of recent preclinical therapeutic trials with neurotrophic factors in mouse models.

NATURALLY OCCURRING MODELS

Mouse Models

Because of a high reproductive turnover, spontaneous mutations are common in laboratory mice. Among many well-known mutants with neurologic diseases, several mouse

Table 17–1. ANIMAL MODELS OF ALS

Naturally Occurring MND Models

Mouse models: Wobbler
mnd
pmn
mnd2

Canine models: Hereditary canine spinal muscular atrophy

Equine models: Equine motor neuron disease

Experimentally Induced Models

Neurotoxin-induced
Excitotoxin
β, β′-iminodipropionitrile
Aluminum
Suicide transport of doxorubicin or lectin
Low-calcium diet

Viral infection
Poliovirus
Retrovirus

Experimental allergic models
Experimental allergic motor neuron disease
Experimental allergic gray matter disease

Transgenic Murine Models

Overexpression of genes
SOD1 transgenic mice
Neurofilament heavy
Mutated murine neurofilament light

Null mutation
Absent ciliary neurotrophic factor

Abbreviations: MND = motor neuron disease, mnd = motor neuron degeneration, mnd2 = motor neuron degeneration 2, pmn = progressive motor neuronopathy, *SOD1* = superoxide dismutase 1.

mutants with MND have been recognized and studied for the model of ALS.[23,92]

THE WOBBLER MOUSE MODEL

The wobbler mouse model, the oldest model among all the mouse MND models, was first reported in the C57BL/Fa inbred strain in 1956 by Falconer,[30] and full details of this animal disease were described by Duchen and Strich.[24] Since then, this animal model has been the most extensively investigated of the natural MND models, and many independent researchers study this model (see review by Mitsumoto and Pioro[79]). However, this MND is obviously not a mouse ALS. Nevertheless, this model provides the opportunity to analyze the mechanisms of motor neuron degeneration producing the key feature of ALS, spontaneous muscle paralysis and denervation atrophy. Because we are most familiar with the wobbler model and use it in our investigations, we will describe it in detail.

Genetic Background

The gene that causes wobbler mouse MND is linked on chromosome 11[48] near *rab* 1[106] and is transmitted by autosomal-recessive inheritance. Junier and colleagues[47] found that the size of the base pair for the glutamine synthetase (*glst*) microsatellite gene is smaller in the original wobbler strain (C57BL) than in the New Zealand black (nzb) mice. This *glst* microsatellite gene is believed to be close to the wobbler gene, which has not yet been determined. A hybrid between the wobbler and nzb strains in which the wobbler gene is transmitted is termed *new* (New Zealand black–elicited wobbler mouse).[47] Affected *new* mice carrying the wobbler gene have a smaller base pair for *glst* microsatellite, as occurs in the original C57BL strain. In the *new* strain, we can make a molecular diagnosis using polymerase chain reaction to identify affected wobbler mice at the preclinical and clinical stages and to separate the heterozygote from the wild type.

Clinical Features

This MND is unique in that forelimb muscles predominantly are affected, but hindlimb muscles are relatively spared. The disease progresses rapidly during age 6 to 8 weeks.[4,24,69] Affected animals develop jitteriness and tremulousness as early as 3 to 4 weeks of age; these are probably the earliest clinical manifestations. A few days after onset, a wobbling gait and front paw weakness develop. The latter is detected as a weak grip reflex when an affected animal is held in the air by the tail and permitted to grip the grid bar of the cage top. Wasting of front paw digits and progressive weakness ensue. The front paws gradually flex and curl, and the gait becomes more wobbly. However, even when the front paws are completely paralyzed and contracted, the hindlimbs apparently function normally, because an affected animal can hop and stand on its hindlimbs alone. After 2 months of age, the disease progression slows, and animals may survive beyond 6 months of age. Electrophysiologic studies show denervation.[38]

Muscles innervated by the lower cranial nerves also are affected in this MND,[24,57] but predominant involvement of the forelimbs is unique among natural MND models, in which disease mostly affects the hindlimbs. In contrast, in ALS the disease begins in any motor neuron region (bulbar, upper extremities, or lower extremities) and generalizes rapidly.

Motor Neuron Pathology

The morphologic changes in the lower motor neurons are characterized by vacuolar degeneration.[2,24,71,72] At the earliest preclinical stage (in a 2-week-old clinically healthy animal), neurons may or may not have vacuoles. Normal-looking neurons without vacuoles contain abundant granular endoplasmic reticulum, whereas neurons with even a few vacuoles (which suggests early neuronal degeneration) have no granular endoplasmic reticulum and fewer free ribosomes. This finding suggests that the endoplasmic reticulum or Golgi apparatus may be a morphologic target of vacuolar degeneration. The contents of these vacuoles are un-

known. Preliminary studies (EP Pioro, MD, unpublished observation) showed that motor neurons in wobbler mice had increased ubiquitin and phosphorylated neurofilament immunoreactivity, suggesting an immunohistologic feature resembling a characteristic of ALS. Vacuolar degeneration similar to that in wobbler mice has been reported in a case of Werdnig-Hoffmann's disease,[50] but not in ALS. Therefore, this pathologic feature of the motor neuron distinguishes the wobbler MND from ALS. Table 17–2 summarizes the similarities and differences between naturally occurring MNDs and ALS.

Dendrites of spinal cord motor neurons in affected animals are shorter, with fewer branches and spines.[60] Similar changes have been described for the smaller interneurons.[61] Whether astrogliosis exists in the cervical spinal cord is controversial. Earlier studies showed none,[2,24,71] but more recent investigations using immunocytochemistry or immunoblotting have revealed significant reactive gliosis in the brain stem and cervical spinal cord neuropil.[37,55] Astrocytes in wobbler mice are abnormal morphologically and in vitro growth characteristics are also different from those of normal littermates,

Table 17–2. **ALS FEATURES FOUND IN ANIMAL MODELS OF MOTOR NEURON DISEASE**

ALS Features	mnd	Wobbler	pmn	HCSMA
Inheritance pattern*	AD	AR	AR	AD
Age of onset	5 to 11 mo	Early	Early	Varied
Location of onset	Hindlimb	Forelimbs	Hindlimb	General
Terminal course	No	Yes	Yes, rapid	Yes, vary
Muscle denervation	Absent	Present	Present	Yes
AHC loss	Late probably	Yes	Yes	No
Chromatolysis	No	Yes	Yes	Unknown
Phosphorylated NF	No	Yes	Unknown	Yes
AHC inclusions	Yes	Yes	No	Yes, spheroids
AHC atrophy	No	Yes	Unknown	Yes
Large axon loss	No	Yes	Unknown	Yes
Upper MN involvement	Unknown	Probably	Unknown	No
Other neurons affected	Unknown	Yes	Unknown	Unknown

*Of all ALS cases, 5% to 10% have AD inheritance.

Abbreviations: AD = autosomal dominant, AHC = anterior horn cells, AR = autosomal recessive, HCSMA = hereditary canine spinal muscular atrophy, MN = motor neuron, mnd = motor neuron degeneration, NF = neurofilaments, pmn = progressive motor neuronopathy, .

suggesting an inherent pathology in wobbler astrocytes.[37]

Histometry of the lower motor neurons and their nerve fibers at the ventral roots shows that a reduction in number begins when clinical disease appears, progresses rapidly from 3 weeks to 6 weeks of age, and slows thereafter.[6,71,83,85] These morphologic studies also indicate that the disease process may be largely completed in the rapidly progressive stage.

In short, the evidence of upper motor neuron involvement in wobbler mice is meager, making this model more suitable for studying lower motor neuron degeneration.

Neuronal Degeneration Outside of Motor Neurons

Vacuolated neurons occasionally are found in the brain cortex, deep gray matter, cerebellum, brain stem, and dorsal horn, but most occur in the cervical anterior horn. As many as 3.5% of all lower motor neurons may be vacuolated.[71,78] In fact, degenerating nerve fibers are widespread in both the descending and ascending nerve tracts of the spinal cord.[11] Thus, neurons other than motor neurons are affected to a minor degree, a feature also seen in ALS.

Muscle Pathology

Skeletal muscles in the forelimbs, particularly flexor muscles, show severe denervation atrophy, but at the same time, axonal sprouting and reinnervation clearly are present.[8,21] In fact, the skeletal muscles of wobbler mice have significantly increased plasminogen activity, which is consistent with increased reinnervation.[8] In an investigation of motor endplates in ocular muscles, neuronal degeneration may begin at the axon terminal.[58]

The Degenerative Process: Neuronopathy vs. Axonopathy

To identify the initial site of the disease in motor neuron degeneration is a critical issue because this question is directly associated with the pathogenesis of MND. Wobbler mice again provide an excellent opportunity to study this issue.

In the entire neuron, from the perikaryon to the axon terminal, the first pathologic change develops in the perikaryon; thus, the pathogenic process is a neuronopathy according to the definition of toxic neuropathies.[98]

When the mice are at 3 weeks of age (1 week after the vacuolar degeneration appears in the perikaryon and when the clinical disease develops), a series of changes occur in the ventral roots of the motor axons.[71,72] These changes include adaxonal vacuole formation, redistribution of the axonal cytoskeleton and rare axonal swelling, adaxonal-Schwann cell profile formation, intra-axonal vacuole formation, and the resulting acute axonal degeneration. As soon as acute axonal degeneration (myelin ovoids) appears in the ventral roots, axonal regeneration occurs, suggesting that proximal axons that undergo wallerian degeneration distal to focal axonal disease regenerate. At a later stage (6 weeks to 3 months of age), small clusters of regenerated axons are found. The axonal pathology, including the axonal regeneration, in this MND is consistent with axonopathy (primary disease of the axon). Therefore, axonopathy develops in the early course of neuronopathy in wobbler MND. This study suggests that the distinction between axonopathy and neuronopathy, although conceptually important and helpful,[98] may be somewhat artificial for clinical diseases.[71] These axonal changes rarely are present in the dorsal root.

The number of axons undergoing such changes at any time is less than several percent of all ventral root axons. Histometry shows that loss of large myelinated fibers progressively decreases the number of motor nerve fibers, an effect seen in motor axons in ALS (see Chapter 11).

Biochemical Abnormalities

Autopsy of patients with ALS has revealed decreased levels of two excitatory amino acids, glutamate and aspartate, in the brain and spinal cord (see Chapter 12); in wobbler mice, levels are normal in the brain but slightly decreased in the spinal cord compared to unaffected mice.[52,53] In contrast to excitatory amino acid levels, however, an inhibitory amino acid, glycine, and its receptor are both significantly reduced in wobbler mice. Also, levels of several neuropeptides—thyrotropin-releasing hormone, substance P, and leucine enkephalin—increase in wobbler MND.[21,101,103]

Neuronal Function

Some questions in ALS, such as whether diseased neurons retain their neuronal function, or whether they have the ability to regenerate after nerve injury, are not easily answered. Such questions are fundamental for a better understanding of the disease process, however.

Axonal Regeneration. Axonal regeneration is a normal reparative process after neuronal injury and an important neuronal function.[64] Spontaneous axonal regeneration occurs in response to proximal axonal degeneration in the ventral roots in wobbler mouse MND, suggesting that diseased motor neurons can support axonal regeneration.[62,71] A study of experimental traumatic axotomy revealed that diseased motor neurons indeed can sustain axonal regeneration.[68] However, the degree of regeneration varied between axons: some axons regenerated at a nearly normal rate, whereas others barely regenerated at all. This range indicates that the ability to support axonal regeneration may substantially differ among individual motor neurons in wobbler MND.

Protein and RNA Synthesis and Axonal Transport. Protein and RNA synthesis decrease in the motor neurons of affected animals,[81,82] which can impair axonal regeneration. Axonal transport also crucially affects axonal regeneration. We have shown that fast axonal transport is abnormal,[77] and slow axonal transport, particularly neurofilament transport, is impaired markedly.[73] The rate of retrograde axonal transport of horseradish peroxidase is unchanged but less is transported to the cell body in affected animals than in unaffected mice.[73] The reduction in slow axonal transport corresponds to the diminished total axonal area of the motor axons.[74]

Difference Between Morphologically Normal and Abnormal Motor Neurons. The impaired slow axonal transport and regeneration are not the direct consequence of morphologically abnormal lower motor neuron perikarya because the impaired functions are more widespread than would be expected if only affected neurons were involved.[68,74,81] This observation suggests that biochemical abnormalities must occur in normal-looking neurons and that the morphologic abnormality follows the biochemical changes. Thus, morphologic normality does not indicate functional normality.

Further studies show that some vacuolated neurons not only maintain axons into the periphery but also can support axonal regeneration, implying that they sustain neuronal protein synthesis and axonal transport.[70] However, the overall functional ability of these vacuolated neurons is marginal compared with the majority of neurons that appear normal in this MND. Morphologic abnormality accompanies impaired function but not complete loss of function.

Selective Neuronal Involvement

In human MNDs, certain groups of motor neurons are affected, but others are spared. Similarly, in wobbler mouse MND, the cervical motor neurons innervating the forelimb muscles are predominantly affected, and the lumbar motor neurons innervating the hindlimb muscles are spared.[71,78] Such selective neuronal involvement in wobbler mouse MND offers the opportunity to investigate the neuronal mechanisms of selective vulnerability in neurodegenerative disorders.

We have searched for differences between these two groups of motor neurons that would account for a selective vulnerability in one group or disease resistance in the other. No axonal pathology exists in the lumbar ventral roots. The frequency of vacuolated neurons in the lumbar motor neurons (0.6%) is less than that in the cervical motor neurons (1.7%), a statistically significant difference.[78] However, whether such a subtle difference in the number of vacuolated neurons creates a marked clinical difference is unclear.

The histometry of motor nerve fibers at the lumbar ventral roots differs from that in the cervical ventral roots, whose abnormalities are described above. In the lumbar roots, the total number of myelinated fibers remains unaffected throughout the disease course because an increased number of small myelinated fibers offsets the loss of large myelinated fibers.[78] Furthermore, in contrast to the cervical motor neurons, all aspects of axonal transport in the lumbar motor neurons are normal.[79] Axonal regeneration after experimental traumatic axotomy is also normal in the lumbar motor neurons.[78] These findings clearly indicate that the cervical and lumbar motor neurons have different susceptibilities to the wobbler gene, producing vulnerability in cervical motor neurons but disease resistance in the lumbar neurons.

Usefulness of the Model

Wobbler mice are best suited to investigate the mechanisms of motor neuron degeneration and the reparative process of degenerating motor neurons, including the response to neurotrophic factors. This animal model also provides a unique opportunity to analyze the mechanisms of selective involvement of motor neurons in MND in general. These questions cannot be easily answered in patients with ALS, and thus this MND is a valuable tool.

MOTOR NEURON DEGENERATION MOUSE MODEL

An autosomal-dominant form of motor neuron degeneration (mnd) has been studied.[65,66] Affected mice develop progressive gait abnormalities by 6 months of age, followed by spastic paralysis and death before age 1 year. Degenerating motor neurons contain ubiquitin-positive inclusion bodies,[63] which are seen in neurodegenerative disorders (see Chapter 11). Recently, cytoplasmic lipofuscin-like material in the motor neurons has been found to contain the subunit c of mitochondrial adenosine triphosphate synthase, which is characteristic of neuronal ceroid lipofuscinosis.[9] The mnd mouse is now considered a model of Batten's disease, the most common human neuronal lipofuscinosis. Although late-onset motor neuron degeneration is a feature of ALS, important morphologic features of ALS are missing in the mnd mouse model, including denervation atrophy of skeletal muscles, significant signs of lower motor neuron involvement, and substantial motor neuron loss (see Table 17–2).

PROGRESSIVE MOTOR NEURONOPATHY MOUSE MODEL

An autosomal-recessive murine mutant characterized by muscle atrophy, rapidly progressive hindlimb and then forelimb paralysis,

and death by 6 to 7 weeks of age was first described by Schmalbruch et al.[91] The sensory system is not involved. Affected animals develop denervation atrophy of skeletal muscles and a moderate decrease in the number of myelinated nerve fibers in the phrenic and peroneal nerves. Because the numbers of motor neurons in the spinal cord and myelinated ventral root fibers do not decrease, the degenerative process may involve a dying-back neuropathy. However, Sendtner and colleagues[93] documented a loss of facial nucleus motor neurons in older progressive motor neuronopathy (pmn) mice. That this finding was not observed in the original report may be a result of an age difference between the animals used in the studies.[94] Ultrastructural observation reveals that granular endoplasmic reticulum is replaced by free ribosomes. This change is consistent with neuronal chromatolysis that possibly is caused by dying-back axonal disease. Although this animal model has been termed pmn, which implies a primary cell body disease, it may actually be an axonopathy (primary disease of the axon).

The progressive motor neuron loss and resulting weakness are features consistent with ALS, but the rapid course and possible axonopathy may not be (see Table 17–2). Identifying the responsible gene is critically important to analyze the mechanism of motor neuron degeneration, and further characterization of the pmn model is necessary.

MOTOR NEURON DEGENERATION 2 MOUSE MODEL

An autosomal-recessive mutation, motor neuron degeneration 2 (mnd2) results in an early-onset MND, usually beginning at 21 to 24 days of age with rapidly progressive paralysis, severe muscle wasting predominantly in the hindlimbs, and death before 40 days of age. Electrophysiologic studies show spontaneous activity in skeletal muscle, consistent with the fibrillation potentials seen in denervated muscles. Motor neurons swell and undergo chromatolysis.[44] The gene is linked on mouse chromosome 6. This animal model has lower motor neuron involvement, which is consistent with ALS, but the disease course is rapid and short, perhaps more closely resembling infantile spinal muscular atrophy.

Hereditary Canine Spinal Muscular Atrophy

Several canine motor neuron diseases have been previously described without detailed investigations.[92] Hereditary canine spinal muscular atrophy (HCSMA) is the only model that has been extensively investigated. The disease was first identified in Brittany spaniels.[18] The disease is transmitted by autosomal-dominant inheritance, and onset is between 6 weeks and 1 year of age. Clinically, the disease is characterized by weight loss, progressive generalized but predominantly proximal muscle weakness and respiratory difficulty. The sensory system is spared. The tendon reflexes are diminished, and electrophysiologic studies show fasciculation and fibrillation potentials. Spinal cord pathology shows prominent axonal spheroids near the anterior horn cell bodies, but the number of anterior horn cells is normal. The cell body is always smaller than in healthy littermates, suggesting that the anterior horn cells in this disease never reach a normal size.[18] Study of the ventral roots support the above findings.[19] Interestingly, no axonal degeneration occurs. A study of large kinships provided an opportunity to investigate the relationship between gene dose and disease severity because the three different forms of HCSMA—slow, intermediate, and rapid—are identified on the basis of gene dose.[17,89] In contrast, human spinal muscular atrophy produces no axonal spheroids, and thus the canine disease is not an adequate model of human spinal muscular atrophy. In human ALS, anterior horn motor neurons are lost, which does not occur in HCSMA. However, this model is useful in studying the mechanisms of spheroid formation in ALS and the relationship between disease severity and gene dose.[86] The gene responsible for canine spinal muscular atrophy is important for further understanding of the mechanisms involved with spheroid formation.

Equine Motor Neuron Disease

A new MND in the horse has been reported.[80] After a rapidly progressive fatigue, affected horses develop a late-onset, non-hereditary, spontaneous progressive generalized weakness, muscle atrophy, fasciculations, and weight loss. Lower motor neurons show neuronal swelling, chromatolysis, and eosinophilic cytoplasmic inclusions, and positive phosphorylated neurofilament accumulation. These features resemble the pathologic features of ALS. Mohammed and colleagues[80] suspect that the incidence of this equine MND is similar to that of ALS. This model is too new to assess whether it is an adequate model for ALS. Further characterization of the disease is important.

EXPERIMENTALLY INDUCED MODELS

Neurotoxic Models

One hypothesis that may explain the pathogenesis of ALS is that the disease is caused by neurotoxin exposure. Various neurotoxins have been given to animals as probes to analyze specific neuronal metabolic and morphologic changes.[100] Several neurotoxins appear to cause morphologic and functional changes similar to those occurring in ALS. Table 17–3 summarizes the primary advantages and disadvantages of toxic models of ALS.

EXCITOTOXINS

A neurotoxicity caused by glutamate or other excitotoxic agents may be associated with ALS (see Chapter 12). Spencer and colleagues[97] in 1987 reported that they produced a neurotoxicity in primates by feeding them a large amount of cycad constituent, beta-methylamino-1-alanine, an *N*-methyl-D-aspartate receptor agonist. Clinically, the animals had corticospinal dysfunction, parkinsonian features, behavioral abnormalities, and histologic evidence of chromatolysis and degeneration in anterior horn cells. This primate model rekindled great interest in excitotoxin as the cause of Guamanian ALS, but several careful epidemiologic and neurotoxicity studies failed to support this excitotoxin as a model for Guamanian ALS.[25,26] Thus, the significance of cycad neurotoxin is diminished for the investigation of ALS. On the other hand, a similar neurotoxin, beta-

Table 17–3. **SUMMARY OF NEUROTOXIC ANIMAL MODELS OF ALS**

Neurotoxin	ALS-like Changes	Mechanism	Disadvantages as a Model for ALS
BMAA	Chromatolytic changes	NMDA agonist	Not supported by epidemiology
BOAA	Chronic spastic paraparesis	Quisqualate agonist	No lower motor neuron signs
IDPN	Axonal swelling	Axonal transport impairment	Nonselective, no motor neuron loss
Aluminum	Axonal swelling	Impaired axonal transport?	Nonselective
Doxorubicin	Neuronal denervation	Suicide retrograde transport	Nonselective

Abbreviations: BMAA = beta-methylamino-l-alanine, BOAA = beta-oxalylamino-l-alanine, IDPN = β, β′-iminodipropionitrile, NMDA = N-methyl-D-aspartate.

oxalylamino-1-alanine, which is found in *Lathyrus sativus* (chickling pea) and is a quisqualate-sensitive glutamate agonist, produces clinical and electrophysiologic evidence of corticospinal deficits in primates after long-term ingestion.[96] This animal model is unusual because signs are only seen in the upper motor neurons.[40] It is useful for studying the lathyrism that occurred in concentration camps during World War II and for investigating the relationship between excitotoxin and upper motor neuron dysfunction. It may be an important model for ALS because few animal models demonstrate upper motor neuron involvement.

β, β′-IMINODIPROPIONITRILE

β, β′-iminodipropionitrile (IDPN) causes hyperactivity characterized by the "waltzing" (continuous circling and head rolling) syndrome and progressive paralysis in rats.[12–14] Histologically, it causes proximal axonal swelling in many different neurons, including motor neurons, red nuclei, vestibular nuclei, cerebellar nuclei, and dorsal root ganglion cells. IDPN interferes with slow axonal transport, resulting in proximal axonal swelling, distal axonal atrophy, and secondary demyelination. The proximal axonal swelling resembles that seen in the proximal segments of motor axons in ALS. Thus, this model is important for studying the relationship between impaired slow axonal transport and axonal swelling.[34] However, evidence is not convincing that the number of motor neurons decreases, as occurs in ALS. Furthermore, many neurons other than the mo-

tor neurons are similarly affected. Thus, this model is not ideal for studying ALS.

ALUMINUM

Direct injection of aluminum chloride in the rabbit cisterna magna causes clinically acute encephalopathy and histologic neurofibrillary changes in perikaryal and neuronal processes.[7,102] Impaired axonal transport is associated with accumulation of neurofilaments and axonal swelling.[7] Chronic repeated injection results in signs of chronic myelopathy and widespread argentophilic inclusions in cell bodies and axons that morphologically resemble those found in ALS.[99,100] Accumulated neurofilaments are either phosphorylated or nonphosphorylated. Ubiquitin-positive skein inclusions occur as well. These pathologic changes are located in spinal cord motor neurons and are diffusely distributed in nonmotor neurons in the brain stem. The distribution of affected neurons in the rabbit brain stem perhaps represents "upper motor neuron involvement" in this animal. Recent studies further show that aluminum inhibits the normal dephosphorylation-dependent reversal of neurofilament heavy molecules that are associated with cross-linkage with microtubules. This model offers an intriguing opportunity to study posttranslational abnormalities of neurofilament processing and impaired slow axonal transport, which may occur in ALS.[102]

SUICIDE TRANSPORT

A large dose of doxorubicin can cause toxic sensory neuropathy because dorsal root ganglion cells, which have no blood-nerve barrier, can be affected. In contrast, motor neurons, which are protected by the blood-brain barrier, are spared. When doxorubicin is injected directly into the intraneural space of peripheral nerves, however, motor neurons undergo subacute degeneration. Doxorubicin is transported retrogradely to motor neurons, where it interferes with DNA processing. This transport is called *suicide* or *lethal retrograde transport*.[29,109] This model provides an interesting paradigm for studying a potential route by which neurotoxins (including viral particles) might be taken up from motor axon terminals and transported to motor neuron cell bodies, resulting in motor neuron degeneration. Lectin, when similarly injected into the peripheral nerves, causes motor neuron degeneration.[110] In these models, however, dorsal root ganglion cells are affected, which does not occur in ALS. In ALS, the suicide transport model is useful for testing the hypothesis that the motor axon terminal may be a port of entry for neurotoxins.

LOW-CALCIUM DIET

Long-term epidemiologic studies indicate that environmental factors have a causative role in the high incidence of ALS and parkinsonism-dementia complex in the Western Pacific[111] (Chapter 16). Low concentrations of calcium and magnesium, combined with high levels of aluminum in the soil and drinking water, have been suspected as a potential cause. On the other hand, the accumulation of calcium, aluminum, and silicon in motor neurons and neurofibrillary-tangle-bearing neurons also suggests that minerals are abnormally metabolized in the brain in the Guamanian ALS-parkinsonism-dementia complex. Juvenile primates fed a low-calcium diet with or without supplemental aluminum and magnesium showed no abnormal behavior but had neuropathologic findings suggestive of those seen in Guamanian ALS, including chromatolysis, accumulation of phosphorylated neurofilaments, neurofibrillary tangles, axonal spheroids, and other inclusion bodies.[33] This primate model may reproduce neuropathologic features of ALS, perhaps supporting the environmental hypothesis for Guamanian ALS.

Viral Models

As discussed in Chapter 14, virus infection has been one of the oldest hypotheses to explain the cause of ALS because poliomyelitis has been known for so many years to induce acute and chronic MND. Researchers have used experimental viral infections to attempt to produce disease in laboratory animals that mimics ALS.

POLIOMYELITIS VIRUS

A persistent poliomyelitis infection occurs when polio virus is directly inoculated into the mouse brain.[67] Another model is produced by direct intracerebral inoculation of diluted poliomyelitis virus after immunosuppression with cyclophosphamide.[45] These models require direct inoculation to the brain and always show lymphocytic infiltration when the disease develops. However, if persistent poliomyelitis infection can cause an ALS-like syndrome, experimental techniques have yet to successfully reproduce a clinical syndrome resembling ALS (see Chapter 14).

MURINE RETROVIRUS

Gardner and colleagues[32] reported a mouse disease causing both hindlimb paralysis and leukemia in the wild mouse; a retrovirus, originally called type C RNA leukemia virus, was the cause. Since then, several similar strains of laboratory-derived murine retroviruses have been identified, and the gene responsible for the neurotropic infection, leukemia, and disease virulence is now clearly mapped.[43] As seen in the wild mouse hindlimb paralysis, only neonatal mice are susceptible to this virus, and older mice become immune. Neonatal mice inoculated with murine retrovirus develop hindlimb paralysis within 4 weeks of inoculation. A marked spongy degeneration occurs in endothelial and glial cells but not in neurons. Virion budding is found at the granular and agranular endoplasmic reticulum.[3] Inflammation is not seen. Neuronal degeneration appears to be indirect and not the result of neuron infection (the viral infection perhaps blocks neurotrophic receptor sites).[105] This model provides an intriguing paradigm for the investigation of retrovirus infection, immune response, and the mechanism of viral neurotropism, but it cannot be considered to be useful for ALS because its pathology differs.

Autoimmune Models

Various humoral and cellular abnormalities in the immune system have been reported extensively in patients with ALS (see Chapter 13). An approach to test the autoimmune hypothesis is to produce experimental models. Engelhardt and Joo[28] successfully demonstrated that guinea pigs immunized with isolated pig motor neurons developed autoimmune MND. Later, Engelhardt and Appel[27] developed an experimental allergic motor neuron disease (EAMND). Isolated bovine motor neurons are inoculated monthly with Freund's adjuvant for 4 months. More than half the guinea pigs immunized against bovine motor neurons develop weight loss, sluggish movement, limb weakness, and footdrop. Electromyography shows a decreased number of firing motor units, but not fibrillation potentials. Pathologic studies show group atrophy and fiber-type grouping, consistent with chronic neurogenic muscle atrophy. Anterior horn cell loss and neuronophagia are seen in the spinal cord. Motor neuron cell depletion is greater in symptomatic than in asymptomatic guinea pigs. Immunohistochemical studies reveal that anterior horn motor neurons stain heavily for guinea pig immunoglobulin G (IgG) in both symptomatic and asymptomatic animals. Abnormal immunostaining against guinea pig IgG also is found at the neuromuscular junction. The serum IgG antibody reacts against only bovine motor neurons and increases markedly after the second antigen injection. In this autoimmune model, researchers suspect that IgG reacts in vivo at the motor axon terminal, neuromuscular junction, or both, and then is transported to the motor neuron cell body in the spinal cord.[95] In contrast to the EAMND model, guinea pigs inoculated with spinal cord gray matter develop more acute and severe paralyzing disease, which is characterized by extensive neuronal damage and lymphocytic inflammatory reactions. Intraneuronal IgG deposits are found not only in anterior horn motor neurons but also in pyramidal motor neurons. This experimental model is termed experimental allergic gray matter disease (EAGMD).

Mice injected with sera or IgG obtained from guinea pigs with EAMND or EAGMD have greater miniature endplate potentials, which suggests that passively transferred IgG alters the physiologic properties of the presynaptic axon terminals, such that acetylcholine release increases.[5] Therefore, the disease process in EAMND and EAGMD appears to be passively transferred. These experiments support the idea that EAMND and EAGMD are true autoimmune disorders.[95] Whether these autoimmune models represent features in ALS is quite uncertain because the autoimmune hypothesis of ALS has been meagerly supported (see Chapter 13).

TRANSGENIC MODELS

Transgenic mice are genetically engineered mice born with multiple copies of a newly introduced gene that is to be tested, along with its promoter, so that the animals express excessive gene products in their cells. These transgenes can be either normal or mutated genes derived from the same or different species. The phenotypic effects of the overproduction of the specific gene product are investigated in the mutant mice. The recent discovery of *SOD1*-linked familial ALS (FALS) (see Chapter 10) has opened a series of new animal models for the investigation of ALS.

Mutated Human Superoxide Dismutase Expression

Gurney and colleagues[36] have produced a transgenic mouse that expresses a human Cu, Zn superoxide dismutase 1 (*SOD1*) mutation found in some patients with FALS.[88] Mice that express mutated human *SOD1* in which alanine is substituted for glycine 93 develop hindlimb weakness, coarse coats that suggest poor grooming, and a shorter stride at 3 to 4 months of age. The disease rapidly progresses, and the mice become moribund at 5 months of age. Mutated SOD is expressed in a large quantity in the brain. Pathologic analysis shows a loss of choline acetyltransferase immunoreactive anterior horn cells. Anterior horn cells contain an increased amount of mutated SOD and also neurofibrillary material probably consisting of phosphorylated neurofilaments. Vacuolar degeneration is marked in axon terminals and dendrites. The vacuoles appear to develop in the mitochondria.[22] Upper motor neurons also are involved. Myelinated axons are severely diminished at the ventral root but relatively spared at the dorsal root. A "butterfly" lesion in the posterior column, which is found in the spinal cord in FALS, is also found in these transgenic mice. In the skeletal muscles, the number of intramuscular myelinated fibers is reduced, but active reinnervation is present.

In these transgenic mice, only one of the several identical transgenic mouse lines develop MND. A valine substitution for alanine 4 is the most common SOD1 mutation in FALS. When this mutation is expressed in transgenic mice, MND did not develop while the animals were observed up to age 3 to 4 months. However, transgenic mice having a glycine 93 to alanine substitution (the second most common SOD1 mutation in FALS) developed MND before 3 to 4 months of age.[36]

Similar transgenic mice have been produced to express different types of mutated human SOD1 found in FALS.[87] These transgenic mice have motor neuron degeneration similar to that found in other SOD1 transgenic mice, but SOD1 activity is not reduced in any tissue, suggesting that an SOD1 mutation may be viewed as a "gain of toxic function" rather than "loss of function" mutation. Wiedau-Pazos and colleagues[107] have recently demonstrated that excessive hydroxy radical production is triggered by the mutated SOD1 enzyme, resulting in "gain of toxic function" neuronal injury in SOD1 mutation.

Transgenic mice expressing the mutated SOD1 gene may provide some of the most exciting information in future human ALS research. Although knowledge from the SOD1 transgenic mouse model may be relevant only to a small proportion of those with ALS (approximately 2% of all ALS patients), this appears to be the first true animal model of ALS because the cause of ALS is transferred to another animal. This animal model offers the opportunity to study the mechanism of how free radical toxicity or how the gain of toxic function mutation in SOD1 causes motor neuron degeneration.[10,86] The answers will be enormously useful for the further understanding of cell death mechanism in both FALS and sporadic ALS (see Chapter 12).

On the other hand, how the gene is regulated in the natural disease and whether the overexpression of mutated SOD1 gene product in transgenic mice truly represents the natural disease condition occurring in ALS are valid questions. We need to know whether analogous phenotypic differences exist between humans and small rodents with the identical genotypic abnormality. More investigations are required to characterize MND in these transgenic mice. Furthermore, preclinical trials with this model should provide important information for treatment of FALS.[35]

Human Heavy Neurofilament Gene Overexpression

Transgenic mice overexpressing the human heavy neurofilament (NF-H) gene develop progressive neuronopathy characterized by tremor, abnormal hindlimb flexion when held suspended, and progressive gait abnormality.[20] Histologically, neurofilamentous swellings develop primarily in the large motor neuron cell bodies and their proximal axons but also occur in dorsal root ganglion cells. Slow axonal transport is significantly disrupted because of an abnormal accumulation of mitochondria in the perikaryon and a relative absence of mitochondria distally. The shortage of mitochondria in axons likely causes a severe energy deficiency that results in further nerve dysfunction.[15] When survival extends beyond 1 year of age, progressive degeneration and loss of spinal cord motor neurons and ventral root axons are seen.[46] Skeletal muscles undergo denervation atrophy. This NF-H transgenic mouse may be another important model of ALS because the neurofilamentous and axon transport abnormalities are essential features of motor neuron dysfunction in ALS.[46] Furthermore, the late onset of these degenerative changes in NF-H transgenic mice reflects the adult onset of ALS. An abnormal expansion of three amino-acid sequences, in the c-terminal region of the NF-H subunit, has been reported in five patients with sporadic ALS.[31] This particular mutation in patients with ALS must be widely confirmed, however.

Murine Light Neurofilament Gene Overexpression

Transgenic mice having proline instead of leucine in codon 394 of the light neurofilament (NF-L) gene develop progressive upper and lower limb weakness beginning at 2 to 3 weeks of age.[59,108] Severity of disease and time of death depend on the amount of abnormal transgene accumulation; death usually occurs between 3 weeks and 5 months of age. The number of large, but not small or medium, spinal cord motor neurons decreases, and the remaining neurons often are filled with neurofilaments, including phosphorylated neurofilaments. Proximal axonal swellings (resembling spheroids seen in ALS) containing neurofilaments also are found in the ventral roots. Axonal degeneration is prominent, with accompanying neurogenic atrophy of skeletal muscle. Degeneration of descending fibers in the ventral and dorsolateral funiculi of the spinal cord implies an upper motor neuron pathology, although cortical regions reportedly are unremarkable. Although dorsal root ganglion sensory neurons and proximal axons contain modest accumulations of neurofilament, no neuronal loss is seen. These findings raise the intriguing possibility that, like the NF-H gene, aberrations of the NF-L gene are responsible for the neuronal pathology in ALS as well.

GENE KNOCKOUT MODELS

In contrast to transgenic mice, *gene knockout* (null mutation) mice are genetically engineered to delete a specific gene so that animals are born without the products normally produced by the gene. Investigators specifically analyze the effects of the lack of gene products to specifically identify the biologic significance of the gene product. Masu and colleagues[62] recently produced mice in

which the gene for ciliary neurotrophic factor (CNTF) was disrupted (CNTF−/−). Four-week-old mutant animals have no morphologic abnormalities in the lumbar spinal cord motor neurons compared to normal mice (CNTF+/+). The expression of the CNTF gene therefore is not necessary for the development of morphologically normal spinal cord motor neurons. However, beginning at 8 weeks of age, CNTF−/− mice have progressive degeneration and loss of motor neurons in the spinal cord and facial nerve nucleus. These changes are clinically apparent by 7 months, although only a 22% reduction of facial motor neurons is seen in mutant animals. A mild but statistically significant muscle weakness can be detected in the forelimbs at this time. These findings indicate that CNTF is essential for normal maintenance and survival of motor neurons in the postnatal period. Whether pathology occurs in the cortex or outside the motor system is unknown.[62] This model may have relevance to human MNDs because recent studies reveal that CNTF is decreased in the spinal cord anterior horns of ALS patients.[1] However, the issues involved with absent CNTF are complicated. Chapter 15 reviews such issues in detail, along with the effects of other gene knockouts.

PRECLINICAL THERAPEUTIC TRIALS

The development of new therapeutic agents begins first in in vitro studies and then proceeds to the preclinical studies, which include in vivo toxicity and pharmacodynamic studies and preclinical trials in experimental animal models (see Chapter 20). In ALS, animal models are not readily available for preclinical trials. The animal model MND in which the preclinical trial is performed should have features seen in ALS, and moreover, its clinical and pathologic features must be thoroughly investigated so that the effects of a therapy can be objectively and quantitatively assessed. Furthermore, a sufficiently large number of affected animals must be available for a reasonably short period. To satisfy these requirements, only a few murine models are available. Although mnd and pmn mice have been used for preclinical

Table 17–4. **SEMIQUANTITATIVE AND QUANTITATIVE ASSESSMENT TECHNIQUES IN WOBBLER MOUSE MOTOR NEURON DISEASE**

General condition
  Body weight
Semiquantitative assessment
  Paw posture abnormalities
  Walking pattern abnormalities
Quantitative assessment
  Grip strength
  Running speed
  Resting locomotion activity
In vivo biceps muscle twitch tension*
Histometric studies*
  Motor neuron
  Cervical ventral root myelinated axons
  Biceps muscle
  Terminal sprouting

*These tests are performed at the end of the study.

studies in a limited degree,[39,90,93] wobbler mice have been far more extensively investigated. Transgenic *SOD1* mice have only recently become available for preclinical testing.[35]

The advantage in using the wobbler mouse model for preclinical trials is that the clinical and histologic features of this MND are well-defined.[56] Semiquantitative and quantitative assessment techniques also have been devised[51,75] (Table 17–4). The effects of biologic agents on motor neurons and skeletal muscles can be tested with histometric analyses at the end of the study. Figure 17–1 illustrates the paw posture abnormalities and the changes during the natural disease course. The paw posture abnormalities, grip strength, and running speed are also assessed in relation to disease progression (Fig. 17–2).

Using these evaluation techniques, several biologic agents have been tested extensively in preclinical trials.[41,42,51,54,56,75,76] Figure 17–3 illustrates how the clinical course of wobbler mouse MND is altered with a treatment intervention using CNTF or brain-derived neurotrophic factor. The results are interesting and provide encouraging data to support future clinical trials. However, it should be remembered that wobbler mouse MND is not a true animal model of ALS and thus results from these animal studies cannot anticipate the results of clinical trials in patients with ALS.

SUMMARY

This chapter reviewed major categories of animal models of MND and ALS: the naturally occurring, experimentally induced, transgenic, and gene knockout models. Preclinical therapeutic trials were briefly discussed.

No naturally occurring model of MND is entirely adequate as a model for ALS. In the murine mnd model, which likely represents neuronal ceroid lipofuscinosis, a late-onset gait abnormality develops but without skeletal muscle atrophy. In a newly recognized model, mnd2, mice develop rapidly fatal motor paralysis. Mice with pmn develop an early-onset rapidly fatal paralysis; the neuronal degeneration may be a dying back axonopathy. In the wobbler model, mice develop an early-onset progressive paralysis, predominantly in the forelimb muscles. Motor neurons undergo vacuolar degeneration and are depleted progressively. Extensive investigations have analyzed mechanisms of motor neuron generation, regeneration, and selective vulnerability of MND. Only one well-established canine model exists, hereditary canine spinal muscular atrophy; progressive lower motor neuron involvement occurs, with the severity depending on the gene dose. Axonal spheroids are a hallmark of this MND, but the number of motor neurons is not reduced. The newly identified equine

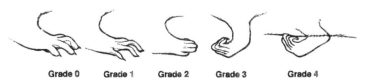

Figure 17–1. Paw position abnormality grading: 0 = normal; 1 = paw atrophy; 2 = curled digits; 3 = curled wrists; and 4 = forelimb flexion contracture.

Grade 0   Grade 1   Grade 2   Grade 3   Grade 4

NATURAL HISTORY OF WOBBLER MOUSE MND

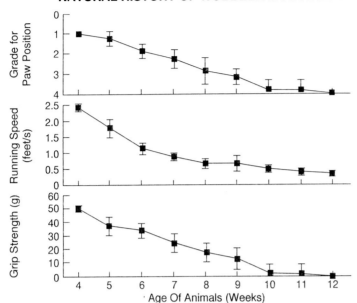

Figure 17–2. Motor neuron disease of the wobbler mouse is clinically diagnosed at the age of 3 to 4 weeks, when paw position abnormality is found to be grade 1. The mean paw position abnormalities of all examined animals at each week are shown in the top graph. The natural history of this motor neuron disease is quantitatively assessed with measurements of running speed and grip strength. Steady decline of motor function is evident.

MND appears to resemble ALS in its incidence and pathology. Identifying the responsible genes in these natural models is crucial to understanding the mechanisms of motor neuron degeneration.

Experimentally induced models of ALS are based on hypotheses of ALS pathogenesis. Potential neurotoxins include glutamate agonists that cause excitotoxic injury on motor neurons; β, β'-iminodipropionitrile and aluminum, which produce neurofilamentous abnormality and axonal swelling; retrograde transport of doxorubicin to neuronal cell bodies; and a diet low in calcium, which

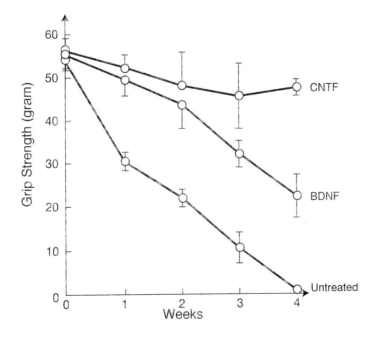

Figure 17–3. Subcutaneous administrations of CNTF (1 mg/day, 6/week) sustain grip strength over 4 weeks. BDNF (5 mg/kg) injections provide benefits but less than CNTF. Compare a steady decline of grip strength in vehicle-treated animals over 4 weeks.

causes neurofilamentous abnormalities. All models have at least one specific feature of ALS pathology, but none have many of the features. Experimental viral infection and autoimmune models were also discussed.

The *SOD1* transgenic mouse model can be considered as the only true animal model of ALS because *SOD1* mutations found in FALS are reproduced in these mice. The clinical and pathologic features resemble human ALS. However, more studies are necessary to understand mechanisms of cell degeneration in these transgenic mice. The hypothesis that the NF-H or NF-L subunits are overexpressed in such mice is being tested. In both types of overexpression, neurofilamentous swelling and neuronal loss occur in motor neurons and to some degree in sensory neurons. Molecular biotechnology allows one to study the "pure" effect of a specific protein because a null mutation can be produced so that affected mice develop without a specific protein.

A number of neurotrophic factors and other pharmacologic agents have been tested in animal models in preclinical trials of ALS. Wobbler mice have been most extensively studied for the preclinical trials. In this MND, the natural disease course is well-delineated and quantitative assessment techniques have been developed to objectively evaluate the effects of medications to be tested. Positive results from preclinical trials are promising but need to be interpreted cautiously because wobbler MND is not ALS.

REFERENCES

1. Anand, P, Parrett, A, Martin, J, et al: Regional changes of ciliary neurotrophic factor and nerve growth factor levels in the post mortem spinal cord and cerebral cortex from patients with motor disease. Nature Med 1:168–178, 1995.
2. Andrews, JM: The fine structure of the cervical spinal cord, ventral root, and brachial nerves in the wobbler (wr) mouse. J Neuropathol Exp Neurol 43:12–27, 1975.
3. Andrews, JM and Gardner, MB: Lower motor neuron degeneration associated with type C RNA virus infection in mice: Neuropathological features. J Neuropathol Exp Neurol 33:285–307, 1974.
4. Andrews, JM, Gardner, MB, Wolfgram, FJ, et al: Studies on a murine form of spontaneous lower motor neuron degeneration—the wobbler (wr) mouse. Am J Pathol 76:63–78, 1974.
5. Appel, SH, Engelhardt, JI, Garcia, J, et al: Im-

6. Baulac, M, Rieger, F, and Meininger, V: The loss of motoneurons corresponding to specific muscle in the wobbler mutant mouse. Neurosci Lett 37:99–104, 1983.
7. Bizzi, A, Crane, RC, Autilio-Gambetti, L, et al: Aluminum effect on slow axonal transport: A novel impairment of neurofilament transport. J Neurosci 4:722–731, 1984.
8. Blondet, B, Barlovatz-Meimon, G, Festoff, BW, et al: Plasminogen activators in the neuromuscular system of the wobbler mutant mouse. Brain Res 580:303–310, 1992.
9. Bronson, RT, Lake, BD, Cook, ERC, et al: Motor neuron degeneration of mice is a model of neuronal ceroid lipofuscinosis (Batten's disease). Ann Neurol 33:381–385, 1993.
10. Brown, RH, Jr: Amyotrophic lateral sclerosis: Recent insights from genetics and transgenic mice. Cell 80:687–692, 1995.
11. Campbell, MJ: Ultrastructural observations on the wobbler mouse [abstract]. J Neuropathol Exp Neurol 31:190, 1972.
12. Chou, SM and Hartman, HA: Axonal lesions and waltzing syndrome after IDPN administration in rats. Acta Neuropathol (Berl) 4:428–450, 1964.
13. Chou, SM and Hartman, HA: Electron microscopy of focal neuroaxonal lesions produced by β, β′-iminodipionitrile (IDPN) in rats. Acta Neuropathol (Berl) 4:590–603, 1965.
14. Clark, AW, Griffin, JW, and Price, DL: The axonal pathology in chronic IDPN intoxication. J Neuropathol Exp Neurol 39:42–55, 1980.
15. Collard, J-F, Côté, F, Julien, J-P: Defective axonal transport in a transgenic mouse model of amyotrophic lateral sclerosis. Nature 375:61–64, 1995.
16. Cork, LC, Altschuler, RJ, Zbruha, PJ, et al: Changes in neuronal size and neurotransmitter marker in hereditary canine spinal muscular atrophy. Lab Invest 61:69–76, 1989.
17. Cork, LC, Griffin, JW, Choy, C, et al: Pathology of motor neurons in accelerated hereditary canine spinal muscular atrophy. Lab Invest 46:89–99, 1982.
18. Cork, LC, Griffin, JW, Munnell, JF, et al: Hereditary canine spinal muscular atrophy. J Neuropathol Exp Neurol 38:209–221, 1979.
19. Cork, LC, Struble, G, Gold, BG, et al: Changes in the size of motor axons in hereditary canine spinal muscular atrophy. Lab Invest 61:333–342, 1989.
20. Côté, F, Collard, J-F, and Julien, J-P: Progressive neuronopathy in transgenic mice expressing the human neurofilament heavy gene: A mouse model of amyotrophic lateral sclerosis. Cell 73:35–46, 1993.
21. Court, JA, McCermott, JR, Gibson, AM, et al: Raised thyrotrophin-releasing hormone, pyroglutamylamino peptidase, and proline endopeptidase are present in the spinal cord of wobbler mice but not in human motor neurone disease. J Neurochem 49:1084–1090, 1987.
22. Dal Canto, MC and Gurney, ME: Development of

munoglobulins from animal models of motor neuron disease and from human amyotrophic lateral sclerosis patients passively transfer physiological abnormalities to the neuromuscular junction. Proc Natl Acad Sci U S A 88:647–651, 1991.

central nervous system pathology in a murine transgenic model of human amyotrophic lateral sclerosis. Am J Pathol 6:1271–1279, 1994.

23. Duchen, LW: Motor neuron diseases in man and animals. Invest Cell Pathol 1:249–262, 1978.

24. Duchen, LW and Strich, SJ: An hereditary motor neurone disease with progressive denervation of muscle in the mouse: The mutant "wobbler." J Neurol Neurosurg Psychiatry 31:535–542, 1968.

25. Duncan, MW: β-Methylamino-ʟ-alanine (BMAA) and amyotrophic lateral sclerosis-parkinsonism dementia of the Western Pacific. Ann NY Acad Sci 648:161–168, 1992.

26. Duncan, MW, Kopin, IJ, Garruto, RM, et al: 2-Amino-3 (methylamino)-propionic acid in cycad-derived foods is an unlikely cause of amyotrophic lateral sclerosis/parkinsonism. Lancet 2:631–632, 1988.

27. Engelhardt, JI and Appel, SH: IgG reactivity in the spinal cord and motor cortex in amyotrophic lateral sclerosis. Arch Neurol 47:1210–1216, 1990.

28. Engelhardt, J and Joo, F: An immune-mediated guinea pig model for lower motor neuron disease. J Neuroimmunol 12:279–290, 1986.

29. England, JD, Asbury, AK, Rhee, EK, et al: Lethal retrograde axoplasmic tansport of doxorubicin (Adriamycin) to motor neurons. A toxic motor neuronopathy. Brain 111:915–926, 1988.

30. Falconer, DS: Wobbler (wr). Mouse News Lett 15:23, 1956.

31. Figlewicz, DA, Krizus, A, Martinoli, MG, et al: Variants of the heavy neurofilament subunit are associated with the development of amyotrophic lateral sclerosis. Hum Molec Genet 10:1757–1761, 1994.

32. Gardner, MB, Henderson, BE, Officer, JE, et al: A spontaneous lower motor neuron disease apparently caused by indigenous type-C RNA virus in wild mice. J Natl Cancer Inst 51:1243–1254, 1973.

33. Garruto, RM, Shankar, SK, Yanagihara, R, et al: Low-calcium, high-aluminum diet-induced motor neuron pathology in cynomologus monkeys. Acta Neuropathol 78:210–219, 1989.

34. Griffin, JW, Hoffman, PN, Clark, AW, et al: Slow axonal transport of neurofilament proteins: Impairment by β, β'-iminodipropionitrile administration. Science 202:633–635, 1978.

35. Gurney, ME, Cutting, FB, Zhai, P, et al: Benefit of vitamin E, riluzole, and gabapentine in a transgenic model of familial amyotrophic lateral sclerosis. Ann Neurol 39:147–157, 1996.

36. Gurney, ME, Pu, H, Chiu, AY, et al: Motor neuron degeneration in mice that express a human Cu, Zn superoxide dismutase mutation. Science 264:1772–1775, 1994.

37. Hantaz-Ambroise, D, Blondet, B, Murawsky, M, et al: Abnormal astrocyte differentiation and defective cellular interactions in wobbler mouse spinal cord. J Neurocytol 23:179–192, 1994.

38. Harris, JB and Ward, MR: A comparative study of "denervation" in muscles from mice with inherited progressive neuromuscular disorders. Exp Neurol 42:169–180, 1974.

39. Helgren, ME, Friedman, B, Kennedy, M, et al: Ciliary neurotrophic factor (CNTF) delays motor impairments in the Mnd mouse. A genetic model for

motor neuron disease. Soc Neurosci Abstr 18:618, 1992.

40. Hugon, J, Ludolph, A, Roy, DN, et al: Clinical and electrophysiologic features of pyramidal dysfunction in macaques fed Lathyrus sativus and IDPN. Neurology 38:435–442, 1988.

41. Ikeda, K, Klinkosz, B, Greene, T, et al: Effects of brain-derived neurotrophic factor (BDNF) on motor dysfunction in wobbler mouse motor neuron disease. Ann Neurol 37:505–511, 1995.

42. Ikeda, K, Wong, V, Holmlund, TH, et al: Histometric effects of ciliary neurotrophic factor in wobbler mouse motor neuron disease. Ann Neurol 37:47–54, 1995.

43. Jolicoeur, P: Retrovirus-induced lower motor neuron disease in mice: A model for amyotrophic lateral sclerosis and human spongiform neurological disease. In Hudson, AJ (ed): Amyotrophic Lateral Sclerosis. University of Toronto Press, Toronto, 1990, pp 53–75.

44. Jones, KR, Farinas, I, Backus, C, et al: Targeted disruption of the BDNF gene perturbs brain and sensory neuron development but not motor neuron development. Cell 76:989–999, 1994.

45. Jubelt, B and Meagher, JB: Poliovirus infection of cyclophosphamide-treated mice results in persistence and late paralysis: I. Clinical, pathologic, and immunologic studies. Neurology 34:486–493, 1984.

46. Julien, J-P: A role for neurofilaments in the pathogenesis of amyotrophic lateral sclerosis. Biochem Cell Biol 73:593–597, 1995.

47. Junier, MP, Coulpier, M, LeForestier, N, et al: Transforming growth factor alpha (TGF) expression in degenerating motor neurons of the murine mutant wobbler: A neuronal signal for astrogliosis? J Neurosci 14:4206–4216, 1994.

48. Kaupmann, K, Simon-Chazottes, D, Guénet, J-L, et al: Wobbler, a mutation affecting motoneuron survival and gonadal functions in the mouse, maps to proximal chromosome 11. Genomics 13:39–43, 1992.

49. Klein, R, Smeyne, RJ, Wurst, W, et al: Targeted disruption of trkB neurotrophin receptor gene results in nervous system lesions and neonatal death. Cell 75:113–122, 1993.

50. Kohn, R: Clinical and pathological findings in an unusual infantile motor neuron disease. J Neurol Neurosurg Psychiatry 34:427–431, 1971.

51. Kozachuk, WE, Mitsumoto, H, Salanga, VD, et al: Effects of daily TRH administration in murine motor neuron disease (wobbler mouse). J Neurol Sci 78:253–260, 1987.

52. Krieger, C, Lai, R, Mitsumoto, H, et al: The wobbler mouse: Quantitative autoradiography of glutamatergic ligand binding sites in spinal cord. Neurogeneration 2:9–17, 1993.

53. Krieger, C, Perry, TL, Hansen, S, et al: The wobbler mouse: Amino acid contents in brain and spinal cord. Brain Res 551:142–144, 1991.

54. Krieger, C, Perry, TL, Hanson, S, et al: Excitatory amino acid receptor antagonists in murine motor neuron disease. Can J Neurol Sci 19:462–465, 1992.

55. Laage, S, Zobel, G, and Jockusch, H: Astrocyte overgrowth in the brain stem and spinal cord of

mice affected by spinal atrophy, wobbler. Dev Neurosci 10:190–198, 1988.

56. Lange, DJ, Good, PF, and Bradley, WG: A therapeutic trial of gangliosides and thymosin in the wobbler mouse model of motor neuron disease. J Neurol Sci 61:211–216, 1983.

57. LaVail, JH, Koo, EH, and Dekker, NP: Motoneuron loss in the abducens nucleus of wobbler mice. Brain Res 404:127–132, 1987.

58. LaVail, JH, Koo, EH, and Irons, KP: Abnormal neuromuscular junctions in the lateral rectus muscle of wobbler mice. Brain Res 463:78–89, 1988.

59. Lee, MK, Marszalek, JR, and Cleveland, DW: A mutant neurofilament subunit causes massive selective motor neuron death: Implications for the pathogenesis of human motor neuron disease. Neuron 13:975–988, 1994.

60. Ma, W and Vacca-Galloway, LL: Reduced branching and length of dendrites detected in cervical spinal cord motoneurons of wobbler mouse, a model for inherited motoneuron disease. J Comp Neurol 311:210–222, 1991.

61. Ma, W and Vacca-Galloway, LL: Spiny interneurons identified in the normal mouse spinal cord show alterations in the Wobbler mouse: A model for inherited motoneuron disease. Restorat Neurol Neurosci 4:381–392, 1992.

62. Masu, Y, Wolf, E, Holtmann, B, et al: Disruption of the CNTF gene results in motor neuron degeneration. Nature 365:27–32, 1993.

63. Mazurkiewica, JE: Ubiquitin deposits are present in spinal motor neurons in all states of the disease in the motor neuron degenerations. Neurosci Lett 128:182–186, 1991.

64. McQuarrie, IG: Axonal transport and the regenerating nerve. In Seil, FJ (ed): Neural Regeneration and Transplantation. Liss, New York, pp 29–42, 1989.

65. Messer, A and Flaherty L: Autosomal dominance in a late-onset motor neuron disease in the mouse. J Neurogenet 3:345–355, 1986.

66. Messer, A, Strominger, NL, and Mazurkiewicz, JE: Histopathology of the late-onset motor neuron degeneration (Mnd) mutant in the mouse. J Neurogenet 4:201–213, 1987.

67. Miller, JR: Prolonged intracerebral infection with poliovirus in asymptomatic mice. Ann Neurol 9:590–596, 1981.

68. Mitsumoto, H: Axonal regeneration in murine motor neuron disease. Muscle Nerve 8:44–51, 1985.

69. Mitsumoto, H: Study of motor neuron disease. An approach with an animal model (the wobbler mouse). In Daroff, RB and Conomy, JP (eds): Contributions to Contemporary Neurology: A Tribute to Joseph M. Foley, M.D. Butterworth, Stoneham, 1988, pp 127–142.

70. Mitsumoto, H and Boggs, AL: Vacuolated anterior horn cells in wobbler mouse motor neuron disease: Peripheral axons and regenerative capacity. J Neuropathol Exp Neurol 46:214–222, 1987.

71. Mitsumoto, H and Bradley, WG: The murine motor neuron disease (the wobbler mouse): Degeneration and regeneration of the lower motor neuron. Brain 105:811–834, 1982.

72. Mitsumoto, H and Bradley, WG: Axonal pathology in the murine motor neuron disease. In Adachi, M,

Mirano, A, and Aronson, G (eds): Current Trends in Neuroscience, Vol 3. Igaku-Shoin Med, Tokyo, 1985, pp. 126–149.

73. Mitsumoto, H, Ferut, AL, Kurahasi, K, et al: Impairment of retrograde axonal transport in wobbler mouse motor neuron disease. Muscle Nerve 13:121–126, 1990.

74. Mitsumoto, H and Gambetti, P: Impaired slow axonal transport in wobbler mouse motor neuron disease. Ann Neurol 19:64–68, 1986.

75. Mitsumoto, H, Ikeda, K, Holmlund, T, et al: The effects of ciliary neurotrophic factor in wobbler mouse motor neuron disease. Ann Neurol 6:142–148, 1994.

76. Mitsumoto, H, Ikeda, K, Klinlosz, B, et al: Arrest of motor neuron disease in wobbler mice cotreated with CNTF and BDNF. Science 265:1107–1110, 1994.

77. Mitsumoto, H, Kurahashi, K, Jacob, JM, et al: Retardation of fast axonal transport in wobbler mice. Muscle Nerve 16:542–547, 1993.

78. Mitsumoto, H, McQuarrie, IG, Karuhashi, K, et al: Histometric and functional characteristics in the subclinical system of wobbler mouse motor neuron disease. Brain 113:497–508, 1990.

79. Mitsumoto, H and Pioro, EP: Animal models of ALS. In Serratrice, G and Munsat, TL (eds): Pathogenesis and Therapy of Amyotrophic Lateral Sclerosis. Lippincott-Raven Press, Philadelphia, 1996, pp 73–87.

80. Mohammed, HO, Cummings, JF, Divers, TJ, et al: Risk factors associated with equine motor neuron disease. Neurology 43:966–971, 1993.

81. Murakami, T, Mastaglia, FL, and Bradley, WG: Reduced protein synthesis in spinal anterior horn neurons in wobbler mouse mutant. Exp Neurol 67:423–432, 1980.

82. Murakami, T, Mastaglia, FL, Mann, DM, et al: Abnormal RNA metabolism in spinal motor neurons in the wobbler mouse. Muscle Nerve 4:407–412, 1981.

83. Papapetropoulos, TA and Bradley, WG: Spinal motor neurones in murine muscular dystrophy and spinal muscular atrophy. J Neurol Neurosurg Psychiatry 35:60–65, 1972.

84. Pioro, EP and Mitsumoto, H: Animal models of ALS. Clin Neurosci (in press).

85. Pollin, MM, McHanwell, S, and Slater, CR: Loss of motor neurons from the median nerve motor nucleus of the mutant mouse "wobbler." J Neurocytol 19:29–38, 1990.

86. Price, DL, Cleveland, DW, and Koliatsos VE: Motor neurone disease and animal models. Neurobiol Dis 1:3–11, 1994.

87. Ripps, ME, Huntley, GW, Hof, PR, et al: Transgenic mice expressing an altered murine superoxide dismutase gene provide an animal model of amyotrophic lateral sclerosis. Proc Natl Acad Sci U S A 92:689–693, 1995.

88. Rosen, DR, Siddique, T, Patterson, D, et al: Mutations in Cu/Zn superoxide dismutase gene are associated with familial amyotrophic lateral sclerosis. Nature 362:59–62, 1993.

89. Sack, GH, Cork, LC, Morris, JM, et al: Autosomal dominant inheritance of hereditary canine spinal muscular atrophy. Ann Neurol 15:369–373, 1984.

90. Sagot, Y, Tan, SA, Hammang, JP, et al: GDNF slows loss of motorneurons but not axonal degeneration or premature death of pmn/pmn mice. J Neurosci 16:2335–2341, 1996.

91. Schmalbruch, H, Jensen, H-J S, Bjaerg, M, et al: A new mouse mutant with progressive motor neuronopathy. J Neuropathol Exp Neurol 50:192–204, 1991.

92. Sellevis Smitt, PAE, and de Jong, JMBV: Animal models of amyotrophic lateral sclerosis and the spinal muscular atrophies. J Neurol Sci 91:231–258, 1989.

93. Sendtner, M, Schmalbruch, H, Stöckli, KA, et al: Ciliary neurotrophic factor prevents degeneration of motor neurons in mouse mutant progressive motor neuronopathy. Nature 358:502–504, 1992.

94. Sendtner, M, Stöckli, KA, Carroll, P, et al: More on motor neurons. Nature 360:541–542, 1992.

95. Smith, RG, Engelhardt, JI, Tajti, J, et al: Experimental immune-mediated motor neuron diseases: Models for human ALS. Brain Res Bull 30:373–380, 1993.

96. Spencer, PS, Ludolph, A, Dwivedi, MP, et al: Lathyrism: Evidence for role of the neuroexcitatory amino acids BOAA. Lancet 2:1066–1077, 1986.

97. Spencer, PS, Nunn, PB, Hugon, J, et al: Guam amyotrophic lateral sclerosis-parkinsonism dementia linked to a plant excitant neurotoxin. Science 237:517–522, 1987.

98. Spencer, PS and Schaumburg, HH: Classification of neurotoxic disease: A morphological approach. In Spencer, PS and Schaumburg, HH (eds): Experimental and Clinical Neurotoxicology. Williams & Wilkins, Baltimore, 1981, pp 92–101.

99. Strong, MJ and Garruto, RM: Chronic aluminum-induced motor neuron degeneration: Clinical, neuropathological and molecular biological aspects. Can J Neurol Sci 18:428–431, 1991.

100. Strong, MJ and Garruto, RM: Experimental paradigms of motor neuron degeneration. In Woodruff, ML and Nonneman, AJ (eds): Toxin-Induced Models of Neurological Disorders. Plenum Press, New York, 1994, pp 39–88.

101. Tang, F, Cheung, A, and Vacca-Galloway, LL: Measurement of neuropeptides in the brain and spinal cord of wobbler mouse: A model for motoneuron disease. Brain Res 518:329–333, 1990.

102. Troncoso, JC, Price, DL, Griffin, JW, et al: Neurofibrillary axonal pathology in aluminum intoxication. Ann Neurol 12:278–283, 1982.

103. Vacca-Galloway, LL and Steinberger, CC: Substance P neurons sprout in the cervical spinal cord of the wobbler mouse: A model for motorneuron disease. J Neurosci Res 16:657–670, 1986.

104. Vrbová, G, Greensmith, L, and Sleradzan, K: Motor neuron disease model. Nature 358:502–504, 1992.

105. Westarp, ME, Westphal, KP, Clausen, J, et al: Retroviral interference with neuronotrophic signalling in human motor neuron disease? Clin Physiol Biochem 10:1–7, 1993.

106. Wichmann, H, Jockusch, H, Guénet, J-L, et al: The mouse homolog to the ras-related yeast YPT1 maps on chromosome 11 close to the wobbler (wr) locus. Mamm Genome 3:467–468, 1992.

107. Wiedau-Pazos, M, Goto, JJ, Rabizadeh, S, et al: Altered reactivity of superoxide dismutase in familial amyotrophic lateral sclerosis. Science 271:515–518, 1996.

108. Xu, Z, Cork, LC, Griffin, JW, et al: Increased expression of neurofilament subunit NF-L produces morphological alterations that resemble the pathology of human motor neuron disease. Cell 73:23–33, 1993.

109. Yamamoto, T, Iwasaki, Y, and Konno, H: Retrograde axoplasmic transport of adriamycin. Neurology 34:1299–1304, 1984.

110. Yamamoto, T, Iwasaki, Y, Konno, H, et al: Primary degeneration of motor neurons by toxic lectins conveyed from the peripheral nerve. J Neurol Sci 70:327–337, 1985.

111. Yase, Y: Metal metabolism in motor neuron disease. In Chen, K-M and Yase, Y (eds): Amyotrophic Lateral Sclerosis in Asia and Oceania. National Taiwan University Press, Taipei, 1984, pp 337–356.

PART 4

Treatment and Management

CHAPTER 18

COMPREHENSIVE CARE

The care of patients with ALS is especially challenging and differs from the care of patients with other neurodegenerative disorders because the disease progresses rapidly and is terminal; its course is predictably short in most cases; patients maintain normal intelligence; and to date, no treatment is effective. Special skills and experience are re-quired for effective care.[8] Caring for ALS patients requires a holistic approach. As Thompson[20] states, "ALS requires a commitment on the part of the patient, family, and health care providers to collaborate in a way that can bring meaning and hope to circumstances that make no sense, and a sense of wholeness in the face of relentless physical disintegration."

Those who provide health care to patients with ALS need to combine their resources creatively to continue care from diagnosis to death. In this chapter, we review how the diagnosis of ALS should be presented to patients and their families and outline the general principles of ALS care. Sexuality and unconventional or unorthodox treatments, issues that are often neglected, are reviewed. We also discuss the benefits of four independent resources that are used in combination: the ALS clinic, home care, alternate care sites, and hospice care. Close communication between these resources is necessary for effective management.

PRESENTING THE DIAGNOSIS

According to Beisecker and colleagues,[1] patients with ALS want physicians to be straightforward and honest but not premature in their diagnosis, to be sensitive to patients' desire for information, and to convey some degree of hope. Addressing these desires when presenting the diagnosis of ALS can be crucial in establishing a good physician-patient relationship. A good relationship is especially important because the diagnosing physician may treat the patient for several years or longer.

When the disease is advanced and clearly manifested, experienced neurologists often suspect the diagnosis of motor neuron disease or ALS while taking the history and need only verify their clinical impression by examining the patient. However, even when the diagnosis is quite evident, the neurologist should order ancillary tests to exclude other conditions[2] and should explain why the tests are necessary. A thorough, if not exhaustive, differential diagnosis is essential when such a devastating disease is suspected, not only because the physician must define the disease medically and detect treatable conditions but also because patients must be prepared for the diagnosis.[3] This diagnostic process is an important factor in presenting the diagnosis and in how the patient reacts. If the physician gives the diagnosis immediately after the examination and before reviewing test results, the patient may wonder whether the diagnosis has been reached prematurely. Further, if the physician states that nothing can be done, the patient may feel that the physician is abandoning him or her. In contrast, if reasons for the tests and the disease process are explained to the patient and family, they may accept the diagnosis with less difficulty. Table 18–1 lists points that should be considered when presenting the diagnosis of ALS to patients and their families.[9]

When neurologists present the diagnosis of ALS, they usually begin by explaining the disease process and then give the diagnosis itself. Patients and their families should be encouraged to ask questions. When questions are invited, the neurologist's responses and explanations are more likely to be accepted. When discussing the prognosis, it is crucial to provide patients with a sense of hope. The neurologist should emphasize that the average duration of ALS is only a statistical determination and that prognosis differs for each individual patient. The prognosis may be better than is described in the literature if a patient has several features associated with a better prognosis (see Chapter 9). Exact estimations of life expectancy for individual patients—a statement like, "You have three years to live"—are almost invariably wrong. Such projections are irresponsible and should never be made. The variability of prognosis and recent advances in the understanding of ALS should be stressed. Additionally, it is important to emphasize the neurologic systems that are spared in ALS.

Nevertheless, physicians who make the diagnosis must be ready to deal with the patient's emotional response, which may range from being overwhelmed emotionally to complete denial. Physicians should not challenge such denial because it is often the patient's defense mechanism. Also, Mulder[9] has pointed out that patients may tend to dislike physicians who present the diagnosis. For this reason, another health-care professional should be involved when the diagnosis is presented. For instance, nurses who specialize in ALS can be highly effective because they can take an approach when discussing the diagnosis that differs from that of the physicians. Goldblatt[5] has suggested a team of two neurologists, one to make the diagnosis and the other to provide care. In many situations, a second opinion is imperative. Pri-

Table 18–1. **SPECIAL CONSIDERATIONS REQURED IN THE DIAGNOSTIC PROCESS AND PRESENTATION OF THE DIAGNOSIS OF ALS**

- Thorough investigation for differential diagnoses
- Involving family and caregivers when presenting the diagnosis
- Sensitive presentation of the diagnosis
- Providing a sense of hope
- Providing information when requested
- Educating patients and families about the disease process and mechanisms
- Obtaining a second opinion
- Discussing clinical trials and research updates

mary neurologists who recommend a second opinion, however, should provide their own opinion of the diagnosis. Some neurologists refer patients who are suspected of having ALS without discussing the possibility of such a diagnosis with them. This lack of discussion unfairly burdens the consulted neurologist, who then must present the diagnosis.

The diagnosis and prognosis are best discussed during an extended meeting scheduled for this purpose—usually during the second appointment, when the test results are discussed. The meeting should not be brief or rushed. Family members and identified caregivers should be involved. If this meeting must occur at another time after discussion of the test results, it should be scheduled generally in a short interval, within a week or two. Such a brief postponement is sometimes beneficial because the patient and family may have time to consider the diagnosis, think of specific questions, and identify potential caregivers. Also, when the diagnosis is given, the patient and family may not be emotionally ready to assimilate large amounts of information. In the meeting, the neurologist should outline what the patient can do and what the ALS team can do. Discussing symptomatic treatment, ALS team care, possible participation in clinical trials, and participation in an ALS support group also provides patients with hope. Thus, the diagnosis, patient care, and disease management should be integrated in this session. Before leaving the meeting, the patient, caregiver, and neurologist should schedule the next appointment, as outlined in the care path (Fig. 18–1).

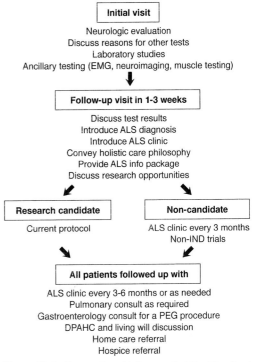

Figure 18–1. Care path guideline used at the Cleveland Clinic ALS Center. DPAHC = durable power of attorney for health care; IND = investigational new drug; PEG = percutaneous endoscopic gastrostomy.

GENERAL PRINCIPLES OF PATIENT CARE

Table 18–2 lists the general principles of caring for patients with ALS. Probably the most important factor for successful care is

Table 18–2. **GENERAL PRINCIPLES OF CARE FOR THE PATIENT WITH ALS**

- Care driven by the patient's decisions
- Thorough understanding of ALS on part of neurologist
- Neurologist strongly committed to care for patients with ALS
- Holistic and team approach at an ALS clinic
- Aggressive symptomatic treatment
- Patient participation in clinical trials
- Effective use of home care and hospice care
- Close communication between patients, caregivers, and health-care providers
- Discussion of patient's advance directives
- Palliative care at the terminal stages

that the patient's care decisions must be central to the overall plan. Care and treatment decisions should not be driven by the desires of the health-care providers or family.

Successful care also requires the neurologist to have strong interest, commitment, and a good understanding of ALS. Although visiting an ALS clinic is advantageous for overall treatment, it is not essential; a neurologist who is committed to caring for these patients can deliver satisfactory care while practicing in a regular office setting. In such a situation, the neurologist can coordinate evaluations by various therapists for comprehensive management. However, a visit to an ALS center is beneficial for both the patient and primary neurologist not only for a second opinion but also for general guidance for ALS patient care. Information on treatment trials and newer medications may be easily available at such centers.

The neurologist must understand the disease thoroughly for a number of reasons. Although prognosis is predictable in most patients, some may live for long periods; rarely, the disease may stabilize or even improve (see Chapter 9). The neurologist must be aware of all such possibilities for prognosis. Also, research activity in ALS is progressing rapidly, and many therapeutic trials are becoming available; the neurologist must keep abreast of such developments. The neurologist must also be able to provide aggressive symptomatic treatment because such treatment reduces patient discomfort (see Chapter 19). As the disease progresses, medications are necessary for respiratory distress, anxiety, insomnia, and pain. The neurologists should be able to discuss alternative, unproven, or unorthodox treatments when necessary. Sexuality is a neglected subject but should not be ignored even in caring for patients with ALS.

A major principle in ALS care is that patients must be followed closely to detect impending problems in nutrition or respiration. When the patient and family have accepted the diagnosis and understand the disease process, the neurologist is responsible for discussing advance directives related to nutritional and respiratory care. Open but sensitive discussion is essential during review of such issues. The patient's decisions must be respected, and to help the patient make decisions, the neurologist must provide all necessary information and answer any questions the patient might have. Appropriate terminal care is of paramount importance for those who decide not to accept any artificial ventilatory support.

THE MULTIDISCIPLINARY ALS CLINIC

The multidisciplinary clinic is not a new concept; it is well established at many muscular dystrophy clinics. Such services also have been developed for patients with ALS at many centers, and the ALS Association and Muscular Dystrophy Association have certified several centers in the United States based on their standards for expertise in diagnosis and management of ALS. The multidisciplinary clinic has several advantages over the regular neurology office setting. Health professionals working at such a center can develop expertise in ALS much faster and in greater depth than therapists elsewhere because of concentrated experience with many ALS patients. Because the ALS clinic uses a team approach, team members will be present at appointments, so the patient's and family's questions and concerns can be answered quickly. Also, the multidisciplinary nature of the ALS clinic enhances patient care. Because the patient's problems often overlap multiple disciplines, they can be best addressed by all therapists involved. The approach to ALS treatment is holistic, and the ALS clinic setting is conducive to such an approach. Finally, patients need not travel from one office to another to see different therapists.

Some shortcomings exist as well. Seeing many therapists in a short time may be exhausting for patients (this is also true for therapists seeing many ALS patients). If a fee is charged for each service provided, the total cost of one ALS clinic visit may be high. Also, the time allocated for appointments with each therapist may be insufficient when patients present with multiple problems, so patients will have to return for further evaluation and treatment.

Table 18–3 lists the services of a typical multidisciplinary ALS clinic. All services are important and ideally should be available at

Table 18–3. **MEMBERS OF THE MULTIDISCIPLINARY ALS CLINIC**

Mandatory On-Site Members	On-Call Members
• Neurologist	• Research nurse coordinator
• Nurse coordinator	• Pulmonologist
• Physical therapist	• Physiatrist
• Occupational therapist	• Gastroenterologist
• Dietitian	• Psychiatrist or psychologist
• Speech pathologist	• Orthotist
• Social worker	• Oral surgeon

the clinic site. One requirement for ALS Association certification is the availability of on-site multidisciplinary services. However, the format of the clinic may vary, depending on the availability of certain services, characteristics of the individual institutions, and the unique nature of each clinic's development. The clinic must be directed by neurologists who have special expertise in ALS and have access to necessary diagnostic laboratories, such as electromyography, neuroradiology, and neuropathology.

The remainder of this section will discuss the roles and responsibilities of the clinic personnel.

Neurologist

The neurologist directs the ALS clinic and is responsible for medical and neurologic investigation to diagnose ALS and to detect underlying or superimposed diseases while patients are followed at the clinic. Neurologists must provide maximum symptomatic treatment (see Chapter 19). They make orders based on recommendations given by the team members and prescribe appropriate equipment and braces. The neurologist should explain the disease, the purposes and side effects of all treatments and medications, progress in ALS research, and proactive treatment plans, such as enteral feeding and noninvasive positive-pressure ventilation (NIPPV). The neurologist's discussions with patients and their families may overlap those of the nurse coordinator and other therapists, but such repetition usually helps patients and families to understand more fully.

Neurologists, along with social workers, also discuss advance directives, ventilatory support, preparation of a living will, and durable power of attorney for health care. Table 18–4 summarizes the responsibilities of neurologists at the ALS clinic.

Nurse Coordinator

The nurse coordinator (Table 18–5) is a key to the successful ALS clinic, having many responsibilities in coordinating the clinic and all health professionals, directing nursing care, coordinating home care or hospice care, and finally functioning as a nurse educator and patient advocate. At the end of the clinic, the nurse coordinator moderates the team conference, discussed later.

An important function of the nurse coordinator is to explain the care path to the patient and family. The patient and family

Table 18–4. **RESPONSIBILITIES OF THE NEUROLOGIST**

- Perform medical and neurologic evaluation.
- Explain the disease.
- Explain treatment modalities.
- Provide maximum symptomatic treatment.
- Make recommendations based on recommendations from the ALS clinic team.
- Discuss research progress.
- Evaluate and explain treatment trials.
- Discuss advance directives.
- Direct the ALS clinic.
- Educate the public about ALS.

Table 18–5. **RESPONSIBILITIES OF THE ALS NURSE COORDINATOR**

- Coordinate the clinic team.
- Explain the disease.
- Provide informative literature.
- Provide emotional and psychological support and discuss advance directives.
- Teach patients how to maximize functional ability and quality of life.
- Assess general medical status, including respiratory and weight status.
- Evaluate current medications.
- Suggest participation in a support group.
- Review care path and suggest changes as the disease progresses.
- Act as a liaison to other therapists and the clinical research team.
- Coordinate alternate-site and home placement.
- Educate home care staff about ALS symptoms.
- Educate the public about ALS.
- Engage in nursing research regarding quality of life and patient satisfaction.
- Act as a patient advocate.

must understand this path so that they will know how, when, and why treatment is given at the clinic; such understanding will help ensure compliance and satisfaction. The patient should receive an information packet that includes ALS literature published by the ALS Association, Muscular Dystrophy Association, or National Institutes of Health; ALS Association chapter and support group information; and the care path. At one of our ALS clinics (Cleveland Clinic Foundation), we individualize the packet by including our own literature, which describes ALS and the disease stage that is appropriate for each patient. The nurse coordinator explains the packet and ensures good communication between patients and families and team members.

Physical Therapist

At the ALS clinic, physical therapists most frequently evaluate lower-extremity muscle strength and motor skills. They develop individualized exercise programs for each patient, and, to maintain existing motor function, they evaluate the need for leg braces (such as the ankle-foot orthosis), neck braces, and wheelchairs. On the basis of the degree of functional impairment, physical therapists also recommend equipment for the home that will ensure patient safety and mobility. Services given by physical therapists are listed in Table 18–6. Chapter 21 describes the physical therapy ALS patients require.

Table 18–6. **RESPONSIBILITIES OF PHYSICAL AND OCCUPATIONAL THERAPISTS**

The Physical Therapist
- Evaluate muscle strength by manual muscle testing.
- Evaluate lower-extremity function and gross mobility skills, such as walking and rising from a chair.
- Teach stretching and flexibility exercises as well as general fitness guidelines.
- Instruct on pain management for periarthritis or other joint pain.
- Recommend bracing (leg braces and neck collars).
- Recommend home equipment (adaptive devices for walking, transferring, or other daily activities, and wheelchairs).

The Occupational Therapist
- Evaluate arm and hand function.
- Evaluate activities of daily living.
- Recommend splinting of extremities.
- Recommend assistive or adaptive devices to improve functional independence.
- Recommend activity modification, energy conservation, and work simplification.

Occupational Therapist

As described in Table 18–6, occupational therapists are concerned particularly with skilled motor function. In the ALS clinic, they evaluate hand and arm function and assess the activities of daily living. Based on the assessment, they give recommendations for splinting and adaptive devices. They also discuss activity modification, energy conservation, and work simplification with the patient (see Chapter 21).

Dietitian

Careful assessment of nutritional status and appropriate recommendations are necessary throughout the disease course and are crucial for patients in whom bulbar dysfunction develops. Table 18–7 outlines the dietitian's key tasks. To follow the patient's nutritional status, the dietitian evaluates the patient's appetite and weight regularly and determines whether the patient is at risk for poor nutrition. The dietitian often works with a speech pathologist to determine the degree of dysphagia and will recommend strategies to modify swallowing and food preparation. Early oral supplementation is important when appetite or weight begins to decline. The dietitian also determines whether enteral feeding is required. For those patients who undergo percutaneous endoscopic gastrostomy (PEG), the dietitian selects an enteral feeding formula based on the patient's daily caloric, protein, and fluid requirements before the procedure, imme-

Table 18–7. **RESPONSIBILITIES OF THE DIETITIAN**

- Assess nutritional status and risks.
- Recommend caloric, protein, and fluid requirements.
- Recommend how to cook and prepare food to facilitate chewing and swallowing.
- Give suggestions for appropriate oral supplementation.
- Educate in swallowing problems and enteral feeding.
- Assess enteral feeding formula and appropriate calories, proteins, and fluid at each enteral feeding.

Table 18–8. **RESPONSIBILITIES OF THE SPEECH PATHOLOGIST**

- Evaluate motor speech and speech intelligibility.
- Clinically evaluate swallowing.
- Perform modified barium-swallow studies.
- Counsel regarding strategies and compensation for communication and swallowing problems.
- Recommend augmentative or alternative communication systems and speech orthoses.

diately afterward, and for the remainder of the disease course. Chapter 24 reviews dietary therapy in detail.

Speech Pathologist

Table 18–8 shows the responsibilities of speech pathologists in evaluating bulbar function in patients with ALS. When office evaluation at the ALS clinic is not sufficient to determine the degree of swallowing impairment, speech pathologists should request a modified barium-swallowing test, which helps to identify less obvious dysfunction and silent aspiration. Speech pathologists work closely with dietitians to recommend effective treatment strategies and compensation for progressive dysphagia. They also counsel patients in regard to augmentative and other communication devices (see Chapter 23).

Social Worker

The social worker assesses health insurance coverage and assists with the application for disability payments, when indicated. Social workers provide referrals for financial resources, community resources, ALS Association chapters, and support groups. Although they evaluate and discuss nonmedical issues with patients and their families, they also often provide emotional and psychological support. When the disease progresses to a stage at which patients require home care or hospice care, the social worker makes the necessary arrangements and applications for patients. In addition, the social worker discusses advance directives, durable power of attorney for health care, and preparation of a living will.

Research Nurse Coordinator

The research nurse coordinator cares for those participating in clinical trials. Research nurse coordinators coordinate appointments for research and ALS clinic visits. Because they establish personal relationships and excellent rapport with patients during clinical trials, research nurses assist the ALS clinic nurse coordinator when research patients visit the ALS clinic. They participate in the team conference at the end of the clinic.

Other Members

PULMONOLOGIST

A pulmonologist usually is not a regular member of the ALS clinic team. However, because respiratory muscle weakness occurs in ALS, impending respiratory impairment may develop, and pulmonary consultation will be necessary. Thus, a pulmonologist should be readily available for consultation, and a close consulting relationship with this pulmonologist should be developed. If impending respiratory distress develops, NIPPV devices should be used when appropriate. For those patients who have decided to undergo permanent ventilatory support, a pulmonary consultation should be obtained long before respiratory distress begins.

In patients without preexisting pulmonary diseases, the forced vital capacity (FVC) should be measured at each clinic visit so that respiratory muscle involvement can be detected early. When the FVC decreases to 60% of normal, a pulmonologist should evaluate the patient, even if he or she has no symptoms of respiratory impairment. The pulmonologist should conduct a full evaluation, treat underlying or superimposed pulmonary diseases, and discuss noninvasive and invasive permanent ventilatory support. For patients who have preexisting pulmonary disease (such as bronchial asthma or chronic obstructive lung disease) or a history of heavy smoking, pulmonary consultation at the early stages of ALS is essential even if the patient has no significant pulmonary symptoms. The pulmonologist should follow these patients carefully, so that impending pulmonary impairment is detected as early as possible. The pulmonologist's role is discussed further in Chapter 22.

PHYSICAL MEDICINE AND REHABILITATION

The physiatrist works directly with physical therapists and occupational therapists to determine specific rehabilitation needs of ALS patients. In some ALS clinics, the physiatrist is a team member who may play a key role.

GASTROENTEROLOGIST

The gastroenterologist is consulted when enteral feeding is necessary, and the patient agrees to undergo PEG. Gastroenterologists evaluate the patient's respiratory status and obtain informed consent for the PEG. The procedure is performed in an outpatient endoscopy suite, and the patient stays overnight for observation. This observation period is particularly important for those who have respiratory symptoms. Both the gastroenterologist and dietitian follow the patient during the immediate postprocedure period. The PEG enteral feeding is discussed further in Chapter 24.

PSYCHIATRIST AND PSYCHOLOGIST

Depression secondary to the disease is highly prevalent in patients with ALS but psychiatric consultation is usually unnecessary, if the depression is properly managed. Severe (suicidal) depression or frank psychosis is rare in these patients but can occur and requires such consultation. Overwhelming catastrophic reaction to the disease, stress-induced adjustment problems, or marital problems stemming from stress may become a serious problem. Psychiatry (or psychology) referral is essential for these patients. In general, all members of the ALS clinic attempt to provide psychosocial support to patients and their families.

ORTHOTIST

The orthotist should be available either within or outside the hospital setting. The ankle-foot orthosis is most frequently used by patients with ALS. For those who develop a relatively restricted paraspinal muscle weakness as manifested by the "drop-head" posture with well-preserved extremity strength, a neck brace is essential. Orthotists and biomechanical engineers may need to work together to design and fabricate a customized neck brace because the commercially available neck braces are disappointingly ineffective (see Chapter 21).

ORAL SURGEON

When patients have predominantly paretic bulbar palsy and velopharyngeal incompetence, a palatal prosthesis (the palatal lift) may significantly improve paretic dysarthria that is caused by air leakage. After evaluation by the speech pathologist, the patient is referred to an oral surgeon, who then fabricates such a prosthesis (see Chapter 23).

The ALS Team Meeting

At the end of each ALS clinic, the team members discuss the patients seen at the clinic. The nurse coordinator facilitates the discussion, and the team reviews the issues and recommendations. The problems and concerns of each patient and family are addressed, and necessary solutions and suggestions are presented. Specific treatment plans, including symptomatic medical treatment, clinical trial participation, necessary consultations, home care, and hospice referral also are discussed. The nurse coordinator records the key points, and the team decides on a treatment plan for each patient, which the nurse then prepares. The nurse or, if necessary, the appropriate individual team members arrange to discuss the recommendations with the patient. Neurologists are asked to write necessary letters to various outside agencies.

This meeting gives the team members the opportunity to discuss patient issues that are of concern to all. Furthermore, unrecognized or innovative ideas and suggestions are frequently raised because of the meeting's collaborative nature. For team members, the meeting can foster camaraderie, provide hope, and boost morale after working with patients afflicted by a devastating disease.

ALTERNATIVE, UNCONVENTIONAL, OR UNORTHODOX TREATMENTS

When patients find they have a rapidly progressive, terminal disease, they naturally begin to explore any treatments that are available. Patients who have ALS are no exception. When Food and Drug Administration–approved clinical trials are available, they participate. However, for some patients, the potential for receiving a placebo control discourages them from entering formal clinical trials, and they instead seek unconventional treatment (Table 18–9). Glasberg[4] has reviewed recent unorthodox treatments reported by patients with ALS.

A snake venom treatment offered by Sanders and Fellows[19] in Florida in the 1970s epitomized a prototypic unorthodox treatment for ALS. Many patients with ALS went to Florida to receive this treatment, at a significant financial cost. Several years passed before Tyler[21] concluded that, based on controlled clinical trials, the snake venom treatment was not effective in ALS.

Yase[22] stated that if ALS is difficult for "western" medicine, it is equally difficult for "oriental" medicine. Treatments including acupuncture and ancient Chinese herbal therapy have not benefitted patients with ALS, with the exception of easing pain in some cases. We do not believe that chiropractic manipulation offers any benefit for ALS. Homeopathic physicians recommend high doses of vitamins and minerals, based on the results of serum vitamin and trace metal levels, but sometimes these treatments cost several hundred dollars a month.

Often patients ask for the physician's opinion about unconventional treatments with which the physician is not familiar. Although neurologists may perceive these treatments as categorically ineffective, they should attempt to obtain information from the available literature, other patients, or voluntary organizations, and even evaluate the data so that they can provide appropriate advice. Our fundamental principle is to "do no harm"; patients should be discouraged from receiving unconventional treatments that have potential side effects, medical risks, unknown risks, and high cost. The patient should be aware of the cost involved in medi-

Table 18–9. UNCONVENTIONAL TREATMENTS*

Treatment	Chief Advocate	Claimed Indications	Comments
Calcium-EAP	Hans Nieper	MS, ALS, cancer, and others	$1,000–2,000 cost
Live cell therapy	Not known; practiced in Philippines	Any diseases including ALS	$13,000 and additional fees for the initial examination, laboratory tests, take-home medications
Interferon/somatomedin	Rajko Medenica	ALS, MS, PD, and others	$2,000 per treatment
Ayurvedic medicine	American Association for Ayurvedic Medicine	Any neurologic diseases	Internal purification, herbs, transcendental meditation
Meditation, wet-cell treatment and massage	William McGarey of the Edgar Cayce Foundation	ALS	
Diet treatment	—	ALS	Aluminum-free diet
Homeopathic Rx	—	Any diseases	Massive vitamins, minerals, and herbs
Allergy injections	—	ALS	Chelating treatment
Chelation Rx	—	Any diseases	Chelating treatments
Psychic healer	Dean Kraft	Any diseases	Vibration from his hands; $250 per session.

*Fuller details of unorthodox treatment are available.[4]
Abbreviations: MS = multiple sclerosis, PD = Parkinson's disease, Rx = therapy.

cally unproven treatments. If patients are asked to pay a substantial amount of money in advance of receiving the treatment, the treatment possibly is fraudulent. Neurologists must be firm in discouraging potentially harmful and costly unorthodox treatments, but tactful and sensitive explanations are essential. Patients may be desperate to try anything, even if the treatments appear unacceptable to the neurologist because they have no obvious benefit and the possibility of at least some risk. When a physician vehemently rejects treatments, patients may feel that they no longer have any chance of becoming better and that the physician is attempting to take away all hope. In such circumstances, patients are not likely to discuss any further alternative treatments with the physician but may obtain such treatments anyway. This behavior may be particularly troublesome when the same patients participate in clinical research trials.

Physicians should be more accepting of the patient's decision to try unconventional treatments when they involve no obvious ma-

jor adverse effects and when the costs are reasonable. Such benign treatments include herbs, fresh air, meditation, yoga, or changing one's habits. The approval of riluzole (Rilutek) as a standard of care for ALS may reduce the likelihood that patients will seek unorthodox or unconventional treatments, but it is unlikely that patients will stop searching for a possible cure, no matter how unconventional or unorthodox. Also, some patients will attempt to buy the hope that physicians cannot offer, regardless of monetary cost.

A 58-year-old woman with ALS who participated in a clinical trial told us that she was spending several hundred dollars a month for "homeopathic treatment." She never came to our ALS clinic because her health-management organization would not pay for the visit. It was disappointing that she was willing to spend so much money for homeopathic treatment but not for a visit to the ALS clinic. We encouraged her to discontinue the homeopathic treatment, but she believed this treatment was her hope for fighting against ALS. As this example illustrates, sometimes patients are determined to try unconventional treatments. Neurologists may need to follow these patients carefully for potential side effects of the treatments. We must continue to discuss the pros and cons of such unproven treatments with the patients and discourage them. Unfortunately, as long as ALS is an incurable disease, unorthodox or unconventional treatments will attract some patients who are desperately seeking a last chance to become well.

SEXUALITY

Sexuality in patients with ALS has seldom been discussed. Because ALS does not affect the autonomic nervous system, sexual function is thought to be well preserved. In patients with ALS, however, various medications used for symptomatic treatment may cause sexual dysfunction. For instance, baclofen (Lioresal) can reduce libido, and the anticholinergic effects of tricyclic antidepressants may cause erectile dysfunction, decreased vaginal lubrication, and decreased clitoral enlargement. Patients with ALS who do not have side effects from medications may still experience problems with sexual function. Muscle weakness, fatigue, spasticity, communication difficulty, respiratory distress, fear, anxiety, and depression may interfere with sexual performance. Furthermore, the loss of a positive body image and self-esteem, losing the affection of one's partner, fear of impotence, loss of interest in sex, and fear that the partner will "look elsewhere" may all be potentially serious issues.[17]

Patients often express the feeling that when everyday survival is an issue, talking about sexuality is not only rather embarrassing but also an inappropriate subject.[18] Pernick[18] twice surveyed patients with ALS and health professionals about sexuality. In 1981, she found that almost no health professionals had discussed ALS and sexuality; in 1988, however, more health professionals were talking about sexuality, although their attitude was essentially the same as that in 1981; many felt that it was not a pressing issue. All the patients and their partners (100%) wanted their diagnosing doctor to discuss the issue, and 75% of them also wanted nurses to discuss it.[18] Health professionals express discomfort with the subject matter, because of inadequate knowledge, insufficient time for meaningful discussion during the clinic visit, and the dismissal of the importance of pleasureful sexual activity.

If one takes a holistic approach to health care, the issue of sexuality must not be ignored. Health professionals may begin the discussion of sexuality directly. One may refer to other patients, saying that "some patients with ALS express concern about continuing to express their sexuality. Do you have any concerns or questions?" Alternatively, the issue can be raised indirectly by providing literature containing information on the issue of sexuality in ALS. The more open the atmosphere, the more comfortable both patients and the health-care professionals will be.

Health-care professionals must understand that patients with ALS who have limited physical ability but normal sexual desire should be able to enjoy sexual intimacy. Health-care professionals can suggest role changes within the partnership, more comfortable positions during intercourse, and other ways to express affection and intimacy, such as mutual masturbation.[17] One of our patients who had moderate respiratory difficulty developed wheezing during sexual intercourse, which frightened both the patient and his spouse and resulted in abstinence. On the next ALS clinic visit, his wife hesitantly expressed her concerns, which led to a frank discussion about the techniques the couple might use to continue a satisfying sexual relationship. We suggested changes in position and the use of an inhaler or bronchodilator before sexual intercourse. The atmosphere of openness and ease helped both us and the couple to discuss their sexual life, and they successfully resumed intercourse. It is important to be willing and ready to discuss sexuality, an issue that patients and health-care professionals both tend to avoid.

HOME CARE

The Need for Home Care

Given the changes that are occurring in the United States health-care system, long-term hospital stays for those with chronic terminal diseases are becoming increasingly improbable. On the other hand, a long-term hospital stay is not necessarily desirable; patients often prefer to remain in their homes rather than in the hospital.

As the disease progresses and motor function decreases, mobility and basic self-care will become increasingly difficult for the patient, and the activities of daily living (ADL) status index will begin to decline. In most instances, patients eventually will be unable to work, require increasing support inside and outside the home, and lose independence. At this point, home care becomes a reality for patients and their families (Fig. 18–2). If the patient, family, and caregiver are unfamiliar with home care, it is essential that the ALS team clearly explain the concepts and goals of such care.

As motor dysfunction progresses, more follow-up visits to the ALS clinic will be required. At this point, the clinic visits become more helpful because patients need symptomatic treatment and the family and caregivers require more information and training in home care. The primary goal is to attain the patient's independence by rehabilitation techniques (see Chapter 21).

The home care nurse plays a key role in educating and training patients and caregivers in home care. The ALS support group is also

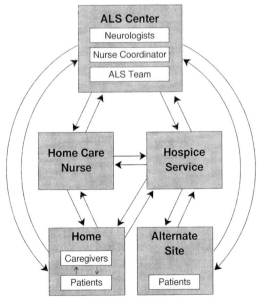

Figure 18–2. A diagrammatic presentation of comprehensive care for patients with ALS. Ensuring close communication is the key to successful care.

Table 18–10. **CONDITIONS FOR SUCCESSFUL HOME CARE***

- Patient desires home care.
- Family desires home care.
- Caregivers are available.
- Patient understands the disease.
- Symptomatic treatments are available.
- Symptomatic treatments are simple.
- More than one caregiver is available.
- Physicians and home care nurses are nearby.
- Family physicians are available.
- Emergency hospital admission, when required, is easily available.

*Translated from Kawagoe, K: Cancer patients who are cared for at home. Medical Friend Publishers (Japan), p. 21, 1991, with permission.

highly effective in helping patients and caregivers achieve effective home care. It is crucial for all involved, including health-care professionals, to understand that patient and caregivers must desire (or at least accept) the idea of home care so that they will be satisfied with the care. Home care decisions must revolve around the patient's desires; care decisions that are driven by the desires of the involved health professionals, family, or caregiver will not produce satisfactory care for the patient. Kowa[6] listed several conditions that should be fulfilled for successful home care (Table 18–10).

Caregiver

Caregivers are usually family members, such as a spouse or children, but can be relatives, close friends, or even neighbors. Initially, home care focuses primarily on maintaining the patient's independence for self-care but gradually changes to assisting patients with mobility, eating, and personal hygiene. Cooking must be modified to prepare forms that the patient can chew and swallow easily. The patient must be frequently repositioned to prevent discomfort and bed sores. As the disease advances, more complex care is required, and sometimes multiple caregivers are necessary for around-the-clock care. In such situations, Norris et al.[14] have suggested that the main caregiver be regarded as a "chief nurse," who establishes a care team and guides the team to achieve effective care. Caregivers need to familiarize themselves with complex equipment: the enteral tube (and gastrostomy button for patients with gastrostomy; see Chapter 24), the saliva and secretion suction device, and ventilation equipment. Furthermore, as the patient's speech becomes more dysarthric, the caregiver must adapt to the changes so that he or she can continue to interpret the patient's speech; familiarity with the communication devices patients might use is essential. When patients choose permanent ventilator care through a tracheostomy or even if they use a noninvasive ventilator, more skilled care is necessary.

Home Care Nurse

The home care nurse may play a major role in successful home care (Table 18–11), but major decisions should rest with the patient and perhaps the main caregiver. When the patient, caregiver, and ALS team realize that home care will soon be needed, a home care or visiting nurse should assess the home environment. Home assessment is important because the safety of the home for the patient and caregivers is evaluated, along with the need for equipment to enhance patient safety and independence. The nurse also identifies the need for home visits by physi-

Table 18–11. **RESPONSIBILITIES OF THE HOME CARE NURSE**

- Understand the disease.
- Communicate frequently with treating neurologists and nurse coordinators.
- Identify medical problems, acute medical diseases, and disease changes in ALS.
- Evaluate the home environment.
- Identify specific therapy and equipment needs.
- Instruct patient and family in using various types of equipment and instruments.
- Provide suggestions, solutions, and education for patient and family.
- Act as liaison between physician, patient, and caregiver.
- Discuss advance directives, life support, and do-not-resuscitate issues.
- Identify psychological strain in the family.

cal therapists, occupational therapists, and speech pathologists. If patients use an NIPPV device, care becomes more specialized and a visiting respiratory therapist should provide necessary care and train caregivers. The nurses are responsible for giving patients and caregivers special instructions, ranging from how to provide personal care to how to use medical equipment.

Home care nurses are crucial also as a liaison between patients and the ALS team (see Fig. 18–2). They assess the patient's medical and neurologic condition and report the findings to the treating physician for necessary orders. Experienced home care nurses also may offer specific medical recommendations that physicians often find useful when deciding what orders are needed. The home care nurse sometimes must discuss advance directives with patients and caregivers, if such a discussion has not occurred previously. The nurse may be key in identifying psychological stress at home and recommend or provide counseling for the patient and family (see Table 18–11).

Social and Psychological Issues at Home

"Home care" may imply that a home is suddenly transformed into a hospital-like setting. This change creates unforeseen stress on all family members living at home, and patients receiving care at home are likely to develop feelings of guilt. If the patient has been the main income generator for the household, the rapid changes will cause anxiety and financial concern,[14] of which the patient will be more aware if he or she receives care at home. The privacy of the family is often jeopardized, and the main caregiver may become exhausted physically and mentally. Also, the need to base the home care on the patient's decisions can seriously strain relationships between the patient, family, and caregiver. All these factors create enormous stress, to the extent that the patient may begin to wish to die quickly, and family members may begin to wish the same. Such feelings can result in hostility and guilt-bound behavior (see Chapter 25).

However, if these issues are resolved, home care provides the most rewarding care to patients and a satisfying experience for caregivers and their families. The home care nurse, and later the hospice nurse, must identify underlying family dynamics and provide counseling; professional psychological or psychiatric counseling should be recommended, too. At the ALS clinic, social workers and nurse coordinators should also discuss these issues with patients, caregivers, and family members (see Fig. 18–1). The ALS support group meeting is ideal for sharing such feelings and learning how other people cope with and resolve such issues.

In addition to the requirements listed in Table 18–11, several other issues must be considered if home care is to be effective and rewarding:

- All those involved should clearly understand that the patient is the key decision maker for all medical care.
- The main caregiver must be identified and should mobilize other caregivers.
- Each capable family member should share some responsibility in the care.
- All those involved must respect the privacy of the patient, the caregivers, and family members.
- Every effort should be made to have open discussions concerning problems that arise.
- Time should be set aside regularly for family gatherings and recreation that includes the patient.
- The family should continue to engage in the social activities in which they participated before the illness.
- The hospital-based ALS care team must not "abandon" patients and caregivers who are at home.

The Role of the ALS Clinic during Home Care

The nurse coordinator usually arranges the initial home care nurse visit. When the patient's condition worsens, routine visits to the ALS clinic become more important because patients need symptomatic treatment, and caregivers need further suggestions, instruction, and support concerning skilled care.[7,13] When visiting the ALS clinic becomes difficult for the patient, the patient's home may become not only an important but perhaps the sole care site. Neurologists or primary physicians, nurse coordinators, and other team members at the ALS clinic must then provide care indirectly through caregivers or a home care nurse, depending on the nature of treatment. Because the home care nurse may not initially be familiar with ALS, educating and instructing these nurses is another important responsibility of the ALS clinic team.

ALTERNATIVE CARE SITES

Some patients with ALS have no family or available caregiver. For these patients, social workers must identify suitable assisted-living facilities, nursing homes, or skilled-care nursing homes (see Fig. 18–2). Medical insurance does not permit certifying patients for placement in such facilities until they become seriously disabled, which greatly frustrates patients and medical personnel alike. When the patient's condition deteriorates such that he or she is expected to survive less than 6 months, hospice care is justified. Hospice care is given at home or at another care site.

HOSPICE CARE

The hospice provides unlimited terminal care for those who are expected to live for less than 6 months. In the United States, such care has progressed greatly in recent years and is available for patients with neurodegenerative disorders such as ALS.[11,12,15,16,20] Government insurance (Medicare) and private health insurance pays the total cost of hospice care for 210 days as a lump sum (see Chapter 26). When patients survive beyond this period, the hospice is responsible for maintaining care until the patient's death. The certifying physician is not penalized for "poor" predictions. Because the hospice is financially responsible for continuing care beyond 210 days, hospice physicians also often evaluate the patient's life expectancy at the initial application and may reject the application that the patient's own physicians had certified. One condition for receiving hospice service is that patients cannot receive life-sustaining measures. In ALS, this means that life-supporting permanent ventilation through tracheostomy is not accepted. NIPPV and enteral feeding are not generally considered as life-sustaining measures, but some hospices may consider them as life-sustaining. The certifying physician must write a "do not resuscitate" order. Patients also must prepare advance directives and a durable power of attorney for health care (see Chapter 26). Once the hospice service is approved, it provides necessary care.

The ultimate goal of the hospice is to provide "holistic care," that is, body, mind, and spiritual care for those with terminal disease and their families.[11,12,15,16] The hospice usually has three different services: home hospice care, day care, and in-hospital care. Home hospice care is essentially an extension of home care, but hospice provides more frequent visits by nurses or volunteers (see Fig. 18–2). The hospice also provides day care for those who can visit the hospice facility so that varied therapies, recreation, and personal counseling can be given to patients and their families. Support group meetings may be available. Day care is directed to maintaining the patient's dignity and functional independence as much as possible. In-hospital hospice care is given to patients close to death. It is also used to temporarily admit patients when the caregivers require respite.

The hospice allows the patient's own physicians to continue making medical orders. In the terminal stages, patients should receive judicious amounts of opioids such as morphine sulfate (or equivalent benzodiazepine) to treat severe insomnia, respiratory distress, excessive anxiety, and pain from joint contracture. Such treatment is safe and highly successful in the home care and hospice settings.[13,16] The final major function of the hospice is to support families and friends during bereavement.[10] Table 18–12 summarizes the main functions of the hospice.

Table 18–12. **CHARACTERISTICS OF HOSPICE CARE**

- Maximizes basic medical care
- Maximizes the patient's motor function
- Maintains the patient's dignity
- Provides no life-sustaining measures
- Provides terminal and comfort care
- Provides patient and family education
- Provides continuous psychological support
- Provides support during bereavement

SUMMARY

The care of patients with ALS is especially challenging and differs from that for other neurodegenerative disorders. ALS requires a commitment on the part of the patients, family, and health-care professionals to work together not only to provide the most appropriate treatment but also to give meaning to a devastating situation. Care of the patient with ALS begins at diagnosis and ends with the patient's death. The diagnostic process should include ancillary tests not only to exclude other diagnoses but also because this process itself is an important step in educating the patient about ALS, preparing the patient for the diagnosis, and in presenting the diagnosis sensitively. The physician who presents the diagnosis of ALS without hesitation or with little sensitivity essentially abandons the patient and family. To break such news, sufficient time should be set aside. Explaining the disease process, stressing the variable prognosis of ALS, vigorous research activities, and opportunities to participate in clinical trials, and obtaining a second opinion may provide patients with hope. A general neurologist can provide good care for patients with ALS, but care and treatment is most effective when provided in ALS clinics run by neurologists who specialize in ALS and having multidisciplinary teams consisting of a nurse coordinator, physical therapists, occupational therapists, dietitians, speech pathologists, and social workers. Pulmonary specialists and other health professionals should at least be on call. Neurologists make the necessary orders based on the ALS team's recommendations. They provide patients with up-to-date research information on ALS and discuss participation in clinical trials, when appropriate. The ultimate goal is to make the patient independent as long as possible and to provide psychosocial support to patients and families in a holistic approach. All caregivers must remember that the patient is the principal decision maker in his or her own care.

Physicians are responsible to protect patients from unconventional or unorthodox treatments that may be financially wasteful and medically risky. However, harsh rejection and discouragement without thoughtful explanation may not be helpful for those who are desperately looking for any therapy to give them hope.

Sexuality is not an issue usually discussed openly because physicians often have little knowledge, and patients and their spouses may feel it is inappropriate to discuss it when facing a terminal disease. As a part of holistic care, however, the discussion of sexuality may greatly improve quality of life.

When the patient's condition deteriorates, home care or admission to an alternative care site is required. Home care nurses are crucial. They evaluate the patient, family situation, and home safety; relay information to physicians for further recommendations; teach and educate patients and caregivers; and even may counsel patients and families. Close collaboration among patients, caregivers, home care nurses, and the entire ALS team will ensure effective and satisfying home care. When a patient has no caregiver, a site other than the home should be chosen for extended care. In the terminal stages, hospice care should be started, with the patient's primary physician certifying the patient's terminal medical status. Hospice provides highly effective comfort care to patients and their families. Judicious use of opioids (or other equivalent medications) is highly recommended to relieve significant discomfort.

REFERENCES

1. Beisecker, AE, Kuckelman-Cobb, A, and Ziegler, DK: Patients' perspectives of the role of care providers in amyotrophic lateral sclerosis. Arch Neurol 45:553–556, 1988.
2. Belsh, JM and Schiffman, PL: Misdiagnosis in patients with amyotrophic lateral sclerosis. Arch Intern Med 150:2301–2305, 1990.
3. Bradley, WG: Amyotrophic lateral sclerosis: The diagnostic process. In Mitsumoto, H and Norris, FH, Jr (eds): Amyotrophic Lateral Sclerosis. A Comprehensive Guide to Management. Demos, New York, 1994, pp 21–28.
4. Glasberg, MR: Amyotrophic lateral sclerosis: Unorthodox treatments. In Mitsumoto, H and Norris, FH, Jr (eds): Amyotrophic Lateral Sclerosis. Demos, New York, 1994, pp 53–62.
5. Goldblatt, D: Caring for patients with amyotrophic lateral sclerosis. In Smith, RA (ed): Handbook of Amyotrophic Lateral Sclerosis. Marcel Dekker, New York, 1992, pp 272–287.
6. Kowa, H: Home care system in amyotrophic lateral sclerosis. Neurol Therapeutics (Tokyo) 10:279–283, 1993.
7. Leigh, PN and Ray-Chaudhuri, K: Motor neuron disease. J Neurol Neurosurg Neuropsychiatry 57:886–896, 1994.
8. Mitsumoto, H, and Norris, FH, Jr (eds): Amyotrophic Lateral Sclerosis: Comprehensive Management and Treatment. Demos, New York, 1994.
9. Mulder, DW: Amyotrophic lateral sclerosis: Pitfalls of the diagnostic interview. In Rose, FC (ed): ALS—From Charcot to the Present and into the Future. Smith-Gordon, London, 1994, pp 1–4.
10. Murphy, NM: Mourning and amyotrophic lateral sclerosis. In Mitsumoto, H and Norris, FH, Jr (eds): Amyotrophic Lateral Sclerosis. A Comprehensive Guide to Management. Demos, New York, 1994, pp 283–294.
11. Murphy, NM and Thompson, B: Hospice: A family approach to amyotrophic lateral sclerosis. In Mitsumoto, H and Norris, FH, Jr (eds): Amyotrophic Lateral Sclerosis. A Comprehensive Guide to Management. Demos, New York, 1994, pp 267–282.
12. Newrick, PG and Langton-Hewer, R: Motor neurone disease: Can we do better? A study of 42 patients. Br Med J 289:539–542, 1984.
13. Norris, FH: Treating the untreated. Br Med J 304:459–460, 1992.
14. Norris, FH, Holden, D, Kandal, K, et al: Home nursing care by families for severely paralyzed ALS patients. In Cosi, V, Kato, AC, Parlette, W, et al: (eds): Amyotrophic Lateral Sclerosis. Plenum, New York, 1987, pp 231–238.
15. Norris, FH, Smith, RA, and Denys, EH: Motor neurone disease: Towards better care. Br Med J 291:259–262, 1985.
16. O'Brien, T, Kelly, M, and Saunders, C: Motor neurone disease: A hospice perspective. Br Med J 304:471–473, 1992.
17. Oliver, D: Ethical issues in palliative care—An overview. Palliat Med 7:15–20, 1993.
18. Pernick, E: Sexuality/intimacy/sensitivity of ALS patients. In Mancall, EL (symposium director): Current Concepts in Managing ALS. ALS Association, Philadelphia, 1994, pp 129–134.
19. Sanders, M and Fellows, ON: Use of detoxified snake neurotoxin as a partial treatment for amyotrophic lateral sclerosis. Cancer Cytol 15:26–30, 1975.
20. Thompson, B: Amyotrophic lateral sclerosis: Integrating care for patients and their families. Am J Hosp Pall Care 7:27–32, 1990.
21. Tyler, HR: Modified snake venom therapy in motor neuron disease: A double-blind study. Neurology 29:77–81, 1979.
22. Yase, Y: ALS treatment. Neurol Therapy (Tokyo) 10:171–176, 1993.

CHAPTER 19

SYMPTOMATIC TREATMENT

SIALORRHEA
PSEUDOBULBAR SYMPTOMS
CRAMPS
FASCICULATIONS
SPASTICITY
PAIN
FEAR, ANXIETY, AND DEPRESSION

The progressive upper and lower motor neuron degeneration in ALS results in many and varied symptoms. Upper and lower motor-neuron-type weakness involving the bulbar musculature leads to sialorrhea; it also contributes to emotional lability, which is part of the pseudobulbar affect. Involvement of spinal lower motor neurons leads to cramps and fasciculations, whereas disease of the corticospinal upper motor neurons causes limb spasticity. Joint contractures caused by weakness and progressive loss of mobility lead to joint and limb pain, which is often severe and sometimes incapacitating. Last, the shock of what for many patients is an unfamiliar and rare disease, the fear of its progressive nature, and the knowledge that there is no cure may contribute to anxiety and depression. In this chapter, we discuss the management of these symptoms and point out that a great deal can be done to ameliorate them.

SIALORRHEA

During the course of ALS, patients develop excessive salivation, or sialorrhea, an often frustrating, uncomfortable, and embarassing problem. In patients with bulbar-onset disease, this symptom tends to occur relatively early. In the setting of dysarthria, dysphagia, and facial weakness, saliva accumulates and drooling ensues. The repeated use of a tissue or handkerchief to wipe the corners of the mouth results in perioral skin irritation that is uncomfortable and unsightly. In addition to its adverse psychological impact on the patient, the accumulated oropharyngeal secretions may spill into the airway, triggering laryngospasm and coughing.[10]

Fortunately, several treatments can ameliorate sialorrhea. Perhaps the most direct treatment is a small portable suction device, although it may be cumbersome or inconvenient. Probably the most efficacious treatment is pharmacotherapy with any of a variety of medications, including tricyclic antidepressants[7] (Table 19–1). The antidepressant action of the tricyclics is mediated by the inhibition of the neuronal uptake of serotonin and norepinephrine. Most relevant to the problem of sialorrhea is the anticholinergic side effect ("dry mouth") that we attempt to exploit; the drugs also have sedating, hypotensive, and cardiac arrhythmogenic effects.[1]

Of all the tricyclics, amitriptyline, doxepin, and imipramine are perhaps the best choices because they have the most potent anticholinergic effects[11] (Table 19–2). In most patients, especially the elderly, we begin with a small dose (10 to 25 mg at bedtime) and gradually increase it every few days until the target dose is reached. These agents may also cause sedation and orthostatic hypotension,

321

Table 19–1. **MEDICATIONS USED TO CONTROL SIALORRHEA**

Medication	Dose/Schedule	Side Effects
Amitriptyline	25–100 mg hs	Anticholinergic—prominent Sedation—prominent Orthostatic hypotension—prominent
Doxepin	25–100 mg hs	Anticholinergic—moderate Sedation—moderate Orthostatic hypotension—moderate
Imipramine	25–100 mg hs	Anticholinergic—moderate Sedation—mild Orthostatic hypotension—moderate
Protriptyline	10–20 mg hs	Anticholinergic—moderate Sedation—mild Orthostatic hypotension—mild
Nortriptyline	20–100 mg hs	Anticholinergic—mild Sedation—mild Orthostatic hypotension—mild
Atropine sulfate	0.4 mg q 4–6 hr	Anticholinergic—mild to moderate
Trihexyphenidyl	2–4 mg tid	Anticholinergic—mild to moderate
Scopolamine transdermal patch	0.5 mg q3d	Anticholinergic—mild to moderate
Glycopyrrolate	1–2 mg tid	Anticholinergic—mild to moderate
Diphenhydramine	25–50 mg tid	Anticholinergic—mild to moderate Sedation—mild

Table 19–2. **ANTICHOLINERGIC EFFECTS OF TRICYCLIC ANTIDEPRESSANTS**

Major Effect Sought
Dry mouth

Unwanted Side Effects
Gastrointestinal
  Sour metallic taste
  Epigastric distress
  Constipation
Genitourinary
  Urinary retention
CNS
  Dizziness
  Confusion
Ocular
  Precipitation of untreated glaucoma
  Blurred vision
Cardiac
  Tachycardia

however, which may not be acceptable for some patients. In these cases, protriptyline or nortriptyline may be better choices, although the latter has less-pronounced anticholinergic effects and may not be as effective. These drugs must be used with great care in the elderly and in patients with cardiac conduction disorders, especially those already receiving antiarrhythmics (such as quinidine), because they exert a quinidine-like slowing of intracardiac conduction.[1] These drugs are contraindicated in patients with bifascicular block, left bundle-branch block, or a prolonged QT interval.

If the use of tricyclic antidepressants is problematic, atropine sulfate or anticholinergic agents such as trihexyphenidyl may be used. Transdermal scopolamine is also effective. These agents must also be used with caution, especially in the elderly, and titrated slowly upward in dose. They may cause other unwanted anticholinergic side effects (see Table 19–2). Glycopyrrolate, a quaternary anticholinergic agent, is also effective. Its limited ability to cross the blood-brain barrier makes its CNS side effects less pronounced than those of the tertiary amines, which readily cross this barrier.[3] Antihistamines, such as diphenhydramine, may also be helpful in reducing sialorrhea; a common side effect is sedation, although this effect tends to diminish after a few days of continued use.

Two other approaches to control sialorrhea have been described, although they are rarely used because of their radical nature: transtympanic neurectomy and irradiation of the parotid gland.[12] The tympanic nerves form a plexus that innervates the parotid glands, whereas the chorda tympani supplies the submaxillary and sublingual salivary glands. The tympanic nerves and chorda tympani pass near each other behind the tympanic membrane, where they can be sectioned through a circumferential incision under local anesthesia. The procedure may provide relief but needs to be repeated if regeneration occurs. The parotid glands have also been irradiated, although the results are unpredictable. Either of these procedures may result in thick saliva that exacerbates the problem of dysphagia.[3]

Sometimes during the management of sialorrhea, excessive dryness of the mouth and tongue—xerostomia—may develop. A combination of medication side effects, mouth-breathing during sleep, and a chronic open-mouth posture caused by muscle weakness contribute to this symptom.[8] Xerostomia interferes with the oral phase of swallowing and should be treated. It may improve with lemon-glycerine swabs or by spraying the mouth with ice water, followed by a rinsing and expectoration.

PSEUDOBULBAR SYMPTOMS

Patients with bulbar involvement may have prominent emotional lability characterized by uncontrollable paroxysms of laughing or crying. These symptoms are thought to be related to damage of the subcortical forebrain white matter tracts (see Chapter 4). The emotional lability may embarrass and demoralize patients and family members. The pseudobulbar symptoms often coexist with sialorrhea, dysphagia, and dysarthria, and in com-

Table 19–3. MEDICATIONS USED FOR PSEUDOBULBAR SYMPTOMS IN ALS

Medication	Dose/Schedule
Amitriptyline	50–150 mg hs
Nortriptyline	50–75 mg hs
Desipramine	50–150 mg hs
Lithium carbonate	300 mg qd, bid, tid*
L-Dopa/carbidopa	25/100 mg tid

*Low doses may achieve desired clinical effect.

bination these symptoms have the potential to become debilitating.

For some patients, amitriptyline ameliorates this emotional lability.[2] Other tricyclics with more favorable side effects may also have a therapeutic effect (Table 19–3). Lithium carbonate in small doses (300 mg qd to tid, with levels less than 0.6 mEq/L) that are not likely to affect the neural pathways involved in manic-depressive psychosis may also be helpful.[10] Finally, levodopa is effective in some patients.[13]

CRAMPS

Cramps are common in ALS, especially in the lower motor neuron form of the illness. The cramp is heralded by muscle twitching or fasciculations, typically develops suddenly, and involves a portion of a muscle in a painful, palpable contraction. During the contraction, electromyographic recordings disclose high-frequency discharges of motor unit potentials (see Chapter 5). (This cramp differs from the pain of contracture, which is related to a defect in carbohydrate metabolism and is associated with a painful shortening of the muscle; in contrast to the neurogenic cramp of ALS, contracture is electrically silent.[6]) Pain from cramps may be intense, simulating angina when occurring in the chest and an attack of cholecystitis when present in the abdominal wall. More commonly, cramps occur in the arms and legs. The occurrence of cramps at night contributes to disturbed sleep.

Despite the lack of definite efficacy for treating cramps, the mainstay of therapy used to be quinine sulfate. Recently, however, numerous reports of life-threatening and fatal reactions to quinine caused the Food and Drug Administration to ban it from the market.[4] As a first-line approach to treatment, we recommend physical therapy, such as muscle stretching and warm compresses, especially at bedtime. We then employ a variety of medications (Table 19–4). The anticonvulsants phenytoin or carbamazepine are sometimes helpful. We aim for blood levels in the range considered therapeutic for seizure control. A benzodiazepine, diazepam, may also ameliorate cramps. The onset of its therapeutic effect is rapid, with blood levels peaking within 1 hour after administration; because of the rapid distribution of the drug, a single dose will be active for a relatively short period. At higher doses, especially in the elderly, sedation may be a problem.

FASCICULATIONS

Fasciculations, like cramps, are seen most often in patients with prominent lower motor neuron involvement. While fasciculations per se are rarely painful, their presence, particularly when they are brisk, widespread, and frequent, is disconcerting for most patients. Avoiding caffeine and nicotine may minimize their occurrence. Explaining that fasciculations do not reflect the activity of the disease often reassures patients. We have found that a high-potency, short-duration benzodiazepine, such as lorazepam, reduces the intensity of the fasciculations and has an anxiolytic effect (see below), which helps patients to cope with these muscle twitches.

SPASTICITY

Like cramps, spasticity is a major cause of discomfort for patients with ALS. It is especially problematic in patients with a primarily upper motor neuron form of the disease. As in the management of cramps, physical measures such as passive stretching of the involved limbs several times a day should be part of all therapeutic regimens. (The clinician must be mindful of the importance of spasticity in helping to maintain a certain posture and that treatment of, or reduction in, spasticity may occasionally result paradoxically in functional impairment.)

Three different drugs are commonly used to manage spasticity (Table 19–5): the benzodiazepines (usually diazepam), baclofen, and dantrolene. Diazepam binds to a specific site on the gamma-aminobutyric acid (GABA) receptor of spinal cord neurons, enhances neuronal hyperpolarization, and promotes motor neuronal inhibition. We begin with a dose of 2 mg tid and increase it gradually as tolerated to 15 mg tid. The most common side effect is sedation; confusion may be seen in elderly patients. Patients with an underlying gait instability may become more unsteady as the dose is increased. If there is accompanying pulmonary disease or respiratory compromise, diazepam (and other benzodiazepines) must be used with care because of their propensity to cause hypoventilation.

Baclofen is an analog of GABA that, like diazepam, inhibits spasticity at the spinal cord level. Treatment begins with 5 mg tid and

Table 19–4. MEDICATIONS USED TO CONTROL CRAMPS

Medication	Dose/Schedule	Side Effects
Phenytoin	300 mg hs*	Gastrointestinal upset, rash[†]
Carbamazepine	200 mg tid[‡]	Gastrointestinal upset, rash, sedation, dry mouth[¶]
Diazepam	2–10 mg tid	Increased weakness, sedation, dizziness, respiratory depression

*Dose will vary; aim to achieve serum level of 10–20 μg/mL.
[†]Other idiosyncratic reactions are rare and include leukopenia, granulocytopenia, thrombocytopenia, aplastic anemia, pseudolymphoma, and lupuslike syndrome.
[‡]Dose will vary; aim to achieve serum level of 4–10 μg/mL.
[¶]Other rare effects include cholestatic jaundice, aplastic anemia, pancytopenia, hyponatremia.

Table 19–5. **MEDICATIONS USED TO CONTROL SPASM AND SPASTICITY**

Medication	Dose/Schedule	Side Effects
Diazepam	2–15 mg tid	Increased weakness, sedation, dizziness, respiratory depression
Baclofen	10–25 mg tid	Increased weakness, sedation, dizziness
Dantrolene	50–100 mg qid	Increased weakness, sedation, dizziness, diarrhea, hepatotoxicity

gradually is increased to a total dose of 30 to 75 mg in three divided doses. We find that combining baclofen with diazepam provides additional therapeutic effect and allows relatively low doses of each agent to be maintained. Side effects of baclofen include increased weakness, sedation, dizziness, gastrointestinal symptoms, tremor, insomnia, headache, and hypotension. If, for some reason, the drug needs to be discontinued, it should be withdrawn slowly to avoid hallucinations and seizures.

Diazepam and baclofen may only partially relieve spasticity. These drugs are most effective in reducing spasticity associated with primary afferent stimulation and are not of major benefit for improving functional activities, which are innervated through the pyramidal or parapyramidal pathways, the situation prevailing in ALS.

Dantrolene suppresses calcium release from the sarcoplasmic reticulum and thus interferes with excitation-contraction coupling (it prevents myofibril contraction). Because it produces weakness proportional to the relief of spasticity, it is infrequently used in ALS. Beginning doses are generally 25 mg qd or bid, which can be increased as tolerated to a total of 100 mg qid. Dantrolene may occasionally cause hepatotoxicity (sometimes severe), so liver function needs to be monitored carefully.

PAIN

Although sensory pathways are spared in the majority of patients with ALS, pain is a troubling symptom for many. It occurs especially in those with prominent upper motor neuron signs in whom joint mobility is severely reduced. In particular, weakness and spasticity lead to a relatively immobile shoulder joint that is exquisitely susceptible to the development of adhesive capsulitis, bursitis, and tendonitis. Cramps and increased muscle tone (with its attendant spasm) are also sources of discomfort. Lack of ability to change body position leads to undue pressure on skin, bone, and joints and causes pain. Episodes of pain may become frequent, and a dominant theme in some patients' lives. Pain may affect the neck, back, and limbs, and is described as diffuse aching, burning, and electric or shock-like in nature.[9]

A major treatment for pain is physical therapy (see Chapter 21). Maintaining joint mobility is important to prevent contractures and to alleviate the discomfort of muscle spasm. Several analgesics, including acetaminophen and the nonsteroidal anti-inflammatory drugs (NSAIDs), anticonvulsants, and tricyclic antidepressants, also have an important role in relieving discomfort (Table 19–6). These drugs are often most useful in combinations.

The NSAIDs produce analgesia mainly by decreasing the production of prostaglandins. Ibuprofen, naproxen, or one of the newer agents (e.g., oxaprozin) may ameliorate discomfort, especially joint pain that has an inflammatory component. They have a variety of side effects, the most common being abdominal discomfort caused by a decrease in production of gastric mucous (which can be improved by misoprostol, a prostaglandin analogue, not by type 2 histamine recep-

Table 19–6. **MEDICATIONS USED TO CONTROL THE PAIN ASSOCIATED WITH ALS**

Medication	Dose/Schedule
Ibuprofen	600 mg tid
Naprosyn	550 mg bid
Oxaprozin	600–1200 mg qd
Phenytoin	300 mg hs
Carbamazepine	200 mg tid
Clonazepam	0.5–2 mg tid
Amitriptyline	50–150 mg hs
Nortriptyline	50–75 mg hs
Desipramine	50–150 mg hs
Codeine	60 mg q4h
Hydrocodone	10 mg q4h
Methadone	20 mg q8h
Morphine*	2–10 mg IV q3–4h
Fentanyl transdermal*	25–75 μg/qh

*To ease suffering for patients in the terminal stages of the disease.

tor–blocking agents). If abdominal discomfort becomes dose-limiting, choline magnesium trisalicylate (Trilisate), which has a lower incidence of gastric irritation, may be better tolerated. With long-term use, liver enzymes and blood urea nitrogen or creatinine should be measured periodically because of the risk (albeit low) of hepatotoxicity and nephrotoxicity. Patients with asthma, nasal polyposis, and aspirin hypersensitivity are at high risk for anaphylaxis when exposed to other NSAIDs.

When the pain has a shooting, electrical, or lancinating component, antiepileptic drugs may be efficacious. Phenytoin, carbamazepine, and clonazepam, in doses that achieve blood levels considered therapeutic for seizure control, are among the drugs we select in patients with this type of pain.

We have already mentioned the tricyclic antidepressants (in particular their anticholinergic side effects) in the context of treatment for sialorrhea, but their major pharmacologic action is to potentiate the effect of the endogenous biogenic amines throughout the brain. In addition to their effects on mood and affect, norepinephrine and serotonin act as neurotransmitters in CNS pain modulating pathways. In contrast to the antidepressant effects, which may take weeks to become noticeable, the analgesic effects may have a rapid onset within days. For some patients, amitriptyline (see Table 19–6) will be an appropriate choice because of the need for both anticholinergic and analgesic effects. Others may be at a stage in their illness when sialorrhea is not an issue and anticholinergic effects can be minimized with the use of nortriptyline or desipramine.

Should the pain fail to respond to these agents, then opioids may be appropriate for selected patients (see Table 19–6). Codeine or hydrocodone is sometimes effective. Methadone is a good choice for moderately severe, chronic pain because of its long analgesic action, low cost, and efficacy comparable to morphine. We avoid oral meperidine because of its many side effects. For some patients in the last stages of the disease, and in the hospice setting, intravenous morphine will provide analgesia, sedation, and relief from respiratory distress. In this terminal situation, patients unable to take tablets may benefit from a fentanyl transdermal patch changed every 48 to 72 hours.

FEAR, ANXIETY, AND DEPRESSION

Receiving the diagnosis of ALS is a major stressor in the life of the patient and commonly leads to symptoms of fear, anxiety, and depression. As a result, the patient's coping mechanisms may be overwhelmed. Our first treatment approaches include developing a supportive, caring physician-patient relationship and counseling by a therapist experienced in working with ALS patients (see Chapter 25). As symptoms of anxiety diminish, ALS support groups may be beneficial in educating the patient and family about the disease and its management. Our second approach is pharmacotherapy, which in many patients plays an important role in alleviating these distressing symptoms (Table 19–7).

Benzodiazepines are helpful for the short-term relief of fear and anxiety. Low-potency, long-acting compounds (chlordiazepoxide, clorazepate, diazepam, flurazepam) are recommended because they have the lowest risk

Table 19–7. **MEDICATIONS FOR FEAR, ANXIETY, AND DEPRESSION IN ALS**

Medication Class	Indication	Specific Drugs (Example)
Benzodiazepine (low potency, long duration of action)	Fear, anxiety	Diazepam (5 mg tid)
Benzodiazepine (short duration of action, not hepatic metabolism)	Fear, anxiety (especially in the elderly or in setting of liver disease)	Lorazepam (0.5–1 mg bid)
Nonbenzodiazepine anxiolytic	Fear, anxiety (intolerance of sedation, tenuous respiratory status)	Buspirone (10 mg tid)
SSRI	Depression	Sertraline (50–100 mg qd)
SSRI and benzodiazepine	Depression and anxiety or depression and insomnia	Sertraline (50–100 mg qd) and diazepam (5 mg tid)
Tricyclic antidepressant	Depression and insomnia	Amitriptyline (100–200 mg qd)

Abbreviation: SSRI = selective serotonin reuptake inhibitor.

of causing dependence and subsequent withdrawal symptoms.[5] For example, we begin with diazepam, 5 mg tid or the equivalent, and gradually increase the dose as needed. We generally do not exceed 30 mg/day of diazepam because this should suffice for most instances of situational anxiety. In general, the approach of frequent (tid or qid) lower doses is preferred over fewer, higher daily doses because it avoids oversedation at peak levels and inadequate treatment at trough levels. In the elderly, or in patients with liver disease, low doses of benzodiazepines not metabolized by the hepatic microsomal enzymes (lorazepam, oxazepam, and temazepam) are preferred to avoid drug accumulation and toxicity. For patients who cannot tolerate the sedating effects of benzodiazepines, or if respiratory status is tenuous and the addition of a benzodiazepine could further compromise it, the nonbenzodiazepine, buspirone, may be indicated.[5] It has a slow onset of action, however, taking 1 to 2 weeks to show initial effects and 4 to 6 weeks to reach full effect. The initial starting dose is 5 mg tid, increasing gradually to 10 mg tid.

The benzodiazepines also alleviate the insomnia that accompanies anxiety. Other benzodiazepines marketed as hypnotic agents (flurazepam, temazepam, triazolam) may also be used.[5] Because of its long elimination half-life, flurazepam (15 to 30 mg at bedtime [hs]) should be used with great care in the elderly and should not be used for more than a few nights in a row. Triazolam (0.125 to 0.25 mg hs) is an effective hypnotic that does not accumulate, but because of its short half-life it may cause rebound insomnia. Temazepam (15 to 30 mg hs), with an intermediate half-life, poses much less risk of accumulation and is uncommonly associated with rebound insomnia.

For some of our patients, counseling alone is insufficient to ameliorate symptoms of depression, and we recommend treatment with an antidepressant. Our first choice, especially in elderly patients, is a selective serotonin reuptake inhibitor (SSRI) because of the absence of anticholinergic, antihistaminergic, anti-alpha-adrenergic, weight gain, and cardiotoxic effects. We initiate therapy with fluoxetine (20 mg qd to begin; target dose 20 mg bid) or sertraline (50 mg qd to begin; target dose 100 mg qd) but do not expect to see an antidepressant effect for 2 to 4 weeks. Potential difficulties with the SSRIs are the side effects of agitation and insomnia. Thus, when insomnia or agitation or both are prominent features of depression, a sedating tricyclic antidepressant (amitriptyline or imipramine) may be used instead of an SSRI. Alternatively, if the adverse side effects of the tricyclic antidepressants must be avoided, a benzodiazepine may be temporarily added to the SSRI[5]; as the SSRI takes effect, and depression lessens, sleep difficulties and anxiety will improve and the benzodiazepine may be discontinued.

SUMMARY

Although there is no specific treatment to reverse the weakness of ALS, many are available to ameliorate the uncomfortable symptoms of this disease. For sialorrhea, tricyclic antidepressants with prominent anticholinergic effects, such as amitriptyline, are particularly beneficial. The embarassment and distress of pseudobulbar symptoms may be relieved in part by amitriptyline; in some patients lithium or L-dopa may be helpful. Painful cramps respond to diazepam as well as to the antiepileptic drugs phenytoin or carbamazepine. Brisk fasciculations may be attenuated with lorazepam. Spasticity, a major problem in the upper motor neuron form of the illness, may be eased by a combination of diazepam and baclofen; dantrolene is reserved for the most severely affected patients. Pain arising from immobilized joints and limbs may be reduced by all classes of analgesic medications, including NSAIDs, antiepileptic drugs, tricyclic antidepressants, and opioids. Fear, anxiety, and insomnia stemming from the diagnosis may be alleviated by benzodiazepines; depression after diagnosis is helped by either an SSRI or a tricyclic antidepressant. The care and love of family and friends; the wisdom of a support group; the educational resources provided by the Muscular Dystrophy Association and ALS Association; the compassion of treating physicians, nurses, and therapists; the knowledge of ongoing therapeutic trials; and their own courage help patients to cope with ALS.

REFERENCES

1. Baldessarini, RJ: Drugs and the treatment of psychiatric disorders. In Gilman, AG, Rall, TW, Nies, AS, et al (eds): The Pharmacological Basis of Therapeutics, ed 8. Pergamon Press, New York, 1990, 383–435.
2. Caroscio, JT, Cohen, JA, and Gudesblatt, M: Amitriptyline in amyotrophic lateral sclerosis. N Engl J Med 313:1478, 1985.
3. Clawson, LL, Rothstein, JD, and Kuncl, RW: Amyotrophic lateral sclerosis. In Johnson, RT and Griffin, JW (eds): Current Therapy in Neurologic Disease. CV Mosby, St Louis, 1993, pp 285–295.
4. Hogan, TT: FDA bans quinine for nocturnal leg cramps. Drug Utilization Rev. October 1995, p 150.
5. Hyman, SE, Arana, GW, and Rosenbaum, JF: Handbook of Psychiatric Drug Therapy, ed 3. Little Brown, Boston, 1995.
6. Layzer, RB: Muscle pains and cramps. In Bradley, WG, Daroff, RB, Fenichel, GM, et al (eds): Neurology in Clinical Practice. Butterworth-Heinemann, Boston, 1996, p 375.
7. Leigh, PN and Ray-Chaudhuri, K: Motor neuron disease. J Neurol Neurosurg Psychiatry 57:886–896, 1994.
8. Mancinelli, JM: Dysphagia and dysarthria: The role of the speech-language pathologoist. In Mitsumoto, H and Norris, FH (eds): Amyotrophic Lateral Sclerosis. A Comprehensive Guide to Management. Demos, New York, 1994, pp 63–75.
9. Newrick, PG and Langton-Hewer, R: Motor neurone disease: Can we do better? A study of 42 patients. Br Med J 289:539–542, 1984.
10. Norris, FH: Care of the amyotrophic lateral sclerosis patient. In Mitsumoto, H and Norris, FH (eds): Amyotrophic Lateral Sclerosis. A Comprehensive Guide to Management. Demos, New York, 1994, pp 29–42.
11. Potter, WZ, Rudorfer, MV, and Manji, H: The pharmacologic treatment of depression. N Engl J Med 325:633–642, 1991.
12. Smith, RA and Norris, FH: Symptomatic care of patients with amyotrophic lateral sclerosis. JAMA 234:715–717, 1974.
13. Ukada, F, Yamao, S, Magata, H, et al: Pathologic laughing and crying treated with levodopa. Arch Neurol 41:1095–1096, 1984.

CHAPTER 20

TREATMENT TRIALS

Neurology is entering an exciting era when the time-honored tradition of localization and accurate diagnosis is met by innovative and promising clinical trials of drug therapy based on the growing understanding of the pathophysiology of a variety of disorders. In ALS, we hope to emulate the approach taken by oncology, where the availability of promising new therapeutic agents has generated sophisticated multicenter trial designs, quantitative measurement techniques, and statistically reliable results. Up to 1980, approximately 800 clinical trials were performed for ALS, but only two were randomized controlled trials.[30] In fact, only in the past several years have extensive therapeutic trials emerged as an important dimension of general clinical neurology.

As clinicians treating patients with ALS, we should not only provide the best available symptomatic treatment but also offer potentially beneficial new therapies, which can be studied and proven efficacious only in the context of controlled clinical trials. Such trials are important not only in developing effective treatments but also in increasing our understanding of ALS. However, conducting clinical trials is not easy. Bradley[15] stated, "A correctly planned trial is of vital importance in order to steer a course avoiding the Scylla of failing to recognize the effectiveness of the therapy, and the Charybdis of raising false hopes about ineffective therapies." McKhann[56] warned of clinical trials, "To subject our patients to unproved treatments based on personal whims or prejudices is

Table 20–1. ALS CLINICAL TRIALS GUIDELINES

Diagnosis

1. The diagnosis should conform to the World Federation of Neurology El Escorial Criteria.

Inclusion

2. Both sporadic and familial ALS can be entered depending on the nature of the trial.
3. Entry should be limited to patients between the ages of 18 and 85.
4. Before entry there should be evidence of progression during a period of 6 months from onset of symptoms but not more than 5 years.

Exclusion

5. Patients with significant sensory abnormalities, dementia, other neurologic diseases, uncompensated medical illness, substance abuse, and psychiatric illness should be excluded. The patient should not be on concurrent investigational drugs.

Endpoints

6. Primary and secondary endpoints should be crisply defined. A change in muscle strength and death or ventilator dependence are at present the most useful primary endpoints for a therapeutic trial.

Use of a Control

7. All trials should include a control group. The type of control used should depend on the trial design and objective.

Quality-of-Life Assessment

8. A specific quality-of-life assessment should be developed and incorporated into every efficacy trial.

Statistical Analyses

9. Trials should be designed with careful and detailed statistical analysis which should begin in the planning phase.

"Compassionate Release" and Treatment IND

10. "Compassionate release" and treatment INDs should only be used when assessment of therapeutic efficacy of the drug is not compromised.

Release of Information and Investigators' Responsibility

11. The manner in which information is released during and after a trial should be an integral part of the protocol. It is recommended that no efficacy results be released until peer review publication is imminent, other than at scientific meetings.
12. It is the investigator's responsibility to assure that commercial concerns do not distort the conduct of the trial.

Clinical Trial Phases

13. ALS trials should be organized in three phases. Phase I trials are conducted to obtain toxicity and pharmacokinetic information. Phase II trials (pilot, exploratory, screening) are performed for dose finding, preliminary efficacy assessment, and further safety observations. Phase III studies are performed to determine definitive efficacy and safety.
14. Phase I trials should incorporate concurrent placebo control and should be conducted for 6 months depending on the design.
15. Phase II trials may use concurrent placebo controls, historic controls or a crossover design. This phase is used to screen agents with potential therapeutic value. If improvement in strength or function is the endpoint, the trial should last at least 6 months. If stabilization or slowing of deterioration is the endpoint, the trial should last a minimum of 12 months depending on the nature of the drug.
16. Phase III trials should be placebo-controlled. This trial should include analysis of time to death, assessment of strength measured by maximum voluntary isometric contraction, pulmonary function, functional performance by the ALS rating scale, and measurement of bulbar function.

Data and Safety Monitoring Board

17. An independent data and safety monitoring board should be established for most studies. This should consist of independent physicians and biostatisticians who periodically review all data during the conduct of the trial and at its conclusion. This committee is also responsible for safeguarding against scientific fraud. It is essential that this committee be free of conflict of interest and acting on the patients' behalf.

Abbreviation: IND = investigational new drug.
Source: Modified from The World Federation of Neurology Research Group on Neuromuscular Disease Subcommittee on Motor Neuron Disease: Airlie House Guidelines. Therapeutic trials in amyotrophic lateral sclerosis. J Neurol Sci 129 (suppl): 1–10, 1995, with kind permission from Elsevier Science - NL, Sara Burgerhartstraat 25, 1055 KV Amsterdam, The Netherlands.

wholly unethical, as is designing and directing a study which is uninterpretable." Therefore, clinical trials must be planned and executed with great care and caution. Recently, the World Federation of Neurology (WFN) Subcommittee on Motor Neuron Disease recommended ALS Clinical Trial Guidelines[83] (Table 20–1). Most clinical neurologists are affected by recent clinical trials in one way or another: some are involved directly in the trials, others may refer their patients to study centers, and all learn the results at national meetings and from medical journals. This chapter discusses the role of therapeutic trials in the treatment of ALS.

DRUG DEVELOPMENT AND FDA REGULATION

Clinical trials are the final stage of the long and complex process of drug development. This process begins with in vitro and in vivo basic research. Preclinical studies include animal pharmacology, pharmacokinetic, and toxicity studies, and then the effects of a new drug are tested in animal models; human clinical trials can start only after all basic studies are completed. ALS is designated as an "orphan" disease by the United States Food and Drug Administration (FDA) because it affects only a small proportion of the population. An "orphan drug" is a drug that is developed to treat a disease with a prevalence in the United States of less than 200,000 individuals. The FDA supports the rapid devel-

Table 20–2. **HIGHLIGHTS OF THE ORPHAN DRUG ACT, 1983**

- An orphan disease is one that affects less than 200,000 Americans.
- There are an estimated 2,000 such diseases.
- A drug company that develops an orphan drug (for the treatment of an orphan disease) has a 7-year exclusive use of license.
- The company will receive a tax credit of two thirds of the product costs.
- Orphan drug applications receive high priority for FDA review.
- Less stringent requirements may be placed for approving such a drug.
- The FDA provides grants to develop orphan drugs.

Abbreviation: FDA = Food and Drug Administration.
Source: Data from Young, FE and Norris, JA: An FDA consumer special report. HHS Publication No. 88-3168. Public Health Service, Rockville, MD, 1988.

opment of orphan drugs and provides special protection to drug companies that develop them (Table 20–2).

The FDA has also formulated guidelines for developing new drugs for human consumption (Table 20–3). All clinical trials of unproven new medications must be approved by the FDA under an Investigational New Drug (IND) application. The clinical trials process includes several phases. In a phase I study, the drug is given for the first time to less than 100 human subjects, usually healthy volunteers. The purpose of a phase I study is to investigate the safety, pharmaco-

Table 20–3. **STAGES OF DRUG DEVELOPMENT FOR HUMAN SUBJECTS UNDER FDA REGULATION**

Component	Phase I	Phase II	Phase III	Phase IV
Subjects	Healthy*	Patients	Patients	Patients
Stage	Preliminary	Preliminary	Pivotal	Post-license
Safety	Yes	Yes	Yes	Yes
Placebo	Yes/no	Yes/no	Usually yes[†]	Yes
Randomization	Yes/no	Yes/no	Yes	Yes
Efficacy	No	Yes	Yes	Yes
FDA license for commercial sale	No	No	No	Yes

Abbreviations: FDA = Food and Drug Administration.
*In phase I trials involving diseases like ALS, AIDS, or terminal cancer, patients are allowed to enter the study and, depending on the trial, a placebo is also allowed.
[†] "Standard" therapy may be used as control.

kinetic characteristics, and clinical toxicity of the drug. However, in certain terminal diseases, such as extensive cancer, AIDS, and ALS, affected patients may participate in the phase I investigation. This accommodation facilitates the drug development and approval process because early indication of efficacy may emerge from such trials. Recent studies with ciliary neurotrophic factor (CNTF) and brain-derived neurotrophic factors (BDNF) exemplify such an approach in ALS.

Phase II studies are still exploratory and generally include 100 to 200 patients. Several outcomes and dose regimens may be tested in this phase to identify the trial design that would best demonstrate the potential benefits of the drug in a phase III trial, the pivotal clinical trial stage, in which by definition the proof of efficacy is sought in several hundred to several thousand patients. Phase IV studies are conducted once a drug has received marketing approval, with the goal of detecting low-frequency, serious side effects that may have escaped detection in phases I, II, and III studies. Although Table 20–3 gives general definitions and guidelines for the four stages, in reality, distinctions between phase I and II, and between phase II and III become less clear, depending on the study design.

In 1988, the FDA introduced new procedures for the use of investigational drugs in the treatment of immediately life-threatening disease, and serious illness, such as ALS. This "treatment IND" allows breakthrough drugs that are still undergoing clinical trials to be used for patients when there are no satisfactory alternative treatments.[85] Riluzole and insulin-like growth factor I (IGF-I) in ALS are such examples.

PATIENT INCLUSION AND EXCLUSION

Although the inclusion and exclusion criteria are chosen to ensure that the designed clinical trial will provide the best possible results, the appropriate criteria depend on the population to whom the treatment is targeted and more generally to the goals of the study. Table 20–4 summarizes key elements of the inclusion and exclusion criteria for

ALS clinical trials. Many issues need to be considered when determining the inclusion and exclusion criteria in ALS. The most fundamental criterion is the accuracy of the diagnosis for the disease under clinical trial consideration. Because there are no diagnostic markers for ALS, the diagnosis of ALS must depend on the uniform diagnostic criteria, such as the widely accepted El Escorial diagnostic criteria for ALS[82] (see Chapter 6, Table 6–3). For the inclusion criteria, patients diagnosed as "definite" or "probable" ALS are usually included. However, Dr. Robert G. Miller (Pacific Medical Center, personal communication, 1995) argues that patients with definite and probable ALS based on El Escorial criteria are already in well-developed stages of ALS, and these criteria may be too strict to enter patients who are in early stages of ALS. Patients with all other subsets of motor neuron disease cannot be included for the study because the subsets of ALS may be different from classic ALS and respond differently to the drug. Familial ALS poses the same question, but these patients are usually not excluded. The lack of diagnostic markers in ALS makes these inclusion and exclusion criteria difficult because a certain degree of arbitrariness may be unavoidable.

Patients for whom a benefit cannot be hypothesized should be excluded from the study. For instance, those who are in very advanced stages of ALS must be excluded. ALS functional scales or muscle strength testing are used to screen the patients for inclusion and exclusion. Active neurologic diseases other than ALS are clearly another example, but a history of minor neurologic diseases, such as resolved stroke, resolved head trauma, or controlled epilepsy, may not require exclusion. Very old age (older than 80 or 85 years) poses a different type of question because of limited life expectancy. Because ALS with a duration longer than 5 years may be different from typical ALS with rapid progression,[45] patients with an extended course of ALS may respond differently to drug treatment, and generally are excluded.

Medical diseases also raise similar concerns. Patients having active, unstable concomitant diseases that require specific treatments, recent major surgery, or a history of significant medical diseases, such as cancer

Table 20–4. INCLUSION AND EXCLUSION CRITERIA FOR ALS CLINICAL TRIALS

Subjects	Inclusion	Absolute Exclusion	Depending on Study Design
Diagnosis	Definite ALS, probable ALS (on El Escorial Criteria)	PLS, PMA, SMA, motor neuropathy; all other active neurologic diseases, including dementia, sensory, bladder, and bowel dysfunction	Familial ALS, controlled epilepsy; history of or inactive neurologic diseases
Age	—	Younger than 18, older than 85	Ages 18–25 and 75–85 may be excluded
Duration of disease	—	Generally more than 5 yr	More than 3 yr
Disease progression	Active progression	No progression	—
Functional level	ALSFRS scores >20 or equivalent	ALSFRS <16 or equivalent	Nonambulatory, tube-feeding, incapable of self-care
Pulmonary function	—	—	Ventilatory support >60% FVC in phase I study
Concomitant medical diseases	Chronic and stable diseases	Unstable, active diseases; recent major surgeries; cancer (except for basal cell skin cancer); history of neurotoxin exposure; porphyria	Gammopathy, metabolic diseases
Concomitant drugs	Usual drugs for common medical diseases, usual antioxidants, vitamins	IND-approved medications, drugs potentially causing effects or side effects mimicking those of the testing drug	Gabapentin Riluzole Drugs used for symptomatic relief for ALS
Laboratory abnormalities	Clinically insignificant changes	Significant abnormalities; CSF protein >100 mg/dL, if done	—
Nonmedical factor	Caregivers available; living an accessible distance from the center	—	—
Drug and alcohol dependency	—	Active dependency	History of dependency
Reproduction	Both sexes with contraception	Pregnant women	—
Informed consent	Understands and signs	Unable to understand or unable to obtain consent	—

Abbreviations: ALSFRS = ALS functional rating scale, CSF = cerebrospinal fluid, FVC = forced vital capacity, IND = investigational new drug, PLS = primary lateral sclerosis, PMA = primary muscular atrophy, SMA = spinal muscular atrophy.

or lymphoproliferative disorders must be excluded. These patients cannot be assumed to respond to experimental treatment for ALS; if they do respond to the trial drug, it would be hard to evaluate such responses. For similar reasons, patients with a history of neurotoxin exposure, metabolic diseases potentially causing neurologic complications such as porphyria, or clinically significant monoclonal gammopathy should be excluded. On the other hand, chronic stable diseases under proper treatment, such as essential arterial hypertension, non–insulin-dependent diabetes mellitus, treated hypothyroidism, and coronary arterial disease, need not be excluded because these diseases are unlikely to interfere with the effects of the drug or the assessment process.

Patients receiving any other investigational drug should be excluded from the study, unless such drugs are discontinued a certain time before entry to eliminate their effects (a "washout" period). Investigational drugs that have unknown or long-lasting "carryover" effects, such as neurotrophic factors or cyclophosphamide, may need to be excluded for long periods. The recent availability of riluzole as a prescribable drug and IGF-1 under a treatment IND certainly forecasts the likelihood that trials with multiple investigational drugs might become a reality.

Some "unlabeled drugs" (FDA-approved drugs for diseases other than ALS, such as gabapentine) cause relatively minor side effects and may not interfere with the main purpose of the investigation. The decision to include or exclude patients receiving such drugs depends on the nature of the medication to be tested. When a test drug is expected to have side effects similar to those of a concomitant medication, or if one drug may mask the side effects of the other, the concomitant medication needs to be discontinued. Some concomitant medications, however, are often crucial because they provide symptomatic relief for patients with ALS. It is medically unacceptable and unethical to discontinue such medications unless there are clear safety reasons for doing so, as described above. These medications include antidepressants, muscle relaxants, antisialorrhea agents, and sedatives or hypnotics.

Unexpected abnormal laboratory results must be investigated for clues to underlying diseases. Only patients with minor abnormal test results without clinical significance should be included. A cerebrospinal fluid protein concentration greater than 100 mg/dL is grounds for exclusion. These restrictions minimize the chance that unrecognized active disease will interfere with the response to the trial drug.

Nonmedical issues, such as the availability of a caregiver and the distance to and from the study center, are important for effective patient care and follow-up. Patients dependent on narcotic drugs or alcohol are prone to develop unexpected medical diseases and to have poor adherence to a protocol and should be excluded from the study. Patients with a history of dependency and recovery may be suitable, however.

The effects of investigational drugs on a fetus or on breast-fed infants are usually unknown, so women of childbearing age must not be pregnant on entering the study and must not risk pregnancy during the study. The recent trials with IGF-I (discussed later) excluded all women of childbearing age, which caused ethical concerns.[50] For the same reasons, sexually active men entered into a study must use appropriate contraception (the effects of a new drug on sperm are also unknown). The last but crucial criterion is the ability of study subjects to understand the informed consent form, which describes the entire trial in full detail in lay language, and to give consent by signing or by proxy.

ASSESSMENT AND MEASUREMENT TECHNIQUES

ALS causes progressive loss of muscle strength, so loss of motor function and deterioration in quality of life are inevitable consequences antedating death by months or years. A variety of assessment and measurement techniques can analyze and document these changes in ALS patients.[22,35] Louwerse and colleagues[55] list 12 important requirements for measurement techniques used in clinical trials for ALS (Table 20–5). Table 20–6 summarizes the techniques used, including ALS global scales and other scales (clinimetrics), semiquantitative and quantitative muscle strength testing, quantitative neuromuscular testing, electrophysiologic testing, and quality-of-life assessment. We will

Table 20–5. REQUIREMENTS FOR ALS ASSESSMENT OR MEASUREMENT

Relevance	• Assessing clinically meaningful key features of ALS
Validity	• Measuring what the test is purported to measure; the test should be validated by other measurement techniques
Reliability or reproducibility	• No or minimal variation in data between test and retest evaluations
Sensitivity to change	• Reflecting even small clinical changes over time
Quantification	• Able to quantify deficits and neurologic changes
Simplicity	• Does not require complicated training or equipment
Communicability	• Methods and results are easily understood by others
Range	• Detecting changes from the begnning to the end of the disease
Ordinal scales	• Providing discrete, definable, mutually exclusive numerical scales in hierarchical order
Statistical analysis	• Lends itself to standard statistical analyses
General acceptance	• Easily transferrable among studies
Variables	• Depending on the purpose of the test

Source: Adapted from Louwerse, ES, de Jong, VJMB, and Kuether, G: Critique of assessment methodology in amyotrophic lateral sclerosis. In Rose, FC (ed): Amyotrophic Lateral Sclerosis. Demos, New York, 1990, pp 151–179.

Table 20–6. TYPES OF ALS MEASUREMENT TECHNIQUES

ALS Global Scales (Clinimetric Tests)
Scores based on subjective or historic data alone
    ALS severity scale
    ALS functional rating scale
Scores based on clinical tests and subjective or historic data
    Norris scale
    Appel scale
    Honda scale
Scales used for ALS and other diseases
    Schwab and England global rating scale
    Ashworth spasticity scale

Muscle Strength Testing
Semiquantitative tests
    Manual muscle testing
Quantitative tests
    Maximum voluntary isometric contraction
    Handheld dynamometer
    Isokinetic muscle strength

Quantitative Neuromuscular Testing
Tufts quantitative neuromuscular examination
Other testing

Electrophysiologic Testing
Compound motor action potentials
Motor unit number estimate

Quality-of-Life Assessment
Sickness impact profile

review the usefulness of these measurement techniques with regard to the requirements.

ALS Global Scales and Other Scales

ALS FUNCTIONAL RATING SCALE

The ALS functional rating scale (ALSFRS) is derived in part from the ALS severity scale (ALSSS) and the unified Parkinson rating scale (UPRS).[2] To evaluate motor function in more detail than the ALSSS, the ALSFRS adds several different motor function tests from the UPRS. The ALSFRS assesses four bulbar-respiratory functions, two upper-extremity functions (cutting food and dressing), two lower-extremity functions (walking and climbing), and two other functions (dressing-hygiene and turning in bed) (Table 20–7). The score ranges from 40 (normal function) to 0 (unable to attempt the task). The test is simple and easily administered. A recent analysis has validated the internal consistency of the individual items and the test-retest reliability. Furthermore, the ALSFRS correlates well with isometric muscle strength and the Schwab and England global scale[2] (Fig. 20–1). The sensitivity of this scale in revealing changes over time is also well documented. A 3-point change in the ALSFRS corresponds with a 0.4-point change in the combined megascore in isometric muscle strength testing, as discussed later. The ALSFRS has been used in recent clinical trials with CNTF[3] (Fig. 20–2) and BDNF. In addition to clinical trials, ALSFRS is also widely used in clinical evaluation at several ALS clinics.

ALS SEVERITY SCALE

Hillel and colleagues[40] developed a simple global ALSSS that can be administered easily by any health-care worker because no tests are required. It assesses speech, swallowing, lower extremities (walking), and upper extremities (dressing and hygiene), each with 10 ordinal scores. This scale is reliable, and

---

Table 20–7. **ALS FUNCTIONAL RATING SCALE**[*]

1. Speech
   - 4   Normal speech processes
   - 3   Detectable speech disturbance
   - 2   Intelligible with repeating
   - 1   Speech combined with nonvocal communication
   - 0   Loss of useful speech

The rest are all similarly graded into 4 (normal) to 0 (complete loss of function):

2. Salivation (4 to 0)
3. Swallowing (4 to 0)
4. Handwriting (4 to 0)
5a. Cutting food and handling utensils (patients without gastrostomy) (4 to 0)[†]
5b. Preparing tube food and handling device (patients with gastrostomy) (4 to 0)[†]
6. Dressing and hygiene (4 to 0)
7. Turning in bed and adjusting bedclothes (4 to 0)
8. Walking (4 to 0)
9. Climbing stairs (4 to 0)
10. Breathing (4 to 0)

*Point scores range from 0 (maximum impairment) to 40 (healthy).

†5a is used for those who take oral food and 5b is used for those who use only gastrostomy tube feeding.

Source: Adapted from the ALS CNTF Treatment Study (ACTS) Phase I-II Study Group: The amyotrophic lateral sclerosis functional rating scale: Assessment of activities of daily living in patients with amyotrophic lateral sclerosis. Arch Neurol 53:141–147, 1996.

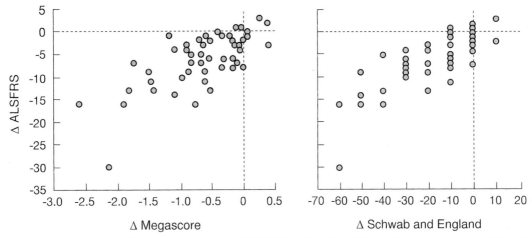

Figure 20–1. Changes in ALS functional rating scale (ALSFRS) as a function of change in the megascore and Schwab and England score. (*Left*) Change in ALSFRS vs change in megascore, maximum voluntary isometric contraction normalized by the average ALS patient muscle strength. (*Right*) Change in ALSFRS vs change in Schwab and England score. ALSFRS correlates well with quantitative muscle strength and Schwab and England global measure of activities of daily living. (From The ALS CNTF Treatment Study (ACTS) Phase I-II Study Group: The amyotrophic lateral sclerosis functional rating scale: Assessment of activities of daily living in patients with amyotrophic lateral sclerosis. Arch Neurol 53:146, 1996, with permission. Copyright © 1996 American Medical Association.)

the changes in the ALSSS have been validated by evaluating patients with ALS over 2 years. However, the ALSSS has not yet been used in clinical trials.

NORRIS SCALE

The Norris scale was proposed by Norris and colleagues[67] in 1979 and modified in 1990 (Table 20–8). This scale involves 28 clinical tests and six subjective evaluations

(e.g., chewing, bowel and bladder pressure, and feeding) to measure neurologic function as well as disability in ALS. The Norris scale is characterized by its simplicity and feasibility and satisfied most requirements listed in Table 20–5. This ALS global scale has been applied in clinical trials.[42,48,69] Although it has been considered the best ALS global scale, it has disadvantages:[20,22] First, the arm subscore is weighted more heavily than other subscores, so this score contributes more

Figure 20–2. The patients who received the placebo during the 9-month CNTF clinical trial showed a steady decline of function and muscle strength. The ALS Functional Rating Scale (ALSFRS) and maximum voluntary isometric contraction (MVIC), expressed as megascore, showed nearly identical changes from the baseline. (Figure prepared by Nancy Stambler, Regeneron Pharmaceuticals Inc., from data supplied by the ACTS Steering Committee, with permission.)

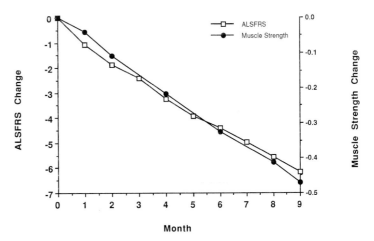

Table 20–8. **THE NORRIS ALS SCALE***

	3 (Normal)	2 (Impaired)	1 (Trace)	0 (No Use)
1. Hold up head (test)				
2. Chewing (history)				
3. Swallowing (test)				
4. Speech (test)				
5. Roll over (test)				
6. Sit up (test)				
7. Bowel/bladder pressure (history)				
8. Breathing (test)				
9. Cough (test)				
10. Write (test)				
11. Buttons, zippers (test)				
12. Feeding (history)				
13. Grip/lift self (test)				
14. Grip/lift book, tray (test)				
15. Grip/lift fork, pencil (test)				
16. Change arm position (test)				
17. Climb stairs (test)				
18. Walk (test)				
19. Walk one room (test 15 ft)				
20. Walk assisted (test only if assist required above)				
21. Stand (test)				
22. Change leg position (test)				
23. Biceps, brachioradialis, triceps muscle stretch reflexes (test)				
24. Quadriceps, Achilles, internal hamstring muscle stretch reflexes (test)				
25. Jaw jerk (test)				
26. Plantar response—right (test)				
27. Plantar response—left (test)				
28. Fasciculation (test)				
29. Atrophy—face (test)				
30. Atrophy—arms, shoulders (test)				
31. Atrophy—legs, hips (test)				
32. Labile emotions (history and observation)				
33. Fatigability (test): Requiring only two grades: 2 (normal) or 0 (present)				
34. Leg rigidity (test): Requiring only two grades: 2 (normal) or 0 (present)				

*Point scores range from 0 (maximum impairment) to 100 (healthy).
Source: Adapted from Norris, FH, Jr: Charting the course in amyotrophic lateral sclerosis. In Rose, FC (ed): Amyotrophic Lateral Sclerosis. Demos, New York, 1990, pp 83–92.

to the overall score. Second, the respiratory score is not weighted heavily enough. Patients with a high score can die abruptly because of undetected respiratory compromise; therefore, the Norris ALS score is not a good prognostic predictor. Third, the meaning of a change in the score of an individual item is not easily interpreted. In this scale, variables such as bladder pressure, which has little clinical relevance to ALS, and muscle stretch reflex, which has no clinical significance in the progression of ALS, are considered equivalent to major variables. The Norris scale has been used in conjunction with pulmonary function tests and manual muscle testing.[68]

APPEL ALS SCALE

The Appel ALS scale (Table 20–9) integrates pulmonary function and manual muscle testing.[8,37] Thus, the disease milestones of individual patients can be easily detected. The scale consists of 16 tests (one pulmonary and 15 extremity tests) and three subjective evaluations. Bulbar function assessment, however, involves two subjective evaluations, and the lack of objective and quantitative measurements of bulbar function can be a disadvantage. Another shortcoming of this scale is the use of manual muscle testing, a technique insensitive to changes over time (see below). Brooks et al.[22] analyzed the differences in the Norris and Appel scales over 12 months in the same 14 patients and found that scores from the Norris scale were linear over time, whereas scores from the Appel scale leveled off after 6 months, suggesting that sensitivity may diminish as the disease progresses. Sensitivity is reduced in patients whose scores reach more than 100 (of a maximum deficit of 164, starting from 30 points indicating healthy subjects). However, the standard deviation of the Appel scores at 12 months was smaller than that of the Norris scale, suggesting that the Appel scale might allow smaller sample sizes in standard placebo-controlled studies to detect the effectiveness of a drug over 12 months. Several clinical trials have used this scale.[7,42,50,51]

HONDA SCALE

Honda[41] describes a scale that gives equal emphasis to cranial nerve and truncal muscle functions, in addition to upper- and lower-

Table 20–9. **APPEL SCALE**[*]

1. Bulbar (6–30)
   - Swallowing (3–15)
   - Speech (3–15)
2. Respiratory—FVC (6–30)
3. Muscle strength—MMT by MRC scales (6–36)
   - Upper extremities (sum of R and L sides) (2–14)
   - Lower extremities (sum of R and L sides) (2–14)
   - Grip (pounds R grip plus L grip divided by 2) (1–4)
   - Lateral pinch (pounds R pinch plus L pinch divided by 2) (1–4)
4. Muscle function—lower extremities (6–35)
   - Standing from chair in seconds (1–5)
   - Standing from lying supine in seconds (1–6)
   - Walking 20 ft (6 m) (1–5)
   - Need for assistive devices (1–5)
   - Climbing and descending four standard steps in seconds (1–6)
   - Hips and legs (behavioral) (1–8)
5. Muscle function—upper extremities (6–33)
   - Dressing and feeding (behavioral) (1–4)
   - Propelling wheelchair 20 ft (6 m) in seconds (1–6)
   - Arms and shoulders (grades the most affected side) (1–6)
   - Cutting Theraplast—dominant hand in seconds (1–6)
   - Purdue pegboard (60 s)—number of pegs R side plus number of pegs L side divided by 2 (1–5)
   - Block (60 s)—number of blocks R side plus number of blocks L side divided by 2 (1–5)

[*]Point scores range from 30 (healthy) to 164 (maximum impairment), derived by totaling scores from all test items (score ranges in parenthesis).
Abbreviations: FVC = forced vital capacity, MMT = manual muscle testing, MRC = Medical Research Council.
Source: Adapted from Appel, V, et al: A rating scale for amyotrophic lateral sclerosis: description and preliminary experience. Ann Neurol 22:328–333, 1987.

extremity functions. It consists of 127 tests and 8 subjective evaluations. This scale involves no major equipment and can be administered at home, although it does require extensive examination, which may pose a problem to patients and examiners. Simplicity, reproducibility, transferability, and general acceptability remain to be established.

SCHWAB AND ENGLAND GLOBAL RATING SCALE

Schwab and England[76] developed a global measure of activities of daily living (ADL) in evaluating surgical outcomes in Parkinson's disease. Thus, the scale is not specific for ALS. This scale consists of 11 points and asks the rater to assess ADL function from 100 (normal) to zero (vegetative functions only). The ALS CNTF Treatment Study Group[2] analyzed the validity of the Schwab and England global rating scale and found it to be highly correlated with ALSFRS and sensitive to changes over time. A 1-point change in the Schwab and England scale is roughly equivalent to a 3-point change in the ALSFRS. This scale has been used in the recent CNTF clinical trials.[3]

ASHWORTH SCALE

The Ashworth scale[9] is a semiquantitative measurement of spasticity (see Table 4–3). Regrettably, the scale has no quantitative measurements to test upper motor neuron signs. This scale has been used in recent clinical trials in ALS.

Semiquantitative and Quantitative Muscle Strength Testing

MANUAL MUSCLE TESTING

Manual muscle testing (MMT) developed by the Medical Research Council (MRC)[58] (see Table 4–5) is a semiquantitative muscle strength testing widely used by practicing neurologists. It has also been used in clinical trials but has several disadvantages.[65] First, MMT produces ordinal scores, which require nonparametric, statistically less powerful analyses. Second, the ordinal scores on the MRC scale are not uniformly distributed. Third, the MRC scale is characterized by a pronounced loss of sensitivity, particularly at the stronger (muscle strength) end of the scale.[65] Figure 20–3 illustrates the problem of sensitivity with MMT. The scores of grade 4 (overcomes passive resistance) and grade 5 (normal) reflect at least 40%[12] and sometimes as much as 97% of the patient's muscle strength.[80] On the other hand, MMT is usually reliable. Testing a total of 34 muscles (16 muscles on one side times two plus neck extensor and flexor muscles) is adequate to improve the low sensitivity of MMT, which may thus serve as a satisfactory muscle strength evaluation method for clinical trials.[22]

MAXIMUM VOLUNTARY ISOMETRIC CONTRACTION

Assessment of maximum voluntary isometric contraction (MVIC) measures isometric muscle strength quantitatively. The techniques were developed as part of the Tufts Quantitative Neuromuscular Evaluation (TQNE).[5] The test requires a strain gauge (a force displacement transducer), a strap to hold the extremity being tested, a special examining table to position the patient's joints and to fix the strain gauge at a proper angle, and a computer to process the data (Fig. 20–4). This technique has been used extensively during the past 10 years by many investigators. MVIC satisfies almost all of the important requirements for measurement techniques (see Table 20–5). Importantly, its range and sensitivity have been validated by several natural history studies[21,22,64,73] (see Chapter 9). However, testing of MVIC has two potential disadvantages: Reliability may be low unless the examiner is well trained, and a need for certain equipment causes its lack of simplicity. Also, the equipment is relatively expensive, probably more than $5,000. Nonetheless, this muscle strength testing technique is most widely used in the clinical trials throughout North America.[3,18,23,60,66] MVIC has not been incorporated in studies done in Europe.

The full TQNE exam tests 26 muscle groups. However, testing a smaller group of muscles can generate equally satisfactory results. The reduced set of muscles tested includes at a minimum shoulder, elbow, hip, knee flexors and extensors, and ankle dorsiflexors. Usually, grip strength is measured by a Jamar hand dynamometer.

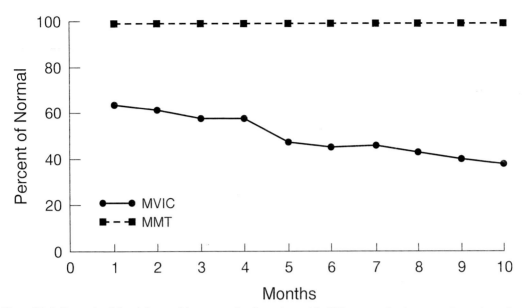

Figure 20–3. Strength of the right quadriceps muscle of a patient with ALS measured using manual muscle testing (MMT) and maximal voluntary isometric contraction (MVIC) during a 10-month period. Note that the MMT indicates that strength remains at 100% while MVIC declines from 64% to 40% of normal during the 10 months. (From Munsat, TL, et al: Therapeutic trials in amyotrophic lateral sclerosis: Measurement of clinical deficit. In Rose, FC (ed): Amyotrophic Lateral Sclerosis. Demos, New York, 1990, p. 70, with permission.)

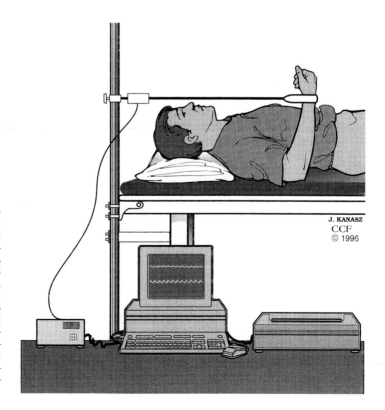

Figure 20–4. Maximal voluntary isometric contraction is measured on a standard examination table with orthopedic aluminum bars and adjustable rings. A nylon strap is placed around the limb. The strap is connected to the strain gauge, which is attached to a ring on an immobile upright bar. The strap and strain gauge remain parallel with the table. The amount of distortion in the strain gauge is transduced into force and then processed on a computer. (Copyright © 1996 Cleveland Clinic Educational Foundation.)

MMT, although low in sensitivity, allows ordinal scores of different muscles to be compared. In contrast, raw scores from MVIC do not allow such comparisons, because normal scores differ from muscle to muscle. Munsat and colleagues[5,64] thus applied a statistical technique called z-score transformation to standardize raw scores into comparative scores relative to a reference population. To use the z-transformation, data from a normative ALS population are required. Such data have been generated by several investigators.[21,64,73] The formula for transforming a raw MVIC score of the muscle tested is as follows:

$$z\text{-score} = \frac{(\text{Raw MVIC score}) - (\text{mean ALS reference population score})}{\text{Standard deviation of the ALS reference population score}}$$

Once the raw scores are standardized, individual z-scores can be averaged by region (right or left arm, arms, right or left leg, or legs) to form "megascore." Figure 20–5 shows a series of mega arm scores in individual patients with ALS. The best-fit curve by linear regression analysis of z-scores over time provides z-slopes, and grouped z-slopes are called "megaslopes." These z-slopes or megaslopes have been used as an outcome variable indicating the rate of progression in ALS. These slopes were used in the recent CNTF clinical trials (see Fig. 20–2).

HANDHELD DYNAMOMETER

The handheld dynamometer is widely available in European countries. Its cost is modest, it is portable, and it provides quantitative, reproducible data (see Table 20–5).[34]

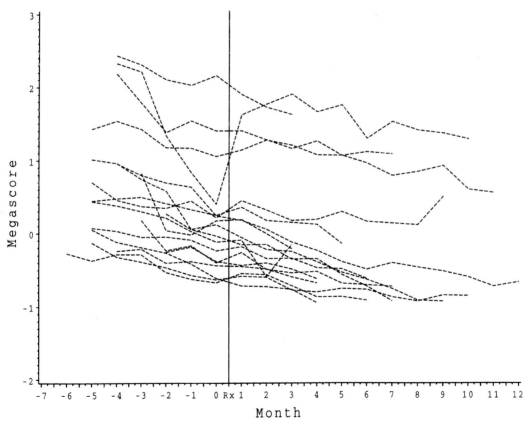

Figure 20–5. Serial, monthly measurements of maximal voluntary isometric contraction (MVIC) expressed as megascore (see text) in patients with ALS who received intravenous immunoglobulin treatment. The patients were followed for 3 to 6 months (−3 to −6) before the treatment. In one patient who had high levels of anti-GM1 antibody along with upper motor neuron signs, strength improved remarkably with the treatment.

However, this technique may depend on the examiner's muscle strength because muscle strength is measured at a "breaking" point when the patient pushes the dynamometer, which is held by the examiner.[65] The potential problem is that MMT and handheld dynamometer strength correlate well only when muscle strength on the MRC scale is between 3 to 5.[34]

ISOKINETIC MUSCLE STRENGTH

In contrast to the MMT and MVIC, isokinetic muscle strength technique does not require immobilizing the joint to be tested, which is a potential source of error in the measurements of MMT and MVIC. Furthermore, large proximal muscles are easily tested by this technique. Isokinetic strength is expressed as peak torque (in foot-pounds), whereas the examined joint is mobilized (in revolutions per minute) with the maximum effort.[61] Sufit and colleagues[79] demonstrated that isokinetic strength testing has a greater sensitivity and reproducibility than MMT. Isokinetic muscle strength testing may show an abnormality long before isometric muscle strength testing reveals weakness.[79] Its limitations include a need for an expensive dynamometer, such as a Cybex dynamometer; difficulty in positioning and transferring patients; and a prolonged testing period. This strength-testing method was used in earlier clinical trials with thyrotropin-releasing hormone.[61,79]

Quantitative Neuromuscular Testing

TUFTS QUANTITATIVE NEUROMUSCULAR EVALUATION

The TQNE, developed by Munsat and his colleagues,[5,64,72] includes:
- The MVIC measurement as the key test of muscle strength
- Pulmonary function tests, such as forced vital capacity (FVC) and maximum ventilatory volume
- Timed bulbar function tests, such as diadochokinetic rates of pa and pata (repetition of the syllables "pa" or "pata" in a given time)
- Timed upper-extremity function tests,

such as the time to dial a 7-digit phone number
- The time to transfer a set of pegs to a Purdue pegboard

In the TQNE, these quantitative tests are grouped into five major categories (megascores): pulmonary function, bulbar function, timed hand activities, isometric arm strength (including grip strength), and isometric leg strength.[5] These timed function tests have been analyzed extensively in ALS patients, and normative data are available to compute z-score.

OTHER QUANTITATIVE MEASUREMENTS

Other timed function tests include respiratory function tests such as negative inspiratory pressure, sometimes called maximum inspiratory pressure (see Chapter 22). For leg function, the time required to walk 5 m can be used. Quantitative bulbar function tests have been limited. The time to drink 5 ounces of water had been incorporated into the previous TQNE, and Mitsumoto et al.[61] applied it as a method of assessment, but it is difficult to perform because of the potential risk of aspiration. Bulbar muscle strength has been assessed by testing masseter strength (bite pressure), orbicularis oris strength (lip closure), and tongue muscle strength.[10,22] The changes of these muscle strengths correlated well with MVIC in extremity muscles over time.[22,65]

Such tests seem to be an important addition to other established methods of quantitative testing. Guiloff[34] pointed out, however, that there is a pronounced learning curve for most timed functional tests, such as FVC and timed bulbar function testings (tongue protrusion, word repetition, and timed walking). Therefore, caution is needed when such tests are used as assessment techniques for clinical trials.

Electrophysiologic Testing

Electrophysiologic methods are probably the most objective quantitative tests available, if crucial requirements are fulfilled[43] (see Table 20–5). Functional disability and prognosis of ALS are well correlated with compound muscle action potential

(CMAP)[26,62] (see Chapter 9). Furthermore, the MVIC and CMAP had been found to change linearly with time for a given patient.[26] This suggests that CMAP amplitude may be used as an additional yardstick in ALS clinical trials. In fact, changes in CMAP have been evaluated in clinical trials with thyrotropin-releasing hormone (TRH).[19,61] Brooke and colleagues[19] found a slight increase of CMAP amplitudes with TRH treatment, whereas our studies[61] showed a steady decline despite treatment. More recently, CMAP amplitudes were tested in the CNTF clinical trials and again showed a steady decline in both CNTF and placebo-treated patients.[4]

Motor unit number estimation (MUNE) is another promising electrophysiologic technique to assess the effects of medications. The number of motor units is expected to decline over time in ALS. A detailed discussion of MUNE techniques can be found in Chapter 5. MUNE was performed in 80 patients during the recent clinical trials with CNTF; the number of the motor units continued to decline in both CNTF-treated patients and controls.[4]

Quality-of-Life Assessment

Quality of life is an important issue in patients who suffer from chronic, debilitating, and often terminal diseases,[36,52] and its assessment is helpful in making clinical decisions about patient management, particularly with regard to withholding or withdrawing care from the terminally ill. Whether or not a new drug improves quality of life is an important factor in ascertaining the value of that drug. In the early phases of clinical trials, investigators may seek medications that slow the progression of ALS or reduce mortality. It is also essential to remember, however, that medication that merely prolongs life without improving quality of life may not be considered an effective medication.

For this reason, quality-of-life assessment is incorporated into current clinical trials. In fact, the WFN Subcommittee on Motor Neuron Disease recommends that all clinical trials should include a quality-of-life assessment. A health status measure called the sickness impact profile (SIP) has been widely

Table 20–10. **SICKNESS IMPACT PROFILE**

- SIP physical domain
    Ambulation
    Body care and movement
    Mobility
- SIP psychosocial domain
    Alertness
    Communication
    Emotional behavior
    Social interaction
- Other SIP domains
    Eating
    Home management
    Recreation and pastimes
    Sleep and rest
    Work

Abbreviation: SIP = sickness impact profile.
Source: Adapted from Bergner, M, et al: The sickness impact profile: Development and final revision of a health status measure. Med Care 19:787–805, 1981.

used and validated.[13] The SIP involves 136 yes or no questions in three different dimensions of life (Table 20–10). The SIP is a prototype for quality-of-life measures, and it has been used in recent IGF-I and BDNF clinical trials. Quality-of-life assessment should address the multiple facets of our daily life, as shown on Table 20–10. At present, however, there is no single, uniformly accepted or widely used assessment instrument. Simple and objective quality-of-life assessment techniques, which fulfill requirements for clinical measurement, need to be developed.

PRIMARY AND SECONDARY OUTCOMES

Successful outcomes of ALS clinical trials may be seen in four spheres: (1) prolonged symptomatic improvement, (2) reduced rate of deterioration in one or more affected functions, (3) prolonged survival time, and (4) reduced disease-related mortality.[34] The primary outcome should be of central clinical relevance to the patient. Ideally, effects of the treatment on the primary outcome should impact medical practice. Therefore, in ALS, loss of muscle strength (and sometimes loss of motor function), respiratory failure, or death are usually chosen as primary outcomes. Which primary outcome the clinical trial selects will affect the sample size and study design.

Secondary outcomes are events or conditions that are related to the primary outcomes but of less clinical or medical importance.[59] They may be measures of loss of motor function as expressed by ALS scales, ADL changes, electrophysiologic changes, or alterations in the quality of life, for example.

Death as a primary outcome poses some questions in ALS trials. Although death appears to be the most distinctive and discerning event, it can be influenced in several ways. Longevity in ALS depends on external health factors,[64] which include not only the level of general medical care and the presence or absence of other systemic diseases but also qualities of the caregiver and of the home, the availability of mobility aids, the provision of services, and a variety of personality factors that determine coping ability[77] (see Chapter 9). The judicious use of antibiotics for bronchitis or presumed aspiration pneumonia, tube feeding, noninvasive positive-pressure ventilation, and aggressive general care may prolong life in ALS. Patients who are involved in clinical trials are generally cared for by highly motivated caregivers, physicians, and other health-care professionals who are interested and concerned about the patient's well-being. Again, such care may affect the outcome. Tracheostomy for permanent ventilator care clearly postpones death, and thus the need for this procedure should be considered as equivalent to death for the purpose of defining an outcome measure in survival analysis.[28] Most of these concerns are in fact applicable not only to other primary outcomes but also to secondary outcomes. The strongest argument against death as the primary outcome may be the greater length of the study required. As noted in Chapter 9, the median duration of ALS ranges from 23 to 52 months, and 50% survival is somewhere between 3 and 4 years after the onset of disease. This time span forces the study to be prolonged over 1 or 2 years, which may increase the difficulty of study design as well as its cost.

Once the primary and secondary outcomes are selected, the results of all relevant analyses should be reported at the end of the study, whether or not they are statistically or clinically significant. Obviously, selective reporting, in which only the desirable findings of the study are presented, must be avoided. In the absence of a statement that the results are from a post-hoc analysis, the reader's only defense against selective reporting is to determine whether the relationships make clinical sense. Thus, all results should be reported accurately, completely, and in context.[49]

STUDY DESIGNS

The Open-Label Study and Its Potential Problems

An open-label study is one in which all patients participating in the study receive the active medication (Fig. 20–6A). Open-label studies appear most desirable to patients who wish to try any potentially beneficial medication in the face of a devastating disease like ALS. However, unless the drug produces overwhelming changes and benefits, a study without a control group is nearly uninterpretable and is not currently acceptable as evidence of efficacy.[17] Even in patients with ALS, an otherwise ineffective drug may produce placebo effects lasting as long as 3 or 4 months.[16,18,19,61] Furthermore, if side effects of an experimental drug mimic symptoms produced during the natural course of ALS (something like weakness, fatigue, or weight loss), they may not be identified correctly as the side effects for a long time. Thus, open-label trials should be used only for exploratory or feasibility studies, such as phase I clinical trials (see Table 20–3).

There may be two possible exceptions to the prohibition against open-label studies. One is to compare the results of open-label studies to historic controls; the other is to use the patient as his or her own control by comparing prestudy and poststudy data. The comparison of changes in primary and secondary endpoints reported during the open trials with those obtained from natural historic controls has been proposed,[72] but there are disagreements on using natural history data as a control. For example, questions of the linearity of disease progression and the

STUDY DESIGN

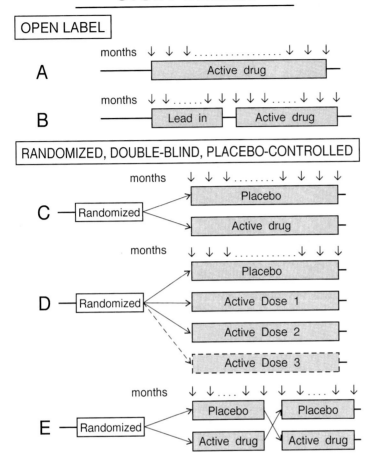

OPEN LABEL

A   months   ↓ ↓ ↓ .... ↓ ↓ ↓
       Active drug

B   months   ↓ ↓ ...... ↓ ↓ ↓ ↓ ↓ .... ↓ ↓ ↓
       Lead in   Active drug

RANDOMIZED, DOUBLE-BLIND, PLACEBO-CONTROLLED

C   Randomized   months   ↓ ↓ ↓ .... ↓ ↓ ↓ ↓
       Placebo
       Active drug

D   Randomized   months   ↓ ↓ ↓ .... ↓ ↓ ↓
       Placebo
       Active Dose 1
       Active Dose 2
       Active Dose 3

E   Randomized   months   ↓ ↓ .... ↓ ↓ ↓ ↓ .... ↓ ↓
       Placebo   Placebo
       Active drug   Active drug

Figure 20–6. Schematic presentations of trial designs. The down arrows indicate months. (A) Open-label study in which patients are compared to historical controls. (B) Open-label study in which patients serve as their own controls: they are followed for a lead-in period of months and then receive the drug. (C) Randomized, double-blind, placebo-controlled parallel study in which one group receives the drug and the other receives a placebo. (D) Randomized, double-blind, placebo-controlled parallel study in which different dose levels are investigated concurrently in multiple parallel groups. (E) Randomized, double-blind, placebo-controlled crossover study design. All subjects receive the drug but one group will receive the active drug first while the other receives the placebo. After a set time, the groups are "crossed over" so that the placebo group receives the drug and the active drug group now receives the placebo.

reliability of natural history data have not been fully answered. The treated patients in a randomized trial often differ from patients in previous natural history studies.[17] Control patients in randomized studies are a specifically selected population (by inclusion and exclusion criteria) and thus are not representative of the general ALS population. In fact, the megaslopes summarizing the decline in muscle strength of control patients who participated in the recent CNTF studies were different from those constituted with natural history data derived from the Wisconsin-Colorado database, supporting this concern[17] (Drs. BR Brooks and JM Cedarbaum, personal communication, 1995). Therefore, the studies involving natural historical data are likely to cause confounding comparisons.[29]

To date, in ALS, such studies have not ma-

terialized. If an ALS population database becomes large enough to enable age, location of onset, duration of disease before entering a study, and the use of placebos in trials to be matched with control data, this study design may be useful. In the meantime, the validity of the natural history controlled design must be tested by using recent clinical trial data. Patient populations completing randomized, controlled studies should be compared against natural history controls to determine whether the results of randomized controlled studies are reproduced by this scheme. Pradas and colleagues[72] proposed not to replace randomized, placebo-controlled, double-blind studies but to use natural history controlled trials to provide an effective gating procedure to screen out drugs with low potential and also to identify drugs that warrant further study in randomized trials. This design, if proven to be acceptable, is certainly cost-effective and solves some of the ethical dilemmas facing patients and physicians, which are discussed later in this chapter.[71]

Figure 20–6B depicts a design in which patients serve as their own controls. The patients are followed for a period of 3 to 6 months to identify the rate of disease progression (a lead-in period) and then receive an open-label drug in the study period. The changes in measured variables between the lead-in period and the treatment period are compared statistically. We[63] conducted such studies with intravenous immunoglobulin treatment in 19 patients. The rate of the deterioration in arm megascore was significantly slower during the immunoglobulin treatment period than in the lead-in period. The question as to whether the lead-in period and the treatment period are medically and biologically comparable cannot be answered. In fact, the preliminary results of recent CNTF studies showed that the natural history data based on monthly examinations for at least 3 months preceding the double-blind phase could not predict the course of the decline in those who received placebo during the treatment phase.[24] This type of study is also limited by the absence of a control group, regression to the mean (the phenomenon whereby an extreme response on the first measurement tends to be closer to the mean at a later measurement), and period effects (progression, regression, or fluctuation in results during the period of investigation). Therefore, the type of design shown in Figure 20–6B may be difficult.

The Randomized, Double-Blind, Placebo-Controlled, Parallel Study

Typically, in this study design, patients are randomly assigned into one of two groups (Fig. 20–6C). One group of patients receives the drug to be tested, whereas the other group receives a placebo, which is usually an inactive vehicle (or the standard treatment). This design is generally considered to be the "gold standard" of therapeutic trial methodology.[54] In a single-blinded study, generally only the patients are unaware of their treatment assignment. In a double-blinded study, the patients and investigators are blinded. In a less common triple-blinded study, the patients, investigators, and biostatisticians (or data analyzers) are blinded. Random assignments can be made from random number tables by computer generation. Unacceptable methods include alternating assignments or assignment by birthday or admission numbers. If assignment can be predicted, patients may be intentionally maneuvered into a particular assignment.

Sometimes, the effects of different dose levels are investigated concurrently, and on such occasions multiple parallel groups are designed in a double-blind, placebo-controlled scheme (Fig. 20–6D).

The Randomized, Double-Blind, Placebo-Controlled, Crossover Study

In contrast to a parallel design, a crossover study provides active medication to all subjects, although not in the same sequence. Patients are randomly assigned to either schedule I (placebo to active drug) or schedule II (active drug to placebo), as shown in Figure 20–6E. All participating patients receive the active drug in either the first or the second phase. Although this design avoids potential ethical pitfalls because everyone receives the medication, it is less than desirable from the standpoint of statistical analysis. The carryover effect in schedule II (i.e., an effect from the active drug that lasts into the placebo stage) adds an element of uncertainty. Thus the evaluation of the placebo in the second stage may not be as valid as in schedule I, in which patients are naive to the study drug. Furthermore, it is not yet clear whether the disease can be considered biologically identical during the first and the second stages. Despite some popularity, this design has been criticized by biostatisticians and generally discouraged because of the potential problems outlined above,[81] although Mitsumoto et al.[61] used it for investigating the effects of TRH.

Potential Problems with the Double-Blind Study

When an active drug produces obvious side effects or adverse reactions, it may be difficult to carry out a study in a blinded fashion. Such a phenomenon has been observed in several controlled clinical studies[18,19,61] and creates an inherit limitation to double-blind, controlled studies.[16,17] In only one controlled study was an "active" placebo (norepinephrine) included to mimic the side effects produced by TRH.[61] Another issue is that at entry the groups of patients must be comparable to ensure that changes occurring in the clinical trial are not the result of imbalance in patient characteristics between treatment groups. Well-designed randomization ensures such balance between the treatment groups at the entry.

It is important to remember that the prospective, randomized, double-blind, controlled design is not foolproof. Clinical investigators must be cautious about potential pitfalls. These include, for example, observing a clinically important difference, but failing to attend to it because the statistical power of the study is inadequate.[25] The more common risk is finding no difference in a study with low power and concluding that the two groups are equivalent, when in fact they are not. Such studies are not negative but inconclusive: not enough data were collected to detect a clinically important difference even if one existed. Careful statistical power calculations should be conducted during the planning stage, which is discussed later.

In many studies, patients who complete a double-blind, placebo-controlled study are allowed to receive open-label medication if they wish, provided the drug appears to be safe. Such procedures resolve ethical dilemmas to some degree, because patients who receive the placebo eventually receive active medication.

PATIENT ADHERENCE

Adherence is an important factor to the success of any therapeutic regimen. For this reason, investigators who conduct treatment trials must consider and deal with a variety of adherence issues in the design of their studies. These issues arise at every stage of execution, from patient selection and allocation through treatment induction and maintenance of follow-up and data analysis.[38] Patients with ALS are generally believed to be highly motivated and adherent, but the situation may change when expected benefits do not occur and instead side effects or adverse reactions develop. Patients may become increasingly depressed and lose interest in the trial. During clinical trials, it is important to monitor adherence and to implement effective adherence-improving strategies.[38] In addition to their involvement in the study, nurses, physicians and investigators should spend time personally with patients, discussing various issues and difficulties patients face while participating in the study. Such practice is always important to improve adherence when a patient's condition deteriorates progressively during the course of clinical trials.

BIOSTATISTICS

In any formal clinical trial, biostatisticians should be involved from the early planning stages (see Table 20–1). Obtaining biostatistical help for the first time only at the completion of the study is too late and may reveal serious flaws that invalidate the study and its results. Biostatistical consultation involves several key areas: control of bias through study design, sample size estimation, database management, data analysis, and interpretation of results. Before estimating sample size, it is important to determine how many groups are involved in the randomized trial; whether the trial aims to look at differences in absolute measures (changes) between the beginning and the end of the study; whether it will look at the rate of change in measures during the study; and how much of a difference in these measures is expected to occur between groups. If expected differences are large, testing differences in absolute measures may require only a relatively short study, whereas examining the rate of change requires a longer study because the longer the analysis, the more reliable the regression curve over time.

Summarizing data collected over time as a slope of the line through the data has some advantages, because the calculation of slope uses all available follow-up data and can be less variable then simply evaluating two data points at the beginning and end of the study. The slope as an overall rate of change also provides a way of using the data from all patients, not simply those who finish the study, because slope can incorporate data from patients lost to follow-up, and even patients who do not complete the study. Slope has disadvantages, however, because it assumes that changes are linear during the study period. Furthermore, the question of how to analyze data from patients who die during the study or drop out of the study, especially in the early stages, may be problematic. The slope of the least-squares line may be estimated for a different portion of the curve for some subjects, if there are incomplete follow-ups.[53] Studies with adequate sample sizes and statistical power can be designed with slope as the primary outcome.

Sample Size Estimation

Sample size for clinical trials is estimated from many components. Sample size requirements differ based on the study design, the level of measurement of the primary outcomes, within- and between-patient variability of the outcome measures, the length of follow-up, the spacing of measurements over time, the length of the trial, the size of the clinically important difference to be detected between groups, the α-level, the required statistical power, and the dropout rate.[1] The study design may involve only one group over time (paired or matched design) or two or more groups (parallel design). Two general types of measurement of the primary outcome should be considered: (1) a continuous variable (i.e., measured on an interval scale, such as MVIC and FVC), or (2) a categorical variable, such as number of deaths or major disability. Examples of sample size calculations are included in an excellent textbook by Altman.[1]

According to Brooks,[22] assuming that an active drug produces more than a 50% difference from placebo in a period of 12 months, with 90% power and an α of 0.05, a study using the total limb MVIC (megascore) as the primary outcome would require 25 patients for each group. In contrast, when MMT is used, 84 patients for each group are required. The sample size changes to 47 for the Norris scale and 33 for the Appel scale, because the standard deviations in these global ALS scales (the variability of the test) are larger than MVIC but smaller than MMT.

Thus, when change of muscle strength is the primary outcome, MVIC requires the smallest sample size when it is combined as the all-limb megascore.

The rate of change (slope) can also be used for sample size calculations. Brooks[22] analyzed the changes of MVIC in 14 patients over 12 months. Based on this study, if one assumes that the total limb megascore declines 18% from baseline to 6 months and the trial follows patients for 6 to 12 months, a sample size of 26 patients is required for each group to have an 80% chance of detecting a true difference of 50% between groups.

When a categorical outcome, such as death, is used, the sample size markedly changes. For instance, when the mortality rate in ALS is chosen as the primary outcome, the sample size for demonstrating a 50% reduction in mortality in the active drug group compared to the control over an 18-month period, with 90% power, an α of 0.05, and a dropout rate of 30%, 130 patients per group are necessary according to Guiloff.[34] This sample size is based on using a Cox proportional hazard regression, a statistical modeling technique used to estimate the risk of a certain event associated with a given characteristic and adjusted for the effects of other characteristics.[34] In contrast, when the time to an event, such as survival time or time to respiratory failure, is used as the primary outcome, the sample size calculation is different. To demonstrate a 50% longer median survival over an 18-month trial, with 90% power, an α of 0.05, and dropout rate 30%, a study would require 692 patients in each group.[34] Therefore, in this case the sample size markedly increases when the time to event rather than the number of events is chosen as the primary outcome measure. However, the time to event may be more appropriate in certain studies despite the large sample size required.

During clinical trials, patients will withdraw from the study for many reasons (disappointment, worsening, being unable to make the trip to the hospital, side effects, and so on). Dropouts also occur because of death, missing a dose, protocol violation (enrolling ineligible patients or administering the wrong dose), nonadherence to the protocol, and withdrawing from the study at any time for any reason. The probable dropout rate is an important factor for sample size estimation.[47] According to Brooks,[22] recent dropout rates have ranged from 30% to nearly 80% for a 1-year study period. A correction for such a potential dropout rate is another important factor for sample size estimation. Sample sizes also depend on many assumptions not fully covered in this section.

Statistical Analyses

The two types of statistical errors, type I and type II, can occur when the hypothesis is testing the framework involved with clinical trials.[46] A *type I error* is committed when one concludes that a treatment is effective when, in fact, it is not. Typical acceptable rates of type I errors are 0.05 or 0.01, usually referred to as the α-level of the study. This error rate can increase rapidly when multiple statistical tests are performed through data dredging or unplanned exploring, because the more variables analyzed, the more likely one is to find a difference by chance alone. Multiple comparison procedures such as the Bonferroni technique are helpful for protecting against this error rate increase, but careful planning is always preferred.

A *type II error* occurs when one concludes incorrectly that a treatment is not effective when in fact it is effective. In planning a study, the acceptable probability of this type of error is referred to as the β-level of the study (typically, 0.2, 0.1, or 0.05). *Statistical power* is the probability of finding a treatment effective when in fact it is effective; power is equal to 1 minus β.[54] Thus, it is clear that the error rates, α and β, should be set as low as possible. When the result of the clinical trial turns out to be negative, it is crucial that there be sufficient power to conclude that the study is negative and not inconclusive.

As for estimation of sample size, patients who drop out during a study present difficult issues related to statistical analysis. Analysis that excludes the dropouts may result in a skewed sample and even cause false results. If patients who died or withdrew from the study were different from those who stayed in the study, excluding them from the analysis may bias the results. In contrast, intent-to-treat analysis includes all patients once they are randomly assigned to a treatment arm.

It is important to recognize that statistical significance is not necessarily synonymous with clinical relevance. When there is sufficient power in the trial, statistical significance may suggest a treatment effect. However, the effect should be clinically important and biologically plausible if it is to be clinically useful. A pitfall in statistical analyses may occur with extensive post-hoc analyses. The more subgroups examined or the more outcomes compared, the more likely a statistically significant difference will be found, which can increase the chance of type I error. Again, clinical relevance becomes a major issue in such studies.[14]

A description of statistical techniques for analyzing data from clinical trials is beyond the scope of this chapter, but many excellent chapters and textbooks are available.[1,46,49,59] However, we recommend that a biostatistician be consulted before the development of the protocol, as well as to assist in analyzing the data and interpreting the results.

THE INSTITUTIONAL REVIEW BOARD AND INFORMED CONSENT

All clinical trials must be approved by the Institutional Review Board (IRB) at the institution where the trial is to take place. The IRB consists of various professionals, such as physicians, lawyers, biomedical ethicists, and members of the lay community. Its primary objectives are to protect patients from any unethical, inhumane clinical research in the name of medical science, as defined by The World Medical Association Declaration of Helsinki in 1979,[84] and to ensure the medical and scientific quality of the study. Its secondary objective is to protect the investigators and institution.

Informed consent must be obtained from all subjects. The consent form must have several key features (Table 20–11). It must be written in plain language, and the investigator must verbally explain the content of the consent form. Patients must understand its content fully before giving their consent by signing. Those who are unable to sign (e.g., because of hand weakness) may sign by proxy.

Table 20–11. **KEY ELEMENTS REQUIRED IN INFORMED CONSENT DOCUMENTS**

- Statement of research purpose
- Information about research
- Potential risks and discomforts
- Expected and potential benefits
- Alternative procedures
- Assurance of confidentiality
- Potential research-related injury
- Questions about the research
- Stipulation of voluntary participation
- Participant costs
- Signature lines

ORGANIZATIONAL STRUCTURE OF CLINICAL TRIALS IN ALS

ALS clinical trials are increasingly likely to be performed as multicenter studies. The larger the sample size, the greater the number of clinical centers required to ensure that the needed number of subjects are entered into the study during an acceptable time period. Multicenter studies are relatively new in ALS. The national TRH study in 1989 involved 14 centers and 108 patients (average less than 8 patients per center) and was the first such large-scale multicenter study in ALS.[66] A recent CNTF study involved 36 centers and 720 patients.[3] This study, the ACTS study, has become a model for multicenter studies in ALS. Table 20–12 summarizes the key components of its organizational structure.

Although the ACTS study was initiated by a pharmaceutical company (Regeneron Pharmaceuticals, Inc.), the study itself was organized and executed by a close collaboration between the study investigators and the pharmaceutical industry. The steering committee, consisting of the director of the coordinating center, the medical director of the company, five clinical investigators who were involved with phase I studies, and one clinical evaluator, took charge of the entire study. All 36 investigators participated in one of the standing committees, as listed in Table 20–12, based on his or her expertise and interest from the planning stages of the study.

Table 20–12. **AN ADMINISTRATIVE MODEL OF MULTICENTER ALS CLINICAL TRIALS**

1. Key structure and organization of the entire program
   Steering committee
   External scientific advisory committee
   External data and safety monitoring board
   Ad hoc committees
      Protocol committee
      Diagnostic and inclusion/exclusion criteria committee
      Quality assurance committee
      Electrodiagnostics committee
      Laboratory and ancillary studies committee
      Writing/Publications committee
      Clinical evaluator committee
2. Coordinating center
   Center director/principal investigator
   Center coordinator
3. Individual clinical centers
   Principal investigator
   Co-investigators
   Nurse coordinators
   Clinical evaluators
4. External data management and analysis center
   Senior biostatisticians
   Biostatisticians
   Database programmers
   Statistical programmers
   Data entry staff
5. External consultants
6. Pharmaceutical company
   Director of clinical affairs
   Medical safety officer
   Monitors
   Regulatory officers
   Biostatisticians

Key clinical evaluators formed a clinical evaluator committee, arranged training sessions, and monitored the internal quality of the evaluations throughout the study.

A coordinating center executed the day-to-day issues, such as patient entry (in conjunction with the data management center and the pharmaceutical company), monitored side effects, and coordinated the entire study throughout its duration. Each clinical center had principal and coprincipal investigators, clinical evaluators, and study coordinators. The study protocol was approved by the IRB at each institution. Each principal investigator was responsible for immediately reporting any major side effects or deaths to the pharmaceutical company, who reported them to the FDA.

Outside consultants provided advice and guidance to the clinical research team of the pharmaceutical company at the early planning stages, particularly on medical, statistical, and pharmacologic issues. An independent external scientific committee was formed to provide opinions on the scientific validity of the study. Most importantly, the ACTS group organized the data management and analysis center (DMAC) and the data and safety monitoring board (DSMB), both of which are independent from any investigators or drug company. The DMAC arranged the randomization, maintained the database, and conducted the final analysis. The DSMB evaluated safety data and study results in a blinded fashion and provided unbiased opinions (see Table 20–3). The importance of the responsibility of the DSMB was recently reviewed by Barnett and Sackett.[11] The company funded the entire study, paying for monitoring each clinical center through frequent site visits by clinical monitors to ensure that the study was being conducted under the "Good Clinical Practice Guide" set by the FDA; immediately reporting to the FDA any major events (including death) occurring during the study; and providing the entire study report to the FDA.

ETHICAL ISSUES

The Ethics of Clinical Research

The objective of the clinical trial is not to deliver therapy; rather it is to answer scientific questions about the safety and efficacy of a drug.[70] In ALS, only one drug, riluzole, has been approved for its treatment, but there is no cure, and thus there is a strong need to investigate any potential treatments that may alter the course of the disease. Unless scientific pursuits are permitted, an effective medication may not be identified.[74] However, regardless of study design, the study is ethical only when there is genuine uncertainty in the expert medical community about the efficacy of a particular drug or treatment. "If a healer's commitment to the patient is attenuated, even for so good a cause as benefits to future patients, the implicit assumptions of the doctor-patient relationship are violated." "The risk of such attenuation by the randomized trial is great."[39] Withholding a drug known to benefit patients with ALS to accomplish a placebo-controlled clinical design clearly violates the ethics of clinical trials. Thus, the ethics of such controlled studies require *equipoise*—a state of genuine uncertainty on the part of the clinical investigator regarding the comparative therapeutic merits of each arm in a trial.[32] On the other hand, there are certainly serious problems in generating a control group. Steiner[77] states, "The concept of equipoise makes no difference: patients envisage only a single chance for themselves. For patients with a life expectancy of a few months, that period on placebo treatment is a sacrifice of everything. The possibility that the treatment may be on trial for safety as well as efficacy has little real meaning in such a context."

There is little doubt that the randomized, double-blind clinical trial is a powerful technique because of the efficiency and credibility associated with treatment comparisons involving randomly assigned concurrent controls.[71] When the studies are properly carried out, with informed consent, clinical equipoise, and a design adequate to answer the questions posed, randomized clinical trials protect physicians and their patients from therapies that are ineffective or toxic.[71] Nevertheless, the new therapy should be offered to patients as soon as they complete the study, if it causes no major toxic side effects. The study design using parallel treatment, where one arm comprises patients meeting inclusion criteria and randomly assigned to treatment, and the other arm of an open-label trial comprises patients who do not meet the inclusion criteria, may be more acceptable to patients who wish strongly to take such medication. This design was used in the recent riluzole trials.

Outcomes such as loss of the ability to walk, loss of speaking ability, or respiratory failure can be used as indicators of treatment failure. In this circumstance, alternative treatments, when available, should be prescribed and symptomatic treatments that might have been withheld because of the trial medication should be resumed. Until "standard" or "alternative" therapies become available in ALS, the issue of treatment failure in clinical trials is a relatively minor problem.

As discussed previously, exclusion criteria may also raise potential ethical dilemmas. For instance, in the recent clinical trial with IGF-I, all women of childbearing age were excluded because of the potential risks to the fetus, should pregnancy have occurred.[50] In contrast, other trials with neurotrophic factors (CNTF and BDNF) allowed nonpregnant women of childbearing age to participate provided "appropriate" contraceptive measures were continued during the study. However, two women (approximately 1%) became pregnant during the CNTF study.*

Another issue is the use of resources. Large multicenter or even multinational trials require enormous amounts of resources and large numbers of eligible patients. The trial being done must be the one that most needs doing; "need" in this context must represent the need of all patients.[77] When several potential therapies become available simultaneously, how can patients judge which is most needed for them? The WFN Subcommittee on ALS Clinical Trials recommends that the results of clinical trials be announced to the public only after the study is reported in refereed journals (see Table 20–1). However, this recommendation may cause conflict between the scientific community, which demands that all scientific data of the trials be made public, and pharmaceutical companies, which require rapid announcement of results to meet their financial responsibility to shareholders. For instance, the recent experience with riluzole and IGF-I (public announcements of "efficacy" were made before the scientific data were presented and analyzed) caused controversy in the neurology community. Furthermore, progress reports of interim analyses may produce bias because preliminary results create

expectations among those who see them. Pharmacoeconomic factors have been analyzed in recent clinical studies, but these valuable data may be more valuable for marketing than for decision making in patient care. How to handle these issues requires serious discussion and agreement among the involved parties.

The Ethics of Clinical Investigators

Randomized clinical trials require doctors to act simultaneously as physicians and as scientists. This requirement puts them in a difficult and sometimes tenuous ethical position.[39] A key question is: Do controlled clinical trials violate the covenant between doctor and patient? Physicians engaged in clinical trials sacrifice the interests of participating patients for the good of all similarly affected patients in the future. The argument is that physicians have a personal obligation to use their best judgment and recommend the best therapy, no matter how tentative or inconclusive the data on which that judgment is based.[71]

Schafer[75] stated, "In other cases, however, the tension between the physician's traditional role as healer and his modern role as scientific investigator may reach the level of outright contradiction. The Hippocratic principle of exclusive commitment to patient welfare, with its corollary of total individualized treatment, may sometimes properly be modified so as to permit randomized clinical trials to proceed with a statistically adequate sample of subjects. The circumstances in which it is ethically permissible to abrogate the Hippocratic principle are in need of careful definition." Society has created mechanisms, such as FDA guidelines, IRB approval, and informed consent, to ensure that the interests of individual patients are served, should they elect to participate in a clinical trial.[71]

Clinical investigators have different ethical responsibilities. Conflict of interest must be avoided in any clinical investigations. Clinical investigators who have financial interest in any drug company that supports drug trials should not participate in that investigation. David A. Kessler,[44] the commissioner of the FDA, has warned of potential ethical pit-

---

*Dr. J. Cedarbaum and the ALS CNTF treatment study group, unpublished observation, 1994.

falls for clinical neurologists in relations with pharmaceutical industries.

In addition to the ethical obligations described above, clinical investigators must adhere to the protocol; that is, no deviation is allowed from the original research plan, unless the study protocol is formally changed after the approval of an institutional IRB and the FDA. There is a legal responsibility to maintain "good clinical practice" and to record all events related to patient care in the medical record and report forms. Investigators are responsible for reporting all major adverse events, including death, to their own IRB and to their sponsoring agency, such as the National Institutes of Health (NIH) or drug companies.

Patient Obligations

Patients who participate in clinical studies have no ethical responsibilities, but they do incur some obligations. In the past several years, however, patients have adopted a much more activist mode.[57] They now use computer-based communication (e.g., the Internet) to share extensive information (and sometimes misinformation) on investigational drugs and advocate multiple medication usage. Patients continue to seek new, ostensibly more effective clinical trials. Under these circumstances, establishing and maintaining the study population becomes increasingly difficult.

Most consent forms do not emphasize the patients' obligations in the clinical trials. No patient, in fact, can be forced to continue in a trial, but the importance of continuing participation adherent to the protocol and follow-up must be stressed at the time of recruitment and throughout the trial.[57]

THE COST-EFFECTIVENESS ISSUE

Over $1 billion per year—only about 0.3% of national health expenditures in the United States—is spent on clinical trials.[31] Although ALS is a relatively rare disease, the socioeconomic impact of this disease on patients and their families is enormous because the disease strikes many when they are most productive. We hope that effective treatments for ALS will change this scenario. The traditional type of cost-effective studies have not been performed in patients with ALS, because they need palliative treatments in this rapidly fatal disease.[27] Therefore, the decisions about the value of clinical trials in such a devastating disease cannot be judged by traditional cost-effectiveness studies. The public awareness of ALS has facilitated therapeutic trials. Clinical investigators must continue to emphasize to policy makers the importance of therapeutic trials in diseases such as ALS.

REVIEW OF RECENT THERAPEUTIC TRIALS AND FUTURE DIRECTION

Table 20–13 summarizes the characteristic features of recent controlled clinical trials in ALS. Data are based on preliminary reports or communications from scientific meetings.[49,78] Clearly an increasing number of phase III trials has been performed in the past few years. They are all multicenter trials, but the endpoint and measurement techniques differ markedly. Resolving these differences would help in comparing these studies and in planning future studies more effectively. As Table 20–13 shows, two therapeutic agents, riluzole and IGF-I, have been found to be beneficial. If the published results confirm these preliminary reports, these medications may be recognized as a "standard of care" for ALS. Studies involving polypharmacy thus may become imperative in the near future, and the randomized, placebo-controlled trial will have to be modified. All enrolled patients will receive two drugs: the same "standard drug therapy" and either an experimental drug or a placebo, depending on group assignment.

SUMMARY

Therapeutic trials may be important not only in developing an effective treatment for ALS but also in increasing our understanding of it. Thus, it is imperative that clinical trials be proper and valid. Practicing neurologists may become involved in such investi-

Table 20–13. **SUMMARY OF RECENT PROSPECTIVE, RANDOMIZED, DOUBLE-BLIND, PLACEBO-CONTROLLED, PARALLEL, MULTICENTER CLINICAL TRIALS**

Components	CNTF (ACTS)	CNTF (CASG)	Riluzole	IGF-I	BCAA
Centers	36	29	31	8	23 (9)*
Patients	730	570	959	236	429 (126)*
Diagnosis	El Escorial	ALSDC	El Escorial	"ALS"	El Escorial by two neurologists
Exclusion	ALSFRS,< 16, >5 yr	FVC < 50%, >3 yr	FVC < 60%, >5 yr	Women of child-bearing age, >115 Appel scores, >3 yr ALS	Wheelchair, tube feeding, ventilator, <FVC 50%, <3 mo, >2 yr, familial ALS
Dose levels	2	3	3	2	1
Lead-in period	3 mo plus	3 mo plus	None	2–3 mo	None
Study period	9 mo	6 mo	18 mo	9 mo	12 mo
Primary outcome	MVIC changes	MVIC changes	Death, tracheostomy, ventilator	Appel scores	Death, loss of independence
Secondary outcomes	FVC/PIF Timed functions ALSFRS SES CGIC	Arm megascore Leg megascore FVC SIP Survival	Muscle scale Modified Norris FVC CGIC VAS	SIP Survival	MRC Norris scale Appel FVC Barthel
Results	No differences	No differences	At 18 months, 50% of placebo-treated patients and 57% of those with 100 mg dose still alive	Appel scores and SIP phycosocial domain deteriorated less with higher dosage	No differences
Other contributions	ALSFRS, prognosis studies	New spasticity scale, natural history study; new diagnostic criteria	Effective multinational studies	—	First SPECIALS study

Continued on following page

Table 20–13.—*continued*

Components	CNTF (ACTS)	CNTF (CASG)	Riluzole	IGF-I	BCAA
Problems	Patients too advanced, unpredicted side effects	Unexpected measurement variability	Use of insensitive measurement techniques, variability in testing	Stringent inclusion criteria, European study was not robust, but supportive	The trial was driven by patients; the Italian group stopped the trials independently because more deaths occurred in BCAA group; limited funding
Publication	The ACTS Group[3]	Miller et al.[60]	Lacombiez et al.[48]	Under preparation	Under preparation

*The number of Italian centers and the number of Italian patients. The Italian group decided to discontinue their study because of increased death in BCAA-treated patients.[42]

Abbreviations: ACTS = ALS CNTF Treatment Study group, ALSDC = ALS diagnostic criteria, ALSFRS = ALS functional rating scale, BCAA = branched-chain amino acids, CASG = CNTF ALS Study Group, CGIC = clinical global impression of changes, CNTF = ciliary neurotrophic factor, El Escorial = WFN El Escorial ALS Diagnostic Criteria, FVC = forced vital capacity, IGF-I = insulin-like growth factor-I, MRC = Medical Research Council, MVIC = maximum voluntary isometric contraction, PIF = peak inspiratory flow, SES = Schwab and England scale, SIP = sickness impact profile, SPECIALS = Scientific pan-European collaboration in amyotrophic lateral sclerosis, VAS = visual assessment scale.

gations by referring their patients to study centers and frequently by interpreting the results of clinical trials.

Drug development in the United States is regulated by a federal agency, the FDA.

Typical ALS clinical trials range from phase I safety and toxicity studies to phase III efficacy studies, which are carried out under the IND application. Patient inclusion and exclusion criteria determine the study population. The next important decision is how to measure changes that may occur with a new treatment. A few well-known ALS scales are available and extensively used in clinical trials. Quantitative testing for muscle strength and other motor functions, such as MVIC and FVC, is crucial because these measurement techniques have proven their sensitivity and reliability. MMT, handheld dynamometer tests, and isokinetic strength tests are also available, but they have shortcomings. Electrophysiologic studies may be added but require further study to demonstrate their validity in clinical trials. In all clinical studies, the issue of quality of life has received more attention because a treatment that prolongs the life of ALS patients without improving the quality of life may not truly be effective. Which primary and secondary outcomes the study chooses to investigate are other key components of the entire study and also help to determine sample size.

Natural history controlled, open-label studies are attractive because they minimize the potential for ethical dilemmas; however, the reliability of the design is uncertain and requires further investigation. At present, the randomized, double-blind, placebo-controlled parallel study is the gold standard in ALS trials design, but it is not foolproof. Biostatisticians who determine sample size and perform later statistical analysis should participate in designing the study from the early planning stages. The informed consent agreement is a crucially important document that must be accepted by both patients and investigators. It should describe the entire protocol in unambiguous lay terms.

To perform a statistically powerful study in a reasonably short time, a multicenter study is imperative. A recent model of an ALS clinical trial with CNTF exemplifies this approach. In such a large study, an independent outside data and safety monitoring board must be established to monitor patient safety and to ascertain the validity of the study. Many ethical issues arise during the process of clinical trial design and implementation and need to be carefully evaluated by the investigator and subjects. Our ultimate goal as clinical investigators is to find therapeutic agents that relieve the suffering of our patients, to improve the quality of their lives, and to halt or at least slow the progress of this illness. Clinical trials must be carried out in an ethical, scientific, and statistically sound fashion. Such an approach will also enhance our understanding of the mysterious and dreaded disease called ALS.

REFERENCES

1. Altman, DG: Practical Statistics for Medical Research. Chapman and Hall, London, 1991.
2. The ALS CNTF Treatment Study (ACTS) Phase I-II Study Group: The amyotrophic lateral sclerosis functional rating scale: Assessment of activities of daily living in patients with amyotrophic lateral sclerosis. Arch Neurol 53:141–147, 1996.
3. ALS CNTF Treatment Study (ACTS) Study Group: A double-blind placebo-controlled clinical trial of subcutaneous recombinant human ciliary neurotrophic factor (rHCNTF) in amyotrophic lateral sclerosis. Neurology 46:1244–1249, 1996.
4. The ALS CNTF Treatment Study (ACTS) Phase II-III Group: Longitudinal electrodiagnostic studies in amyotrophic lateral sclerosis patients treated with recombinant human ciliary neurotrophic factor [abstract]. Neurology 45(suppl 4):A448, 1995.
5. Andres, PL, Finison, LJ, Conlon, T, et al: Use of composite scores (megascores) to measure deficit in amyotrophic lateral sclerosis. Neurology 38:405–408, 1988.
6. Angell, M: Patients' preferences in randomized clinical trials. N Engl J Med 310:1385–1387, 1984.
7. Appel, SH, Stewart, SS, Appel, V, et al: A double-blind study of the effectiveness of cyclosporine in amyotrophic lateral sclerosis. Arch Neurol 45:381–386, 1988.
8. Appel, V, Stewart, SS, Smith, G, et al: A rating scale for amyotrophic lateral sclerosis: Description and preliminary experience. Ann Neurol 22:328–333, 1987.
9. Ashworth, B: Trial of carisoprodol in multiple sclerosis. Practitioner 192:540–542, 1964.
10. Barlow, SM and Abbs, JH: Force transducers for the evaluation of labial, lingual, and mandibular motor impairments. J Speech Hear Res 26:616–621, 1983.
11. Barnett, HJM and Sackett, DL: Monitoring clinical trials. Neurology 43:2437–2438, 1993.
12. Beasley, WC: Quantitative muscle testing: Principles and applications to research and clinical service. Arch Phys Med Rehabil 42:398–425, 1961.
13. Bergner, M, Bobbitt, RA, Carter, WB, et al: The sick-

ness impact profile: Development and final revision of a health status measure. Med Care 19:787–805, 1981.

14. Bland, JM, Jones, DR, Bennett, S, et al: Is the clinical trial evidence about new drugs statistically adequate? Br J Clin Pharmacol 19:155–160, 1985.

15. Bradley, WG: Therapeutic trials in neuromuscular diseases [editorial]. Muscle Nerve 4:185, 1981.

16. Bradley, WG: Critical review of gangliosides and thyrotropin-releasing hormone in peripheral neuromuscular diseases. Muscle Nerve 13:833–842, 1990.

17. Bradley, WG: The need for double-blind controlled trials in amyotrophic lateral sclerosis. In Rose, FC (ed): ALS—From Charcot to the Present and into the Future. Smith-Gordon, London, 1994, pp 263–265.

18. Bradley, WG, Hedlund, W, Cooper, C, et al: A double-blind controlled trial of bovine brain gangliosides in amyotrophic lateral sclerosis. Neurology 34:1079–1082, 1984.

19. Brooke, MH, Florence, JM, Heller, SL, et al: Controlled trial of thyrotropin releasing hormone in amyotrophic lateral sclerosis. Neurology 36:146–151, 1986.

20. Brooks, BR: The Norris ALS score: Insight into the natural history of amyotrophic lateral sclerosis provided by Forbes Norris. In Rose, FC (ed): ALS—From Charcot to the Present and into the Future. Smith-Gordon, London, 1994, pp 21–29.

21. Brooks, BR, Lewis, D, Rawling, J, et al: The natural history of amyotrophic lateral sclerosis. In Williams, AC (ed): Motor Neuron Disease. Chapman & Hall, London, 1994, pp 131–169.

22. Brooks, BR, Sufit, RL, DePaul, R, et al: Design of clinical therapeutic trials in amyotrophic lateral sclerosis. Adv Neurol 56:521–546, 1991.

23. Brooks, BR, Sufit, RL, Montgomery, GK, et al: Intravenous thyrotropin releasing hormone in patients with amyotrophic lateral sclerosis: Dose-response and randomized concurrent placebo-controlled pilot studies. Neurol Clin 5:143–158, 1987.

24. Bryan, WW, Barohn, RJ, Murphy, JR, et al: Placebo versus natural history in an ALS clinical trial [abstract]. Neurology 45(suppl 4):A280–A281, 1995.

25. Chalmers, TC, Smith, H Jr, Blackburn, B, et al: A method for assessing the quality of a randomized control trial. Control Clin Trials 2:31–49, 1981.

26. Daube, JR: Electrophysiologic studies in the diagnosis and prognosis of motor neuron disease. Neurol Clin 3:473–493, 1985.

27. Detsky, AS: Are clinical trials a cost-effective investment? JAMA 262:1795–1800, 1989.

28. Drachman, DB, Chaudhry, V, Cornblath, D, et al: Trial of immunosuppression in amyotrophic lateral sclerosis using total lymphoid irradiation. Ann Neurol 35:142–150, 1994.

29. Ellison, GW, Mickey, MR, and Myers, LW: Alternatives to randomized clinical trials. Neurology 38:73–75, 1988.

30. Festoff, BW and Crigger, NJ: Therapeutic trials in amyotrophic lateral sclerosis: A review. In Mulder, DW (ed): The Diagnosis and Treatment of Amyotrophic Lateral Sclerosis. Houghton Mifflin, Boston, 1980, pp 337–366.

31. Fletcher, RH: Editorial. The costs of clinical trials. JAMA 262:1842, 1989.

32. Freedman, B: Equipoise and the ethics of clinical research. N Engl J Med 317:141–145, 1987.

33. Guiloff, RJ and Eckland, DJA: Observations on the clinical assessment of patients with motor neuron disease. Neurol Clin 5:171–192, 1987.

34. Guiloff, RJ and Goonetilleke, A: Longitudinal clinical assessments in motor neurone disease. Relevance to clinical trials. In Rose, FC (ed): ALS—From Charcot to the Present and into the Future. Smith-Gordon, London, 1994, pp 73–82.

35. Guiloff, RJ, Modarres-Sadeghi, H, and Rogers, H: Motor neuron disease: Aims and assessment methods in trial design. In Rose, FC (ed): Amyotrophic Lateral Sclerosis. Demos, New York, 1990, pp 19–31.

36. Guyatt, GH, Feeny, DH, and Patrick, DL: Measuring health-related quality of life. Ann Intern Med 118:622–629, 1993.

37. Haverkamp, LJ, Appel, V, and Appel, SH: Natural history of amyotrophic lateral sclerosis in a database population. Validation of a scoring system and a model for survival prediction. Brain 118:707–719, 1995.

38. Haynes, RB and Dantes, R: Patient compliance and the conduct and interpretation of therapeutic trials. Control Clin Trial 8:12–19, 1987.

39. Hellman, S and Hellman, D: Sounding board of mice but not men. Problems of the randomized clinical trial. N Engl J Med 342:1585–1589, 1991.

40. Hillel, AD, Miller, RM, Yorkston, K, et al: Amyotrophic lateral sclerosis severity scale. In Rose, FC (ed): Amyotrophic Lateral Sclerosis. Demos, New York, 1990, pp 93–97.

41. Honda, M: Clinical appraisal of progression of amyotrophic lateral sclerosis: A Japanese ALS Scale. In Rose, FC (ed): Amyotrophic Lateral Sclerosis. Demos, New York, 1990, pp 77–82.

42. The Italian ALS Study Group: Branched-chain amino acids and amyotrophic lateral sclerosis: A treatment failure? Neurology 43:2466–2470, 1993.

43. Kelly, JJ, Thibodeau, L, Andres, PL, et al: Use of electrophysiologic tests to measure disease progression in ALS therapeutic trials. Muscle Nerve 13:471–479, 1990.

44. Kessler, DA: Drug promotion and scientific exchange. N Engl J Med 325:201–204, 1990.

45. Kondo, K and Hemmi, I: Clinical statistics in 515 fatal cases of motor neuron disease. Neuroepidemiology 3:129–148, 1984.

46. Kurtzke, JF: Neuroepidemiology. Part II: Assessment of therapeutic trials. Ann Neurol 19:311–319, 1986.

47. Lachin, JM: Introduction to sample size determination and power analysis for clinical trials. Control Clin Trial 2:93–113, 1981.

48. Lacombiez, L, Bensimon, G, Leigh, PN, et al: Dose-ranging study of riluzole in amyotrophic lateral sclerosis. Lancet 347:1425–1431, 1996.

49. Lang, T and Secic M: Reporting statistical information in biomedical publications. A guide for authors, editors, and reviewers. American College of Physicians, Philadelphia, 1997.

50. Lange, D: Experience with myotrophin. In Armon, C and Rowland, LP (eds): Clinical issues in ALS trials: Update, consensus and controversies. American Academy of Neurology, Minneapolis, 1995, pp 27–28.

51. Lange, D, Murphy, PS, Diamond, B, et al: A double-

blind placebo-controlled study to assess the effects of deprenyl on the clinical course of ALS. Neurology 44(suppl 2):A256, 1994.

52. Lawton, MP: Quality of life in Alzheimer disease. Alzheimer Dis Assoc Disord 8(suppl 3):138–150, 1994.

53. Lindstrom, MJ and Bates, DM: Newton-Raphson and EM algorithms for linear mixed-effects models for repeated-measures data. J Am Stat Assoc 83:1014–1022, 1988.

54. Longstreth, WT, Koepsell, TD, and van Belle, G: Clinical neuroepidemiology. Arch Neurol 44:1196–1202, 1987.

55. Louwerse, ES, de Jong, VJMB, and Kuether, G: Critique of assessment methodology in amyotrophic lateral sclerosis. In Rose, FC (ed): Amyotrophic Lateral Sclerosis. Demos, New York, 1990, pp 151–179.

56. McKhann, GM: The trials of clinical trials. Arch Neurol 46:611–614, 1989.

57. McKhann, GM: Clinical trials in a changing era. Ann Neurol 36:683–687, 1994.

58. Medical Research Council: Aid to the investigation of peripheral nerve injuries. War Memorandum, ed 2 (revised). His Majesty's Stationery Office, London, 1943, pp 11–46.

59. Meinert, CL: Clinical Trials. Oxford University Press, New York, 1986.

60. Miller, RG, Petajan, J, Bryan, WW, et al: A placebo-controlled trial of recombinant human ciliary neurotrophic factor (rhCNTF) in amyotrophic lateral sclerosis. Ann Neurol 39:256–260, 1996.

61. Mitsumoto, H, Salgado, ED, Negroski, D, et al: Amyotrophic lateral sclerosis: Effects of acute intravenous and chronic subcutaneous administration of thyrotropin-releasing hormone in controlled trials. Neurology 36:152–159, 1986.

62. Mitsumoto, H, Schwartzman, M, Levin, KH, et al: Electromyographic (EMG) changes and disease progression in ALS. Neurology 40(suppl 1):318, 1990.

63. Mitsumoto, H, Kumar, S, Levin, KH, et al: Intravenous immunoglobulin treatment in ALS. Ann Neurol 32:252, 1992.

64. Munsat, TL, Andres, PL, Finison, L, et al: The natural history of motoneuron loss in amyotrophic lateral sclerosis. Neurology 38:409–413, 1988.

65. Munsat, TL, Andres, P, and Skerry, L: Therapeutic trials in amyotrophic lateral sclerosis: Measurement of clinical deficit. In Rose, FC (ed): Amyotrophic Lateral Sclerosis. Demos, New York, 1990, pp 65–76.

66. The National TRH Study Group: Multicenter controlled trial: No effect of alternate-day 5 mg/kg subcutaneous thyrotropin-releasing hormone (TRH) on isometric-strength decrease in amyotrophic lateral sclerosis [abstract]. Neurology 39(suppl):322, 1989.

67. Norris, FH Jr, U, KS, Sachais, B, et al: Trial of baclofen in amyotrophic lateral sclerosis. Arch Neurol 36:715–716, 1979.

68. Norris, FH Jr: Charting the course in amyotrophic

lateral sclerosis. In Rose, FC (ed): Amyotrophic Lateral Sclerosis. Demos, New York, 1990, pp 83–92.

69. Olarte, MR and Shaffer, SQ: Levamisole is ineffective in the treatment of amyotrophic lateral sclerosis. Neurology 35:1063–1066, 1985.

70. Palca, J: AIDS drug trials enter new age. Science 246:19–21, 1989.

71. Passamani, E: Clinical trials—Are they ethical? N Engl J Med 324:1589–1592, 1991.

72. Pradas, J, Finison, L, Andres, PL, et al: The natural history of amyotrophic lateral sclerosis and the use of natural history controls in therapeutic trials. Neurology 43:751–755, 1993.

73. Ringel, SP, Murphy, JR, Alderson, MK, et al: The natural history of amyotrophic lateral sclerosis. Neurology 43:1316–1322, 1993.

74. Robinson, I: Ethical issues and methodological problems in the conduct of clinical trials in amyotrophic lateral sclerosis. In Rose, FC (ed): Amyotrophic Lateral Sclerosis. Demos, New York, 1990, pp 195–213.

75. Schafer, A: The ethics of the randomized clinical trial. N Engl J Med 307:719–724, 1982.

76. Schwab, R and England, A: Projection technique for evaluating surgery in Parkinson's disease. In Gillingham, J and Donaldson, L (eds): Third Symposium on Parkinson's Disease. Livingstone, Edinburgh, 1969, pp 152–157.

77. Steiner, TJ: Clinical trials. In Williams, AC (ed): Motor Neuron Disease. Chapman and Hall, London, 1994, pp 701–724.

78. Steiner, TJ: Multinational trial of branched-chain amino acids in amyotrophic lateral sclerosis [abstract]. Muscle Nerve (suppl 1):S166, 1994.

79. Sufit, R, Clough, JA, Schram, M, et al: Isokinetic assessment in ALS. Neurol Clin 5:197–212, 1987.

80. Van der Ploeg, RJO, Oosterhuis, HJGH, and Reuvekamp, J: Measuring muscle strength. J Neurol 231:200–203, 1984.

81. Woods, JR, Williams, JG, and Tavel, M: The two-period crossover design in medical research. Ann Intern Med 110:560–566, 1989.

82. The World Federation of Neurology Research Group on Neuromuscular Diseases Subcommittee on Motor Neuron Disease: El Escorial World Federation of Neurology criteria for the diagnosis of amyotrophic lateral sclerosis. J Neurol Sci 124(suppl):96–107, 1994.

83. The World Federation of Neurology Research Group on Neuromuscular Diseases Subcommittee on Motor Neuron Disease: Airlie House Guidelines. Therapeutic trials in amyotrophic lateral sclerosis. J Neurol Sci 129(suppl):1–10, 1995.

84. The World Medical Association Declaration of Helsinki. In Beauchamp, TL and Childress, JF (eds): Principles of Biomedical Ethics. Oxford University Press, New York, 1979, pp 289–293.

85. Young, FE, Norris, JA, Levitt, JA, et al: The FDA's new procedures for the use of investigational drugs in treatment. JAMA 25:2267–2270, 1988.

CHAPTER 21

PHYSICAL REHABILITATION

The main goal of rehabilitation for patients with ALS is to maximize function and independence. To achieve this goal, rehabilitation techniques are aimed at using education, psychological support, and proper equipment to maintain optimal function as long as possible and prevent complications caused by disuse of muscles. Although a rehabilitation program is more effective in those who have slowly progressive ALS, maintaining functional independence in those who have rapidly progressive ALS is equally important. Thus, appropriate and effective rehabilitation is essential in any patient with ALS.

Effective rehabilitation in patients with ALS has several essential requirements: The patient and caregiver must understand the nature of the disease and the disease process; they must be highly motivated and participate actively in the rehabilitation program; and they need to be part of goal-setting and treatment planning from the onset, to ensure a quality of life that will have meaning for the patient.[7,29]

Physical rehabilitation is accomplished most effectively by a multidisciplinary team of neurologists, physiatrists, pulmonologists, nurses, physical therapists, occupational therapists, orthotists, speech pathologists, dietitians, and social workers. The responsibilities of individual health professionals in ALS clinics have been discussed in Chapter 18. In this chapter, we discuss the staging of the disease, which provides a basic guide for rehabilitation; the patient's psychological issues; the use of therapeutic exercise and physical modalities; the use of assistive and adaptive equipment; and educational resources for patients and family.

STAGING OF MOTOR DYSFUNCTION IN ALS

Sinaki[28] and Sinaki and Mulder[29] have divided ALS into six stages based on functional impairment in axial and appendicular muscle, which are the primary concerns of rehabilitation (Table 21–1).

In stage I, the patient is in the early stages of the disease and thus is fully independent.

Table 21–1. **REHABILITATION OF PATIENTS WITH ALS AT DIFFERENT STAGES OF THE DISEASE**

Stages of ALS	Characteristic Clinical Features	Activities to Maintain Motor Function	Equipment
I	Ambulatory, no problems with ADL, mild weakness	Normal activities; moderate exercise in unaffected muscles, active ROM exercise	None
II	Ambulatory, moderate weakness in certain muscles	Modification in living; modest exercise; active, assisted ROM exercise	Assistive devices
III	Ambulatory, severe weakness in certain muscles	Active life; active, assisted, passive ROM exercise; joint pain management	Assistive devices, adaptive devices, home equipment
IV	Wheelchair-confined, almost independent, severe weakness in legs	Passive ROM exercise, modest exercise in uninvolved muscles	Assistive devices, adaptive devices, wheelchair, home equipment
V	Wheelchair-confined; dependent; pronounced weakness in legs, severe weakness in arms	Passive ROM exercise, pain management, decubitus prevention	Adaptive devices, home equipment, wheelchair
VI	Bedridden, no ADL, maximal assistance required	Passive ROM exercise, pain management, prevention of decubitus ulcers and venous thrombosis, pulmonary toilet	Adaptive devices, home equipment

Abbreviations: ADL = activities of daily living, ROM = range-of-motion exercise.
Source: Data from Sinaki, M: Rehabilitation. In Mulder, DW (ed): The Diagnosis and Treatment of Amyotrophic Lateral Sclerosis. Houghton Mifflin, Boston, 1980, pp 169–193.

The patient can perform normal life activities with only mild limitations. A focal or limited group of muscles may show mild weakness. In this stage, the patient is often incorrectly advised to perform excessive strengthening exercises to build weakened muscles. In general, excessive exercise in weakened muscles may need to be discouraged, whereas active strengthening exercises for unaffected muscles to substitute for the weak muscles may be useful. Normal physical activities and active range of motion (ROM) exercise are recommended to maintain or improve mobility. Any exercise, however, should be moderate to avoid undue fatigue.

Stage II is characterized by independent ambulation with moderate weakness in certain muscles. The patient may have muscle imbalances, decreased mobility and function, and increased energy expenditure. For example, a patient in this stage may have a mild footdrop on one or both sides or weakness in one hand. Selection and application of assistive devices to support weak muscles, to reduce energy expenditure, and to improve the patient's safety is the primary goal of rehabilitation. The patient should be encouraged to perform gentle stretching (active or passive ROM) exercises.

Various types of exercises are acceptable to prevent disuse atrophy in unaffected muscles. Isotonic exercise can be done using a light weight or the patient's own body part as resistance. Similarly, isometric exercises are acceptable. Energy conservation and work modification strategies must be incorporated into daily activities.

In stage III, the patient remains ambulatory but has severe weakness in certain muscles. For instance, the patient may have severe footdrop, a markedly atrophied and weakened hand, or may be unable to stand from sitting without help. In addition to the recommendations in stage II, home equipment should be considered so that the patient can maintain independence at home. At this stage, the patient may or may not have respiratory symptoms, but Sinaki and Mulder[29] recommend deep-breathing exercises to strengthen the auxiliary muscles of respiration for when the patient's weakness progresses. Active respiratory exercises with an incentive spirometer may help to maintain functional capacity. The caregiver can learn supportive coughing techniques. If the patient develops joint contracture causing pain, appropriate pain management may be indicated. A wheelchair may become necessary to avoid undue exhaustion.

By stage IV, the patient has become confined to a wheelchair but the arms are only mildly affected. The patient is able to perform most activities of daily living independently. A proper wheelchair that allows the patient to be functional and independent is essential. A motorized wheelchair may be necessary to avoid excessive fatigue. Skin care should be addressed for those who remain in a wheelchair. In this stage, passive ROM exercises by the caregivers or physical therapist are particularly important in weakened muscles that do not have full antigravity ROM. The patient can participate actively in exercising distal joints, such as fingers, wrists, and elbows. Such exercises should not cause fatigue. The activities of daily living should be regularly and carefully reviewed, and any home equipment that maintains the patient's independence at home should be obtained.

The patient in stage V is wheelchair-bound and is now dependent on others for care. Upper-extremity muscle weakness becomes severe. Because transferring the patient to and from a wheelchair is now a major effort for the caregiver, instruction in the proper body mechanics of transferring and positioning is important. A transfer board or raised seat may be insufficient because of the patient's generalized weakness, and a body lift, such as a Hoyer lift, may be necessary. Patients become unable to roll themselves in bed to change their position, and thus frequent repositioning by the caregiver is necessary to minimize uncomfortable positions and to maintain skin integrity. To protect certain body parts susceptible to pressure in the wheelchair and bed, pressure-relief surfaces (i.e., alternating air pressure pads and pressure-relief cushions containing air, water, gel, or foams) must be available. Pain may become a major problem in immobilized joints and at pressure points, and pain management may be necessary (see Chapter 19). Head drop may become a serious problem. The application of a neck brace, such as a Philadelphia collar, and a tall-back seating system in a wheelchair must be considered. When the shoulder girdle muscles become weak, the arm becomes dependent and the humerus may subluxate from the shoulder joint, causing a painful "frozen shoulder." An arm trough (gutter splint) is helpful in supporting the arm while the patient is in a wheelchair. Such adaptive positioning is essential for patients in wheelchairs to provide adequate support for all body parts.

In stage VI, patients are bedridden and need full assistance for the activities of daily living. The fundamental care is identical to that given to quadriplegic patients, although decubitus ulcers and bowel and bladder dysfunction are generally rare in patients with ALS. Proper mattresses and beds, such as hospital beds, should be available. Frequent repositioning of the body, padding to prevent uneven pressure to certain parts of the body, and prevention of venous stasis in the legs are crucial. Caregivers should familiarize themselves with proper positioning techniques, assistive coughing techniques, special feeding techniques, and the use of respiratory assistive devices. Pain management is important because the patient may have severe pain in the joints and extremities. Progressive respiratory distress develops in this stage; a suction machine should be available. Respiratory and nutritional care are discussed in Chapters 22 and 24.

PSYCHOLOGICAL STATUS AND REHABILITATION

Although a medication, riluzole, has been approved by the Food and Drug Administration for the treatment of ALS to modestly prolong life, ALS remains a disease without a cure. This fact has a profound psychological impact on patients. Kelemen[9] pointed out that it is the person and not the person's disease that must be treated. Therefore, holistic approaches become increasingly important (see Chapter 18). Chapter 25 also discusses the psychosocial aspects of ALS in detail. Patients with ALS may attempt to maintain a stoic exterior because the venting of frustration, anger, and hopelessness may be perceived by loved ones and caregivers (and professionals on whom the patient ultimately depends) as discontent or as a reflection of the quality of the care they receive.[4] Therefore, these patients need psychological support probably more than any other patient group.

Hunter and colleagues[7] studied the relationship between functional and psychological status in patients with ALS and found that severity of functional impairment is significantly correlated with psychological distress. They suggested that the rehabilitation of ALS patients must take into account the high incidence of psychological difficulties. From the early stages of the disease, the patient's psychological well being must be monitored because psychosocial status will have a strong impact on any treatment. Unless early intervention with psychological counseling and support is actively sought, rehabilitation (with exercise and assistive or adaptive equipment) may not be effective.[15]

THERAPEUTIC EXERCISE

Types of Exercise

Therapeutic exercise is used as part of a program of treatment under medical supervision. It includes the initial evaluation of the patient's needs, and constant re-evaluation of those needs. Goals of therapeutic exercise include strengthening weakened muscles, increasing muscle bulk, maintaining ROM, preventing disuse atrophy, and most importantly, optimizing patient function. In patients with ALS, exercise is an important part of rehabilitation, which needs to be appropriate, individualized, and adapted to the stage of disease. Table 21–2 summarizes the type of exercises that can be used therapeutically. An excellent review is also available on this subject.[8]

Table 21–2. THERAPEUTIC EXERCISE

- Strengthening exercise
    - Isotonic exercise
        - Concentric
        - Eccentric
    - Isometric exercise
    - Isokinetic exercise
- Endurance exercise
    - Single muscle or muscle group
    - General body (pulmonary-cardiovascular endurance)
- Range-of-motion exercise
    - Active
    - Active assisted
    - Passive

STRENGTHENING EXERCISES

Strength is the dynamic or static ability of a muscle or muscle group to produce tension and the resulting force during one maximal effort.[21] There are three different types of strengthening exercises: isotonic, isometric, and isokinetic exercises. Isotonic exercise involves movement (muscle shortening or lengthening causing joint movement) during contraction with a fixed resistance and variable speed. Tension or force develops throughout the muscle as it contracts, but the tension changes with the total length of the muscle and the angle of the joint. Isotonic exercise involves concentric and eccentric muscle contractions. Concentric contractions occur during a natural shortening of the muscle (e.g., the biceps contract when bending the elbow), whereas eccentric contraction accompanies a lengthening of the contracted muscles (e.g., the biceps remain contracted when slowly extending the elbow). Although an eccentric contraction can generate more tension than a concentric contraction, it carries a greater risk of muscle trauma, which is manifested by an increase in creatine kinase levels. Thus, precautions need to be taken when prescribing eccentric exercises for patients with ALS. In stage I of the disease, resistance may be added to isotonic exercises for strengthening unaffected muscles. These exercises may be accomplished with free weights, such as dumbbells, barbells, sand bags, or cuff weights; weighted pulleys; or, for home use, plastic 1-gallon milk jugs with varying amounts of water.[8]

Isometric exercise is a static exercise with muscle contraction but no joint movement. Thus, there is no change in the total length of the muscle. These exercises consist of exertion against an immovable object, manual resistance, or holding the joint in a static position. Isometric exercise does not require any special equipment and is useful for maintaining muscle strength around joints with limited motion caused by pain or immobilization. Commonly prescribed isometric exercises are muscle "setting" exercises, such as gluteal setting (squeezing the buttocks) and quadriceps setting (tightening the quadriceps muscle with the leg extended). These muscle-setting exercises help maintain strength and perhaps retard atrophy in immobilized patients, but they will not appreciably increase muscle strength. They may be prescribed for a patient with ALS when concentric contractions cannot be performed or when immobilization has resulted from the disease or from complicating medical conditions. Because isometric exercises may increase blood pressure and cause cardiovascular changes if the breath is held during contraction (the Valsalva maneuver), patients should be instructed to exhale on exertion.[10]

Isokinetic exercise involves moving the joint at a constant angular velocity with changing resistance. This exercise requires special equipment, such as the Cybex machine, which may be available in physical therapy departments. Several authors have indicated that isokinetic exercise may strengthen muscles more effectively than isotonic exercise.[10] Isokinetic exercise may be appropriate for patients in the early stages of ALS who maintain good muscle strength in certain muscle groups, but in the latter stages, difficulty in transferring the patient to and from the equipment prohibits its use.

ENDURANCE EXERCISE

There are two types of endurance exercises: those for single muscles or muscle groups and those for the general body (the pulmonary and cardiovascular systems). Muscular endurance is the ability of a muscle (or muscle group) to contract repeatedly or to sustain tension over time. General endurance is the ability of an individual to sustain low-intensity exercise over time.[10] Muscular endurance training is not indicated in the patient with ALS, but general body endurance exercise, such as walking or swimming, if possible, may be beneficial, especially in the early stages of the disease, as long as it is not sustained and is nonfatiguing.

ROM EXERCISE

ROM exercise is probably the most important exercise for patients with ALS at any stage of the disease. ROM exercise prevents the development of contractures that result from muscle shortening and tightening of joint capsules, ligaments, and tendons. When a joint is kept in one position, the collagen tissue on the relaxed side of the joint shortens and becomes fixed unless stretched. Immobilization also triggers collagen deposition in the joint capsule, periarticular structures, and even intra-articular structures. Such reorganization of connective tissue in the joint has been noted within 1 week after immobilization in experimental animals.[1] Muscles also shorten around the immobilized joint, contributing to contracture formation by the periarticular soft tissues. Contractures obviously interfere with vital activities of daily living because they cause pain on movement and thus limit movement.[8]

Even when patients have good muscle function, ROM exercise is still important and should be performed actively to maintain joint mobility, muscle strength, and endurance. In patients with limited muscle function or spasticity, ROM exercise can be performed in an "active-assisted" fashion; that is, part of the exercise is done actively by the patient and part of it is helped by the physical therapist or caregiver.[30] In patients who are unable to move a body part, ROM exercise must be done passively.

Passive ROM is defined as exercise performed by manual or mechanical means on a person who produces no voluntary muscle contraction.[22] Passive ROM is used when the patient is unable to move voluntarily to maintain joint range and flexibility, to prevent joint contracture, and when active movement increases spasticity. Passive ROM can be performed by the patient who has unilateral weakness by using the other extremity to produce the motion. Passive ROM exercise can be performed by health-care professionals, caregivers who have been trained by professionals, or both. During passive ROM exercise, the body segment should be supported with a gentle but firm grip. Hand placement should allow movement through the full available ROM, with minimal hand repositioning. Body segments distal to the joint being moved should be fully supported. All available planes of motion of a joint should be exercised with slow, controlled movements.[14,22]

Tight or spastic muscles should be stretched slowly for prolonged periods. "Ballistic" or bouncing movements should be avoided because such movements stimulate the stretch reflex in antagonists, aggravating spasticity, and are more likely to produce injury. Patients with leg spasticity tend to develop heel-cord tightening, so stretching the Achilles tendon is advised. Progressive shoulder girdle muscle weakness tends to result in contractures around the shoulder. The use of pulleys or a shoulder wheel may improve shoulder ROM.

It is important to be able to determine whether ROM is decreased as a result of weakness, joint and muscle contracture, spasticity, joint instability, or pain. Many different types of ROM and stretching exercises can be prescribed, so the guidance of a physical therapist or occupational therapist is important, especially because each patient with ALS has unique problems.

The Effects of Exercise

The effects of strengthening and endurance exercises in patients with ALS have not been sufficiently investigated and thus are not well understood. More specifically, the effects of exercise on degenerating motor neurons is not known. Strenuous exercise, either for strength or endurance, has been associated with a rise in creatine kinase in patients with muscular dystrophy or chronic denervated muscles, indicating that muscle fibers may degenerate with excessive exercise.[17] Excessive exercise may impair recovery of degenerated muscle fibers. Animal studies have shown that muscle fiber degen-

eration may exacerbate motor neuron denervation.[17]

Moxley[16] investigated the effect of individualized, monitored, endurance and specific muscle-group exercise training in patients with ALS. Patients who participated in the exercise training achieved important functional benefits, but an individual approach and careful monitoring were essential to deliver such exercise programs properly, particularly to avoid overexertion. In the past, physicians have discouraged active exercise of weakened muscles[28] for fear of exacerbating the disease. However, many believe patients with ALS should be encouraged to engage in active exercise short of fatigue. Therapeutic exercise is believed to be psychologically beneficial, to prevent disuse atrophy, and even to improve muscle strength in some patients with ALS.[19] Nevertheless, there have been no prospective studies in this area.[2] Further studies are needed to establish the effects of exercise in patients with ALS, with the focus on "how much of what kind" of exercise is beneficial.[20]

Fatigue from Exercise

Fatigue is the inability of a muscle to continue generating force, or the loss of endurance, and has been shown to occur at any force level greater than 15% of maximum voluntary contraction.[13] The mechanism of fatigue in patients with ALS has not been investigated until recently. One study[24] investigated fatigue after progressive and prolonged exercise in patients with ALS. These patients showed decreased work capacity, an increased oxygen cost of submaximal exercise, and abnormalities in plasma and muscle lipid metabolism. These lipid metabolism abnormalities appear to be unique because, unlike patients with carnitine palmitoyl transferase deficiency who show the plasma lipid abnormalities identical to those found in patients with ALS, patients with ALS can perform prolonged exercise.[24] Another study[27] found that fatigue is not caused by a lack of central activation, an impaired neuromuscular junction, or muscle membrane abnormalities in patients with ALS. Rather, it is apparently caused by activation impairment, in part secondary to an alteration at the level of excitation-contraction coupling.[27] Although fatigue can result from therapeutic exercise in patients with ALS, it mostly occurs from regular daily activities. Therefore, activity modification, energy conservation, and work simplification are important to help the patient conserve energy (see Chapter 18).

PHYSICAL MODALITIES

Thermal Agents

Heat, which can be either superficial or deep, is frequently used in physical rehabilitation for the reasons listed in Table 21–3. Superficial heat modalities include hot packs, hot-water bottles, heating pads, paraffin wax, and infrared lamps. Diathermy and ultrasound are deep-heat modalities because they affect deeper tissues.[5] In patients with ALS, heat agents can be used for the management of pain and can be used before ROM exercises so that exercises may be performed without excessive pain.

Electrical Stimulation

Percutaneous electrical stimulation of sufficient amplitude and duration elicits a muscle contraction. Electrical stimulation has been used to maintain or increase muscle strength and to produce joint movement. Electrical stimulation in patients with Duchenne's muscular dystrophy produced a marked increase in the maximal voluntary contraction in stimulated muscle.[26] However, the effects of electrical stimulation in denervated muscles, particularly in patients with ALS, is unknown. Some patients may find electrical stimulation to be uncomfortable,

Table 21–3. BENEFICIAL EFFECTS OF HEAT ON PATIENTS WITH ALS

- Analgesia
- Sedation
- Increased blood flow
- Increased nonelastic and muscle tissue extensibility
- Increased metabolic rate to promote healing
- Decreased muscle spasms

and because of generalized weakness in ALS, many muscles would require stimulation. Furthermore, electrical stimulation may produce intense muscle contraction, which raises the question of whether such intense muscle contractions may cause degeneration of denervated muscles and motor neurons.[17]

Transcutaneous Electrical Nerve Stimulation

Transcutaneous electrical nerve stimulation (TENS), a form of electrical stimulation, has been used in physical rehabilitation for many years to provide symptomatic relief and management of a variety of acute and chronic pain conditions.[31] There are six primary "modes" or types of TENS: conventional strong, low-rate, brief-intense, pulse-burst, modulated, and hyperstimulation.

The application of electrical stimulation is based on the gate theory of pain.[13] Small A-delta myelinated fibers conveying mechanical and thermal stimuli or C-nociceptive unmyelinated fibers are involved in the production of pain. The gate theory suggests that stimulating large A-alpha fibers activates interneurons in the dorsal horn of the spinal cord, which inhibits the smaller A-delta and C-fiber input. The conventional TENS mode is believed to activate the large A-alpha fibers, thus closing the gate to pain.[18] A more recent and accepted theory, however, has centered on the production of endogenous opiates, resulting in the inhibition of pain.[12]

Patients with ALS often report pain caused by joint contracture, adhesive capsulitis, tendinitis, back strain, and other musculoskeletal problems. TENS may be an effective adjunctive modality in these patients.[6,31]

ASSISTIVE AND ADAPTIVE EQUIPMENT

The ultimate goal of rehabilitation with any patient is to achieve the highest level of independence possible. To achieve this goal, bracing, splinting, and adaptive equipment may be used. In general, most adaptive and assistive equipment must be prescribed by a physician, usually after an occupational or physical therapy evaluation.

Assistive equipment includes a variety of orthoses that fixate or support a weak or deformed part of the body, such as an ankle-foot orthosis or a wrist extensor splint. Assistive equipment also includes mobility-enhancing devices, such as canes, walkers, and regular or powered wheelchairs. Adaptive equipment includes items or instruments such as button hooks or built-up handles for utensils that are used with activities of daily living but not necessarily placed on the body.

When prescribing adaptive equipment, the least-restrictive device that maintains the highest level of independence without sacrificing safety is preferred. Team members involved in recommending equipment include occupational therapists, physical therapists, speech pathologists, nurses, and physicians. The prescription for an elaborate and expensive piece of equipment, such as an electric wheelchair, requires consultation by more specialized team members, such as a specialist at a wheelchair seating clinic.

For any piece of equipment to be effective, the patient and caregiver must be committed to using it properly. Training in the use of the equipment is usually necessary and ideally should be provided by a licensed professional who works with the equipment.

Lastly, it is important to remember that most equipment, particularly durable medical equipment, requires a physician's written prescription, which should include the specific name of the equipment, the medical indications, the duration of use, a catalog number, and other specifications if applicable. For permanent use, a duration of 12 months should be written in the prescription.

Upper-Extremity Weakness

ASSISTIVE EQUIPMENT

Volar Cock-up Splint (Wrist Extensor Splint). Wrist extensor muscle weakness and the accompanying finger extensor weakness prevent grasping an object with the hand. Wrist position at a neutral or slightly extended position maintained with a wrist-support splint allows flexed fingers to extend in a slightly open position for gripping. Usually, hand flexor muscles are preserved better than extensor muscles in patients with ALS.

Volar Opponens Splint (Thumb-Shell, or Short-Thumb Splint). When the abductor pollicis brevis and thumb extensor muscle are weak, the thumb lies in the same plane as the other fingers. This position precludes grasping with the thumb against the other fingers. A volar opponens splint places the thumb in a position opposing the rest of the fingers so that a grasping action becomes possible. A volar cock-up splint and a volar opponens splint can be combined to make grasping more effective.

Dynamic Finger-Extension Device. When the patient has marked atrophy and weakness in the hand, intrinsic muscles and finger extensor muscles, all the fingers tend to remain flexed. A dynamic finger-extension device extends all the fingers at the level of metacarpophalangeal joints so that extended fingers can flex and grasp an object when flexor muscle strength is still well maintained.

Resting Hand Splint. When the patient's fingers tend to remain flexed, wearing this splint at night prevents flexion contractures. Maintaining muscle length allows the hand to be used in dynamic splints and keeps the palm of the hand clean (Fig. 21–1).

Anti-Claw-Hand Splint. Marked atrophy of the intrinsic hand muscles causes the hand to rest in an intrinsic-minus or claw position, where metacarpophalangeal joints are hyperextended and interphalangeal joints are flexed. A claw-hand splint positions the metacarpophalangeal joints in flexion, improving the grasp of objects (Fig. 21–2).

Mobile Arm Support or Balanced Forearm Orthosis. When the shoulder abductors and elbow flexors are weakened but the shoulder adductors are sufficiently powerful, patients can feed themselves independently using the balanced forearm orthosis. The arm's weight is neutralized by the support, which greatly increases arm mobility. The mobile arm support can be attached to a wheelchair arm.

Arm Trough (Gutter Splint). If, while sitting in a wheelchair, the arm slips off the arm rest, the shoulder joint and surrounding capsules can be painfully stretched. The arm trough supports the arm in a resting position and prevents it from subluxing from the shoulder joint.

Slanted Arm Rest. A slanted arm rest is used not only for resting the arm while in a

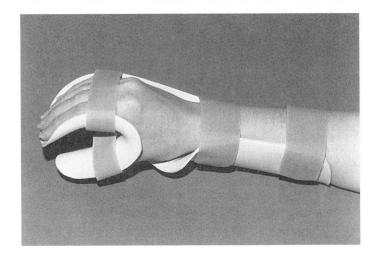

Figure 21–1. A resting hand splint is used to support wrist extensor and finger extensor muscles.

wheelchair but also for preventing dependent edema in the distal part of the arm.

Arm or Shoulder Sling. The arm sling has been used to reduce shoulder subluxation, although radiologic studies suggest that it is ineffective. A Bobath axillary roll may compress the brachial plexus if the sling is placed improperly in the axilla. Humeral cuffs are also available. A hemi-sling may reduce subluxation, but the use of this sling is controversial.

ADAPTIVE EQUIPMENT FOR MODIFYING EVERYDAY TOOLS

The equipment described here can be purchased without a prescription. However, a prescription from a physician may allow third-party reimbursement for part of the cost, depending on the policy. Medicare, however, does not reimburse the cost of this equipment.[23]

Eating

Foam or cork tubes for utensils: Increases the size of handles, making utensils easier to grip

Plastic utensils: The modified shapes and sizes make them easier to grip or to reach (Fig. 21–3)

Universal cuff with palmar pocket: Holds a utensil so that a patient can manipulate utensils without grasping them (see Fig. 21–3)

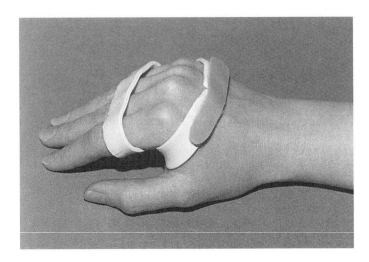

Figure 21–2. An anti-claw-hand splint repositions the metacarpophalangeal joints during flexion, improving a patient's ability to grasp objects.

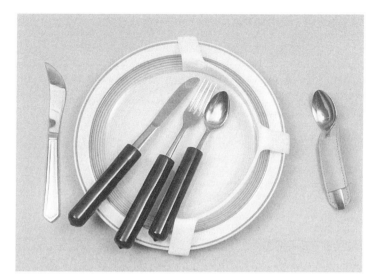

Figure 21–3. Several examples of common adaptive equipment. Eating utensils with enlarged plastic grips (on the plate), or a universal cuff with spoon attached (to the right of the plate) help the patient grasp and handle them more easily. A rocker knife (to the left of the plate) is handy to cut food by rocking motions rather than cutting motions. A plate guard is attached to the plate so that food is easily scooped with one utensil.

Swivel spork: A spoon and fork that are functionally combined in one utensil

Serrated knife *and* Rocker knife (see Fig. 21–3)

Extended straws (for easy reach)

Straw holder: Keeps the straw stationary

Dinnerware with its own built-in guards: Allows food to be scooped with one utensil

Plate guards: A clip-on guard that allows food to be scooped with one utensil (see Fig. 21–3)

Lightweight, large-handled cups (for a better grip)

Dycem pads: Prevent food trays or dishes from slipping

Electric can opener

Jar or bottle opener

Self-care and dressing

Zipper pulls or hooks

Button hooks (Fig. 21–4)

Hair brush and universal cuff: A cuff holding a hair brush so that a patient can brush hair without grasping a brush

A long-handled sponge

Rechargeable electric toothbrush with a rotary brush

Lightweight electric shaver

Velcro fastener: A patient does not need to manipulate shoe laces, buttons, buckles for fastening

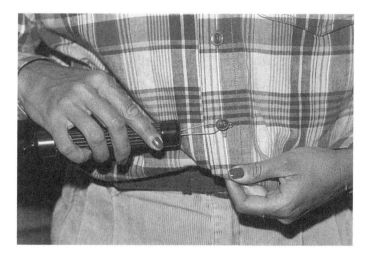

Figure 21–4. A button hook is used to catch a button through a button hole.

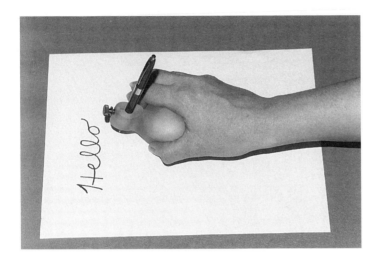

Figure 21–5. A writing bird. This device holds a pen to allow writing as the patient moves the device.

Writing, reading, and desk work

Rubber thumb
Pencil grips
Wanchik writer splint *or* writing bird (Fig. 21–5)
Head and mouth sticks for typing
Slip-on typing aid attached to a universal cuff: A hand cuff with attachment to hold a typing aid
Book holder
Automatic page turner
Tilttop overbed table
Lap-style Able Table with adjustable angle: A portable table positioned on the lap; the table angle can be adjusted
Self-opening scissors
Card holders

Communication

Voice enhancer (Fig. 21–6)
Portable phone, speaker phone
Telecommunication device for the deaf

Others

Key holders
Lightweight reachers
Command center of switches with microprocessor

Neck Weakness

Forward head drop, a common and serious problem in ALS, is caused by weakness

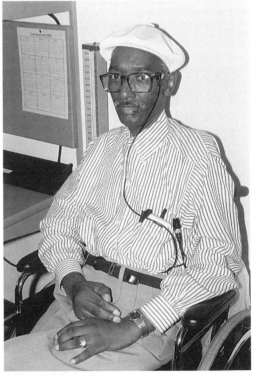

Figure 21–6. A simple voice enhancer is sometimes very helpful for the patient who has reduced voice volume. This patient, a priest who is only able to whisper, resumed preaching every Sunday with such a voice enhancer (this one is from Radio Shack).

in neck extensor and cervical paraspinal muscles (see Chapter 4). Head drop can develop in the early stages of ALS, although it usually occurs after stage III. Initially, the patient experiences heaviness and fatigue in holding the head up; later, posterior neck pain develops. Patients may also complain of low back pain caused by postural changes that begin in the cervical region. Walking, driving, or any activity requiring a static upright head position becomes difficult. The head-drop position also accentuates drooling.

Cervical orthoses can support the head, protect weakened neck muscles, and prevent further deformity. An orthosis may facilitate breathing, eating, and seeing by returning the head to a neutral position.

When the problem is minor, a soft collar may be sufficient. Although this type of collar limits the patient's neck movement to a certain degree, it is the least restrictive of the collars. As the disease progresses and supporting the head becomes increasingly difficult, a semirigid cervical collar, such as the Philadelphia collar, Miami collar, or a New-

port collar, becomes necessary. Although these collars effectively prevent neck flexion, some patients cannot tolerate them because of excessive warmth, throat compression, obstruction of respiration, and general discomfort. In addition, semirigid cervical collars may not provide sufficient support because they are ineffective for paralyzed extensor muscles. For patients with a tracheostomy who require access to the anterior neck, an Executive collar is one option. The Miami collar (Fig. 21–7) and Malibu collar, which is a modified Philadelphia collar, also have tracheostomy access. If a patient does not have success with these prefabricated orthoses, a customized brace can be devised by orthotists and biomechanical engineers.

Trunk Weakness

A corsetlike lumbosacral orthosis has been used for chronic back pain without substantial benefits in otherwise healthy patients. A similar orthosis, a thoracolumbosacral orthosis, can help in rare patients with ALS who

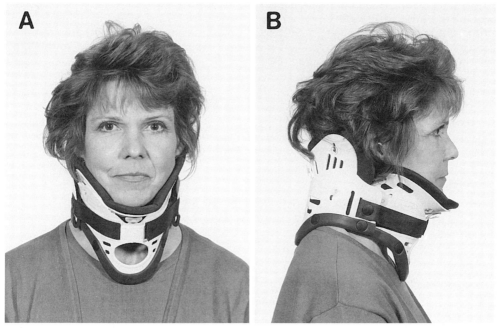

Figure 21–7. Several cervical collars are available for patients with neck extensor muscle weakness. This woman wears a Miami collar. (*A*) Front view; (*B*) side view.

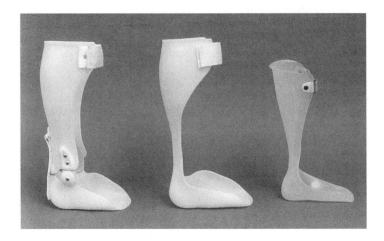

Figure 21–8. Three different ankle-foot orthoses (AFO) are shown. The right is a ready-made AFO, the middle is a custom-made solid AFO, and the left is a custom-made, articulated (hinged) AFO.

develop a prominent kyphosis. However, it may interfere with the patient's mobility.

Lower-Extremity Weakness

ANKLE-FOOT ORTHOSES

Ankle-foot orthoses (AFOs) are probably the most commonly used assistive device in patients with ALS (Fig. 21–8). They can be used for patients in whom spasticity is predominant or those with pure lower motor neuron symptoms. The specific reasons for applying AFOs are listed in Table 21–4.[11]

All AFOs to be used for an extended period (when the disease is slowly progressive) should be custom-made. A plaster cast is made of the foot, ankle, and lower leg to obtain a positive mold that is then used to fabricate the AFO. A team of physical therapists, physiatrists, and orthotists is essential to fab-

ricate an effective AFO. In patients with rapidly progressive ALS who are likely to use their AFOs only for a few months, an off-the-shelf brace may be adequate because of the substantially lower costs. However, such ready-made AFOs come in only three sizes and may consequently produce pain at pressure points and may provide insufficient support. Thus, their purchase may be a waste (Fig. 21–9).

The posterior leaf spring AFO (Teufel or VA Prosthetics Center shoe-clasp) assists dorsiflexion during swing but is unsuitable for a patient with ALS because it does not provide mediolateral support. The double-upright shoe brace provides a strong mechanical support by using metal attachments, but it is not proper for a patient with ALS because it is heavy and obtrusive.

A solid AFO (the Seattle AFO) is best for patients who have both mediolateral instability of the ankle and quadriceps weakness

Table 21–4. **POTENTIAL BENEFITS OF ANKLE-FOOT ORTHOSIS FOR PATIENTS WITH ALS**

- Provides mediolateral stability during standing
- Provides ankle dorsiflexion during swing or the initial contact
- Simulates push-off
- Increases knee stability by stabilizing the ankle
- Approximates a normal gait pattern and thus reduces energy expenditure
- Prevents the development of foot deformities

Source: Data from Lehmann, JF, de Lateur, BJ, and Price R: Ankle-foot orthoses for paresis and paralysis. Physical Medicine and Rehabilitation Clinics of North America 3:139–159, 1992.

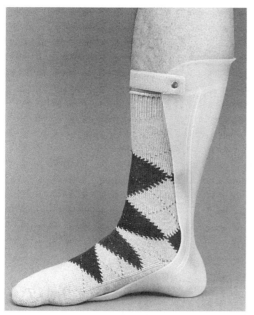

Figure 21–9. A ready-made ankle-foot orthosis (AFO) often does not fit the individual foot, resulting in pain. This particular ready-made AFO is too large at the heel and does not fit at the sole.

For individuals with spasticity and foot drag during the swing phase, a hinged AFO is again beneficial. Special antispasticity modifications, such as a full foot plate, a buildup under the metatarsal head, a medial longitudinal arch buildup, and a peroneal ridge, can be added.

Theoretically, the patient who develops knee extensor weakness may benefit from a knee-ankle-foot orthosis. However, this brace is not well accepted by patients with ALS because excess energy is required to walk with this relatively heavy brace.

AMBULATORY AIDS

Ambulatory aids are used to improve a patient's stability by increasing balance in standing, to compensate for reduced balance and strength, and to improve the ability to bear weight. Canes provide the least amount of support and walkers, the greatest (Fig. 21–12).

(Fig. 21–10). Its disadvantage is the fixed ankle dorsiflexion position, which prevents anterior displacement of the knee over the foot, making rising from sitting, ascending or descending stairs, and ascending inclines difficult.

If a patient has enough quadriceps strength to keep the knee stable while walking, a hinged AFO can be prescribed. A hinged AFO provides unlimited dorsiflexion, but has a plantar flexion stop to control footdrop (Fig. 21–11). This articulated orthosis is made of two plastic pieces, a foot piece and a calf piece, which are connected by a hinge to allow plantar flexion and dorsiflexion. Plantar flexion is limited by a posterior stop and dorsiflexion is limited, if necessary, by an anterior stop. Howell[6] recommends this type of AFO in patients with ALS who still have only mild loss of ankle strength. Patients readily accept such an orthosis because it allows a certain degree of ankle motion. Furthermore, the degree of dorsiflexion and plantar flexion can be adjusted, depending on the patient's stability and need for support.

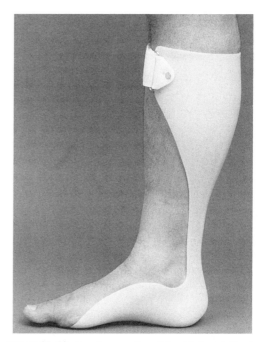

Figure 21–10. A custom-made solid ankle-foot orthosis (AFO) nicely fits the foot and leg. Before the AFO was fabricated, casts of the patient's foot and leg were made. (For the purpose of this picture, the AFO is put on the bare foot. Normally the patient should wear a sock underneath the AFO.)

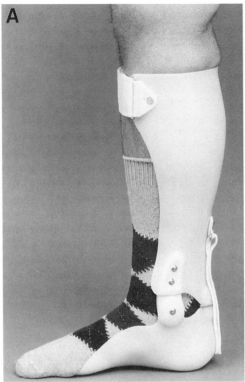

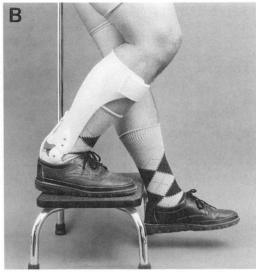

Figure 21–11. (*A*) A custom-made, articulated ankle-foot orthosis (AFO) is used to prevent foot drop by using a posterior stop. When going up or down stairs or an incline, the foot needs to be dorsiflexed. A solid AFO would not give this freedom, causing difficulty and some reluctance to use such a rigid AFO. A hinged AFO allows the foot to dorsiflex to the degree that the patient can handle. (*B*) This hinged AFO used a posterior strap that controls the degree of dorsiflexion.

Cane

A cane decreases the load on an affected leg, increases the base of support to decrease pain, increases balance, and compensates for motor weakness. In general, the cane is used when there is good upper-extremity strength. It should be carried in the hand opposite that of the affected leg.

A standard straight cane is recommended when there is a mild balance deficit resulting from lower-extremity weakness or mild spasticity. The most common type is a C-handle or crook-top cane. Other types have functional grips of varied shapes and texture to make grasping easier. An aluminum cane of adjustable height is also used (see Fig. 21–12).

A quad cane serves as an intermediate between a standard cane and a walker and is also widely used by patients who are primarily hemiplegic. The four prongs provide greater stability than a standard cane, and the quad cane can be left standing alone if the patient is engaged in two-handed activi-

ties. The difficulty with this type of cane is the weight. Patients with ALS who have hand weakness may fatigue quickly because of its eccentric weight. The quad cane may cause instability if only one or two tips touch the ground, although this should not happen if the patient is trained properly (see Fig. 21–12). Such instability is particularly problematic when the ground surface is irregular. Because the greatest stability occurs when all four prongs are in contact with the ground, patients should reduce their stride length to ensure this contact.

A unique quad cane is the Gatorade flexible-base quad (or triple) cane. A flexible attachment to the cane allows all the tips to come in contact with the ground, even when the shaft of the cane makes a sharp angle with the ground. This cane therefore provides more stability than a regular quad cane. Some of these canes have a small base and are relatively light weight and are therefore suitable for patients with ALS (see Fig. 21–12). A cane can be attached to a forearm cuff (a Loftstrand top) to help reduce hand

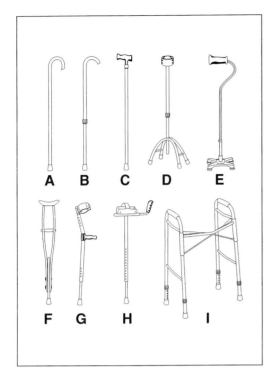

Figure 21–12. Various ambulatory aids are shown. (*A*) C-handle or cock-top cane, (*B*) adjustable aluminum cane, (*C*) functional grip cane, (*D*) adjustable wide-base quad cane, (*E*) Gatorade flexible-base quad cane, (*F*) adjustable wooden axillary crutch, (*G*) adjustable aluminum Lofstrand crutch, (*H*) forearm support, or platform, crutch, and (*I*) collapsible, adjustable aluminum walker.

fatigue by allowing the patient to compensate for a weakened wrist by shifting control of the cane's base to the elbow and shoulder (see Fig. 21–12).[6] This cane, however, is not well known and may be difficult to find.

Crutches

Crutches are generally not used for patients with ALS. If they are, they are usually Lofstrand or Canadian crutches. They leave the hands free for functional tasks while standing and without having to release the crutch. Unlike a walker, they can be used on stairs (see Fig. 21–12).

Walkers

A walker provides maximum support during ambulation. Properly used, all four points of contact are either on the ground

when bearing the patient's weight or in the air when the patient is taking a step (see Fig. 21–12). The disadvantages of a walker are that it takes up increased floor space, cannot be used on multiple steps, promotes a flexed posture, and is generally cumbersome. Special features allow certain designs to be adjusted for height, to fold, to be used to climb stairs, and to be rolled rather than lifted between steps. Various attachments are available at additional cost to suit the patient's walking environment, such as forearm platforms and carrying bags.

When the patient has moderate trunk weakness, decreased standing balance, or hand and wrist weakness, a wheeled or rolling walker is usually best. Patients with greatly decreased endurance may also benefit from this walker because they do not have to lift it. Patients with good side-to-side stability can handle a walker with swivel front casters that allow them to change directions easily. Because of safety concerns, patients who have marked spasticity or poor positional stability should not use the swivel casters.

The rear wheel brake or spring-loaded retractable rear glide minimizes drag of the rear wheel when walking on carpet and provides additional stability while stepping. When the patient transfers weight to the walker, the rear legs drop to the ground, thus providing a braking action.

When the patient has weakness or pain in the arms, forearm troughs are a useful addition to the walker, to allow its control through the upper arm and shoulder. However, this type of walker may be more difficult to manage because the patient needs to have good standing balance to adjust the forearm troughs.

WHEELCHAIRS

When the disease progresses to stage III (see Table 21–1), patients who are still ambulatory may experience undue exhaustion from walking short distances. Such patients benefit from the use of a wheelchair on a part-time basis and are likely to be pushed by caregivers. When a person propels a wheelchair on hard surfaces independently, energy consumption is approximately the same as walking an equal distance. Cardiovascular load is greater, presumably from increased upper-extremity use. Patients with ALS may not be able to propel their own wheelchair because of upper-extremity weakness and decreased endurance.

The choice of a wheelchair and options for a patient's particular need presents difficult questions. Table 21–5 summarizes specific options for manual wheelchairs. Because a wheelchair is generally expensive, the patient's insurance coverage should be reserved for the optimal wheelchair, when trunk and neck weakness develop. The best solution is to rent a lightweight wheelchair until motor loss progresses to where a recliner chair or a motorized wheelchair is required.

Choosing a wheelchair requires a multi-disciplinary assessment by physical therapists, physiatrists, occupational therapists, and sometimes even speech pathologists, to meet the patient's specific needs. Furthermore, wheelchair specialists from vendors can meet with the team and the patient to provide specific recommendations. The most effective way to order a wheelchair is to have access to a wheelchair showroom, where the patient can try a variety of chairs and cushion models to see which combination provides the most comfort and optimal function (see Table 21–5). Seating clinics at large medical centers usually offer such opportunities. Encouraging patients to participate actively in this laborious task of choosing a wheelchair has the benefit of easing acceptance of such

Table 21–5. **OPTIONS FOR MANUAL WHEELCHAIRS**

Arm Function

Removable arm rest—essential for transferring the patient

Desk arm—low enough to go up under ordinary desks or tables

Slanted arm rest—prevents dependent edema

A mobile arm support or balanced forearm orthosis attachment—makes the patient's upper extremity mobile and functional while in the chair

Adjustable-height arm rest—prevents subluxation of a weakened shoulder

Lap tray—provides a work or eating place and prevents shoulder subluxation

Leg Function

Adjustable seat—a lower seat allows the patient to propel the chair with the feet

Adjustable leg rest length—allows optimal knee and hip angles

Swing-away removable leg rest—essential for transferring the patient

Elevating leg rest—prevents dependent edema

Seating

Seat options—sling seat is lightweight and foldable but promotes poor posture; solid seats result in better posture but are more difficult to fold

Cushions—allow for optimal positioning and comfort and help to prevent skin breakdown

Adaptive seating—uses custom molding to the body; highly expensive, provides optimal seating system

Safety belts—lumbar belts and chest belts provide maximal trunk support and alignment, as well as safety

Reclining Option

Reclining back support—used with extreme trunk and neck weakness; important to combine with head, neck, and lumbar supports to prevent aspiration

Head and neck support—for weak neck muscles

Lumbar support—for weak back muscles and to promote optimal lumbar posture

Other Options

Ventilator tray—for a noninvasive or permanent ventilator

A small communication device

an adaptive device by allowing the patients a measure of control in its selection.

MOTORIZED WHEELCHAIRS

There are two kinds of motorized wheel-chairs. The first has an internal motor and battery system, and the second is a standard wheelchair that converts into a motorized one with an external power pack.

When the patient becomes unable to propel a manual wheelchair, an electric wheelchair may be the next consideration. A motorized wheelchair increases the patient's ability to remain independent. However, the patient and family should consider two major issues before choosing a motorized wheelchair: cost and transportation. Any motorized wheelchair is expensive, and thus the patient and family should investigate all possible financial resources, with the help of a social worker, if possible. The second issue deals with transportation and the need for a van, because an electric wheelchair with an internal motor does not fold down. This wheelchair requires installing restraint systems for the wheelchair and the patient and a ramp or electric lift to get the wheelchair in and out of the van. These requirements necessitate additional space, high expense, and substantial planning.

A wheelchair with a power pack is advantageous for people who cannot afford a van and disability access. The power pack can be disassembled, and the wheelchair can be folded to fit inside a large trunk. The drawbacks include the increased time needed for assembly and disassembly, a certain level of mechanical skill by the caregiver, and enough strength to lift a heavy battery, power pack, and chair into the trunk. Furthermore, a wheelchair with an external power pack has limited power and serious space constraints when it comes to installing options, such as a ventilator unit.

For those whose capacity for long-distance ambulation is limited or whose endurance is low, commercially available city-going electric carts or scooters may be practical alternatives for travel within reasonable proximity to home. Many models are available. Some models can be disassembled and transported in a regular car. The cost is also reasonable,

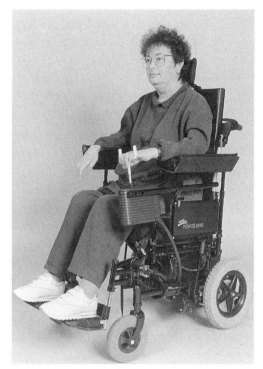

Figure 21–13. A typical motorized wheelchair for a patient who is unable to ambulate but can use a joy stick control to operate the wheelchair.

ranging from $1,500 to $5,000. The one major disadvantage is that when the patient has truncal weakness, sitting balance is poor and falls from the scooter may happen. Furthermore, a regular scooter cannot accommodate a ventilator. Thus, the scooter has clear limitations, requiring continuous adjustments and new installations.

The power wheelchair can become increasingly elaborate with additional options (Fig. 21–14). Prices range from $5,000 to $25,000. Therefore, the type of wheelchair best suited for the patient should be carefully evaluated by the entire multidisciplinary treatment team (Figs. 21–13 and 21–14).

Home Equipment

Most patients with ALS are cared for at home (see Chapter 18). It is crucial to make the home environment safe. Depending on the stage of the disease, a variety of home

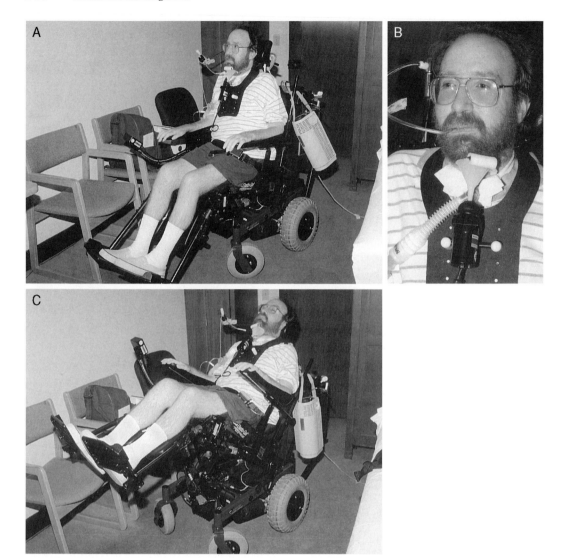

Figure 21–14. A highly elaborate motorized wheelchair. The patient is on a permanent ventilator through a tracheostomy. The ventilator unit is not seen because it is placed at the back of the wheelchair. (*A*) A general view of the wheelchair. The patient controls the wheelchair by using a chin-operating system. He also uses a sophisticated voice enhancer to communicate. A control unit for the entire system is located near the right leg. (*B*) A close-up view of the patient. (*C*) A semi-reclined position for comfort and rest.

equipment is necessary to allow the patient to be as safe and independent as possible. Routine home equipment can be purchased easily (if necessary, by prescription). A home assessment by home-care nurses, physical therapists, and occupational therapists often yields important recommendations for effective equipment.[25] A catalog from a medical supply company is helpful for patients and physicians to review options, as well as current prices (see Chapter 26). Table 21–6 lists standard home equipment options.

RESOURCES FOR PATIENTS AND FAMILIES

Excellent books have been published for patients with ALS and their caregivers. Some catalogs are also surprisingly informative.

Table 21–6. **STANDARD HOME EQUIPMENT OPTIONS FOR PATIENTS WITH ALS**

Transfers

Sliding board—for sliding a patient who is able to sit but not stand from bed to wheelchair and vice versa

Lift (Universal or Hoyer)—for transferring a patient who sits in a mobile sheet which is lifted by hydraulic power. Easily operated by a caregiver with limited strength.

Gait belt (or guard belt)—a broad waist belt easily grabbed by caregivers to help a patient to stand, transfer, or walk

Beds

Gel and foam mattresses

Contour neck pillows

Foam boots for pressure relief

Elbow and heel pads

Blanket support

Toilet

Toilet grab bars

Adjustable elevated toilet seat

Horizontal support rails on both sides of the toilet

Buzzer with pull-chain

Bedside commode

Bathroom

Grab bars—vertical and horizontal rails

Bath bench

Handheld shower head

Home Installations

Ramp for wheelchair access

Light switch extension knobs and levers

Special hinges to widen doorway

Electric stair glider or stair elevator

The ALS Association and the Muscular Dystrophy Association constantly update literature for the patient and caregiver.

- The ALS Association: Managing Amyotrophic Lateral Sclerosis Manual I. Managing Muscular Weakness (in press). The ALS Association. 21021 Ventura Blvd., Suit 321, Woodland Hills, CA 91364-2206.
- Appel, V: ALS: Maintaining Mobility. Houston: Muscular Dystrophy Association, 1987. Department of Neurology, Baylor University, 6501 Fannin NB 302, Houston, TX 77030.
- NCM After Therapy Catalog. Functional Solutions for Independent Living, 1995. P.O. Box 6070, San Jose, CA 95150.
- Sears Health Care Catalog. 1995–1996. Sears Roebuck and Co. Dept. 742 BSC 18-38, P.O. Box 5544, Chicago, IL 60680
- Hold Everything Catalog. P.O. Box 7456, San Francisco, CA 94120-7456
- Bruce Medical Supply. 411 Waverly Oaks Road, P.O. Box 9166, Waltham, MA 02254-9166.
- Cleveland Clinic ALS Care Manual 1996. ALS Coordinator, CCF-Department of Neurology, 9500 Euclid Ave., Cleveland, OH 44195.

SUMMARY

The main goal of rehabilitation for patients with ALS is to improve their ability to live with the disease. The treatment should keep the patient as active and as independent as possible for as long as possible. To achieve this independence, the functional impairment in ALS must be clearly defined. Based on the degree of impairment in axial and appendicular muscles, ALS can be divided into six stages, ranging from stage I, in which the patient is ambulatory and has only mild weakness in some muscles, to stage VI, in which the patient is bedridden and totally dependent. Such staging provides guidance for the type of rehabilitation appropriate for the patient. At any stage, rehabilitation techniques are aimed at maintaining the patient at an optimal functioning level and at preventing the complications secondary to disuse of muscles and immobilization.

For ALS rehabilitation to succeed, the patient and caregiver must understand the nature of the disease and be motivated to participate in the rehabilitation program. From the early stages of disease, the patient's psychologic needs must be addressed. Unless early intervention with psychologic counseling and support is implemented, rehabilitation may not be effective.

Various types of exercise, including those that maintain or enhance strength, endurance, and range of motion, are critical for the rehabilitation of patients with ALS. Although the effects of strengthening and endurance exercises in patients with ALS are not well understood, excessive exercise appears to injure muscle fibers and may injure remaining motor neurons. Nevertheless, the physiologic basis for such concerns is not clear. Strengthening exercises short of fatigue, such as isometric exercise of unaffected muscles or accessory muscles, should be encouraged. The mechanism of fatigue in patients with ALS has only recently begun to be investigated. The avoidance of fatigue, not only from exercise but also from ordinary daily activities, is important. In contrast to controversial strengthening or endurance exercises in patients with ALS, ROM exercise is critically important for these patients throughout all stages of the disease. With proper education, and monitored by physi-

cal therapists, an exercise program can be carried out effectively by the patient and caregivers.

To maintain a patient's independence, rehabilitation also uses assistive and adaptive equipment judiciously and effectively. Arm and hand function is essential for many activities of daily living. Several orthoses, such as wrist extensor supports, mobile arm supports, thumb-shell splints, and so forth, are all highly effective for patients with hand and arm weakness. A wide array of modified tools is available for the patient to enhance daily function.

Poor head support causing head drop frequently occurs in patients with ALS and can be difficult to manage. For a mild head drop, a soft cervical collar is often effective; several types of rigid cervical orthoses are also available. As the problem becomes more pronounced, custom-made braces may be required but not all are effective.

The ankle-foot orthosis is probably the most frequently used brace in patients with ALS. Some patients, however, find it inconvenient because of the lack of any plantar or extensor movement. For such patients, a plastic articulated orthosis made of two pieces is available. For the early stages of gait difficulty, a cane is often helpful. When the problem progresses, a walker may be required. When independent walking becomes too fatiguing or impossible, a wheelchair becomes an important adaptive device. Whether the patient should have a regular manual wheelchair or a motorized wheelchair, and what type of special features and options should be chosen for the wheelchair are difficult and serious questions. Successful rehabilitation also should include an evaluation of the home environment. Home equipment can easily enhance the home environment to help preserve patient independence and safety. The education of patients and caregivers is another important aspect of rehabilitation.

Rehabilitation promotes psychologic well-being with an exercise program and a variety of assistive and adaptive devices. Rehabilitation for patients with ALS requires a comprehensive approach and is best achieved by a multidisciplinary, patient-centered team consisting of physical and occupational therapists, physiatrists, orthotists, nurses, speech pathologists, dietitians, social workers, pulmonologists, and neurologists.

REFERENCES

1. Akeson, WH, Amiel, D, and Woo, SLY: Immobility effects on synovial joints: The pathomechanics of joint contracture. Biorheology 17:95–110, 1980.
2. Bohannon, RW: Results of resistance exercise on a patient with amyotrophic lateral sclerosis. Phys Ther 63:965–968, 1983.
3. Bigland-Richie, B and Woods, JJ: Changes in muscle contractile properties and neural control during human muscular fatigue. Muscle Nerve 7:691–699, 1984.
4. Gould, BS: Psychological aspects of ALS. In Mulder, DW (ed): The Diagnosis and Treatment of Amyotrophic Lateral Sclerosis. Houghton Mifflin, Boston, 1980, pp 157–167.
5. Hecox, B, Mehreteab, TA, and Weissberg, J: Physical Agents, A Comprehensive Text for Physical Therapists. Appleton & Lange, Norwalk, 1994.
6. Howell, CM: Physical therapy interventions in the management of amyotrophic lateral sclerosis. In Mitsumoto, H and Norris, FH (eds): Amyotrophic Lateral Sclerosis. A Comprehensive Guide to Management. Demos, New York, 1994, pp 93–118.
7. Hunter, MD, Robinson, IC, and Nelson, S: The functional and psychological status of patients with amyotrophic lateral sclerosis: Some implications for rehabilitation. Disabil Rehabil 15:119–126, 1993.
8. Joynt, RL, Findley, TW, Boda, W, et al: Therapeutic exercise. In DeLisa, JA, Gerber, LH, McPhee, MC, et al (eds): Rehabilitation Medicine. JB Lippincott, Philadelphia, 1992, pp 526–565.
9. Kelemen, J: Coping with ALS. In Charash, LI, Wolf, SG, Kutscher, AH, et al (eds): Psychosocial Aspects of Muscular Dystrophy and Allied Diseases. Commitment to Life, Health and Function. Charles C Thomas, Springfield, 1983, pp 127–147.
10. Kisner, C and Colby, LA: Therapeutic Exercise: Foundations and Techniques, ed 2. FA Davis, Philadelphia, 1990.
11. Lehmann, JF, de Lateur, BJ, and Price, R: Ankle-foot orthoses for paresis and paralysis. Physical Medicine and Rehabilitation Clinics of North America 3:139–159, 1992.
12. Mayer, DJ and Price, DD: The neurobiology of pain. In Snyder-Mackler, L and Robinson, A (eds): Clinical Electrophysiology: Electrotherapy and Electrophysiologic Testing. Williams & Wilkins, Baltimore, 1989, pp 141–201.
13. Melzack, R and Wall, PD: Pain mechanisms: A new theory. Science 150:971–979, 1965.
14. Minor, MA and Minor, S: Patient Care Skills, ed 2. Appleton & Lange, Norwalk, CT, 1995.
15. Montgomery, GK and Erikson, LK: Neuropsychological perspectives in amyotrophic lateral sclerosis. Neurol Clin 5:61–81, 1987.
16. Moxley, RT: The role of exercise. In Mulder, DW (ed): The Diagnosis and Treatment of Amyotrophic Lateral Sclerosis. Houghton Mifflin, Boston, 1980, pp 195–216.
17. Munsat, TL: Discussion in the paper by Moxley, RT: The role of exercise. In Mulder, DW (ed): The Diagnosis and Treatment of Amyotrophic Lateral Sclerosis. Houghton Mifflin, Boston, 1980, pp 214–215.
18. Nelson, RM and Currier, DP: Clinical Electrotherapy, ed 2. Appleton & Lange, Norwalk, CT, 1991.
19. Norris, FH Jr: Discussion in the paper by Moxley, RT: The role of exercise. In Mulder, DW (ed): The Diagnosis and Treatment of Amyotrophic Lateral Sclerosis. Houghton Mifflin, Boston, 1980, pp 215–216.
20. Norris, FH, Jr: Exercises for patients with neuromuscular diseases: Physical therapy. Phys Ther 142:261, 1985.
21. Ostering, L: Isokinetic and isometric torque force relationships. Arch Phys Med Rehabil 58:254, 1977.
22. Pierson, FM: Principles and Techniques of Patient Care. WB Saunders, Philadelphia, 1994.
23. Preston, W, Donhoe, K, Pandya, S, et al: Managing Amyotrophic Lateral Sclerosis. MALS Manual II. Managing Muscular Weakness. The ALS Association, Sherman Oaks, CA, 1986.
24. Sanjak, M, Paulson, D, Sufit, R, et al: Physiologic and metabolic response to progressive and prolonged exercise in amyotrophic lateral sclerosis. Neurology 37:1217–1220, 1987.
25. Schmitz, TJ: Environmental assessment. In O'Sullivan, SB and Schmitz, TJ (eds): Physical Rehabilitation. Assessment and Treatment. FA Davis, Philadelphia, 1994, pp 209–223.
26. Scott, OM, Vrbova, G, Hyde, SA, et al: Responses of muscles of patients with Duchenne muscular dystrophy to chronic electrical stimulation. J Neurol Neurosurg Psychiatry 49:1427–1434, 1986.
27. Sharma, KR, Kent-Braun, J-A, Majumdar, S, et al: Physiology of fatigue in amyotrophic lateral sclerosis. Neurology 45:733–740, 1995.
28. Sinaki, M: Rehabilitation. In Mulder, DW (ed): The Diagnosis and Treatment of Amyotrophic Lateral Sclerosis. Houghton Mifflin, Boston, 1980, pp 169–193.
29. Sinaki, M and Mulder, DW: Rehabilitation techniques for patients with amyotrophic lateral sclerosis. Mayo Clin Proc 53:173–178. 1978.
30. Sullivan, PE and Markos, PD: Clinical Decision Making in Therapeutic Exercise. Appleton & Lange, Norwalk, CT, 1995.
31. Walsh, NE, Dumitru, D, Ramamurthy, S, et al: Treatment of the patient with chronic pain. In DeLisa, JA, Gerber, LH, McPhee, MC, et al (eds): Rehabilitation Medicine. JB Lippincott, Philadelphia, 1992, pp 973–1017.

CHAPTER 22

PULMONARY FUNCTION AND RESPIRATORY FAILURE

Lisa S. Krivickas, MD

Dr. Krivickas is Instructor, Department of Physical Medicine and Rehabilitation, Harvard Medical School, Boston, Massachusetts.

Respiratory failure in ALS presents many dilemmas for both patients and physicians. This chapter briefly reviews respiratory physiology and then explores the pathophysiology and presentation of respiratory failure in ALS. The remainder of the chapter focuses on ventilatory support and the difficulties it presents. We attempt to provide a framework for discussing impending respiratory failure with patients and their families, for assisting patients in making decisions concerning ventilatory support, and for managing respiratory failure in accordance with the patient's decisions. Noninvasive and invasive (i.e., via tracheostomy) ventilatory techniques, along with quality-of-life issues, are discussed. Finally, we present a case history of a patient who electively underwent tracheostomy for permanent ventilation, to highlight many of the difficult decisions that must be made concerning ventilatory support.

NORMAL RESPIRATORY MECHANICS AND PULMONARY FUNCTION

Neural Control

The neuroanatomy of the central pathways involved in respiratory control is not fully understood. Figure 22–1 depicts areas of the brain stem thought to be responsible for respiratory control. Two groups of respiratory neurons are located bilaterally in the medullary reticular formation: the dorsal respiratory group is chiefly associated with inspiration and the ventral respiratory group with expiration. Neurons from these respiratory groups descend in the ventral and lateral quadrants of the contralateral spinal cord white matter (ventral to the corticospinal tracts) and project to respiratory motor neurons in the ventral horn of the spinal cord. The descending inspiratory and expiratory neurons are spatially separated, with the expiratory neurons lying more medially. The phrenic motor nuclei are located in the third

through fifth segments of the cervical cord; the nuclei of other muscles involved in respiration primarily are located in the thoracic cord segments. The medullary respiratory neurons receive input from two groups of pontine neurons that are, in turn, influenced by higher cortical neurons via pathways that are not clearly understood. The pontine respiratory neurons project from the pneumotaxic center (driving respiration) in the upper pons and the apneustic center (inhibiting respiration) in the lower pons. Neurons from the apneustic center excite neurons in the dorsal respiratory group of the medulla, thus stimulating inspiration, and the neurons from the pneumotaxic cen-

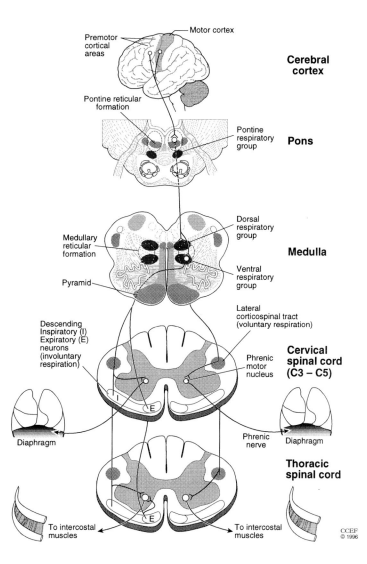

Figure 22–1. Neuroanatomy of respiratory muscle control. The respiratory muscles are controlled by the dual control systems: the brain-stem respiratory centers and the cerebral motor cortex. (Copyright © 1996 Cleveland Clinic Educational Foundation.)

ter inhibit the neurons in the dorsal respiratory group.[8,58]

Inspiratory and Expiratory Muscle Activity

In healthy individuals at rest, inspiration is an active process and expiration a passive process. The diaphragm is the major inspiratory muscle, with the external intercostal, parasternal intercostal, scalene, and sternocleidomastoid muscles acting as the major accessory inspiratory muscles. Table 22–1 shows the innervation of the muscles involved in respiration. The diaphragm contains 55% type I fibers, 25% type IIa fibers, and 20% type IIb fibers; thus, 80% of its muscle fibers (types I and IIa) are fatigue-resistant.[15] With diaphragmatic contraction, the central portion of the diaphragm moves down, and the peripheral portion elevates the lower ribs, which move outward; both movements increase the thoracic cage size. The enlargement of the thoracic cage creates a negative pressure with respect to the atmosphere, which permits air to move passively through the airways and into the lungs.

Expiration occurs passively as the diaphragm relaxes and resumes its initial dome shape. In healthy individuals, expiration becomes active during heavy exertion, resulting in increased ventilatory demand. The abdominal and internal intercostal muscles then become active in respiration as accessory muscles of expiration. With normal respiration, the chest and abdominal walls move together; the movement is outward with inspiration and inward with expiration.

A cough, which is necessary for secretion clearance and prevention of aspiration, occurs with a quick inspiration followed by glottic closure and then expiratory muscle contraction. The expiratory muscles create an intrathoracic pressure of 50 to 100 mm Hg, which, acting against the closed glottis, produces the cough. A weak cough occurs when glottic closure is poor and expiratory muscles are weak, resulting in the inability to generate adequate intrathoracic pressure. In ALS, the cough becomes so weak that a patient cannot prevent aspiration or clear secretions.

Lung Volumes

The lung volume can be determined in several ways by measuring different variables (Fig. 22–2). Total lung capacity depends on both inspiratory muscle strength and elasticity of the chest wall and lung parenchyma. It can be determined from the vital capacity and residual volume. The vital capacity is the maximum volume of air that the individual can voluntarily move in and out of the lungs. Vital capacity can be measured easily with a handheld spirometer as the maximal volume an individual can expel from the lungs; when measured in this manner, it is called the *forced vital capacity* (FVC). The FVC is determined by both inspiratory and expiratory muscle strength as well as chest wall and parenchymal elasticity. The residual volume

Table 22–1. INNERVATION OF RESPIRATORY MUSCLES

Muscle Group	Spinal Level	Nerves
Inspiratory Muscles		
Diaphragm	C3–C5	Phrenic
Parasternal intercostals	T1–T7	Intercostal
External intercostals	T1–T11	Intercostal
Scalenes	C4–C8	
Sternocleidomastoid	C1–C2	Spinal accessory
Expiratory Muscles		
Internal intercostals	T1–T12	Intercostal
Abdominal	T7–L1	Lumbar

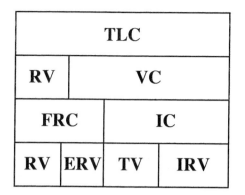

TLC			
RV	VC		
FRC	IC		
RV	ERV	TV	IRV

TLC: Total Lung Capacity
RV: Residual Volume
VC: Vital Capacity
FRC: Functional Residual Capacity
IC: Inspiratory Capacity
ERV: Expiratory Reserve Volume
TV: Tidal Volume
IRV: Inspiratory Reserve Volume

Figure 22–2. Measurements of lung volume.

is the amount of air remaining in the lungs after a maximum expiration; it can only be measured indirectly by sophisticated methods such as body plethysmography and a nitrogen washout technique.[11] Total lung capacity can also be regarded as the combination of inspiratory capacity and functional residual capacity. The functional residual capacity is the amount of air remaining in the lungs after a normal quiet expiration; the diaphragm is in the resting position. Inspiratory capacity reflects inspiratory muscle strength as well as chest wall and parenchymal elasticity. The inspiratory capacity can be subdivided into the tidal volume (controlled by voluntary muscle action) and the inspiratory reserve volume. Functional residual capacity can be subdivided into expiratory reserve volume and residual volume. The expiratory reserve volume is determined by expiratory muscle strength. To evaluate expiratory reserve volume, the forced expiratory volume in 1 second (FEV_1) is routinely measured when pulmonary function tests are performed. Normally, it is approximately 75% of the FVC, but in obstructive lung disease, the FEV_1 is less than 70% of the FVC.

Pulmonary Function Tests

Pulmonary function tests are generally a sensitive indicator of obstructive lung disease, which must be differentiated from the restrictive disease seen in patients with ALS. Obstructive lung disease occurs in processes that narrow the airways (i.e., asthma and chronic obstructive pulmonary disease), thus increasing the resistance against which the expiratory muscles must work to expel air. In restrictive processes, however, the lungs have difficulty expanding because of stiffening and loss of compliance. Inspiratory muscle weakness eventually causes the lungs to stiffen because the chest wall muscles develop contractures from a decrease in the range of motion. For any measure of lung volume, values less than 80% of those predicted or greater than 120% of those predicted for a normal individual, based on age, height, and weight, are considered abnormal.

Several methods are available to measure respiratory muscle strength. Maximum voluntary ventilation measures both respiratory muscle strength and endurance. It is the volume of air that can be inhaled and expelled when breathing as quickly and forcefully as possible for 1 minute. It is generally measured over a 12 second period and converted to units of volume per minute. The maximum inspiratory and expiratory pressures produced at the mouth also measure inspiratory and expiratory muscle strength. Maximum inspiratory pressure is usually measured after maximum expiration, and maximum expiratory pressure after maximum inspiration. Respiratory pressures are useful for identifying respiratory muscle weakness in patients with ALS and concomitant chronic obstructive pulmonary disease; FVC and maximum ventilatory volume often decrease in patients with chronic obstructive pulmonary disease, but maximum inspiratory pressure and maximum expiratory pressure are unaffected. In addition, a normal maximum expiratory pressure with a markedly reduced FVC suggests a nonmuscular cause of impaired pulmonary function. In motor neuron disease, the FVC, maximum ventilatory volume, and inspiratory and expiratory pressures are all reduced (Table 22–2). Respiratory pressures also are useful in differentiating between neuromuscular

Table 22–2. PULMONARY FUNCTION TEST AND BLOOD GAS CHANGES DURING ALS

Early Changes
Decreased maximum ventilatory volume

Middle Changes
Decreased maximum expiratory pressure
Decreased maximum inspiratory pressure
Decreased FVC
Decreased FEV_1
No change in FEV_1/FVC ratio

Late Changes
Decreased Pao_2
Increased $Paco_2$

Abbreviations: FEV_1 = forced expiratory volume in 1 second, FVC = forced vital capacity.

disease and restrictive parenchymal processes, such as pulmonary fibrosis.

RESPIRATORY FAILURE IN ALS

Pathophysiology

Respiratory failure is the failure to deliver adequate amounts of oxygen and remove carbon dioxide. Strictly speaking, respiratory failure can be diagnosed only by arterial blood gas measurement. However, patients with ALS have normal arterial blood gas levels until very late in respiratory failure; thus, arterial blood gas measurements generally are not useful for monitoring pulmonary function in this population.[16,36,51] A Pao_2 less than 60 mm Hg or a $Paco_2$ greater than 50 mm Hg indicates respiratory failure. Respiratory failure can be caused by muscle weakness, airway obstruction, loss of pulmonary compliance, respiratory muscle fatigue, or by central depression of the respiratory drive resulting in hypoventilation. Malnutrition, hypoxia, and loss of compliance all exacerbate respiratory muscle fatigue.

In ALS, respiratory failure is entirely mechanical. In patients with ALS who do not have any underlying intrinsic pulmonary disease, such as chronic obstructive pulmonary disease or pulmonary fibrosis, the lungs themselves are normal and exchange gas normally. However, because of muscle weakness, the lungs do not fully inflate during inspiration, resulting in alveolar hypoventilation. After a period of chronic underinflation, the lungs begin to lose their compliance and stiffen. Atelectasis and possibly a redistribution of surfactant in the alveoli contribute to this stiffening,[11] and patients eventually develop restrictive pulmonary disease.

Respiratory failure in ALS is progressive.[54] Muscle weakness causes atelectasis and decreased pulmonary compliance, which, in turn, increase the work of breathing. The increased respiratory workload produces diaphragmatic fatigue, triggering hypoxemia and acidosis, which further weaken the respiratory muscles. Bulbar dysfunction causes aspiration and malnutrition that further increase respiratory muscle weakness. If aspiration pneumonia develops, the work of breathing increases, causing even greater diaphragmatic fatigue. Clinical factors that increase expiratory resistance, such as mucus, infection, and bronchospasm, can cause acute failure, superimposed on the chronic failure.

Signs and Symptoms

In many patients with ALS, the first signs and symptoms of respiratory failure occur at night because vital capacity is much lower in the supine position. The diaphragm is weakened to a greater extent than the abdominal and intercostal muscles in most ALS patients.[44] When a patient is seated, gravity assists the weakened diaphragm in depressing the abdominal contents during inspiration. In the supine position, the abdominal contents are high in the peritoneal cavity, and the weak diaphragm is unable to depress them to allow maximal inspiration; thus, FVC is reduced. A drop in FVC on moving to a supine position from a seated position can cause ventilation perfusion mismatch; perfusion remains unchanged, but ventilation decreases. In addition, hypoxemia is most likely to develop during rapid eye movement sleep, when tidal volume is maintained primarily by the diaphragm.[35]

Occasionally, obstructive respiratory failure develops in patients with ALS because pharyngeal muscle weakness causes hypopharyngeal collapse or an inability to maintain vocal cord abduction; both can produce inspiratory stridor or signs similar to those seen with laryngeal spasm. This form of respiratory failure is also most prominent at night because the patient may experience episodes of sleep apnea, and the supine position encourages hypopharyngeal collapse. Robbins and coworkers[50] reported on two patients with recumbent apnea caused by contact between the epiglottis and the posterior pharyngeal wall.

Pulmonary Function Tests

Lung volume measurements in patients with ALS at various disease stages reveal that, in general, the most striking abnormalities are decreases in FVC and increases in residual volume.[16,25,36,44,51] Total lung capacity is slightly decreased and functional residual capacity slightly increased. In early ALS, pulmonary function test results may suggest emphysema rather than ALS because residual volume is increased and FVC decreased in both diseases.[11] Residual volume is increased in ALS because of expiratory muscle weakness, but in emphysema it increases because of air trapping. In ALS, the FEV_1-to-FVC ratio is normal (greater than 0.75) unless superimposed obstructive disease is present.[14]

Fallat and colleagues[16] reported the largest series of ALS patients in which pulmonary function tests were performed. Of 218 patients with motor neuron disease, 192 had classic ALS; 103 of these patients were followed serially. Initially, the maximum ventilatory volume was most severely affected: the mean maximum ventilatory volume was only 67% of predicted, while the FVC was still 80% of predicted. Residual volume increased markedly, to almost 200% of predicted, over time in those patients who died during the study period, but it remained relatively constant in survivors. In contrast to Nakano and colleagues' report[44] that FVC decreases linearly over time, Fallat found that the decline was curvilinear, becoming more rapid as death approached. He suggested that this increased rate of FVC decline has prognostic significance, indicating that death from res-

piratory failure is imminent. Interestingly, 29 of 45 patients with either an FVC or a maximum ventilatory volume less than 50% of the predicted had a clinical assessment of "normal breathing."

Kreitzer et al.[36] divided 32 patients with ALS into two groups based on their maximum expiratory flow volume curves. One group had normal curves, and the second group had abnormal curves with a steep drop off in flow as the residual volume was approached. The group with the abnormal curves had a significantly higher residual volume (197% predicted vs. 135% predicted), lower FVC, and lower maximum expiratory pressure with similar maximum inspiratory pressure and total lung capacity. Expiratory muscle weakness has a major role in determining the residual volume, but the residual volume was even higher than that predicted by the maximum expiratory pressure in the group with abnormal flow volume curves. Clinically, the patients with abnormal curves were weaker. They tolerated added expiratory resistance poorly, and the authors suggest that increased expiratory resistance may be a factor in acute (superimposed on chronic) respiratory failure.

Measurement of the static respiratory pressures (maximum inspiratory and expiratory pressures) is one of the most sensitive methods for detecting respiratory muscle weakness.[9,10,25,51] Maximum inspiratory pressure and maximum expiratory pressure may be abnormal while lung volumes are still normal. In patients with ALS, the maximum expiratory pressure is more severely affected than the maximum inspiratory pressure. In the series by Kreitzer et al.[36] of 32 ALS patients, mean values for FVC, maximum inspiratory pressure, and maximum expiratory pressure were 73%, 62%, and 37% of predicted, respectively. The values for maximum inspiratory pressure and maximum expiratory pressure in patients with ALS depend on the lung volume at which they are measured.[51] In contrast, in patients with bilateral diaphragmatic paralysis, these measurements are independent of lung volume.

Braun and Rochester[10] devised a respiratory muscle strength index in which the maximum inspiratory and expiratory pressures are averaged and expressed as a percentage of the predicted value. In myopathic patients, the index correlated highly with maximum ventilatory volume, and all hypercapnic patients had an index of less than 30% of normal. This index may be useful for following respiratory muscle strength in patients with ALS.

Patients with ALS have normal arterial blood gas levels until very late in respiratory failure[16,36,51] (see Table 22–2). Fallat and coworkers[16] observed that arterial blood gas, $Paco_2$, did not rise until FVC fell below 20% of predicted, and at this point, Pao_2 was still normal. Again, these findings contrast with those of patients with bilateral diaphragmatic paralysis who develop resting hypercapnia in arterial blood gas ($Paco_2$ >45 mm Hg). A substantial difference between the supine and seated vital capacity predicts significant diaphragmatic weakness.

Clinical Presentation

Most patients with ALS remain asymptomatic until the FVC has declined to approximately 50% of predicted. The lack of symptoms results from the gradual loss of FVC and the tendency for patients to reduce their level of physical activity because of concomitant loss of strength in the extremities. Signs and symptoms of respiratory failure are outlined in Table 22–3.

Nocturnal symptoms often occur early, but patients may not associate them with respiratory difficulty. Patients report poor sleep with frequent awakening, often because of nightmares. They develop early morning headaches because of hypoxia and often experience excessive daytime fatigue and sleepiness. They may also experience orthopnea because of diaphragmatic weakness and be unable to sleep supine. Exertional dyspnea is common in patients who remain ambulatory or who can manually propel a wheelchair.

Dyspnea is an uncomfortable sensation of shortness of breath.[38] Although the neural pathways for this sensation have not been identified, it is believed that the sense of muscular effort associated with dyspnea comes from activation of the sensory cortex simultaneously with respiratory muscle contraction. In patients with ALS, an increased neural drive is required to activate weakened respiratory muscles; this may also produce

Table 22–3. SIGNS AND SYMPTOMS OF RESPIRATORY FAILURE DURING ALS

Early Signs

Poor sleep
    Frequent awakening
    Nightmares
    Early morning headaches
    Excessive daytime fatigue and sleepiness
    Orthopnea
Frequent sighing
Weak cough
Inability to clear lung secretions

Middle Signs

Dyspnea with exertion
Truncated speech
Respiratory paradox
Dyspnea while eating
Rapid, shallow breathing
Flaring of the nasal alae
Accessory muscle contraction

Late Signs

Increased hematocrit
Hypertension
Acidosis, low serum chloride levels
Drowsiness, to coma

---

dyspnea. Hypercapnia triggers dyspnea in both normal individuals and in patients with no respiratory muscle activity, such as those who are C1–C4 tetraplegic on ventilators. On the other hand, hypoxia has not been proven to produce dyspnea. The ability of opioids, phenothiazines, and benzodiazepines to relieve the sensation of dyspnea has been investigated, but only opioids were found to be effective.[34]

Other signs of respiratory failure include rapid shallow breathing, flaring of the nasal alae, an abnormal speech pattern consisting of shortened phrases, and respiratory paradox in which the chest and abdominal walls no longer move together in the same direction; instead, the chest wall moves out, while the abdominal wall moves in with inspiration (see Chapter 4). Contractions of the accessory respiratory muscles in the anterior neck, as well as shoulder movement, may be visible during respiration. Early in the course of the disease, patients may also have a weak cough, frequent sighing, and difficulty managing secretions because of expiratory muscle weakness. A maximum expiratory pressure greater than 40 cm H_2O (300 mm Hg) is needed to generate a cough adequate for secretion clearance.[35] Shortness of breath while eating is a sign of impending acute respiratory failure.[32]

Late in the progression of respiratory failure, the hematocrit may rise as the body attempts to compensate for chronic nocturnal hypoxia. Patients may also develop hypertension from pulmonary vasoconstriction and right heart failure.[54] If the patient does not receive mechanical ventilatory support, CO_2 retention eventually leads to acidosis, coma, and respiratory arrest. Cardiac arrhythmia resulting from a combination of acidosis and hypoxia may also cause death.

Although respiratory failure is usually insidious and appears after extremity or bulbar weakness develops, several case reports describe patients with ALS in whom respiratory failure was precipitous or was the initial manifestation of the disease.[18,31,39,48] In two reports, three patients who presented with respiratory failure had extremely malignant courses of disease.[18,39] All died within a few months of respiratory failure despite being placed on ventilatory support. On autopsy, all three had marked loss of anterior horn cells in the C3–C7 region of the spinal cord. On the other hand, Hill and coworkers[31] described two patients presenting with acute respiratory failure who, after aggressive respiratory support, remained stable on nocturnal ventilatory support only for an extended period of time. Their acute respiratory failure was blamed on inspiratory muscle fatigue that was alleviated by nocturnal ventilation.

Natural History

Historically, respiratory failure has directly or indirectly caused death in most patients with ALS. In fact, some clinical drug trials have used the need for tracheostomy and death as equivalent endpoints. With the increasing availability of home mechanical ventilation and noninvasive ventilation tech-

niques, some patients with ALS are choosing to live beyond the point of respiratory failure. The natural history of progressive respiratory failure in ALS has been described, but limited information[30] is available concerning the disease course in patients who live beyond respiratory failure.

Pulmonary function usually declines linearly, but the rate of decline varies substantially from one patient to the next.[42,52] Figure 22–3 illustrates the decline in FVC over 20 months in 12 ALS patients followed in our clinic. In the Western ALS Group study, pulmonary function was most closely associated with survival, and the 3-month slope of decline in vital capacity was a reliable gauge of the rate of disease progression that might be used to measure outcome in clinical trials.[49] Those with dyspnea at onset had a statistically shorter survival time. In a prospective study of 21 ALS patients over a period of 18 months, maximum ventilatory volume and maximum inspiratory pressure were the most sensitive predictors of respiratory failure, while FVC was most specific. No patient with a maximum inspiratory pressure of less than 60 cm H_2O and maximum ventilatory volume of less than 80% of predicted values survived 18 months.[19]

Schiffman and Belsh[52] followed pulmonary function in 36 patients with ALS until death or institution of mechanical ventilation. Only 7 (19%) of the patients com-

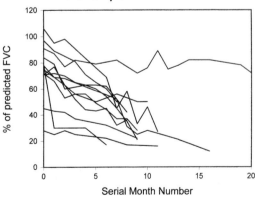

Figure 22–3. FVC changes over time in 12 patients with ALS followed at the Cleveland Clinic. Note markedly variable rates of decline in individual patients.

plained of respiratory symptoms initially, despite having significant decreases in FVC, maximum inspiratory pressure, and maximum expiratory pressure. Overall, FVC declined by 3.5% of its predicted value, maximum inspiratory pressure by 2.9 cm H_2O, and maximum expiratory pressure by 3.4 cm H_2O per month. Although the overall pattern was linear, the rate of decline in pulmonary function seemed to be somewhat greater in the early stages of the disease. Fallat et al.[16] reported a somewhat slower decline in FVC of 1.6% of predicted per month.

LONG-TERM VENTILATION

Hayashi and colleagues[29,30] have studied the largest series of ALS patients on long-term mechanical ventilation. They followed 49 patients on ventilatory support. One-year survival was 80%, and 5-year survival was 26%. Seven patients developed total paralysis of the extraocular muscles at 1 to 5 years after the institution of full-time ventilation, rendering them totally "locked in" and unable to communicate. Several others developed partial limitation of extraocular movements, intermittent spasmodic gaze fixation, or both, which was presumed to be of supranuclear origin. Impairment of cranial motor function is thought to occur in the reverse of the ontogenic sequence, with the relatively older functions being preserved the longest.[27] Patients who become totally locked in seem to deteriorate rapidly, becoming ventilator-dependent within 1.5 years of disease onset.[28]

The reported cause of death in 25 ventilator-dependent patients with ALS was respiratory tract infections in 12, sudden death during sleep in 6, accidental ventilator disconnection in 3, myocardial infarction in 2, renal failure in 1, and gastric ulcer perforation in 1.[30] Autonomic instability was noted in several patients and may have contributed to sudden death during sleep or predisposed patients to myocardial infarction.

Oppenheimer[45] reported survival data on patients with ALS participating in Kaiser Permanente's home mechanical ventilation program from 1985 to 1992. Of 31 patients discharged home on mechanical ventilation, 27 were alive 1 year after discharge, 18 at 3 years,

and 10 at 5 years. No data were reported on their functional or communication status.

MONITORING PULMONARY FUNCTION

Pulmonary function should be monitored regularly. In most cases, the primary physician can do this during routine office visits. A crude method for assessing respiratory muscle strength is to ask the patient to count as high as possible in one breath. Those with normal respiratory function can count to at least 15. The patient may also be asked to cough as hard as possible so a subjective assessment of expiratory muscle strength can be obtained. Table 22–4 gives recommendations for pulmonary function monitoring.

After the initial diagnosis, a complete set of baseline pulmonary function tests (FVC, FEV_1, maximum ventilatory volume, maximum inspiratory pressure, and maximum expiratory pressure) is recommended in both the seated and supine positions. Depending on the patient's psychological status, it may be best not to perform these tests during the same visit in which the patient is given the ALS diagnosis; however, pulmonary function testing should be performed at the next visit and ideally before any respiratory signs or symptoms develop. Baseline studies allow de-

Table 22–4. RECOMMENDATIONS FOR PULMONARY FUNCTION MONITORING

Evaluation at Diagnosis
Forced vital capacity, seated and supine
Forced expiratory volume in 1 second
Maximum ventilatory volume
Maximum inspiratory pressure
Maximum expiratory pressure
Arterial blood gas levels, if pulmonary function testing abnormalities suggest disease that is not purely restrictive
Peak flow rate

Follow-up Evaluations
Forced vital capacity, seated and supine
Peak flow rate

tection of any underlying pulmonary disease, such as chronic obstructive pulmonary disease or asthma, that would affect future management. If pulmonary function test results indicate only restrictive disease, arterial blood gas evaluation is unnecessary. After this baseline set of pulmonary function tests, patients with no underlying pulmonary disease may be followed by measuring FVC with a handheld spirometer at each office visit or at least every 3 to 6 months, depending on the rate of disease progression. Peak flow rate can be measured with disposable peak flow meters such as those used in emergency rooms for evaluating patients with asthma exacerbation. A peak flow of at least 5 L/s or 300 L/min is necessary for adequate clearance of secretions.[3]

If the patient reports nocturnal signs or symptoms, or if the supine FVC is less than 1 L, home monitoring to detect nocturnal hypoventilation is useful. Both O_2 saturation and end-tidal CO_2 can be monitored noninvasively in the home. Nocturnal hypoventilation is present if the O_2 saturation is less than 95% for more than 1 hour or if end-tidal CO_2 is greater than 50 mm Hg at any time during the night.[6]

A patient whose respiratory function appears to be acutely decompensating may have a superimposed pulmonary infection and should have a complete pulmonary evaluation including arterial blood gas measurement, chest radiographs, sputum cultures, and any other appropriate diagnostic tests.

PREVENTING RESPIRATORY FAILURE

Several steps can be taken to prevent exacerbating respiratory failure or hastening its onset in the patient with ALS. These include preventing aspiration and infection, assisting the patient with secretion clearance, and judiciously using pharmacotherapy. These interventions are outlined in Table 22–5. Once respiratory failure has occurred, both noninvasive and invasive respiratory support can be used to relieve symptoms and prolong life.

Aspiration can be avoided by evaluating the swallowing mechanism and then recommending compensatory strategies, such as

Table 22–5. GUIDELINES FOR PREVENTING RESPIRATORY FAILURE

Prevent aspiration
    Swallowing evaluation
    Modified swallow techniques
    Diet consistency modification
    Oral suctioning
    Percutaneous gastrostomy tube
Prevent infection
    Pneumococcal vaccination
    Influenza vaccination
Assist in secretion clearance
    Suction machine
    Assisted coughing
    In-Exsufflator
Provide judicious pharmacotherapy
Avoid supplemental oxygen

the chin tuck, changing the food consistency, or both. If dysphagia and aspiration are already present, nutritional support should be recommended (see Chapter 24). A bedside swallowing evaluation, even when performed by an experienced speech pathologist, is inadequate for detecting aspiration: the bedside evaluation misses aspiration in 40% of patients with neurologic disabilities who aspirate.[57] A videofluoroscopic swallowing study is the best method for assessing patients for both dysphagia and aspiration. If fluoroscopy is not available, an otolaryngologist (and speech pathologist) can perform fiberoptic endoscopic evaluation of swallowing, a new technique for swallowing assessment; it is as specific and sensitive as videofluoroscopy for detection of aspiration.

A portable oral suction machine can be used to remove food or secretions that cause difficulties for the patient. If a patient continues to aspirate more than 10% of the food taken in despite using compensatory techniques and modifying food consistency, a percutaneous endoscopic gastrostomy tube should be strongly encouraged. This approach will reduce the likelihood of food aspiration but does not prevent aspiration of oral secretions or regurgitated tube feedings. Some patients have undergone laryngeal diversion procedures to prevent continuous aspiration.[12]

All patients with ALS should receive a pneumococcal vaccination and a yearly influenza vaccination. If FVC is less than 60% of predicted, patients should also avoid close contact with people who have upper respiratory tract infections.

Effective oral and pulmonary secretion management is important in preventing aspiration pneumonia. As previously mentioned, a peak expiratory flow rate of 5 L/s is required for a cough that is strong enough to clear secretions. If the expiratory muscles are too weak to generate an adequate cough, patients can be helped with either manually assisted coughing or with a suction device called the In-Exsufflator (JH Emerson Co, Cambridge, MA).[3]

The In-Exsufflator (Fig. 22–4) is a machine with a vacuum cleaner motor that can be used to deliver positive pressure (insufflation) to inflate the lungs fully and negative pressure (exsufflation) to suction secretions from the lungs. Pressure is delivered via an anesthesia face mask, and cycling can be done either automatically or manually. After exsufflation, secretions and mucus plugs are carried into the mouth and face mask where they can be removed with oral suction. The In-Exsufflator can generate a peak flow rate of 7 to 11 L/s, which is better than that achieved with manually assisted coughing.

The In-Exsufflator can also be used in place of tracheal suctioning in patients who have tracheostomies; the anesthesia face mask is not used, and the hosing is attached directly to the tracheostomy tube.

Caregivers can manually assist the patient in coughing by providing an abdominal thrust and anterior chest compression synchronized with the patient's attempts to cough. This technique can generate a peak flow of 5 to 7 L/s.[6] If the patient's vital capacity is less than 1.5 L, cough force can be improved by providing the patient with an insufflation using a manual resuscitator, an intermittent positive-pressure breathing machine, a portable ventilator, or the In-Exsufflator.

Appropriate use of medications also can help prevent premature respiratory failure. For example, calcium channel blockers, aminoglycosides, steroids, and benzodiazepines can decrease the ventilatory response to hypoxia and hypercarbia and thus exacerbate chronic alveolar hypoventilation,[6] these medications should be avoided if possible. Theophylline may increase diaphragmatic contractility and prevent diaphragmatic fatigue, but no reports clearly show that this occurs in the ALS population. Schiffman and Belsh[53] found that theophylline slightly increased negative inspiratory pressure and vital capacity in patients with ALS after resistive inspiratory muscle exercise, but it did not

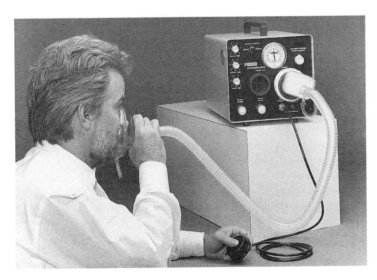

Figure 22–4. In-Exsufflator being used for secretion clearance. (Courtesy of J. H. Emerson Co., Cambridge, MA. Photograph by Hutchins Photography, Inc.).

significantly affect pulmonary function during rest.

Providing patients with supplemental oxygen can relieve symptoms of air hunger and dyspnea but also may suppress respiratory drive, exacerbate alveolar hypoventilation, and ultimately lead to CO_2 narcosis and respiratory arrest. Supplemental oxygen is only recommended for patients with concomitant pulmonary disease or as a comfort measure for those who decline assisted ventilation. Severe hypercapnia developed in eight patients with neuromuscular disease (including two with ALS) who were placed on low-flow oxygen therapy at 0.5 to 2.0 L/min via nasal cannula.[20] All patients in this group had vital capacities less than 45% of predicted values. The mean baseline $Paco_2$ rose from 58 to 86 mm Hg within 1 to 42 hours of oxygen administration, and three patients required intubation. Thus, the standard "2 L O_2/min via nasal cannula" order may not be safe in ALS patients with chronic respiratory failure.

Some have suggested that the diaphragm can be strengthened by resistive inspiratory muscle exercise. There is too little research on the role of exercise in ALS to make a clear statement as to whether overuse weakness occurs. One study in which six patients with motor neuron disease (two with ALS) performed inspiratory muscle training for 10-minute sessions three times daily for 3 months showed significantly improved maximum ventilatory volume, maximum inspiratory pressure, and FVC.[26] In general, patients may be able to minimally improve the strength of moderately weak muscles with an exercise program. Schiffman and Belsh,[53] however, found that many patients do not tolerate resistive inspiratory muscle exercise. Using an incentive spirometer does not constitute resistive exercise and does little to prevent alveolar hypoventilation or improve pulmonary function.

MANAGING RESPIRATORY FAILURE

The clinician's approach to managing respiratory failure depends on the patient's desires concerning ventilatory support. Discussion concerning the possibility of respiratory failure should be initiated soon after the diagnosis of ALS so that patients and their families can learn about their choices and, ideally, make a decision about ventilator use in a noncrisis situation. The best time to initiate such a discussion will depend on the psychological state of the patient. The noninvasive respiratory muscle aids listed in Table 22–6 are not a permanent solution to respiratory failure but do provide many patients with additional time to make a decision concerning tracheostomy. In addition, noninvasive ventilation techniques, when initiated before acute respiratory failure, allow patients to adjust gradually to ventilator use and make a more informed decision regarding tracheostomy.

Ventilation issues must be discussed regularly because many patients change their views concerning life-sustaining therapy as the disease progresses.[55] Introducing the patient to another ventilator-dependent individual, whether with ALS or another diagnosis, may provide the patient with a clearer sense of what life is like with ventilatory support. Ultimately, fewer than 5% of ALS patients choose long-term ventilatory support.[41] Patients not choosing ventilatory support should be reassured that, with appropriate medications and oxygen administration, death by respiratory failure can be a painless, peaceful experience for both patient and family.

Table 22–6. NONINVASIVE VENTILATION OPTIONS FOR MANAGING RESPIRATORY FAILURE

Negative-pressure ventilation
    Iron lung
    Wrap-style ventilator (poncho)
    Chest shell (cuirass)
Intermittent abdominal pressure ventilation
    Exsufflation belt
Positive-pressure ventilation
    Oral interface
    Nasal interface
    Custom-molded mask
    Oral-nasal interface

Noninvasive Ventilation: Negative-Pressure Techniques

Noninvasive ventilatory assistance can be provided by both negative- and positive-pressure devices, although positive-pressure methods are more commonly used because they present fewer difficulties. Negative-pressure ventilation is achieved with body ventilators, chest shells, or wrap-style ventilators.[13] The iron lung was the first negative-pressure ventilation device and is primarily of historic interest. The patient's entire body, except the head and neck, is enclosed in an airtight chamber. Air is withdrawn from the chamber, creating a subatmospheric pressure around the chest. Air passively flows into the lungs via the patient's mouth and nose to expand the chest and equalize pressure on either side of the chest wall. The patient then passively exhales when air at atmospheric pressure is allowed to return to the chamber. Disadvantages of the iron lung include immobilization of the patient, lack of access to the patient for nursing care, and incomplete pulmonary expansion when compared with positive-pressure ventilation. A more compact version of the iron lung, the Porta Lung (Lifecare International, Westminster, CO), weighing only 110 pounds, is currently manufactured and is used for a small number of postpolio syndrome patients.[1]

The wrap-style ventilator, also known as the poncho or pulmowrap, operates by the same principle as the iron lung and is slightly less cumbersome. It is a nylon or Gore-Tex garment covering a firm plastic grid that is attached to a rigid backplate. The garment is sealed around the patient's neck, wrists, and legs. It can be time consuming and difficult to put on and remove and has the same drawbacks as the iron lung.[1]

The chest shell, or cuirass, is slightly more practical and is used by some patients with ALS for nocturnal ventilation. It works best when the patient is supine but can be used in the sitting position if the spine is straight. A subatmospheric pressure is created under the shell by a negative-pressure ventilator, causing air to flow passively into the lungs. All negative-pressure devices use room air and act merely as mechanical aids to assist with lung inflation.[1]

Intermittent abdominal pressure ventilation requires a positive-pressure portable ventilator but works more like negative-pressure ventilation. An abdominal corset (or exsufflation belt) containing an inflatable bladder is attached to a positive-pressure ventilator. The ventilator inflates the bladder to compress the abdominal contents, move the diaphragm upward, and expel air from the lungs. When the bladder deflates, gravity pulls the diaphragm downward, and air passively enters the lungs. The exsufflation belt must be used in the seated position. It is useful during the daytime for patients who use positive-pressure ventilation nocturnally with an oral or nasal interface; it frees the mouth for speech, use of a mouthstick, and other activities. In addition, the exsufflation belt can be worn under street clothing and is cosmetically acceptable. On average, tidal volume can be increased by 300 mL using this method.[1]

Noninvasive Ventilation: Positive-Pressure Techniques

Noninvasive positive-pressure ventilation (NIPPV) can be delivered through a variety of oral or nasal masks and interfaces using portable volume-cycled or pressure-cycled ventilators. Oral interfaces include mouthpieces that must be held in place using voluntary lip seal and those held in place by straps placed over the head when voluntary lip seal alone is inadequate. For patients with adequate head and neck muscle control, the mouthpiece can be mounted on a wheelchair frame using a gooseneck clamp adjacent to other mouth controls, such as a sip-and-puff or chin-operated switch; this position also enables the patient to speak when not inhaling from the ventilator. Patients will not be able to speak or take food by mouth when wearing an oral interface that is held in place by straps. Nasal interfaces include standard continuous positive airway pressure (CPAP) or bilevel positive airway pressure (BiPAP) masks as well as custom-molded devices; these interfaces are preferred by most patients for nocturnal and even daytime ventilation[3] (Fig. 22–5). If air leakage from the mouth is excessive, a chin strap can be used

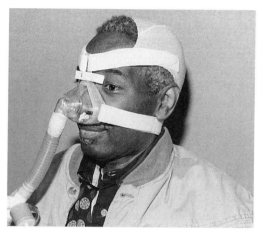

Figure 22–5. A patient using noninvasive positive pressure ventilation via nasal interface.

to hold the mouth closed. When an oral interface is used, air leaks from the nostrils can be prevented by blocking them with cotton pledgets. Combined oral and nasal interfaces are also available, but they tend to make patients feel claustrophobic, and adequate ventilation can usually be provided through a single orifice. Many patients need to experiment with several interfaces before they find the one that works best and is most comfortable. In addition, some patients require that two or three interfaces be used on a rotating basis to prevent pressure-related skin breakdown over the bridge of the nose or other areas.

Volume-cycled ventilators are more commonly used than pressure-cycled ventilators for noninvasive ventilation in the home. If airway resistance is increased by mucous plugging, pressure-cycled ventilators may not deliver adequate volumes. Pressure-cycled ventilators also use three to eight times more electricity than volume-cycled ventilators.[1] With volume-cycled ventilators, the tidal volume is adjusted as needed to compensate for any air leakage. In general, tidal volumes are greater than those used for a patient with a tracheostomy, which is essentially a closed system. The goal of ventilatory support is to generate an intrapulmonary pressure of 20 cm H_2O, which is adequate for full lung inflation. Either an assist-control or intermittent mandatory ventilation mode may be used, and the ventilator rate should be set to maintain $Paco_2$ between 30 and 40 mm Hg. Periodically, a few breaths can be delivered at an increased tidal volume to hyperinflate the lungs and provide the chest wall with range of motion. Theoretically, providing range-of-motion exercise to the chest wall helps prevent atelectasis and loss of lung compliance.

The BiPAP machine is a type of pressure-cycled ventilator used for some patients with ALS. With BiPAP, the tidal volume plateaus when a pressure of 15 cm H_2O is reached, so the lungs cannot be inflated as fully as with a volume-cycled ventilator. Inspiratory and expiratory pressures can be set independently; for the most effective ventilation, the inspiratory pressure should be set at maximum and the expiratory pressure as low as possible unless the patient tends to have apneic episodes caused by hypopharyngeal collapse. BiPAP provides adequate inspiratory muscle assistance only to those with mild alveolar hypoventilation. BiPAP machines cannot adequately ventilate patients with no vital capacity, whereas volume-cycled ventilators can. In addition, most BiPAP units cannot deliver a large enough volume for effective assisted cough.

Guidelines as to when to initiate NIPPV vary.[6,54] Symptoms of respiratory distress or the presence of nocturnal hypoventilation, as indicated by nocturnal oxygen saturation and end-tidal CO_2 monitoring, are certainly indications for NIPPV. Some[54] recommend that NIPPV be initiated when the supine FVC falls below 1 L, whereas others[6] suggest initiation when the FVC falls below 50% of predicted values. Beginning regular insufflation treatments when the FVC falls to 50% to 60% of predicted values may help prevent loss of pulmonary compliance. The rate of the patient's disease progression must also be considered in deciding when to initiate NIPPV. Initially, NIPPV is used only at night. As patients continue to lose vital capacity, ventilator use extends into the day for varying periods and eventually becomes continuous. It often takes several weeks for patients to become comfortable using the ventilator and be able to sleep through the night with it. If NIPPV is started before respiratory distress occurs, the patient can become slowly accustomed to the equipment by using it intermittently and gradually extending the night period of use until overnight use is tolerated.

Ventilation via Tracheostomy

Most patients with ALS who choose assisted ventilation will eventually require a tracheostomy because of progressive bulbar muscle dysfunction.[56] Bach[2] studied 50 patients with ALS who learned to use NIPPV and found that success depended on the patient's residual bulbar muscle strength, not the vital capacity or amount of ventilator-free time. Specifically, patients with peak cough expiratory flow rates greater than 3 L/s and maximum insufflation capacities (the amount of air which can be held against a closed glottis) greater than their vital capacities were successful noninvasive ventilation users. When they became dependent on NIPPV full time, the successful group had a mean seated FVC of 580 mL, supine FVC of 545 mL, maximum insufflation capacity of 1010 mL, and peak cough expiratory flow of 4.1 L/s. Half the successful users eventually underwent tracheostomy, at which time mean seated FVC was 160 mL and maximum insufflation capacity was 460 mL.

When tracheostomy is performed, the tracheostomy tube cuff should be kept deflated if possible to prevent tracheal damage, such as tracheomalacia, tracheal erosion, and tracheal rupture. In some patients, cuff deflation is not possible because the patient will aspirate secretions or food. If the patient is not severely anarthric or dysarthric, to preserve speech, a fenestrated tracheostomy tube or speaking valve can be used. All tracheostomy tubes should have outer and inner cannulas; the inner cannula is left in place except when it is cleaned. The inner cannula prevents secretion buildup in the outer cannula, which could occlude the tracheostomy.

Comparison of Noninvasive Ventilation and Tracheostomy

The major advantage of noninvasive ventilation in the ALS population is that it allows patients to make educated decisions concerning their desire for ventilatory support, and it serves as a transition to permanent ventilation with a tracheostomy for those choosing that route. Patients and their families find learning to use noninvasive ventilatory aids in the home much less stressful and less threatening than learning to manage a tracheostomy. Also, most patients have never known anyone who used a ventilator in the home, and using noninvasive techniques gives them an idea of what ventilatory support entails. Noninvasive ventilation is less costly than ventilation by tracheostomy because fewer expensive supplies are needed, and a less costly level of skilled home help can be used. If the patient with a tracheostomy hires home assistance through an agency, a registered nurse will be required because of liability issues. In contrast, licensed practical nurses and nurse's aides are often provided for patients on noninvasive ventilation. Other advantages of noninvasive ventilation include more natural speech, a decreased risk of infection because the normal mucosal barriers are not bypassed, and sometimes, greater patient comfort.

The most significant disadvantage of noninvasive ventilation is that it does not prevent aspiration. In fact, if an oral or nasal interface is used and held in place by head straps, aspiration risk increases during emesis episodes. Another disadvantage is that many hospital medical personnel are unfamiliar with the equipment used for noninvasive ventilation; thus, if patients develop an acute medical problem requiring hospitalization, they may not be allowed to use their own equipment in the hospital and may have to accept intubation. When initially learning to use NIPPV, some patients experience aerophagia and abdominal discomfort. This problem generally resolves with continued use. Some patients also find full-time use of an oral or nasal mask uncomfortable and may opt for tracheostomy once they have no ventilator-free time. Table 22–7 outlines the pros and cons of both noninvasive ventilation and ventilation through a tracheostomy.

Successful Home Ventilation

Use of either invasive or noninvasive ventilation in the home requires considerable patient and family training and education. The patient and family may benefit from a short

Table 22–7. **COMPARISON OF NONINVASIVE VENTILATION AND VENTILATION WITH TRACHEOSTOMY**

Ventilation	Advantages	Disadvantages
Noninvasive	Allows informed decisions about long-term ventilation Less threatening to caregivers Comfort Lower cost Decreased infection risk Allows normal speech	Does not prevent aspiration Medical personnel unfamiliar with equipment Aerophagia
Tracheostomy	Less risk of aspiration May be more comfortable when required 24 h	Increased risk of infection Risk of tracheal erosion and hemorrhage Frequent suctioning increases secretions Higher cost Speech alteration

inpatient stay to receive intensive training in home ventilator management. Rehabilitation admission has been reimbursed by insurance carriers if the patient has other rehabilitation goals such as family training for transfer assistance, wheelchair and adaptive home medical equipment prescription, and evaluation for an augmentative communication system.

Table 22–8 lists the minimum equipment necessary for successful home ventilation, particularly using tracheostomy. An attachment that allows the ventilator to be plugged into the cigarette lighter of a car and be powered by the car's battery is useful for travel. (Most importantly, the patient needs an effective communication system, as discussed in Chapter 23).

QUALITY-OF-LIFE AND PSYCHOLOGICAL ISSUES RELATED TO VENTILATORY SUPPORT

In the United States, 4,000 to 11,000 patients with neuromuscular disease are on long-term mechanical ventilation,[33] but only a fraction of those have ALS. The decision to pursue long-term ventilatory support has many ramifications for both the patient and the family. Mechanical ventilation provided at home or in a long-term care facility is extremely costly. Ventilation given at home is emotionally draining for caregivers because of an overwhelming number of responsibilities (Table 22–9). On the other hand, it can

Table 22–8. **EQUIPMENT NEEDED FOR HOME VENTILATION**

Portable ventilator with battery	Extra ventilator tubing
Backup ventilator*	Extra tracheotomy tube*
Backup battery	Tracheotomy supplies*
Manual resuscitation bag	Ventilator tray for wheelchair or walker
Supplemental oxygen for emergency*	Effective communication system
Suction machine	

*Required for the use of a permanent ventilation and tracheostomy.

Table 22–9. CAREGIVER RESPONSIBILITIES FOR THE VENTILATOR-DEPENDENT PATIENT

Tracheostomy care	Bathing the patient
Ventilator monitoring and troubleshooting	Dressing the patient
Medication administration	Coordinating medical care
Problem solving related to emergencies (i.e., power failure)	Seeking information on financial assistance resources
Feeding the patient	Obtaining services from agencies

provide the patient with added months or years of quality time with family and friends. Table 22–10 summarizes several attributes of successful users of ventilation at home, based on the previous studies.[46,47,56]

When patients consider mechanical ventilation, they must understand that their decision is reversible.[23] In all reported series of ALS patients on ventilators, a few individuals have chosen to withdraw from permanent ventilation.[4,41,47] Patients have withdrawn for a variety of reasons, ranging from dissatisfaction with their quality of life to not having a willing caregiver. Moss and coworkers[40] surveyed 50 permanent ventilator users with ALS concerning conditions under which they would wish to withdraw from ventilation. Of the 50, 34 stated that they would wish to withdraw if permanently unconscious, 21 if they were unable to communicate, 12 if they were a burden to their family, and 9 if they were unable to pay for the ventilation.

Table 22–10. CHARACTERISTICS OF SUCCESSFUL HOME VENTILATOR USERS

Positive attitude

Executive personality in patient or caregiver

Maintaining some independent mobility

Maintaining some activities of daily living

Enjoyment of daily activities

Good communication skills

Slowly progressing ALS

Adequate financial resources

Supportive family or other caregiver

Multiple caregivers in the home

Availability of multidisciplinary medical team experienced in home ventilation

Patients must be encouraged to discuss with both their families and their physicians the situations in which they would no longer wish to continue ventilation. All patients should have a durable power of attorney for health care that should be reviewed periodically, because patients' wishes and their perceptions of quality of life often change as their disease progresses.

The quality of life of the ventilator-dependent patient requires discussion because many physicians use "poor quality of life" as a reason to avoid discussing options concerning ventilatory support, or they present the options negatively. In a 1992 survey of 273 Muscular Dystrophy Association clinic directors from 167 clinics who treat a large number of patients with ALS, only 26% recommended the elective use of ventilatory assistance to prevent respiratory failure; 41% discouraged the use of ventilatory assistance, and 33% did not discuss the issue. Of the clinic directors who discouraged ventilator use, 64% did so because they believed the patient's quality of life would be poor.[5] A recent review[21] of 75 studies on quality-of-life measures revealed that most measurements focus on the wrong target, the opinions of the "experts" rather than those of the patient. Only 17% of the instruments reviewed asked patients to rate their own quality of life, and no distinction was made between overall quality of life and health-related quality of life. Bach[7] has stated:

It is remarkable that there should be the need to discuss as an ethical issue physician intervention to prolong the lives of mentally competent individuals who in most cases desperately want to live, but the traditional stereotypes concerning individuals using ventilators and the general lack of knowledge about noninvasive management options make this necessary.

The work of Bach and others indicates that able-bodied individuals indeed are unable to adequately judge the quality of life of those with disabilities.[5] In a survey of nonambulatory, ventilator-dependent patients with muscular dystrophy, both the patient and health-care professionals who cared for them were asked to rate their own quality of life using a 7-point scale with a score of 1 indicating complete dissatisfaction and a score of 7 indicating complete satisfaction. The patients gave themselves a mean overall score of 4.9, and the health-care providers gave themselves a mean score of 5.4, which did not significantly differ from what the patients had given themselves. However, the health professionals rated the patients' quality of life as 2.5.[5]

Although the research is limited, most ALS patients receiving ventilatory support seem to be satisfied with their choice and with their quality of life. In one series of 89 patients receiving noninvasive or invasive ventilatory support for a mean of 4.4 years, only 2 patients regretted their choice of ventilation. In this series, an effective communication system was associated with higher perceived quality of life and longer survival.[4] In one series of 19 ventilator-dependent ALS patients, 16 of whom had tracheostomies, 17 of the patients and 16 of their caregivers said they would make the same decision again,[41] but only 10 of the caregivers said they would choose home ventilation for themselves if in a similar situation. Oppenheimer and colleagues[47] found quite similar results for 38 patients, all with tracheostomies, on home mechanical ventilation: more than 95% of the patients would opt for home mechanical ventilation again, but only 50% of their caregivers would choose it for themselves.

The experience of Sam Filer, a Canadian judge with ALS who has been ventilator-dependent for several years, highlights the positive aspects of life on a ventilator.[22] He was diagnosed with ALS at age 51 and became ventilator-dependent at age 54 but continued to work as a judge. At age 56, he was tetraplegic, had a gastrostomy tube, and used an electronic voice synthesizer to communicate when he said the following:[22]

Throughout the process of my ALS, I have learned many things. I have learned that having ALS does not necessarily mean a death sentence, that I am not living with a life-threatening disease, but rather with a life-enhancing condition. I have learned, moreover, that it is possible to continue to live a life of quality. . . . I have learned that I have much to offer.

At the same time, his wife described her experience with physicians' perceptions of her husband's potential quality of life:[22]

Sam went into respiratory failure while in the hospital . . . Six attending physicians encircled me, offering assurance that it would be inhuman to not let him die with dignity; that his care would become financially ruinous; that I had an infant at home to whom I owed my devotion; that there is, not could be, but is, no quality of life once ventilated; and that I had 10 minutes within which to make a decision.

Having a family member on home mechanical ventilation is extremely stressful. Ninety percent of the primary caregivers are women, usually a wife or an adult daughter.[41] Even with assistance from nurses and aides, the primary caregiver cares for the patient an average of 9 hours daily. Major stressors identified by caregivers include the inability to leave patients alone, financial strain, and having to deal with nurses, insurers, and suppliers. Many patients go through periods of depression and times during which they may contemplate discontinuing ventilation, which places further stress on the caregiver. Almost 50% of the primary caregivers in one study felt that their own health was suffering because of their responsibilities for the patient's care.[41] Some family members who did not participate in the decision to have home mechanical ventilation have felt trapped.[46] Families function best when the caregiver acts from a sense of devotion, rather than duty, to the patient (ED Sivak, MD, Upstate New York University, unpublished data, 1996). Temporary hospitalization of the patient can provide caregivers with needed respite, but this often is difficult to arrange under the current insurance coverage systems.

The financial cost of home mechanical ventilation is considerable. In one series, the average yearly cost was $153,000 with tracheostomy and $19,200 with NIPPV; the monthly cost was $12,800 for those with tracheostomies and $1600 for those using noninvasive ventilation. On average, insurance paid for 83% of the costs and, for some patients, paid 100%.[41] Obviously, without full insurance coverage, the financial burden on the family is heavy. Most of the costs incurred by patients with tracheostomies are for skilled nursing assistance. These costs can be reduced considerably by hiring aides privately instead of through an agency and having family members train them in tracheostomy management. The cost of home mechanical ventilation with skilled nursing assistance 16 hours per day is still considerably less than caring for a ventilator-dependent patient in a skilled nursing facility.[17] This fact could be used by physicians and family members to bargain with insurance case managers to increase home-care coverage.

Case Study

We present a case study of a patient we have followed. The case illustrates how permanent ventilatory support and nursing home care can be a good option for the right patient when a case is managed well, discussion between all involved is open and ongoing, and caregivers are devoted and well trained.

This patient is a 58-year-old woman who was diagnosed with ALS at age 55 after developing right-leg weakness. Weakness rapidly developed in all four extremities, along with dysarthria and dysphagia. Four months after the onset of the leg weakness, pulmonary function testing revealed an FVC of 50% of predicted values in the seated position. At that time, she could walk short distances with a cane and did not notice any respiratory symptoms. She agreed to percutaneous gastrostomy tube placement 6 months after the onset of ALS because of progressive dysphagia and a 14-kg weight loss.

When she was initially diagnosed with ALS, this patient stated that she would not want to live on a ventilator but was afraid of dying of respiratory failure because she would feel like she was smothering. Noninvasive ventilation alternatives were discussed with her. At 7 months after onset, her supine FVC had fallen to 25% of predicted. She was not sleeping well and constantly felt fatigued, but she did not complain of dyspnea or orthopnea. She decided to try nocturnal NIPPV. After experimenting with several interfaces, it was determined that an oral mask with a lipseal delivered the best ventilatory support. The mask was secured by headstraps, and cotton balls and a piece of tape were used to plug her nostrils to prevent excessive air leaks. A volume-cycled ventilator was used, along with a home suction machine and pulse oximeter to monitor blood oxygenation. She initially felt claustrophobic wearing the oral interface and could tolerate it for only 15 minutes at a time. Over the next few weeks, she gradually increased her time on the ventilator until she could tolerate it all night. Once she was using the ventilator every night, she began to sleep better and felt less fatigued during the day. Her devoted husband became adept at problem solving and at adjusting the ventilator settings. A nurse's aide was hired to assist her while her husband was at work.

Over the next 3 months, she began to use the ventilator for progressively longer periods during the day. She became wheelchair-bound and began to use a spelling board because severe dysarthria had developed. Eventually, she was using the NIPPV continuously with only 15-minute periods of ventilator-free time. Her oral interface was uncomfortable when worn for such long periods, and she began to consider a tracheostomy. She briefly tried using an exsufflation belt for daytime ventilation but felt anxious and inadequately ventilated. One evening, she had been off the ventilator for 10 minutes when she experienced a respiratory arrest, most likely because of CO_2 retention. Her husband revived her by applying the oral interface and ventilator. After this experience, she decided to undergo tracheostomy.

At 10 months after the onset of ALS, the patient was hospitalized for an elective tracheostomy. The procedure was without complications, and she remained in the hospital 2 weeks while her husband was trained to care for the tracheostomy, and a home care system was established. She returned home and had private nurse's aides 12 hours daily. They were trained in tracheostomy management by her husband. She remained medically stable at home but gradually became completely dependent for all transfers and activities of daily living. The aides and her husband began to have difficulty making one-person transfers. Her husband found managing her care to be extremely stressful and physically draining because he continued to work full time. Three months after the tracheostomy procedure, she and her husband realized that she could no longer safely be cared for at home. She became depressed about the idea of going to a nursing home and considered refusing her enteral feedings.

The patient moved to a nursing home a few miles from her own home. Her husband spends every evening with her, and she has private aides to serve as companions and assist with personal care 12 hours each day. Her children, who live out of state, visit frequently. After a period of adjustment lasting approximately 2 months, she befriended several of the nursing home staff, accepted her disability, and was no longer depressed. She has remained in the nursing home for 2.5 years without any acute hospitalizations. All voluntary muscles except the extraocular muscles are paralyzed, and she uses a computer with a voice synthesizer and an eye-blink switch to communicate. She enjoys spending time with her family, visiting with friends, watching television and movies on videotape, and listening to books on audiotape. She maintains a keen interest in the lives of her family and friends as well as in the world at large. She knows that she can choose to withdraw from ventilation at any time if she no longer finds her quality of life acceptable. She has discussed with her primary physician how withdrawal would be done and has reaffirmed that she is happy to be alive, even with her disability.

This case study highlights several of the issues discussed in this chapter. When the patient was first diagnosed with ALS, she did not consider life on a ventilator to be an acceptable quality of life; as she became more disabled, she changed her views and voluntarily underwent tracheostomy. The shift in viewpoint began when she noted better sleep and less fatigue when using noninvasive ventilation. Because she began using nocturnal noninvasive ventilation before she was aware of any respiratory symptoms, she was able to gradually become accustomed to the equipment over a period of several weeks; this prolonged period of adjustment probably contributed to her acceptance of noninvasive ventilatory support. The patient's change in wishes concerning life support demonstrates why physicians caring for ALS patients must regularly review and discuss their patients' views about ventilatory support. The patient reconsidered her ideas again when she could no longer remain in her home. If she had known that when she requested tracheostomy, she would ultimately have to live in a nursing home, she might not have undergone the procedure. However, after a period of adjustment to this further progression of disability, she once again accepted her present quality of life. Having her family's and physician's support for her request to be able to withdraw from ventilation at any time gave her a sense of control over her destiny and made it easier for her to choose tracheostomy.

This family had private insurance coverage that paid for nursing home care and all medical supplies. However, the insurance did not cover hiring aides either at home or in the nursing home. This patient's quality of life and feelings about long-term ventilation might have been quite different if she had not been able to afford private aides.

This case illustrates the advantages of using noninvasive ventilation techniques as a transition to tracheostomy. The patient experienced full-time respiratory support before undergoing tracheostomy and thus did not have to make the decision in a crisis situation. She was adequately ventilated noninvasively 24 hours daily and chose tracheostomy for reasons that she perceived as being improved comfort and security. Each patient must weigh for himself or herself the relative advantages and disadvantages of noninvasive ventilation techniques and tracheostomy; no single choice is right for everyone.

WITHDRAWAL FROM VENTILATION

One of the most difficult situations for physicians, family, and caregivers occurs when a patient wishes to terminate ventilatory support. Withdrawal of ventilatory support is not assisted suicide, mercy killing, or euthanasia; rather, the patient is merely allowed to die from the natural course of ALS. Withdrawal of ventilation is fully supported by legal precedent. For competent patients who are not suffering from depression, the decision to die once their quality of life has deteriorated beyond the point they consider acceptable can be perfectly rational and appropriate. Goldblatt[24] has suggested that the decision to die restores the power to patients that their illness has stolen from them (see Chapter 26).

Little has been written about how to withdraw ventilation from the patient with ALS so that death is peaceful and without suffering. The patient should not be weaned from the ventilator to the point of loss of consciousness, as this will be extremely uncomfortable and will provoke anxiety. Sedative medication should be provided but not in such a dose that it would independently cause the patient's death.

A few case reports in the literature may be

helpful to physicians facing this dilemma. The patient and family's wishes must be considered in deciding whether to withdraw ventilation in the hospital or the home. Goldblatt[23] describes one case in which a hospitalized patient was given sodium thiopental as if for induction of anesthesia. Once the patient lost consciousness, the ventilator was turned off, and the patient's heart stopped in 8 minutes. In the home, patients have been given a combination of diazepam and meperidine,[23] intravenous morphine,[17] or a combination of liquid pentobarbital and subcutaneous morphine,[43] until they lost consciousness, at which time the ventilator was either turned off or the patients were weaned from it. Their deaths were described as peaceful. Two patients spent their last days happily visiting with family and friends who had traveled long distances to share memories and say good-bye.[17,43] Libby,[37] a home care nurse with experience in ventilation withdrawal in the home setting, recommends a trial disconnection before the actual withdrawal of ventilation, to provide feedback to the patient and reduce fear;[37] this trial disconnection is performed by a physician and terminated before the patient becomes apneic or has a respiratory arrest.

SUMMARY

Respiratory failure, directly or indirectly, causes death in most patients with ALS. The decline in pulmonary function is generally linear over the course of the disease but tends to accelerate just before death. In a few patients, respiratory failure is the presenting symptom of ALS. Patients who choose mechanical ventilation can live beyond the point of respiratory failure; the natural history of this group has not been clearly delineated, but some patients eventually lose all voluntary movement, including that of the extraocular muscles, and become totally "locked in."

Respiratory failure in ALS is purely mechanical, with patients developing restrictive lung disease. Vital capacity is lowest in the supine position because the diaphragm is generally weakened more than the abdominal and intercostal muscles. Occasionally, patients develop obstructive respiratory problems because of hypopharyngeal collapse. Lung volume abnormalities include a decrease in FVC and increase in residual volume with a normal FEV_1/FVC ratio. Maximum inspiratory pressure, maximum expiratory pressure, and maximum ventilatory volume are abnormal even before the FVC drops. Blood gas levels usually remain normal until the FVC is less than 20% of predicted values, so blood gas measurements will not reveal respiratory failure. Patients often do not have any signs or symptoms of respiratory failure until the FVC is less than 50% of predicted values. The earliest symptoms often occur at night and impair sleep. Pulmonary function can be monitored in the office with regular FVC measurements and possibly peak flow measurements, once a more complete initial evaluation has been performed.

Managing respiratory failure encompasses both preventive measures and the provision of mechanical ventilatory support. Attention must be given to the prevention of aspiration and infection, aggressive management of secretions, and the judicious use of medications. Patients may be offered both negative- and positive-pressure noninvasive ventilatory support when they begin to experience signs or symptoms of nocturnal hypoventilation. If they wish to continue ventilatory support, most ALS patients using noninvasive ventilatory support will eventually require a tracheostomy because of bulbar dysfunction.

Less than 5% of ALS patients choose home mechanical ventilation. It is costly and requires supportive caregivers. The physical and emotional strain on family members can be great. However, patients who have chosen home mechanical ventilation are, for the most part, satisfied with their choice and with their quality of life. One reason that few patients elect home mechanical ventilation may be inadequate patient and family education concerning ventilatory support. Able-bodied physicians are unable to assess the quality of life of ventilator-dependent individuals accurately and should attempt to present information concerning ventilatory support in as neutral a manner as possible. Each patient with ALS deserves the right to make his or her own informed decision about respiratory support. Patients and physicians must also realize that no decision is permanent: withdrawal of the competent patient with ALS from ventilatory support is both ethical and legal.

REFERENCES

1. Bach, JR: Pulmonary rehabilitation: The obstructive and paralytic conditions. Hanley and Belfus, Philadelphia, 1995.
2. Bach, JR: Amyotrophic lateral sclerosis: Predictors for prolongation of life by noninvasive respiratory aids. Arch Phys Med Rehabil 76:828–832, 1995.
3. Bach, JR: Respiratory muscle aids for the prevention of pulmonary morbidity and mortality. Semin Neurol 15:72–83, 1995.
4. Bach, JR: Amyotrophic lateral sclerosis: Communication status and survival with ventilatory support. Am J Phys Med Rehabil 72:343–349, 1993.
5. Bach, JR: Ventilator use by Muscular Dystrophy Association patients. Arch Phys Med Rehabil 73:179–183, 1992.
6. Bach, JR: Pulmonary rehabilitation considerations for Duchenne muscular dystrophy: Prolongation of life by respiratory muscle aids. Critical Reviews in Physical Medicine and Rehabilitation 3:239–269, 1992.
7. Bach, JR: Perspectives, indications, and the ethics of prolonging "meaningful life" for individuals with progressive neuromuscular disease. Journal of Neurologic Rehabilitation 6:61–66, 1992.
8. Berger, AJ: Control of breathing. In Murray, JF and Nadel, JA (eds): Textbook of Respiratory Medicine. WB Saunders, Philadelphia, 1994, pp 199–210.
9. Black, LF and Hyatt RE: Maximal static respiratory pressures in generalized neuromuscular disease. American Review of Respiratory Disease 103:641–649, 1971.
10. Braun, NMT and Rochester, DF: Muscular weakness and respiratory failure. American Review of Respiratory Disease 119:123–125, 1979.
11. Braun, SR: Respiratory system in amyotrophic lateral sclerosis. Neurol Clin 5:9–31, 1987.
12. Carter, GT, Johnson, ER, Bonekat, HW, et al: Laryngeal diversion in the treatment of intractable aspiration in motor neuron disease. Arch Phys Med Rehabil 73:680–682, 1992.
13. Corrado, A, Gorini, M, and DePaola, E: Alternative techniques for managing acute neuromuscular respiratory failure. Semin Neurol 15:84–89, 1995.
14. Data from American Thoracic Society: Evaluation of impairment/disability secondary to respiratory disorders. American Review of Respiratory Disease 133:1205–1209, 1986.
15. Epstein, SK: An overview of respiratory muscle function. Clin Chest Med 15:619–639, 1994.
16. Fallat, RJ, Jewitt, B, Bass, M, et al: Spirometry in amyotrophic lateral sclerosis. Arch Neurol 36:74–80, 1979.
17. Farrell, AM and Obert-Thorn, ME: The amyotrophic lateral sclerosis client and the issues surrounding mechanical ventilation. Holistic Nurse Practitioner 7:1–7, 1993.
18. Fromm, GB, Wisdom, PJ, and Block, AJ: Amyo-
19. Gay, PC, Westbrook, PR, Daube, JR, et al: Effects of alterations in pulmonary function and sleep variables on survival in patients with amyotrophic lateral sclerosis. Mayo Clin Proc 66:686–694, 1988.
20. Gay, PC and Edmonds, LC: Severe hypercapnia after low flow oxygen therapy in patients with neuromuscular disease and diaphragmatic dysfunction. Mayo Clin Proc 70:327–330, 1995.
21. Gill, TM and Feinstein, AR: A critical appraisal of the quality of quality-of-life measurements. JAMA 272:619–626, 1994.
22. Goldblatt, D: A life-enhancing condition: The Honorable Mr. Justice Sam N. Filer. Semin Neurol 13:375–379, 1993.
23. Goldblatt, D and Greenlaw, J: Starting and stopping the ventilator for patients with amyotrophic lateral sclerosis. Neurol Clin 7:789–806, 1989.
24. Goldblatt D: Caring for patients with amyotrophic lateral sclerosis. In Smith, RA (ed): Handbook of ALS. Marcel Dekker, New York, 1994, pp 271–288.
25. Griggs, RC, Donohoe, KM, Utell, MJ, et al: Evaluation of pulmonary function in neuromuscular disease. Arch Neurol 38:9–12, 1981.
26. Gross, D and Meiner, Z: The effect of ventilatory muscle training in respiratory function and capacity in ambulatory and bed-ridden patients with neuromuscular disease. Monaldi Arch Chest Dis 48:322–326, 1993.
27. Hayashi, H, Kato, S, Kawada, T, et al: Amyotrophic lateral sclerosis: Oculomotor function in patients on respirators. Neurology 37:1431–1432, 1987.
28. Hayashi, H and Kato, S: Total manifestations of amyotrophic lateral sclerosis: ALS in the totally locked-in state. J Neurol Sci 93:19–35, 1989.
29. Hayashi, H, Kato, S, and Kawada, A: Amyotrophic lateral sclerosis patients living beyond respiratory failure. J Neurol Sci 105:73–78, 1991.
30. Hayashi, H: Long-term in-hospital ventilatory care for patients with amyotrophic lateral sclerosis. In Mitsumoto, H and Norris, FH (eds): Amyotrophic Lateral Sclerosis: A Comprehensive Guide to Management. Demos, New York, 1994, pp 127–138.
31. Hill, R, Martin, J, and Hakim, A: Acute respiratory failure in motor neuron disease. Arch Neurol 40:30–32, 1983.
32. Hillel, AD and Miller, R: Bulbar amyotrophic lateral sclerosis: Patterns of progression and clinical management. Head Neck 11:51–59, 1989.
33. Hotes, LS, Johnson, JA, and Sicilian, L: Long-term care, rehabilitation, and legal and ethical considerations in the management of neuromuscular disease with respiratory dysfunction. Clin Chest Med 15:783–795, 1994.
34. Johnson, MA, Woodcock, AA, and Geddes, DM: Dihydrocodeine for breathlessness in "pink puffers." Br Med J 286:675–677, 1983.
35. Kaplan, LM and Hollander, D: Respiratory dysfunction in amyotrophic lateral sclerosis. Clin Chest Med 15:675–681, 1994.
36. Kreitzer, SM, Saunders, NA, Tyler, HR, et al: Respiratory muscle function in amyotrophic lateral sclerosis. American Review of Respiratory Disease 117:437–447, 1978.
37. Libby, BL: ALS nursing care management: State

of the art. In Mitsumoto, H and Norris, FH (eds): Amyotrophic Lateral Sclerosis: A Comprehensive Guide to Management. Demos, New York, 1994, pp 183–196.

38. Manning, HL and Schwartzstein, RM: Pathophysiology of dyspnea. N Engl J Med 333:1547–1552, 1995.
39. Meyrignac, C, Poirier, J, and Degos, JD: Amyotrophic lateral sclerosis presenting with respiratory insufficiency as the primary complaint. Eur Neurol 24:115–120, 1985.
40. Moss, AH, Oppenheimer, EA, Cazzolli, PA, et al: Advance directives, quality of life, and cost of long-term mechanical ventilation for patients with amyotrophic lateral sclerosis. Paper presented at the ALS Association National Conference, Current Concepts in ALS, Philadelphia, August, 1994.
41. Moss, AH, Casey, P, Stocking, CB, et al: Home ventilation for amyotrophic lateral sclerosis patients: Outcomes, costs, and patient, family, and physician attitudes. Neurology 43:438–443, 1993.
42. Munsat, TL, Andres, PL, Finison, L, et al: The natural history of motoneuron loss in amyotrophic lateral sclerosis. Neurology 38:409–413, 1988.
43. Murphy, P: Helping Joanne die with dignity: A nursing profile in courage. Nursing 20:45–49, 1990.
44. Nakano, KK, Bass, H, Tyler, HR, et al: Amyotrophic lateral sclerosis: A study of pulmonary function. Diseases of the Nervous System 37:32–35, 1976.
45. Oppenheimer, EA: Respiratory management and home mechanical ventilation in amyotrophic lateral sclerosis. In Mitsumoto, H and Norris, FH (eds): Amyotrophic Lateral Sclerosis: A Comprehensive Guide to Management. Demos, New York, 1994, pp 139–166.
46. Oppenheimer, EA: Decision-making in the respiratory care of amyotrophic lateral sclerosis: Should home mechanical ventilation be used? Palliat Med 7(suppl 2):49–64, 1993.
47. Oppenheimer, EA, Baldwin-Myers, AS, Fuller, JA, et al: Ventilator use by patients with amyotrophic lateral sclerosis, 1985–1992, in the Kaiser Permanente home care program in California. Abstract present-

ed at the Fourth International Conference on Home Mechanical Ventilation, Lyon, France, March, 1993.
48. Parhad, IM, Clark, AW, Barron, KD, et al: Diaphragmatic paralysis in motor neuron disease. Neurology 28:18–22, 1978.
49. Ringel, SP, Murphy, JR, Alderson, MK, et al: The natural history of amyotrophic lateral sclerosis. Neurology 43:1316–1322, 1993.
50. Robbins, J, Scanlan, K, and Brooks, BR: Recumbent apnea in amyotrophic lateral sclerosis patients caused by mesopharyngeal closure due to epiglottic obstruction [abstract]. Neurology 38(suppl 1):425, 1988.
51. Saunders, NA and Kreitzer, SM: Diaphragmatic function in amyotrophic lateral sclerosis. American Review of Respiratory Disease 119:127–130, 1979.
52. Schiffman, PL and Belsh, JM: Pulmonary function at diagnosis of amyotrophic lateral sclerosis. Chest 103:508–513, 1993.
53. Schiffman, PL and Belsh, JM: Effect of inspiratory resistance and theophylline on respiratory muscle strength in patients with amyotrophic lateral sclerosis. American Review of Respiratory Disease 139:1418–1423, 1989.
54. Sherman, MS and Paz, HL: Review of respiratory care of the patient with amyotrophic lateral sclerosis. Respiration 61:61–67, 1994.
55. Silverstein, MD, Stocking, CB, Antel, JP, et al: Amyotrophic lateral sclerosis and life-sustaining therapy: Patient's desires for information, participation in decision making, and life-sustaining therapy. Mayo Clin Proc 66:906–913, 1991.
56. Sivak, ED, Gipson, WT, and Hanson, M: Long-term management of respiratory failure in amyotrophic lateral sclerosis. Ann Neurol 12:18–23, 1982.
57. Splaingard, ML, Hutchins, B, Sulton, LD, et al: Aspiration in rehabilitation patients: Videofluoroscopy vs. bedside clinical assessment. Arch Phys Med Rehabil 69:637–640, 1988.
58. West, JB: Respiratory Physiology—The Essentials, ed 4. Williams & Wilkins, Baltimore, 1987, pp 116–118.

CHAPTER 23

SPEECH AND COMMUNICATION MANAGEMENT

"Communication of our feelings, needs, and intentions is the essence of being human. Now, imagine if you could no longer communicate through neither the spoken nor the written word . . . For the most neurologically impaired individuals, this is a devastating and frustrating reality."

—**Communication Independence for the Neurologically Impaired, Inc., 1994.**

MOTOR CONTROL IN NORMAL SPEECH
Lower Brainstem Nuclear Control
Neuromuscular Control of Speech
SPEECH ABNORMALITIES IN ALS
Pathophysiology of Dysarthria in ALS
Pathology of Dysarthria in ALS
Clinical Features of Dysarthria in ALS
ASSESSING DYSARTHRIA IN ALS
The Initial Evaluation
Ongoing Evaluation
Evaluating the Oral Mechanism
MANAGING DYSARTHRIA IN ALS
A Six-Step Approach
Orofacial Exercises
Augmentative and Alternative
   Communication Intervention

In ALS, speech is affected in most patients at some stage of the disease. Progressive dysfunction of the muscles of the face, throat, and neck—the so-called lower cranial nerve–innervated muscles—causes an increasing degree of speech abnormality (dysarthria). In some patients, this dysfunction can progress to a complete inability to speak (anarthria). Dysarthria results when the motor control of speech is disturbed, and it differs from disorders of language (dysphasias) or of speech sequencing and construction (apraxias). As defined by Darley et al.,[10] dysarthria is speech dysfunction resulting from paralysis, weakness, or incoordination of the speech musculature that is neurologic in origin.

For the patient with ALS who is experiencing speech and communication difficulties and is not prepared both psychologically and functionally to adapt, dysarthria or anarthria can be emotionally and socially devastating. Because the speech dysfunction is usually accompanied by progressive difficulties in swallowing (dysphagia), these additional symptoms further contribute to patient discomfort and frustration. Evaluation and management of dysphagia and nutrition are presented in Chapter 24.

Before discussing the management of speech and communication dysfunction in patients with ALS in this chapter, we review the pertinent neuroanatomy and physiology

405

of normal speech, as well as the pathophysiology and clinical characteristics of dysarthria in ALS. The approaches we discuss for evaluating and managing dysarthria primarily represent our approach to the ALS patients we treat. Presently, the treatment of speech dysfunction in ALS is symptomatic and compensatory in nature. Nonetheless, improving communicative abilities in ALS has a significant impact on overall disease management, patient comfort, and quality of life.

MOTOR CONTROL IN NORMAL SPEECH

"We cannot state exactly the number of muscles that are necessary for speech and that are active during speech. But if we consider that ordinarily the muscles of the thoracic and abdominal walls, the neck and the face, the larynx, and pharynx and the oral cavity are all properly coordinated during the act of speaking, it becomes obvious that over 100 muscles must be controlled centrally."

—Eric H. Lenneberg, Biological Foundations of Language, 1967.

Normal speech is a complex and precisely executed action requiring split-second motor control of facial, nasopharyngeal, and oropharyngeal muscles by specific cortical, subcortical, cerebellar, and brainstem centers. Feedback sensory information from muscle activity and the sounds produced constantly influence this motor activity. All these intricate sensorimotor actions are performed almost automatically and without conscious effort until something perturbs normal function. In ALS, speech dysfunction results from pathology of motor neurons in both the cortical (upper motor neuron) and brainstem (lower motor neuron) control centers; sensory feedback function is unaffected.

The muscles used in speech (and swallowing) are innervated by five cranial nerves. Three arise in the medulla oblongata: hypoglossal (cranial nerve XII), vagal (X), and glossopharyngeal (IX), and two arise in the pons: facial (VII), and the trigeminal motor nerve (V). Because the medulla was originally referred to as the "bulb" (from the Latin, *bulbus*), the medullary nuclei giving rise to

the three lower cranial motor nerves are known as the *bulbar nuclei* and the muscles they innervate are termed the *bulbar muscles*. This is the reason patients with ALS who have dysarthria or dysphagia are said to have bulbar symptoms. This is not to say that pathology is only present in brainstem nuclei or begins there, but rather that the functional impairment is bulbar.

Lower Brainstem Nuclear Control

Nuclear origins of the brainstem nerves innervating the muscles of the face, mouth, and throat involved in speech are listed in Table 23–1. All these lower brainstem nuclei are under the control of several cortical areas, in particular the primary motor cortex, where speech is initiated; this control is effected via the corticobulbar tract[5] (Fig. 23–1).

Hypoglossal (XII) nerve fibers, arising from motor neurons in the hypoglossal nucleus of the lower medulla, innervate the nine paired intrinsic and extrinsic muscles of the tongue (see Table 23–1). Normal function of these muscles is essential not only for speech but also for chewing and swallowing. Normal tongue movement and control are essential to form all labial (e.g., "l") and fricative (e.g., "t") consonants.

The glossopharyngeal (IX) and vagal (X) nerves are closely related anatomically and functionally. They arise from the ambiguus nucleus in the reticular formation of the mid medulla to innervate the voluntary muscles of the pharynx (including the soft palate), larynx, and upper esophagus. Each nerve probably differentially innervates the pharyngeal muscles (see Table 23–1). One of these muscles, the levator palati, is essential for velopharyngeal closure to prevent nasal speech and nasal regurgitation of liquids during swallowing. Descending corticobulbar tract input onto the neurons of the ambiguus nucleus is not direct but occurs via interneurons.

The facial (VII) nucleus lies just rostral to the nucleus ambiguus in the lower pons near the pontomedullary junction and sends motor fibers to the muscles controlling facial expression and eye and mouth closure, among other functions (see Table 23–1). Not only is

Table 23–1. **LOWER CRANIAL NERVES INNERVATING
THE BULBAR MUSCLES[5]**

Cranial Nerve	Brainstem Origin	Muscles Innervated	Functions
Hypoglossal (XII)	Hypoglossal nucleus (lower medulla)	Intrinsic tongue: Inferior longitudinal, superior longitudinal, transverse, and vertical	Alters tongue shape
		Extrinsic tongue: Genioglossus, chondroglossus, hyoglossus, palatoglossus, styloglossus	Controls tongue movement
Vagal (X)	Ambiguus nucleus (lower medulla)	X: Soft palate (levator palati, tensor palati), laryngeal and upper esophagus	Velopharyngeal closure (levator palati) Vocal cord control
Glossopharyngeal (IX)	Ambiguus nucleus (mid medulla)	IX: Pharyngeal	Vocal cord control
Facial (VII)	Facial nucleus (lower pons)	Orbicularis oris, orbicularis oculi, buccinator, zygomaticus, frontalis, occipitalis	Facial expression, eye and mouth closure
		Levator palati, stylohyoid, posterior belly of digastric, platysma	Velopharyngeal closure (levator palati)
Motor trigeminal (V)	Trigeminal nucleus (mid pons)	Masseter, temporalis, internal and external pterygoids	Mastication
		Tensor palati, mylohyoid, anterior belly of digastric	

lip movement and control essential to normal speech production, but facial expression also plays an important nonverbal role in communication.

The motor component of the trigeminal (V) nucleus is situated in the mid pons and primarily innervates muscles controlling mouth opening and closure. As such, it is critical to both speech and chewing. Nerve fibers to the tensor palati influence soft palate position and tone, which are important in adjusting the internal shape of the upper oropharynx (see Table 23–1).

Neuromuscular Control of Speech

Better understanding of the motor control of normal speech has improved the evaluation and treatment of speech dysfunction. Netsell[21] has discussed speech motor control at length, and three important concepts are summarized here in relation to ALS.

Generation of meaningful sounds requires forming precise vocal tract shapes at exact points in time, so-called spatial-temporal goals. For example, to produce the sound [pa], as in "papa," the [p] sound occurs when

there is a coordinated, rapid opening of the velopharynx and glottis before lip release, all occurring within 100 ms. Subsequently, the glottis must quickly close again to produce the [a] sound. Weakness or abnormal tone (e.g., spasticity or flaccidity) in the muscles of these structures, as occurs in ALS, will compromise these spatial-temporal goals and result in dysarthria.

Motor equivalence refers to attaining the same spatial-temporal goal through a variety of other motor actions, a type of redundancy in the vocal mechanism. The initial lip closure needed to produce the [p] sound of [pa], discussed above, can also be accomplished by a number of movements of the upper lip, lower lip, and jaw. In another example, the tongue, lips, and lower jaw are involved in forming the sound [i]. Experiments in healthy individuals showed that when jaw movement was prevented (with a bite block), the tongue compensated by automatically changing position and shape to form the appropriate vocal tract shape and same [i] sound as before jaw immobilization. Such compensation explains how speech can sound normal in patients with ALS who have relatively advanced bulbar dysfunction.[12]

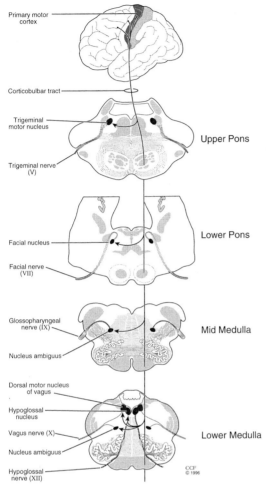

Primary motor
cortex

Corticobulbar tract

Trigeminal
motor nucleus

Upper Pons

Trigeminal nerve
(V)

Facial nucleus

Lower Pons

Facial nerve
(VII)

Glossopharyngeal
nerve (IX)

Mid Medulla

Nucleus ambiguus

Dorsal motor nucleus
of vagus

Hypoglossal
nucleus

Vagus nerve (X)

Lower Medulla

Nucleus ambiguus

Hypoglossal
nerve (XII)

CCF
© 1996

Figure 23–1. The descending corticobulbar motor pathway. Upper motor neurons in the primary motor cortex project along the corticobulbar tracts onto lower motor neurons in the motor trigeminal nucleus, facial nucleus, nucleus ambiguus, dorsal vagal motor nucleus, and hypoglossal nucleus. The motor neurons of these cranial nerve nuclei innervate the muscles of the jaw, face, pharynx, larynx, and tongue. Degeneration of these nuclei in ALS results in speech (and swallowing) dysfunction. (Copyright © 1996 The Cleveland Clinic Foundation.)

Afferent influences coordinate the timing of muscle contraction and vocal tract shape changes through complex feedback and feedforward mechanisms.[1] The feedback system returns information on muscle movement and position to the neural structures controlling the action, whereas the feedforward system relays such information to other vocal tract structures to achieve the spatial-temporal goal. Abbs and Cole[1] hypothesize

that these systems can make adjustments and regulate movements within milliseconds of performing them. Although sensory functions remain generally intact in ALS and do not affect feedback mechanisms, motor degeneration disrupts the efferent feedforward system and compromises the nearly instantaneous control that motor neurons normally exert over muscle activity of the vocal tract during speech.

SPEECH ABNORMALITIES IN ALS

Pathophysiology of Dysarthria in ALS

Bulbar dysfunction causing dysarthria in patients with ALS is usually the result of pathology in both upper motor neuron (motor cortex) and lower motor neuron (lower brainstem nuclei) centers controlling muscles of the face, tongue, and throat. In ALS, the lesion can be situated anywhere along the descending corticobulbar motor pathway: the primary motor cortex, descending axonal pathways (corticobulbar tracts) through which motor axons project, and the lower motor neurons in cranial nerve nuclei V, VII, IX, X, and XII of the pons and medulla (see Fig. 23–1). However, involvement of either the upper or lower motor neuron regions may predominate at any stage of the disease, resulting in characteristic clinical features.

Predominant degeneration of motor neurons in the cortical motor areas and their corticobulbar projections produces the clinical features of upper motor neuron dysfunction—spasticity and weakness of bulbar muscles. When the upper motor neuron pathology is bilateral, as is usually the case in ALS, bulbar dysfunction may appear to be a result of pathology in the brainstem nuclei themselves and has therefore been termed *pseudobulbar*. These characteristics of upper motor neuron dysfunction in ALS have been discussed in detail in Chapter 4. A characteristic spastic dysarthria results when bulbar dysfunction is caused primarily by an upper motor neuron lesion.

Motor neuron degeneration in nuclei of the medulla or pons (the neurons and their axons) results in denervation of muscles of the face, oropharynx, nasopharynx, and tongue. Clinically, this denervation manifests as fasciculations, weakness, and atrophy of these muscles, all characteristics of lower motor neuron involvement in ALS (see Chapter 4). A predominantly lower motor neuron lesion that causes loss of strength and tone in these muscles will result in flaccid dysarthria.

Pathology of Dysarthria in ALS

Muscles of the tongue (lingual), soft palate (velar), lips (labial), and jaw (masticatory) are affected to varying degrees. The severity may, in part, depend on the disease stage, although both pathologic and pathophysiologic evidence suggests differential involvement of cranial motor nuclei XII, IX, X, VII, and V, in that order of severity.

Several studies have found that cranial nerve nucleus XII is the most frequently affected and cranial nerve motor nucleus V the least frequently affected. For example, of 53 patients studied clinically and anatomically, Lawyer and Netsky[17] found that 94% had pathologic changes in the hypoglossal nucleus, whereas only 8% had trigeminal motor nucleus involvement. Quantitative measurements of lip, mandible, and tongue function performed by DePaul et al.[12] in 25 men with ALS revealed the greatest dysfunction in hypoglossal motor neurons. Tongue weakness was detected not only in patients with only bulbar ALS but also in those with only limb muscle symptoms and no discernible dysarthria. Pathologic changes in the nucleus ambiguus and dorsal motor nucleus of the vagus were second in frequency only to those detected in the hypoglossal nucleus, occurring in 81% of the 53 ALS patients studied by Lawyer and Netsky.[17]

A magnetic resonance imaging study of 16 patients with ALS by Cha and Patten[8] also revealed tongue abnormalities. Compared to 20 control individuals, the tongues of all the patients were 30% smaller, more rectangular, and situated more posteriorly and ventrally in the oral cavity. In addition, the internal structure showed an abnormal loss of the radial, curvilinear bands of the intrinsic tongue muscles. Based on clinical findings in the patients, the authors interpreted all the changes to be the result of lower motor neuron degeneration except for the change in tongue position. The tongue abnormalities seen with magnetic resonance imaging were more frequent and more severe than had been suspected clinically.

Clinical Features of Dysarthria in ALS

Dysarthria can be the presenting problem in up to 35% of patients with ALS,[6,17,19,24] particularly in those with bulbar-onset ALS. Reviewing the clinical features of 441 patients with ALS, Carpenter et al.[6] found that 28% presented with head and neck symptoms and 82% had speech difficulties. Most patients (67%) had symptoms and signs of tongue weakness. Another study of 272 patients with ALS revealed that 76% had some orofacial muscle dysfunction, including dysarthria and dysphagia.[15] Carrow et al.[7] found that 83% of patients with moderate to severe loss of intelligible speech had dysphagia and tongue atrophy. Pulmonary function and dyspnea played little or no role in the loss of intelligibility.[7]

At any one time, more than 50% of patients experience bulbar dysfunction,[22] and at death, as many as 75% will be either severely dysarthria or anarthric, as found in a retrospective study of 100 hospice patients with ALS.[25] In our experience, nearly all patients will develop some degree of dysarthria during the course of their illness.

TYPES OF DYSARTHRIA IN ALS

Depending on the degree of involvement of the upper and lower motor neuron components that control speech, dysarthria in ALS can be of three types: *spastic* or *pseudobulbar* (upper motor neuron involvement), *flaccid* or *bulbar* (lower motor neuron involvement), or *mixed* (combined upper and lower motor neuron involvement). Mixed dysarthria is common early in ALS and is present in almost all patients at some point during the disease.[11,13] Characteristics of the different types of dysarthria are listed in Table 23–2.

Table 23–2. CHARACTERISTICS OF THE THREE TYPES OF DYSARTHRIA IN ALS

Spastic Dysarthria	Flaccid Dysarthria	Mixed Dysarthria*
Strained-strangled quality	Nasal air emission	Prolonged intervals
Slow rate	Hypernasality	Prolonged phones
Reduced stress	Audible inspiration	
± Excess and equal stress	Abnormally short phrases	
Low pitch	Monotonous pitch and intensity	
Imprecise consonants	Diplophonia	
Vowel distortion	Wet speech	
Pitch breaks		

*Also includes some or all features of spastic and flaccid dysarthria.

Source: Based on information from Mancinelli, JM: The role of the speech-language pathologist in the diagnosis and treatment of the ALS patient. Syllabus from Toward Effective Management of ALS: The Team Approach, May 30–June 2, 1991, The Cleveland Clinic Foundation, p. 54.

STAGES OF SPEECH DYSFUNCTION IN ALS

The severity of dysarthria can extend from mild articulation difficulties to anarthria. Hillel et al.[16] have outlined 10 stages of speech dysfunction in ALS, ranging from no abnormality (high score) to complete loss of speech (low score) (Table 23–3). In our experience, not all stages will be experienced by any one patient, and some stages may be skipped. It is essential that counseling to maintain effective communication be initiated as early as possible, preferably when speech abnormalities are first perceived.

ASSESSING DYSARTHRIA IN ALS

We encourage early and comprehensive assessment of speech and communication dysfunction in patients with ALS. Assessment is best accomplished by an expert in speech-language function and evaluation, such as a speech-language pathologist. However, because ALS is a relatively rare disorder, speech-language pathologists may have limited experience in evaluating and managing patients with this disease. Consequently, all caregivers, including physicians, need to become better educated in identifying and managing the problems of speech dysfunction in ALS.

In our ALS clinic, the speech-language pathologist works closely with the neurologist and other members of the team (nutritionist, physical therapist, occupational therapist, and social worker) to help the patient to maintain independent communication for as long as possible. The speech-language pathologist has several roles in this regard, including determining the type and extent of neuromuscular weakness, evaluating the patient's ability to communicate effectively, educating the patient and caregiver in alternative and augmentative means of communication, and counseling the patient and caregiver concerning disruptions of personal and family life brought on by the communication difficulties. It must be remembered that the caregivers—especially family members—are instrumental to the successful management of patients with ALS, particularly in the area of speech dysfunction.

The Initial Evaluation

In our ALS clinic, the speech-language pathologist and nutritionist evaluate the patient together because bulbar muscle dysfunction usually affects both speech and swallowing. This approach minimizes duplication of the interview process, lessens the likelihood that the patient will receive conflicting information, and allows immediate coordination of an individualized program for each patient. During the joint interview, a speech-language pathologist familiar with

Table 23–3. **STAGES OF SPEECH DYSFUNCTION IN ALS**

Stage	Symptoms	Signs
10. Normal speech	None	None
9. Nominal abnormality	Noticed only by patient or close caregiver	Normal rate and volume
8. Perceived changes	Noticed by others, especially when patient is fatigued or stressed	Rate essentially normal
7. Obvious abnormalities	Consistent impairment but easily understood	Rate, articulation, and resonance affected
6. Repeats messages on occasion	Specific words must be repeated in adverse listening situations, but complexity or length of message not limited	Rate much slower than normal
5. Frequent repeating required	Extensive repetition or "translator" needed and complexity or length of message probably limited	Speech slow and labored
4. Speech plus augmentative communication	Speech only for responding to questions	Writing or spokesperson required to resolve intelligibility problems
3. Limits speech to one-word response	One-word responses other than yes/no	Initiates communication nonverbally
2. Vocalizes for emotional expression only	Vocal inflection to express emotion, affirmation, and negation	
1. Nonvocal	Vocalization is an effort, limited in duration, and rarely attempted	May vocalize to cry or express pain

Source: Adapted from Hillel, AD, Miller, RM, Yorkston, KM, et al: ALS Scale. Neuroepidemiol 8:142–150, 1989.

ALS will be able to determine quickly the presence or absence of dysarthria, the type of dysarthria, natural compensations made, the patient's communication style and its effectiveness, and the degree to which caregivers are involved in communication functions. Furthermore, the assessment and extent of evaluation will depend on the type of communication disorder; the time available for assessment; the patient's level of understanding, cooperation, and tolerance; and the goals of the patient and family.

Discretion and sensitivity on the part of the speech-language pathologist are paramount in evaluating and managing patients with dysarthria. It is important not to overwhelm the patient and caregiver with too much information or too many details, especially at the first visit. However, because ALS is progressive, addressing communication problems is an urgent matter, and the speech-language pathologist should begin the individualized program as soon as the patient and caregivers accept the reality of bulbar dysfunction. Denial of bulbar difficulties (or even the disease itself) significantly limits the effectiveness of speech management and may result in undue stress to the patient and all concerned when appropriate adaptive steps have not been taken early in the disease. A frank and tactful discussion of the patient's bulbar dysfunction, emphasizing methods of maximizing remaining communicative function (see below) helps the patient with ALS to overcome the fear of being unable to express needs and desires.

Ongoing Evaluation

Unlike static conditions such as strokes or more slowly evolving neurodegenerative diseases such as multiple sclerosis or Parkinson's disease, the motor dysfunction in ALS is progressive, so the evaluation and management of dysarthria in ALS is ongoing. The communication needs of the patient will change as the disease progresses, and it is essential that patient and caregiver be prepared for such changes with appropriate education. Therefore, continued follow-up care after the initial evaluation is of paramount importance. The frequency of this re-evaluation must be individualized because the course of ALS is unpredictable and unique to each patient. In our experience, quarterly reassessment of the patient's communicative abilities is usually reasonable. The management approaches can be adjusted as ability levels decline.

Ideally, the speech-language pathologist provides the follow-up care, preferably in the ALS clinic or other outpatient facility. If the patient is unable to travel outside the home and the speech-language pathologist is unable to travel to the patient's home, home-care providers can be trained in the basic principles of dysarthria management.

Evaluating the Oral Mechanism

ELEMENTS OF SPEECH

Several factors influence the intelligibility of speech, including rate, voice quality, articulation, and phrase groupings. However, intelligibility is very difficult to assess because nonverbal factors such as facial expression, emotion, and intonation may enhance functional intelligibility even when intelligibility of single words or sentences is poor. Various vocal characteristics and their components that are assessed include vocal quality, pitch, prosody, intensity, and resonance (Table 23–4).

For the purpose of evaluating dysarthria, the upper airway can be divided into three functional regions: articulatory (lips, tongue, mandible), velopharyngeal (palate, pharynx), and phonatory (larynx).

To evaluate articulatory ability, labial strength and mobility are assessed by the patient's ability to retract quickly (smile) and protrude quickly (pucker) during a 5-second period. Lingual protrusion, lateral movement, elevation, and depression in a 5-second period are also tested. Consonants that are formed by firm contact between the lips and the tongue and hard palate are particularly important to test; these include plosives such as "p," "t," and "k," and fricatives such as "f" and "s." Vocalization of the sounds "puh," "tuh," "kuh," singly and in rapid succession, is useful in testing both labial and lingual functions. Weakness of the lip muscles (e.g., orbicularis oris) is important (probably as significant as lingual weakness) in causing dysarthria.

In the velopharyngeal region, opening and closing of the passage between the oropharynx and nasopharynx (or valving) is assessed by diadochokinesis (sequential alternating movement) testing. The patient vocalizes "ah," at first in a sustained and then in a rapidly repetitive fashion. This maneuver will accentuate hypernasality and nasal emission of air caused by velopharyngeal weak-

Table 23–4. **VOCAL CHARACTERISTICS EVALUATED IN ALS**

Vocal Component	Features or Characteristics
Quality	Harsh, hoarse, strained or strangled, breathy
Pitch	Habitual or fundamental frequency Range
Prosody	Excess and equal stress (inappropriate stress on monosyllabic words and the usually unstressed syllables of polysyllabic words) Insufficient stress
Intensity	Diminished (hypophonic)
Resonance	Hypernasality or nasal air emission Palatal movement

ness and flaccidity. The soft palate normally elevates during vocalization of "ah" to effect velopharyngeal closure. Such palatal mobility is compromised by lesions in ALS affecting the upper or lower motor neurons.

Hoarseness, a phonation problem, commonly results from laryngeal weakness in ALS. Flaccid weakness of laryngeal muscles causes a weak, breathy voice (hypophonia) that is monotone in pitch. In contrast, spasticity of these muscles produces a harsh, strained voice with varying pitch and loudness; these changes are caused by hyperadduction of the true vocal cords. Two other features unique to flaccid laryngeal weakness include "wet speech" and diplophonia (see Table 23–2). In the former, pooling of secretions in the tonsillar fauces at the base of the oropharynx gives the speech a gurgling quality. In the latter, two frequencies are produced simultaneously (the astute listener can detect them) because of differing rates of vibration of the true vocal cords.

ELECTROMYOGRAPHY

The needle electrode examination of selected head and neck muscles is a useful adjunct to the overall evaluation of the ALS patient with bulbar dysfunction. It is particularly useful when early dysarthria is not accompanied by clear signs of lower motor neuron degeneration such as atrophy and fasciculations. The two most helpful changes on needle electrode examination of facial or lingual muscles are loss of motor unit potentials, resulting in a rapid (neurogenic) firing pattern, and the presence of fibrillation potentials, signifying ongoing motor axon loss. However, it is difficult to assess spontaneous activity in facial and bulbar muscles (especially the tongue) because most individuals are unable to relax and suppress firing of all motor units sufficiently. These and other electromyographic features of ALS are discussed in Chapter 5.

MANAGING DYSARTHRIA IN ALS

Although speech dysfunction in ALS cannot be "cured" at present, speech therapy will minimize symptoms and alter speaking behavior so that intelligibility and communica-

tion can be optimized for as long as possible. Many of the therapeutic techniques are simple modifications of the individual's innate ability to compensate for speech dysfunction, but others involve the use of mechanical or sophisticated electronic devices.

A Six-Step Approach

In our ALS clinic, the speech-language pathologists use a sequential, six-step approach to managing communication abnormalities in patients (Table 23–5). The number of steps introduced at the initial evaluation and the rate of progress through subsequent steps varies with each ALS patient. Usually we initially introduce the patient and caregivers to concepts in at least the first two steps and proceed to subsequent steps at follow-up visits depending on the rate of speech deterioration.

Step 1. The patient is instructed in strategies to maximize intelligibility, including communicating face to face, speaking slowly, overarticulating consonants, holding onto vowels, overexaggerating facial movements, and organizing sentence structure to cue the listener to topic or key words.

Step 2. The patient is taught how to minimize effort and conserve energy to improve or prolong periods of speech production. These changes can be accomplished by using telegraphic (or monosyllabic) speech; having periods of vocal rest before meals, planned visits, telephone calls, and so forth; and using emergency alerting systems such

Table 23–5. **SIX STEPS IN MANAGING COMMUNICATIVE DYSFUNCTION IN ALS**

Step 1. Maximize intelligibility strategies
Step 2. Introduce energy-conserving techniques
Step 3. Train listener or communication partner
Step 4. Introduce multimodality approach
Step 5. Incorporate assistive and augmentative communication devices and techniques
Step 6. Complete augmentative and alternative communication evaluation

as intercoms, bells, and buzzers. Refraining from gum chewing is a simple way to minimize bulbar fatigue.

Step 3. The listener is instructed to assist in the communication process by asking the patient yes or no questions, giving the patient multiple choices, repeating the part of the sentence understood and ending with a question of what was not understood, asking for repetition, and speaking face to face.

Step 4. A multimodality approach is emphasized, which incorporates nonverbal techniques to enhance communication, including the use of gestures or sign language and writing or pointing to key words or the first letter of words.

Step 5. Assistive or augmentative communication devices are introduced, which mechanically or electronically aid intelligibility. These aids can be as simple as notebooks or magic slates for writing, alphabet boards, and picture or word charts. More complex devices include palatal lifts (a dental prosthesis that lifts the soft palate to prevent air from escaping from the nose during speech), personal amplifiers that increase speech volume, and telephone relay services that enable a patient to make a telephone call. The patient types messages on a special keyboard that are transmitted to a trained communication assistant who then verbalizes the messages to a listener.

Step 6. The patient is referred for a full augmentative and alternative communication evaluation by a speech-language pathologist. This evaluation is beneficial for all ALS patients with speech dysfunction, not only those with severe deficits. Its purpose is to instruct patients in the use of assistive communication devices, particularly electronic communication devices such as personal computers equipped with voice synthesis software. Technological advances in electronic voice synthesis are constantly improving the quality and speed of electronic communication, such as producing more realistic speech information and more accurate word prediction.

Orofacial Exercises

There is little or no evidence that bulbar muscle–strengthening exercises are beneficial for the dysarthria of ALS.[14] The progressive nature of the motor neuron degeneration precludes any lasting benefit. Further, although clinical data are lacking, there are numerous anecdotal accounts of dysarthric ALS patients experiencing fatigue and worsening symptoms after extended use of bulbar muscles. Energy conservation, as discussed above, is a key component in managing bulbar function in ALS. However, the value of exercise per se in ALS is debatable, with one side promoting no exercise except for normal daily activities that can be easily performed[26] and the other supporting vigorous daily exercise.[23]

Augmentative and Alternative Communication Intervention

Augmentative and alternative communication is "an area of clinical practice that attempts to compensate (either temporarily or permanently) for the impairment and disability of individuals with severe expressive communication disorders (i.e., the severely speech-language and writing impaired)."[2] As mentioned, communication devices vary in sophistication and complexity, ranging from simple alphabet boards to prostheses (e.g., palatal lift) to portable computer-based voice synthesizers. One or more of these devices may be appropriate for each patient with ALS, depending on his or her speech adequacy, hand function, and mobility. By grouping patients according to these three criteria, Yorkston et al.[27] have developed a useful approach to determine the augmentative communication needs in the ALS population (Table 23–6). Generally, patients with bulbar-predominant ALS develop speech impairment before hand function and mobility are significantly compromised. In contrast, those with generalized ALS have varying degrees of impaired hand function and mobility with or without speech impairment. The task of matching each ALS patient who requires speech assistance with the proper augmentative and alternative communication

Table 23–6. **SELECTION OF AUGMENTATIVE COMMUNICATION DEVICES FOR PATIENTS WITH ALS**

Speech Function	Hand Function	Mobility	Communication Device
Adequate	Adequate	Adequate	None—monitoring and provision of information
Adequate	Poor	Adequate	Alternative to handwriting (e.g., electronic keyboard)
Poor	Adequate	Adequate	Handwriting, alphabet board, attention-getting devices (e.g., buzzer); portable electronic devices (e.g., digital recorders, voice synthesizers)
Poor	Adequate	Poor	As above for electronic devices but portability not essential
Poor	Poor	Adequate	Portable augmentative devices with alternative access (e.g., switches and scanning systems)
Poor	Poor	Poor	Augmentative devices with alternative access but portability not essential

Source: Based on information from Yorkston, KM, Strand, E, Miller, R, et al: Speech deterioration in amyotrophic lateral sclerosis: Implications for the timing of intervention. J Med Speech-Language Pathol 1:35–46, 1993.

system is a challenge requiring keen observational skills, a broad knowledge of the available devices, experience, continued patient evaluation, and a sensitivity to the patient's needs and preferences. In our ALS clinic setting, the speech-language pathologist works closely with the physician, occupational therapist, and physical therapist in this evaluation process.

MECHANICAL DEVICES

Relatively simple and inexpensive mechanical means of communication include all forms of writing devices, picture communication symbols, and alphabet boards. These require adequate upper-extremity function to write or point. Patients unable to write or point can use gaze communication in the form of an eye transfer (ETRAN) board (Fig. 23–2). This device, a transparent board with engraved letters, is placed between the patient and observer. By observing which letter or number the patient's eyes are directed toward, the observer can, with practice, reliably determine the selected symbol. Not only do ETRAN boards require a skilled

observer to interpret the patient's message, but also the number of symbols and speed with which they can be communicated are limited.

Patients with hypernasality and nasal emission because of velopharyngeal weakness will occasionally benefit from a palatal lift. This mechanical device, which is inserted into the oropharynx, elevates the soft palate to occlude the nasopharynx and prevent escape of nasal air or nasal regurgitation of liquids. A hyperactive gag reflex, present in most patients with mixed dysarthria, generally limits its use to ALS patients with flaccid dysarthria, even if tactile desensitization techniques are employed.

ELECTRONIC DEVICES

Numerous electronic devices that assist and augment communication in a variety of ways are now available at a range of prices. Although computer-assisted communication does not prolong survival of patients with ALS, it substantially improves quality of life.[3] Most augmentative and alternative communication systems are dedicated devices, de-

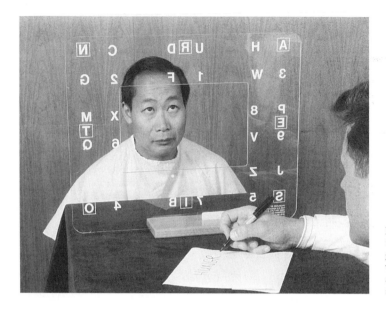

Figure 23–2. A transparent eye transfer (ETRAN) board with engraved letters is used by a patient who gazes at individual letters to spell out words identified by a skilled observer.

signed for this sole purpose. These include portable amplifiers that increase the volume of the patient's voice to improve intelligibility, digital recorders that play back prerecorded words and phrases on command, and keyboard-activated printout- or sound-producing communicators (Fig. 23–3). In addition, dedicated voice synthesizers are available in a variety of models, levels of sophistication, and price ranges. Too numerous to discuss here, a comprehensive list of portable communication devices is available from Applied Science and Engineering Laboratories (Appendix A). Most of these devices can be activated by alternate means, such as specialized switches (e.g., a switch activated by eye blink) or by visual scanning. Increasingly, speech synthesis software is becoming available for use in desktop and laptop computers. Some companies producing augmentative and alternative communication devices are listed in Appendix A.

Caregivers must provide ongoing support in the use of augmentative communication systems. This support may involve technical instruction for using the device, assistance in modifying stored or selected messages, and altering the switch type or position as the patient's motor capabilities change with disease progression.[4] A sampling of organizations for communicative assistance is listed in Appendix B.

Although augmentative and alternative communication systems are reimbursed by Medicaid and by some private insurers, availability of such equipment from a "lending bank" would be ideal. A communication systems bank would circumvent the delays experienced in obtaining these devices when waiting for approval by insurers and would make such equipment more accessible for patients who are unable to afford it. Furthermore, it would maximize the utility of the equipment by making it available to more than one patient with ALS. Patients, their families, or medical device companies could be potential donors of the communication systems. This would provide a general sense of hope and support to ALS patients experiencing speech and communication difficulties.

SUMMARY

Dysarthria occurs in most patients with ALS because of progressive weakness of face, throat, and neck muscles. Speech dysfunction causes discomfort and frustration and can be emotionally and socially devastating. Although treatment for dysarthria in ALS is only symptomatic and compensatory, improving the patient's communicative abilities

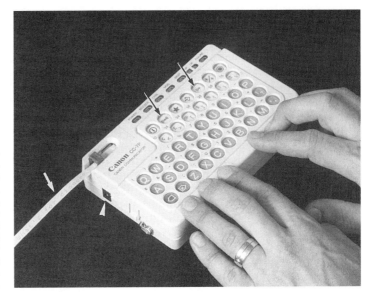

Figure 23–3. Example of a keyboard-activated communication device with a message printout (short arrow). The QWERTY keyboard can be used to type letters, words, or symbols as well as activate preprogrammed messages. Specific buttons (long arrows) are assigned for alert sounds (e.g., buzzer or beep). This lightweight portable device is powered by either a 9V battery or an AC adapter (arrowhead).

has an impact on overall disease management, patient comfort, and quality of life.

Normal speech involves precise motor control of numerous muscles by specific brain centers. The muscles of speech are innervated by cranial nerves arising from brainstem nuclei in the pons and medulla oblongata (previously called the bulb). These muscles are termed the *bulbar muscles,* and ALS patients with dysarthria are said to have *bulbar symptoms.* The brainstem nuclei, which receive input from the primary motor cortex via the corticobulbar tract, include the hypoglossal nucleus, innervating the tongue; ambiguus nucleus, innervating the pharynx and larynx via the glossopharyngeal and vagal nerves; facial nucleus, innervating the face; and motor trigeminal nucleus, innervating the mouth and soft palate. Speech dysfunction in ALS results when the motor control of bulbar muscles is disrupted because of degeneration of upper motor neurons in the cortex and lower motor neurons in the brainstem. The hypoglossal nucleus is affected most frequently and the trigeminal nucleus least frequently. Abnormal tongue size, shape, and position have been observed on magnetic resonance imaging, even when dysarthria is not advanced.

Approximately one-third of patients with ALS present with dysarthria, and over half

have bulbar dysfunction at some stage. Predominantly upper motor neuron dysfunction causes spastic dysarthria, whereas predominantly lower motor neuron dysfunction causes flaccid dysarthria. Each type has distinguishing features. A combination, or mixed, dysarthria occurs most frequently because of coexisting upper and lower motor neuron abnormalities. The severity ranges from very mild dysarthria, noticeable to only the astute listener, to anarthria, when essentially no sound can be produced.

Speech and communication dysfunction in the patient with ALS should be assessed as early as possible, preferably by a speech-language pathologist. Assessment involves evaluating the type and degree of neuromuscular weakness, introducing alternative and augmentative means of communication, and counseling the patient and caregiver concerning disruptions in personal and family life that may occur. Although the initial evaluation is important in laying the groundwork, ongoing evaluations are essential in adjusting care as the patient's needs change. It is advisable not to overwhelm the patient with too much information during the initial evaluation, but the progressive nature of the dysarthria in ALS makes initiating appropriate management an urgent matter. Dysarthria is evaluated by testing articulatory, velopharyngeal, and phonatory function. This can be done relatively quickly in a clinic or bedside setting. Electromyography of bulbar muscles is useful in establishing or confirming the presence of lower motor neuron (motor axon) degeneration in ALS patients with dysarthria.

The goal of management is to help the patient with ALS maintain independent communication for as long as possible. We use a six-step approach that includes maximizing the patient's speaking ability and conserving energy, actively involving the listener in the communication process, introducing assistive or augmentative communication devices, and fully evaluating their usefulness in appropriate cases. Numerous communication devices are available that vary in sophistication and complexity. They range from simple and relatively inexpensive mechanical devices, such as alphabet or picture boards, to specialized and more expensive electronic devices such as voice synthesizers. More patients would have access to the more expensive devices if these were available for use through lending banks.

REFERENCES

1. Abbs, J and Cole, K: Consideration of bulbar and suprabulbar afferent influences upon speech motor coordination and programming. In Grillner, S, Lindblom, B, Lubker, J, et al (eds): Speech Motor Control. Pergamon Press, New York, 1982, pp 159–186.
2. American Speech-Language-Hearing Association: Competencies for speech-language pathologists providing services in augmentative communication. ASHA 31:107–110, 1989.
3. Bach, JR: Amyotrophic lateral sclerosis. Communication status and survival with ventilatory support. Am J Phys Med Rehabil 72:343–349, 1993.
4. Beukelman, DR and Mirenda, P: Adults with acquired physical disabilities. In Augmentative and Alternative Communication. Management of Severe Communication Disorders in Children and Adults. Paul H. Brookes, Baltimore, 1992, pp 309–330.
5. Brodal, A: Neurological Anatomy in Relation to Clinical Medicine, ed 3. Oxford University Press, Oxford, 1981.
6. Carpenter, RJ III, McDonald, TJ, and Howard, FM. Jr: The otolaryngologic presentation of amyotrophic lateral sclerosis. Otorhinolaryngology 86:479–484, 1978.
7. Carrow, E, Rivera, V, Maudlin, M, et al: Deviant speech characteristics in motor neuron disease. Arch Otolaryngol–Head Neck Surg 100:212–218, 1974.
8. Cha, CH and Patten, BM: Amyotrophic lateral sclerosis: Abnormalities of the tongue on magnetic resonance imaging. Ann Neurol 25:468–472, 1989.
9. CINI: Communication Independence for the Neurologically Impaired, Inc. Publication, New York, 1994.
10. Darley, F, Aronson, A, and Brown, J: Differential diagnostic patterns of dysarthria. J Speech Hear Res 12:246–269, 1969.
11. Darley, FL, Aronson, AE, and Brown, JR: Motor Speech Disorders. WB Saunders, Philadelphia, 1975.
12. DePaul, R, Abbs, JH, Caligiuri, M, et al: Hypoglossal, trigeminal, and facial motoneuron involvement in amyotrophic lateral sclerosis. Neurology 38:281–283, 1988.
13. Dworkin, J, Aronson, A, and Mulder, D: Tongue force in normals and in dysarthric patients with amyotrophic lateral sclerosis. J Appl Speech Hear Res 23:828–837, 1980.
14. Dworkin, JP and Hartman, DE: Progressive speech deterioration and dysphagia in amyotrophic lateral sclerosis: Case report. Arch Phys Med Rehabil 60:423–425, 1979.
15. Gubbay, SS, Kahana, E, Zilber, N, et al: Amyotrophic lateral sclerosis: A study of its presentation and prognosis. J Neurol 232:295–300, 1985.
16. Hillel, AD, Miller, RM, Yorkston, KM, et al: ALS Scale. Neuroepidemiol 8:142–150, 1989.
17. Lawyer, T and Netsky, MG: Amyotrophic lateral sclerosis: A clinicoanatomic study of fifty-three cases. AMA Arch Neurol Psychiatry 69:171–192, 1953.
18. Lenneberg, EH: Biological Foundations of Language, Wiley, New York, 1967.
19. Mackay, RP: Course and prognosis in amyotrophic lateral sclerosis. Arch Neurol 8:117–127, 1963.
20. Mancinelli, JM: The role of the speech-language pathologist in the diagnosis and treatment of the ALS patient. Syllabus from Toward Effective Management of ALS: The Team Approach, May 30–June 2, 1991, The Cleveland Clinic Foundation, pp 48–62.
21. Netsell, R: A neurobiologic view of the dysarthrias. In Netsell, R: A Neurobiologic View of Speech Production and the Dysarthrias. College-Hill Press, San Diego, 1986, pp 53–88.
22. Newrick, PG and Langton Hewer, R: Motor neuron disease: Can we do better? A study of 42 patients. Br Med J 289:539–542, 1984.
23. Norris, FH, Sang, K, Denys, EH, et al: ALS [letter]. Mayo Clin Proc 53:544, 1978.
24. Rosen, AD: Amyotrophic lateral sclerosis: Clinical features and prognosis. Arch Neurol 35:638–642, 1978.
25. Saunders, C, Walsh, T, and Smith, M: Hospice care in the motor neuron diseases. A review of 100 cases of motor neuron disease. In Saunders, C, and Teller, J (eds): Hospice: The Living Idea. Edward Arnold Publishers, London, 1981, pp 126–147.
26. Sinaki, M and Mulder, DW: Rehabilitation techniques for patients with amyotrophic lateral sclerosis. Mayo Clin Proc 53:173–178, 1978.
27. Yorkston, KM, Strand, E, Miller, R, et al: Speech deterioration in amyotrophic lateral sclerosis: Implications for the timing of intervention. J Med Speech-Language Pathol 1:35–46, 1993.

APPENDIX A: SOURCES FOR COMMUNICATION DEVICES

Picture Communication Symbols and Displays

- Mayer-Johnson Co.
  P.O. Box 1579
  Solana Beach, CA 92075-1579
  Telephone: 619-550-0084
  FAX: 619-550-0449

- Innocomp
  Innovative Computer Applications
  Suite 302, 26210 Emery Road
  Warrensville Heights, OH 44128
  Telephone: 800-382-8622
  or 216-464-3636
  FAX: 216-464-3638

Portable Voice Amplifiers

- Radio Shack (local store franchise)
  Various models available, from small battery-powered to AC line-powered and wireless FM microphone systems

- Luminaud, Inc.
  8688 Tyler Blvd
  Mentor, OH 44060
  Telephone: 216-255-9082
  FAX: 216-255-2250
  Wide range of models available, from pocket-sized Rand Voice Amplifier to all-weather powerful Minivox

- Park Surgical Company, Inc.
  5001 New Utrecht Ave
  Brooklyn, NY 11219
  Telephone: 800-633-7878
  FAX: 718-854-2431
  Deluxe speech amplifier (microphone purchased separately)

- Electronic Speech Enhancement, Inc.
  1115 Ridge Road
  St. Louis, MO 63021
  Telephone: 800-600-9819
  or 314-394-0770
  FAX: 314-394-9442
  Speech Enhancer systems, separate Proximity Microphone and accessories for wheelchair or ambulatory use. Demonstration videotape available.

Telephone Communication

- Telephone Relay Services
  Available in every state and listed in directory assistance

- Hitech Group International, Inc.
  8160 Madison
  Burr Ridge, IL 60521
  Telephone: 800-433-8505
  Amplifier Telephone (for home use and business use)
  FAX: 630-654-9219

- Luminaud, Inc.
  8688 Tyler Blvd
  Mentor, OH 44060
  Telephone: 216-255-9082
  FAX: 216-255-2250
  Vocaid from Texas Instruments, a lightweight and portable, battery- or line-powered electronic communication board

Voice Synthesizers and Computer Software

- Canon USA, Inc.
  Medical Products Division
  One Canon Plaza
  Lake Success, NY 11042
  Telephone: 516-328-4628
  FAX: 516-328-4639
  Canon Communicator for printout of typed messages (CC-7P) or playback of sound recordings (CC-7S)

- Don Johnston, Inc.
  1000 N. Rand Rd, Building 115
  P.O. Box 639
  Wauconda, IL 60084-0639
  Telephone: 800-999-4660 or
  708-526-2682
  FAX: 708-526-4177
  Voice synthesis and writing software for Macintosh computer systems (e.g., Ke:nx); Alternative input devices and switches

- Innocomp
  Innovative Computer Applications
  Suite 302, 26210 Emery Road
  Warrensville Heights, OH 44128
  Telephone: 800-382-8622 or
  216-464-3636
  FAX: 216-464-3638

Say-It-All digital speech recorder and voice synthesizer
Scan-It-All text-to-speech system for visual scanning or light pointing
Gus! Multimedia Speech System computer software (for Windows/DOS computer system)
Speaking Dynamically computer software (for Macintosh computer system)
Head-mounted Baton laser light pointer with "sip-puff" on-off switch
BlinkSwitch infrared eye blink on-off switch

- Sentient Systems Technology, Inc.
2100 Wharton Street
Pittsburgh, PA 15203
Telephone: 800-344-1778
FAX: 412-381-5241
DynaVox 2 augmentative communication device or software (for Macintosh or DOS-based computer systems)
DigiVox augmentative communication device or software (for Macintosh or DOS-based computer systems)

- Technical Aids and Systems for the Handicapped (TASH), Inc.
Unit 1—91 Station Street
Ajax, Ontario L1S 3H2, Canada
Telephone: 800-463-5685
or 905-686-4129
FAX: 905-686-6895
Alternative keyboard control (WinKing or MacKing plug-ins)
Alternative mouse control (MouseMover)
Switches (Buddy Button) and mounting kits

- Zyco Industries, Inc.
P.O. Box 1008
Portland, OR 92707-1008

Telephone: 800-234-6006
or 503-684-6006
FAX: 503-684-6011
Digital voice recording (Macaw series, Parrot words)
Handheld keyboard display and speech synthesizer (LightWRITER)
Page turners and switches
Hands-free telephone access (Infra-Link speaker telephone)

APPENDIX B: ORGANIZATIONS FOR COMMUNICATIVE ASSISTANCE

- Communication Independence for the Neurologically Impaired, Inc.
250 Mercer Street, Suite B1608,
New York, NY 10012
Telephone: 516-981-3394
FAX: 516-472-9016
Internet address:
73523.151@COMPUSERVE.COM
Compuserve online address: 73523.151
Prodigy online address: XKBG36A

- Augmentative Communication, Inc.
One Surf Way, Suite 237
Monterey, CA 93940
Telephone: 408-649-3050
FAX: 408-646-5428

- Applied Science and Engineering Laboratories (ASEL)
University of Delaware/A.I. duPont Institute
1600 Rockland Road
Wilmington, DE 19899
Telephone: 302-651-6830
FAX: 302-651-6895

CHAPTER 24

NUTRITIONAL MANAGEMENT

Involvement of the brain-stem motor nuclei of cranial nerves V, VII, IX, X, and XII, the loss of upper motor neuron innervation to these nuclei, or both, inevitably leads to dysphagia, a common problem in ALS. Indeed, in 10% to 30% of patients with ALS, dysphagia is the presenting symptom, and eventually almost 100% of patients experience at least some degree of dysphagia[28]; if not managed effectively, dysphagia will lead to weight loss and malnutrition. Because normal swallowing is critical to adequate nutrition, we begin our discussion with a review of the physiology and anatomy that underlie this complex function. We then analyze the pathophysiology of swallowing in ALS and present our approach to the swallowing evaluation, which allows us to ascertain the in-

tervention most appropriate for the degree of dysphagia. As dysphagia progresses, the patient is at risk for weight loss and malnutrition; therefore, we also discuss the evaluation for suspected malnutrition, nutrition assessment techniques used to determine its severity, and approaches to maintain adequate nutrition.

NORMAL SWALLOWING

Normal swallowing is accomplished by a series of finely tuned neural and muscular events modulated through the brain-stem center that controls swallowing.[28] It can be divided into four phases: the oral preparatory, the oral, the pharyngeal, and the esophageal[28] (Table 24–1). During these four phases, the food bolus is confined to a specific pathway in the upper aerodigestive tract. It passes through anatomic structures that may be conceptualized as a series of valves that direct the bolus along the appropriate route[28,30] (Fig. 24–1).

During the voluntary oral preparatory phase, the bolus is created for swallowing: solids are masticated, food is manipulated in the mouth, and saliva is produced to form a cohesive bolus. This phase involves the coordination of lip closure, rotary and lateral jaw motion, facial muscle tone, and anterior bulging of the soft palate; this latter movement widens the nasal airway and narrows the oropharyngeal inlet, allowing breathing while chewing and reducing the possibility of premature spilling of food into the phar-

421

Table 24–1. **PHASES OF NORMAL SWALLOWING**

Phase, Type, and Duration	Event	Cranial Nerve Innervation
Oral preparatory (Voluntary)	• Bolus prepared for swallowing	V, VII, IX, X, and XII
Oral (Voluntary, 1 s)	• Bolus transported to anterior faucial arches	V, VII, IX, X, and XII
Pharyngeal (Involuntary, <0.5 s)	• Closure of soft palate against pharyngeal wall	V, IX, and X
	• Closure of the vocal cords and protection of laryngeal inlet	
	• Pharyngeal peristalsis	
	• Elevation of the larynx, and lowering of epiglottis over laryngeal inlet	
	• Relaxation of cricopharyngeus muscle	
Esophageal (Involuntary, 8 to 20 s)	• Bolus transported to stomach	X

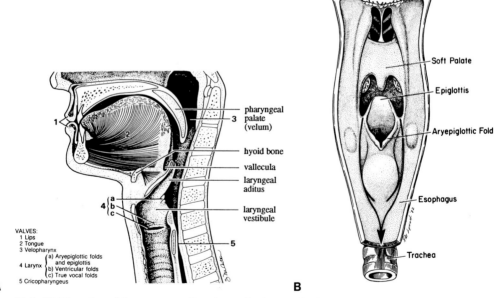

A

VALVES:
1 Lips
2 Tongue
3 Velopharynx
4 Larynx { (a) Aryepiglottic folds and epiglottis
(b) Ventricular folds
(c) True vocal folds
5 Cricopharyngeus

pharyngeal palate (velum)

hyoid bone

vallecula

laryngeal aditus

laryngeal vestibule

B

Soft Palate

Epiglottis

Aryepiglottic Fold

Esophagus

Trachea

Figure 24–1. (*A*) The valves of the upper aerodigestive swallowing mechanism (From Robbins, J: Swallowing in ALS and motor neuron disorders. Neurol Clin 5:216, 1987, with permission.) (*B*) Human larynx and pharynx viewed from behind. Note the role of the epiglottis and aryepiglottic folds in directing swallowed matter around the laryngeal inlet into the upper esophagus posteriorly. (From Sasaki, CT and Isaacson, G: Functional anatomy of the larynx. Otolaryngol Clin North Am 21:598, 1988, with permission.)

ynx.[20] Much of the pleasure from eating is derived from the oral preparatory stage.[20]

The oral phase is also voluntary and is completed in about 1 second. The tongue moves upward and backward, propelling the bolus to the anterior faucial arches where the swallow reflex is triggered (see below). During the oral phase, the nasopharynx is closed off by simultaneous constriction of the tongue, pharyngeal palate (velum), and pharyngeal walls to prevent food from escaping into the nasal passages.[4,33] The oral phase ends when the bolus arrives at the posterior tongue,[28] at which point essentially no food or liquid should remain in the mouth.[20] Receptors in the tongue base and faucial arch area, activated by tongue action and the food bolus, then send impulses carried along cranial nerves IX and X to the brain-stem reticular formation, which generates the appropriate neuromuscular response, marking the onset of the pharyngeal phase.[20]

Normal neurologic function during these first two phases of swallowing depends on the actions of cranial nerves V, VII, IX, X, and XII.[4] Cranial nerve VII, innervating the orbicularis oris, maintains lip closure and prevents food from falling out of the mouth. The sensory division of cranial nerve V relays information about the position of the food bolus in the mouth. The motor division of cranial nerve V controls mastication. Cranial nerve XII innervates the tongue, a muscle critical in controlling the bolus, moving it upward and backward against the palate and with a squeezing and rolling action, propelling the bolus into the oral pharynx. Sensory fibers in cranial nerves IX and X signal the arrival of the bolus at the oropharyngeal region.

The third phase, the pharyngeal swallowing, is involuntary and is triggered by oropharyngeal stimuli. It begins at the anterior faucial arch and is rapid, completed in less than 0.5 seconds. Five motor events occur in the pharyngeal phase to ensure that the bolus enters the esophagus and does not follow other potential pathways.[20] *Velopharyngeal closure* (closure of the soft palate against the pharyngeal wall) prevents food from refluxing into the nose. *Laryngeal closure,* including true vocal cord closure and folding of the epiglottis down over the laryngeal aditus, prevents material from entering the larynx; the combined force of the larynx elevating and the tongue moving backward acts to tilt the epiglottis from upright to transverse to protect the laryngeal inlet.[33] During this phase, vocal cords adduct to protect the airway and respiration ceases momentarily. *Pharyngeal peristalsis* cleans the pharynx with a wave of contraction that follows the bolus. *Laryngeal elevation and anterior movement* carry the larynx up under the tongue out of the path of the bolus. *The cricopharyngeal region opens* (relaxation of the cricopharyngeus muscle, which is the upper esophageal sphincter), an event related in part to laryngeal elevation and anterior movement during the swallow.

Normal function during the pharyngeal phase depends on the actions of cranial nerves V, IX, and X. The motor division of cranial nerve V innervates the mylohyoid, which pulls the hyoid up and forward to bring the larynx beneath the back of the tongue. Cranial nerve IX, innervating the stylopharyngeus, assists the hyoid elevators and lifts the larynx forward. Cranial nerve X generates four motor activities in sequence: it elevates the palate to occlude the nasopharynx, folds the epiglottis over the top of the larynx, initiates pharyngeal peristalsis, and dilates the hypopharynx, allowing the bolus to fall back into the esophagus.

In the esophageal phase, peristalsis of the esophagus is triggered by the swallowing reflex and continues until the bolus reaches the stomach. This phase lasts from 8 to 20 seconds. Cranial nerve X is responsible for innervation of the esophagus.

SWALLOWING ABNORMALITIES IN ALS

Pathophysiology of Dysphagia

For the patient with ALS, symptoms usually result from some combination of spasticity and flaccid muscular weakness and wasting,[28] which leads to abnormalities in the oropharyngeal phases of swallowing (Table 24–2). In the oral preparatory phase, orbicularis oris and buccinator weakness lead to a poor lip seal and pocketing of food particles in the buccal sulcus, respectively. Masseter, pterygoid, and temporalis muscle weakness

Table 24–2. **ABNORMAL SWALLOWING IN ALS**

Phase Involved	Symptom or Sign	Pathophysiology
Oral preparatory	Poor lip seal; food particles collect in buccal sulcus	Weakness of orbicularis oris, tongue, and buccinator
Oral preparatory	Reduced ability to chew	Weakness of muscles of mastication
Oral	Coughing, choking *before* swallowing	Weak, poorly coordinated tongue movement, spilling of food into open airway
Pharyngeal	Nasopharyngeal reflux of food and liquid *during* swallowing	Soft palate fails to close against the pharyngeal wall
Pharyngeal	Coughing and choking *during* swallowing	Reduced or absent laryngeal movement (upward and forward); impaired epiglottic folding over larynx
Pharyngeal	Coughing and choking *after* swallowing	Food collects in pharyngeal recesses because of reduced peristalsis; leads to aspiration during inhalation after swallowing

results in poor chewing and impairs the patient's ability to form a normal bolus. During the oral phase, weakness or poor coordination of the tongue muscles impairs the tongue's ability to propel the bolus and may cause food particles to spill prematurely into the pharynx when the airway is still open and before pharyngeal swallowing.[20]

Because normal tongue movement is one trigger for the pharyngeal swallow, reduction in the tongue's range and force of motion delays this phase.[20] Impaired tongue movement may also allow the bolus to fall over the back of the tongue and into the pharynx after the oral transit phase but before the pharyngeal swallow is elicited; liquids are even more likely to enter the open airway because they can splash into it. Once the pharyngeal stage has begun, reduced soft-palate closure leads to reflux of food and liquid into the nose. Attenuated pharyngeal peristalsis allows food to collect throughout the pharynx from the valleculae to the piriform sinuses after the swallow; the patient is then in danger of aspirating during inhalation after the swallow. Reduced or absent laryngeal elevation leads to incomplete epiglottic closure over the laryngeal vestibule and increases the chance of aspiration during the pharyngeal swallow. Abnormal cricopharyngeal muscle

tone that may occur in patients with ALS also causes an impairment of the last stage of swallowing, which moves the bolus into the esophagus. The esophageal phase is normal in patients with ALS.

The Experience of Dysphagia

During the course of ALS, swallowing changes may occur in five stages[12] (Table 24–3):

1. Normal eating habits
2. Early eating problems, such as difficulty chewing
3. Dietary consistency changes
4. A need for tube feedings
5. Nothing by mouth

Early in the disease, eating habits are essentially normal. Patients may notice occasional difficulty because food becomes lodged in the gingival buccal mucosa as a result of minimal facial weakness, but otherwise swallowing is normal and intervention is not needed. Although conventional wisdom holds that oropharyngeal dysphagia leads to more early difficulty swallowing liquids than solids, the second stage may be heralded by the sensation that solids are sticking in the throat.[28] Thereafter, patients begin to notice cough-

Table 24–3. **PROGRESSION OF SWALLOWING DISTURBANCE IN ALS**

1. Normal eating habits
2. Early eating problems
   - Fatigue of muscles of mastication
   - Lodging of food in buccal gingival mucosa
   - Sense of solids sticking in throat
   - Leaking of liquids from mouth
3. Need for dietary consistency changes
   - Difficulty initiating a swallow
   - Hoarseness, "wet" voice, aspiration
   - Loss of the pleasure of eating
   - Transition to soft or blenderized diet
4. Need for enteral feedings
   - Aspiration of foods and liquid
   - Increasing fatigue during meals
   - Prolonged meal times because of efforts to avoid choking
5. Nothing by mouth
   - Aspiration of saliva

ing after ingesting thin liquids, especially room-temperature water. Patients are in danger of inadequate fluid intake as difficulties with manipulating liquids increase. At this stage, problems include difficulty chewing, leaking of liquids from around the lips, eating slowly, accumulation of saliva because of fewer spontaneous swallows, thickening of saliva, and postnasal congestion.[28]

As the disease progresses, patients may enter the third stage, requiring changes in food consistency. Initially, the patient usually changes to a soft diet, but a blenderized or liquid diet might be needed. Patients with oropharyngeal dysphagia and difficulty transferring food into the pharynx describe trouble initiating a swallow. More specifically, pharyngeal paresis with pooling of secretions in the valleculae and piriform sinuses after swallowing will lead to a variety of symptoms, including dyspnea while swallowing, stridor, hoarseness, wet voice, and possibly episodes of aspiration pneumonia.[18] Patients may report associated phenomena such as dysarthria or nasal speech arising from palatal weakness, changes in sleep patterns, sleep apnea, or an increase in snoring.[6]

As the patient progresses through the lat-ter portion of the third stage of dysphagia, a critical nutritional event occurs[12]—the patient loses the sense of enjoyment associated with eating. The loss of enjoyment and the need for special food preparation signals the onset of significant weight loss and failure to thrive.

The fourth stage begins when tube feedings are needed to prevent repeated aspiration, food spillage, prolonged mealtimes, and respiratory fatigue during meals. Rarely, we encounter patients who aspirate their own saliva, and therefore enter the fifth stage, designated as "nothing by mouth" (NPO) because all oral ingestion is unsafe.

Evaluation of Dysphagia

All evaluations should begin with a careful history followed by a physical examination, bedside swallowing evaluation, and modified barium swallow with videofluoroscopy (Table 24–4). We inquire about weight loss and whether the patient has changed dietary habits. We try to elicit symptoms caused by a misdirected bolus, such as nasal regurgitation, coughing, or choking.

Table 24–4. **EVALUATION OF DYSPHAGIA IN ALS**

Physical Examination
- Check weight
- Check skin turgor
- Examine muscles of face, mouth, tongue, and oropharynx

Evaluate Swallow During a Meal
- Inspect for food collections under tongue, in buccal sulci, and on palate
- Look for food or liquid released from mouth
- Check for elevation of hyoid bone and thyroid cartilage
- Scrutinize for coughing, choking *before, during,* and *after* swallow
- Test swallowing performance

Administer Modified Barium Swallow with Videofluoroscopy
- Use different bolus consistencies
- Examine for motor incoordination of oral and pharyngeal muscles
- Look for aspiration

The physical examination should include evaluation of skin turgor and weight measurements (see below). The mouth and oropharynx should be inspected. The muscles of mastication can be assessed for atrophy and weakness by palpation of masseters and temporalis during biting, and the pterygoids can be evaluated by examining lateral jaw movement. As the disease advances, the weak jaw is pulled down by gravity, resulting in mouth breathing and dehydration of the mouth and lip mucosa.[12] Tongue movements are tested by asking the patient to move the tongue up, down, and sideways and to touch the soft palate with the tip of the tongue.[29]

A swallowing evaluation can be carried out at the outpatient office while the patient is eating. For the oral preparatory and oral phases, we look for pocketing of food in the lateral sulcus and collecting of food under the tongue and on the hard palate. We observe whether food is released from the mouth during chewing, and we scrutinize tongue movements for coordination and forcefulness. Swallowing performance may be evaluated with two bedside assessments: swallowing a 5- to 10-mL bolus of water or swallowing as fast as possible without any liquid or solid in the mouth.[33] The normal patient should be able to swallow water on command without tipping the head back, drooling, choking, or delaying, and in the second test, should swallow 3 to 5 times in 10 seconds. In the pharyngeal stage, we observe for elevation of the hyoid bone and thyroid cartilage, assessing whether it is absent or delayed. We note whether coughing or choking occurs before, during, and after a swallow. We listen carefully for a wet voice after swallowing, look for increased secretions while eating, and observe for expectoration or regurgitation of liquids or solids.

In modified barium-swallow videofluoroscopy, both anteroposterior and lateral views are scrutinized. In our institutions, the test is coadministered by a speech pathologist and radiologist. It focuses on the physiology of the oropharynx, especially the details of oropharyngeal bolus transit.[33] In particular, the study identifies motor incoordination of oral and pharyngeal muscles, nasal regurgitation, and aspiration.[29] The study differs from the traditional barium swallow, which is designed to fill the pharynx with barium and delineate potential structural lesions.[29] A small bolus is adequate to stimulate the interactions that occur during normal swallowing and is safer than a standard barium swallow for patients who are at risk for aspiration. The study helps to assess the location and severity of a swallowing disorder because various bolus consistencies (thin liquid, paste, and solid) are used, and it helps to identify those patients who aspirate small amounts of material not detectable by visual inspection.[5] This study helps the speech pathologist and neurologist estimate the degree to which a patient is at risk for aspiration. For some patients, aspiration may be texture-specific;[5] for example, although a patient may aspirate thin liquids, a puree consistency may be well tolerated.

NUTRITIONAL STATUS IN PATIENTS WITH ALS

Types of Malnutrition

There are three major types of malnutrition: marasmus, kwashiorkor-like or hypoalbuminemic, and mixed.[10] Each has its own clinical and biochemical characteristics and a distinctive pathogenesis. *Marasmus* is seen with prolonged starvation. Although the diet has an acceptable protein-to-calorie ratio, total dietary intake is inadequate. Patients begin to use their endogenous energy reserves of fat and protein, resulting in weight loss, muscle wasting, and loss of fat stores. With progressive weight loss, immunocompetence may decline so that patients have a depressed total lymphocyte count and anergy to common antigens. In the *kwashiorkor-like* state, ingestion of calories is adequate, but they are derived almost entirely from carbohydrates, with little or no protein. Salt retention, hypoalbuminemia, or both may lead to pitting edema, ascites, and anasarca. Muscle mass is usually normal or only slightly reduced. As in marasmus, immuno-incompetence may develop. In addition, the levels of liver-dependent transport proteins, such as albumin, transferrin, and thyroxine-binding globulin, are depressed. Finally, a large group of medical and surgical patients have a *mixed nutritional disorder* that has aspects of both marasmus and kwashiorkor.

In ALS, a variety of factors may reduce total dietary intake and contribute to marasmus-type malnutrition. These include difficulty eating because of weakness in the hands and arms, difficulty swallowing and fear of choking, embarrassment over drooling during mealtime, and depression.[5]

Body Composition

To aid in nutritional assessment, the body can be divided into six compartments:[10] fat, skin and skeleton, extracellular, plasma protein, viscera, and skeletal muscle (Fig. 24–2). When total dietary intake becomes inadequate, the body begins to use its organic materials to provide energy for essential metabolic processes. A variety of anthropometric and biochemical measurements are available to evaluate several of the compartments at risk.

Assessment of Nutritional Status

To evaluate nutritional status, a nutritional history, physical examination, and anthropometric and biochemical measurements should be obtained (Table 24–5). The history should ascertain current nutrient intake

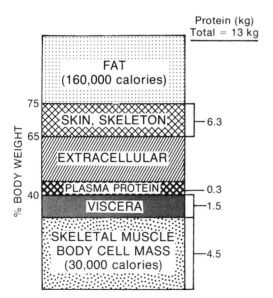

Figure 24–2. Compartments of body composition. (From Grant, JP, Custer, PB, and Thurlow, J: Current techniques of nutritional assessment. Surg Clin North Am 61:441, 1981, with permission.)

based on a verbal recall by the patient or family member of the foods typically eaten over 24 hours.[32] The recommended dietary allowance for protein is 1 to 1.5 g/kg; 20% to 30% of calories should be provided by fat, and the remainder by carbohydrates. Protein provides 4.1 kcal/g; fat, 9 kcal/g; and carbohydrate, 3.4 kcal/g. For each individual, the basal energy requirements are estimated using the Harris-Benedict equation:[17]

Women	$655 + (9.6 \times$ weight, kg$)$ $+ (1.8 \times$ height, cm$)$ $- (4.7 \times$ age, years$)$
Men	$66 + (13.7 \times$ weight, kg$)$ $+ (5.0 \times$ height, cm$)$ $- (6.8 \times$ age, year$)$

The resting energy expenditure is approximately 25 to 35 kcal/kg body weight. Stress and activity require a 10% to 20% increase in energy expenditure.

Signs of nutritional depletion detected on physical examination in patients with ALS may include fat wasting as well as muscle atrophy, the latter being an expected result of progressive motor neuron loss. Less common are signs of protein deficiency, such as changes in skin turgor, interstitial fluid, ascites, and hepatomegaly.

The anthropometric measurements used to assess nutritional status in ALS include weight, skinfold thickness, and mid-upper arm circumference. Weight is perhaps the best measure of malnutrition and is the easiest measure to ascertain. It estimates skeletal muscle or somatic protein mass.[10] The baseline should be the patient's healthy or usual body weight, which is usually obtained from patient recall; however, such recall may be associated with as much as a 3.6-kg error in either direction.[24] The percent usual body weight is calculated as follows:

$$\text{Percent usual body weight} = \text{current weight/usual weight} \times 100$$

Ideal body weight (IBW), in pounds, is estimated by the following formula:

Women	IBW $= 100 + 5 \times$ in. ($>$5 ft)
Men	IBW $= 105 + 6 \times$ in. ($>$5 ft)

Table 24–5. **NUTRITIONAL ASSESSMENT TECHNIQUES IN ALS**

Technique	Purpose
Obtain nutritional history based on 24-h verbal food recall	Allows assessment of major nutrient and caloric intake
Physical examination	Ascertain signs of nutritional deficiency and degree of muscle atrophy and fat loss Detect signs of protein deficiency
Weight measurements (assessing weight loss)	Best measure of malnutrition, easiest to ascertain Indicator of skeletal muscle or somatic protein mass
Measurement of triceps skinfold thickness	Reliable index of total body fat
Measurement of mid-upper arm circumference	Indicator of skeletal muscle protein mass
24-h urinary creatine excretion and creatinine-height index	Reflection of total muscle mass
Measurement of serum albumin	Reflection of visceral protein mass
Measurement of total lymphocyte count	Indication of immune competence

A current weight of 85% to 95% of the usual body weight indicates mild caloric malnutrition, 75% to 84% indicates moderate malnutrition, and less than 75%, severe caloric malnutrition.[10] Weight loss is more serious if a decrease is noted over less than a few weeks.[17] A body weight loss of 10% or more in patients who have unintentionally lost weight but who may still be above their ideal weights is a good indicator of nutritional risk.[32]

Weight is also used to calculate the body mass index, which is the ratio of weight (W) to the square of the height (H):

$$\text{Body mass index} = W\,(\text{kg})/H\,(\text{m})^2$$

A normal body mass index is 20 to 24.9 and values less than 20 suggest undernutrition.[31] Weight loss carries an adverse prognosis in ALS. Patients with a body mass index of less than 20 have reduced forced vital capacity and maximum voluntary ventilation.[19]

The triceps skinfold thickness is a reliable index of total body fat because nearly half the body's fat stores are in the subcutaneous layer, and subcutaneous fat losses caused by dietary change occur proportionately throughout the body.[10] Fat is a valuable energy source during periods of inadequate dietary

intake, and measurements of body fat deposits serve to estimate the duration and severity of malnutrition. The triceps skinfold thickness is measured on the posterior upper arm at the midpoint between the acromion and olecranon while the patient is sitting or standing. Lange calipers are applied gently and left in place for 3 seconds before the value is read (Fig. 24–3). The procedure is repeated three times, and an average thickness is recorded.[10] The percentile within which the skinfold thickness value falls is determined by referring to established tables that list the skinfold thickness value according to patient age and sex.[1] In general, mild fat depletion is assumed if measurements fall within the 35th to 40th percentile, moderate if within the 25th to 34th, and severe if below the 25th percentile.[10]

The mid-upper-arm circumference, like weight, is an indicator of skeletal muscle protein mass. It is measured in centimeters, at the same level in the upper arm as the triceps skinfold thickness. The measuring tape should encompass the perimeter of the arm and not pinch the skin. The mid-upper-arm circumference percentile can be determined from established tables of values for a normal population.[1] Arm circumference percentiles between the 35th and 40th represent mild

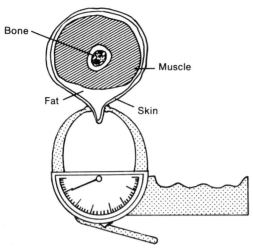

Figure 24–3. This cross-sectional diagram shows the technique for measuring a skinfold, a double layer of subcutaneous fat and skin. In this case, the triceps skinfold is being measured with Lange calipers. The procedure is done three times and an average is obtained. (From Grant, JP, Custer, PB, and Thurlow, J. Current techniques of nutritional assessment. Surg Clin North Am 61:445, 1981, with permission.)

marasmus, 25th to 34th suggest moderate marasmus, and below 25th percentile indicate severe marasmus.[10]

Supplementing these anthropometric techniques are a variety of biochemical measurements that may be used to evaluate nutritional status in ALS. Body muscle mass may be estimated by 24-hour urinary creatinine excretion, because creatinine is derived from the spontaneous dehydration of creatine, which is synthesized in the liver but concentrated mainly in the body muscle mass.[10] The 24-hour urinary creatinine will therefore be directly related to total body creatine and, hence, to total muscle mass. The creatinine-height index is the ratio of the patient's 24-hour creatinine excretion to that of a normal adult of the same sex and height.[2,11] Creatinine-height index values between 60% and 80% are thought to represent moderate somatic protein depletion, and less than 60%, severe depletion.[3]

Malnutrition leads to reduced hepatic biosynthesis of transport proteins. Therefore, visceral protein mass is usually evaluated by measuring the serum concentration of transport proteins synthesized in the liver.[10] The four liver-dependent proteins that have been studied in ALS are albumin, transferrin, thyroxin-binding prealbumin, and retinol-binding protein. Because obtaining, storing, and assaying albumin is simple, we measure and follow the albumin level in our ALS patients. If serum albumin is depressed in the absence of stress, or if it remains depressed for more than 7 days during stress, a protein-to-calorie, kwashiorkor-type malnutrition is present.[10] An albumin concentration between 2.8 and 3.5 g/dL indicates mild visceral protein depletion; between 2.1 and 2.7 g/dL, moderate depletion; and less than 2.1 g/dL, severe depletion.[10]

Immunologic depression is another consequence of malnutrition of all types and may be occasionally encountered in ALS patients. A variety of reversible immunologic disturbances have been described, including a decrease in the total lymphocyte count, impaired cell-mediated immunity, and deficiencies of IgG and complement component C3.[23] We evaluate immune competence with the total lymphocyte count because it is the most convenient measure, requiring only a routine complete blood count and a differential count. A total lymphocyte count between $1200/mm^3$ and $2000/mm^3$ represents mild depletion; $800/mm^3$ to $1199/mm^3$, moderate; and less than $800/mm^3$, severe depletion.[10]

Nutritional Studies

Three studies have highlighted the precarious state of nutrition in patients with ALS. First, Slowie and colleagues[32] evaluated a group of 20 randomly selected ambulatory patients with ALS between 44 and 70 years of age (mean, 57 years) and disease duration ranging from 6 months to 11 years (mean, 4 years), among whom 14 patients had a caloric intake below the recommended daily allowances based on 24-hour dietary recall. Patients reporting the lowest caloric intakes had the greatest weight loss. Five patients had at least a 10% loss of body weight. Four patients had moderately severe dysphagia when consuming semisolid, pureed foods and liquids; in this group, the mean caloric intake was 1400 kcal versus a mean intake of 1600 kcal for the group as a whole. Mean weight loss was 5% for patients with mild dysphagia, and 25% for those with more advanced dysphagia. Hence, the degree of dysphagia corresponded to the reduction in caloric intake and percent weight loss. The reduction in caloric intake was usually a result of dysphagia caused by bulbar impairment. In those patients with lower intake and minimal or no dysphagia, the reduction may have been related to physical inability to prepare food and feed oneself, or to psychologic upset. Five patients had triceps skinfold and arm muscle circumference measurements indicating moderate-to-severe malnutrition. Low serum albumin levels were unusual, occurring in only one patient. Reduced total lymphocyte count values were found in six patients. These biochemical values did not necessarily correlate with the anthropometric data.

In a second study, the nutritional status of 16 ALS patients was followed serially on three occasions over a 6-month period.[19] The study group was representative of the ALS population, with equal numbers of men and women, a mean age of 58 years, and a mean duration of weakness before the study of 24 months for men and 31 months for women (range, 7 to 75 months). Patients ate their accustomed diet as they desired, did not receive nutritional supplementation during the study period, were not on an experimental drug protocol, and received no ventilatory support. Over the course of the study, patients needed to modify the consistency of their diet to accommodate progressive dysphagia. Energy intake expressed as a percentage of recommended dietary allowance decreased in 15 patients (94%). Body mass index, creatinine-height index, and arm muscle area progressively declined, reflecting loss of muscle bulk. Although body fat stores were predicted to increase in the preterminal phases of ALS because of steadily increasing weakness, body fat progressively decreased in relation to the patient's time of death; this decline was more apparent in men than in women. The reduction in body fat could have been a result of increased metabolic requirements, reduction in energy intake, or both. Indeed, it is likely that advancing and spreading muscle atrophy and weakness impose increasing metabolic demands on the remaining functional muscles to maintain mobility and ventilation. Based on dietary logs, the total energy consumed

consistently declined as the disease progressed, but this decline was not associated with a concomitant reduction in protein or micronutrients.

In the third study, nutritional changes early in the course of ALS were studied for 6 months in 12 ambulatory patients without breathing difficulties. Their mean age was 51.3 years (standard deviation, 12.7 years) and mean duration of symptoms was 17 months (standard deviation, 9 months) at the onset of the investigation.[25] A control group consisted of six healthy men. Body composition (bone, fat, and soft tissue) was measured twice in 6 months using dual-photon absorptiometry, and basal energy expenditure was measured by indirect calorimetry. During the study period, patients had an average 2-kg loss of lean mass but at the same time an average gain of 0.55 kg of fat mass, resulting in an average 1.45-kg loss in total body mass. When this loss was converted to energy equivalents, ALS subjects lost an average of 1800 kcal of energy stored in lean mass but gained 4900 kcal in fat mass, resulting in a net increase of 3100 kcal in stored energy. Also notable was that patient caloric intake did not differ from energy expenditure at the beginning of the study, but at the study's end, intake was 130 kcal greater than expenditure, indicating that patients were consuming more calories than needed. Thus, the increase in fat mass can compensate for the energy loss that occurs when denervation and subsequent muscle atrophy reduce lean mass. The amount of energy stored can be preserved even when losses in lean and overall body mass are significant. However, maintaining usual body weight for as long as possible may not be appropriate in ALS. It may result in excessive accumulation of fat without affecting the rate or extent of muscle atrophy. Excessive accumulation of fat on an already weakened muscular structure can negatively affect functional ability and independence.

MAINTAINING ADEQUATE NUTRITION IN PATIENTS WITH ALS

Our goals are to meet the energy, fluid, vitamin, and mineral needs of our patients and to prevent aspiration.[5] As we have seen, in the early stages of ALS, before dysphagia becomes problematic, the loss of muscle or lean mass is more than adequately compensated for by an increase in fat mass. It may be beneficial, therefore, for ALS patients to lose a moderate amount of total body mass over time.[25] A well-balanced diet should include enough calories to meet the individual's metabolic needs plus a little extra to allow just enough fat accumulation to compensate for energy lost in muscle mass.

Dietary Modifications

As dysphagia progresses and patients have increasing difficulty handling a regular diet, dietary changes become necessary to maximize caloric intake and minimize aspiration. We recommend smaller and more frequent (than usual) meals of nutrient-dense conventional foods that are high in calories and protein, as well as multivitamins and minerals. We also suggest that the patient sit upright during the meal and for an hour afterward. Information from the modified barium swallow often aids in identifying the head and neck positions that will promote swallowing. Eating in small bites and sips, often alternating solids and liquids, is important.

The foods should be easy for the tongue to manipulate into a smooth bolus. Given this requirement, the best foods are soft, moist, smooth solids.[5] Meats should be pureed to the appropriate texture. Bread is one of the most difficult foods for a dysphagic patient to handle; it is most easily swallowed if toasted and then dunked in a beverage. Fresh fruit is handled best if pureed; canned fruit, because it is usually soft and moist, is an excellent substitute. Thicker liquids are consumed more easily; various thickeners include pudding, applesauce, mashed potatoes, milkshakes, yogurt, and ice cream.[5] Unmoistened and unchewed food particles; dry, crumbly foods; and tough meats should be avoided. Water and other thin liquids are difficult to handle and may enter the airway, causing choking and coughing. Swallowing in a head-down position (the chin tuck), which tucks the inlet to the larynx under the tongue base, and using a straw, which facilitates placing food in the mouth while in this position, may prevent these difficulties.[12] The chin tuck is helpful also because it narrows the pharyngeal space and slows pharyngeal bolus transit.[14] Swallowing of liquids may be improved by changing the taste (juice or soda), temperature (cooling), and texture (carbonation).[12]

Enteral Tube Feedings

With increasing dysphagia, the patient will find eating to be increasingly tiring and may take an hour to consume a single meal because of efforts to avoid choking.[19] At this point, the patient needs to discuss options for nutritional support (specifically enteral tube support) with the neurologist, speech-language pathologist, and dietitian. In contrast to parenteral nutritional therapy, enteral feeding retains the digestive and absorptive functions of the gastrointestinal tract and sustains the immunologic barrier provided by the gut.[15] There are two methods for delivering enteric feedings, the nasogastric or nasoenteric tube, and the percutaneous endoscopic gastrostomy (PEG) and jejunostomy tube.[15]

NASOGASTRIC TUBE

The familiar nasogastric tube can be used for enteral feeding in ALS. Insertion is usually accomplished easily by medical personnel who thread a well-lubricated tube into a nostril and down into the esophagus and stomach; the length of tube required is estimated by adding the distance between the tip of the nose and earlobe and that between the earlobe and xiphoid.[7] The risk of aspiration may be lowered by advancing the tube into the duodenum under fluoroscopic guidance. Radiologic confirmation should be obtained to ensure the tube is appropriately positioned (in either the stomach or duodenum). The nasogastric tube is a short-term measure to maintain adequate nutrition in the cooperative patient, generally being used for several weeks, although occasionally tubes may be used for months, especially if they are removed and replaced regularly. Nasogastric tubes may pose difficult problems to the patient, including discomfort; frequent tube blockage; pulmonary aspiration; gastroesophageal reflux; and irritation, bleeding, or stricture of the nasopharynx and the esophageal-gastric junction.[5,7,15] These problems may undermine the goal of nasogastric tube feeding, leading to the unintended consequence of inadequate nutrition.[34] The nasogastric tube may also adversely affect the morale of the patient and relatives.[34] On rare occasions, however, we use the nasogastric tube for long-term support if for some reason, such as patient choice, markedly reduced vital capacity, or a major contraindication to the PEG placement procedure, a PEG tube cannot be used.

PERCUTANEOUS ENDOSCOPIC GASTROSTOMY

Because of the problematic nature of nasogastric tube feeding, PEG is recommended for long-term maintenance of good nutrition. The technique, usually carried out fairly easily, was introduced in 1980 as an alternative to traditional operative methods of creation of a feeding gastrostomy.[27] When compared with operative gastrostomy or jejunostomy, PEG significantly reduced costs and length of hospital stay (E. Davis-Carr and H. Mitsumoto, unpublished observation). It permits safe, effective, long-term simplified access to the gastrointestinal tract for enteral nutrition when swallowing is impaired.[21,27] In a randomized study of inpatients requiring long-term enteral nutrition, PEG tube feeding showed important advantages over nasogastric tube feeding, including a lower incidence of blocked or displaced tubes and more effective nutritional support and weight gain.[26] In addition to the situations mentioned above, we recommend a PEG when the patient is no longer eating enough to maintain an adequate level of nutrition, when eating has become exhausting, and when the patient is willing to undergo minor surgery. It is important that the vital capacity be adequate, usually greater than 50% of the predicted value, because of increased pulmonary risks,[16] although experienced gastroenterologists in our centers have performed PEG placements in ALS patients with much lower vital capacities. Ideally, body weight loss should be less than 10% of the usual body weight,[22] but we have had successful PEG placements even if more weight loss has occurred. When the patients can still take nourishment safely by mouth but in less

than adequate amounts, we find that PEG placement enhances quality of life. Table 24–6 lists the indications and contraindications of PEG and summarizes the methods for PEG procedures and feeding.

There are three main techniques of PEG tube insertion, which are equivalent in regard to ease of insertion, patient tolerance, and complications; they compare favorably to the traditional surgically placed gastrostomy.[13] The Ponsky-Gauderer (pull technique)

Table 24–6. FEATURES OF PERCUTANEOUS ENDOSCOPIC GASTROSTOMY

Indications
- Patient no longer able to maintain a healthy level of nutrition by eating
- Patient willing to undergo minor surgery
- No contraindication
- Vital capacity preferably greater than 50% of predicted, but can be less

Contraindications
- Obstructing lesion in pharynx or esophagus
- Marked obesity
- Portal hypertension and ascites
- Active peptic ulcer disease
- Advanced diaphragmatic weakness

Methods
- Pull technique used most often, but push and Russell techniques can be used
- Done in an endoscopy suite; overnight stay
- Feeding begins 24 h after procedure
- Feeding is done as a continuous infusion or bolus

Usefulness
- Percutaneous endoscopic gastrostromy can improve survival and quality of life for ALS patients

*Complications**
- Wound infections (4%)[†]
- Aspiration (3%)[†]
- Overall complication (14%)[†]

---

*In patients with ALS who have progressive malnutrition and impending respiratory failure, percutaneous endoscopic gastrostomy procedures are not benign and are associated with high morbidity and even mortality (H. Mitsumoto, personal experience).

[†] The data are based on the study of Mamel, JJ: Percutaneous endoscopic gastrostomy. Am J Gastroenterol 84:703–710, 1988.

and Sachs-Vine (push technique) methods use a guide wire to position the gastric tube. A needle and series of peelaway catheters are used for the Russell technique.[8] The pull-through technique is used most often and so is described below. Exclusion criteria for PEG include the rare instance of an obstructing abnormality in the pharynx or esophagus, marked obesity or prior surgery making it impossible for the endoscopic light to be seen through the abdominal wall, portal hypertension with ascites, active peptic ulcer, a bleeding diathesis, or advanced diaphragmatic weakness.[8,34] Of these contraindications, the possibility of advanced diaphragmatic weakness is of most concern in ALS.

For our ALS outpatients, the PEG procedure is performed in the endoscopy suite, and thereafter they are admitted to the hospital short-stay unit. Although rarely necessary or indicated in ALS patients, the PEG feeding tube can also be inserted in the intensive care unit, operating room, and at the bedside.[21] Whether the patient has an allergy to the medications used during the procedure should first be determined. The patient should be kept NPO for at least 8 hours before the procedure. Antibiotic prophylaxis to reduce wound infection is provided with intravenous cefazolin, 1 g given 30 minutes before the procedure. The procedure is performed with the patient supine and the head of the bed elevated 30°. The head of the bed may be raised further to improve respiratory function. The endoscopist anesthetizes the pharynx, provides a small dose of rapidly acting, short-lived intravenous sedation to minimize respiratory depression, and then passes the gastroscope into the stomach. Air is insufflated through the gastroscope and the stomach is kept distended with air throughout the procedure to appose the stomach to the abdominal wall.[8] The site for PEG insertion is located by finding the point where the endoscopic light maximally transilluminates the abdomen and determining satisfactory indentation of the gastric wall by pressing on the abdomen with the index finger. This point is usually one-third the distance from the middle left costal margin to the umbilicus. Next, lidocaine is injected into the subcutaneous tissue, a 1-cm incision is made through the skin, and a 14- to 16-gauge needle with a cannula is passed through the incision and into the stomach. The needle is then removed from the cannula, a guide wire is passed into the stomach, and an endoscopic snare is used to capture the guide wire. At this point, the guide wire is brought out through the mouth by withdrawing the endoscope. The gastric tube is attached to the guide wire, lubricated, and then pulled into position by applying traction through the endoscope to the guide wire at the level of the abdominal wall.

The standard PEG leaves a single tube protruding from the abdomen approximately 25 cm long with an adaptor on the end to permit feeding with a feeding pump or a syringe. Because these tubes further disrupt the patient's body image, low-profile feeding tubes have been developed. These tubes are often referred to as button gastrostomy tubes.[9] Although an extension tube must be attached to the button tube when the patient is fed, it may be removed at other times. These button gastrostomy tubes may be placed at the initial procedure or can be inserted as a replacement tube through a mature fistulous tract.

After the PEG is placed, the patient is usually kept NPO and given intravenous fluids to maintain hydration until the next day, when feeding is initiated as a continuous infusion at 30 mL/h if bowel sounds are present. The rate of infusion may be gradually increased and length of feeding time decreased over 3 days; in this way patients can be "cycled" to allow for 12-hour feeding periods overnight so that they are free from the inconvenience of tube feeding during the day. Feeding formulas provide 1 cal/mL, so that an infusion rate of 150 mL/h will deliver 1800 calories in 12 hours. Bolus feeding by attaching a syringe to the feeding tube is an alternative, although it may increase the risk of aspiration. Feeding formulas contain the recommended daily allowances of vitamins and minerals in a volume of 1.0 to 1.5 L. If the total volume infused is less than 1 L, then nutritional supplements may be needed.

The PEG procedure and subsequent nutritional management requires a short hospital stay of 1 or 2 days. The PEG has low risks and costs, and a very short operating time. In our experience, however, respiratory status may suddenly worsen in patients with advanced ALS, and therefore in this subset of the ALS population, PEG may be a high-risk procedure. The better the patient's preoperative nutritional and respiratory status, the more favorable the postoperative course. Careful follow-up after PEG placement is critical.

Other complications after PEG placement have been described. Of 1,338 patients undergoing PEG for a variety of indications, 53 (4%) had wound infections and 40 (3%) had aspiration.[21] Less frequent complications included stoma leaks, pneumoperitoneum, dislodged tubes, perforation or peritonitis, bleeding, gastrocolic fistula, failure to place a PEG, and ileus; in total, approximately 14% of procedures resulted in complications.[21] Mortality reported in the first 30 days after the procedure is reported to range from 9% to 15%[13] and is often associated with underlying disease.

The decision to feed into the stomach or small intestine is based on the patient's inability to sense reflux from the stomach and history of reflux or aspiration of gastric contents. In the setting of one or both of these conditions, the enteric tube should be placed distal to the pylorus. A jejunostomy allows feedings to be infused downstream from the pylorus.[21] To convert a standard PEG into a feeding jejunostomy, the gastrostomy tube is used as a conduit for a long Silastic jejunal feeding tube, which is grasped through the endoscope and carried into the duodenum.

In patients with ALS, PEG nutritional support is generally well accepted and effectively provides adequate nutrition. In a study of 31 ALS patients undergoing PEG, patients were observed at 3-month intervals for 2 years after PEG tube placement.[22] These 31 patients were compared to a control group of 35 ALS patients who declined PEG. In patients who had PEG, the body mass index showed a slight but statistically significant improvement after tube insertion; in the control group, it decreased significantly to a level indicating malnutrition. The mean duration of disease (from first neurologic deficit to death or tracheostomy) was 38 months (standard deviation, 17 months) in patients with PEG and 30 months (standard deviation, 13 months) in the controls ($p <$ 0.03). The cumulative survival showed that mortality did not differ significantly between the two groups of patients during the first 6 months of observation, but after this period

it decreased in the PEG group. This difference was significant at 12 months, 18 months, and 24 months after tube placement.

SUMMARY

Normal swallowing is a complex act with four phases: the oral preparatory, oral, pharyngeal, and esophageal. In ALS, weakness, loss of coordination, or both in muscles supplied by cranial nerves V, VII, IX, X, and XII lead to abnormalities in the two oral phases and in the pharyngeal phase. Swallowing abnormalities include difficulty in forming and propelling the bolus, nasal regurgitation, delayed initiation of swallowing, residue in the pharynx after swallowing, and aspiration. Evaluation of swallowing includes physical examination of cranial nerves used in swallowing, and a modified barium swallow with videofluoroscopy to help assess the location and severity of the swallowing disorder.

Progressive dysphagia leads to weight loss and, if nutritional support is not provided, may lead to malnourishment. There are three types of malnutrition. Marasmus results from inadequate intake of total calories and leads to muscle wasting and loss of fat stores. Kwashiorkor is caused by a diet profoundly deficient in protein, despite adequate calories, and leads to marked fluid retention with little attenuation in muscle mass. The mixed type has characteristics of the other two. The type of malnourishment seen in ALS more closely resembles marasmus. To assess nutritional status, both anthropometric and biochemical techniques are used. The anthropometric techniques include body weight and body mass index, triceps skinfold thickness as a reliable index of total body fat, and mid-upper-arm circumference as an indicator of skeletal muscle protein mass. The biochemical measurements employed are the creatinine-height index (a reflection of total muscle mass), the concentration of serum albumin (synthesized by the liver and a measure of visceral protein mass), and total lymphocyte count (a reflection of immune competence).

Nutritional studies of patients with ALS indicate that inadequate caloric intake and weight loss correlate with severity of dysphagia. As the disease advances toward the terminal stage in patients without ventilatory support, body fat and lean body mass progressively decrease and resting energy expenditure increases. In the early stages of ALS, loss of motor neurons contributes to loss of lean body mass, but there is a corresponding gain of fat mass, leading to a net increase in total calories stored even as total body mass drops. This pattern suggests that early in the disease, a controlled degree of weight loss might be appropriate to avoid potentially deleterious increases in fat accumulation.

As dysphagia develops and worsens, a variety of strategies are used to maintain adequate nutrition in ALS. First, when oral feeding is still possible, the diet is changed to maximize caloric intake and minimize aspiration. Thin liquids should be avoided; the best foods are soft, moist, smooth solids. When oral feeding becomes painfully slow, exhausting, and dangerous because of aspiration, enteral feeding is instituted. The nasogastric tube is familiar to medical and nursing staff and easy to insert. However, it is only a short-term measure for most patients because of problems, including frequent blockages resulting, paradoxically, in inadequate nutrition. The PEG tube provides long-term access to the gastrointestinal tract and is placed during an endoscopic procedure requiring only local anesthesia. Contraindications such as esophageal obstruction, ascites, obesity, and bleeding diathesis are uncommon in our clinical practice. Occasional complications of the procedure include wound infection and stomal leaks. If aspiration proves to be problematic, the PEG can be converted to a jejunostomy. The PEG is well accepted by patients with ALS, improving their nutritional status and enhancing quality of life.

REFERENCES

1. Bishop, BW, Bowen, PE, and Ritchey, FJ: Norms for nutritional assessment of American adults by upper arm anthropometry. Am J Clin Nutr 34:2530–2539, 1981.
2. Bistrian, BR, Blackburn, GL, Sherman, M, et al: Therapeutic index of nutritional depletion in hospitalized patients. Surgery, Gynecology, and Obstetrics 141:512–516, 1975.
3. Blackburn, GL, Bistrian, BR, Maini, BS, et al: Nutritional and metabolic assessment of the hospitalized patient. Journal of Parenteral and Enteral Nutrition 1:11–22, 1977.
4. Bosma, JF, Donner, MW, and Tanaka, E: Anatomy of the pharynx, pertinent to swallowing. Dysphagia 1:23–30, 1986.
5. Carr-Davis, EM: Nutritional maintenance in amyotrophic lateral sclerosis. In Mitsumoto, H and Norris, FH, Jr (eds): Amyotrophic Lateral Sclerosis. A Comprehensive Guide to Management. Demos, New York, 1994, pp 77–91.
6. Castell, DO and Donner, MW: Evaluation of dysphagia: A careful history is crucial. Dysphagia 2:65–71, 1987.
7. Cogen, R and Weinryb, J: Tube feeding. Providing the most nutrition with the least discomfort. Postgrad Med 85:355–359, 1989.
8. Deveney, KE: Endoscopic gastrostomy and jejunostomy. In Rombeau, JL and Caldwell, MD (eds): Clinical Nutrition. WB Saunders, Philadelphia, 1990, pp 217–229.
9. Ferguson, DR, Harig, JM, Kozarek, RA, et al: Placement of a feeding button ("one-step button") as the initial procedure. Am J Gastroenterol 88:501–504, 1993.
10. Grant, JP, Custer, PB, and Thurlow, J: Current techniques of nutritional assessment. Surg Clin North Am 61:437–463, 1981.
11. Heymsfield, SB, Arteaga, C, McManus, C, et al: Measurement of muscle mass in humans: Validity of the 24-hour urinary creatinine method. Am J Clin Nutr 37:478–494, 1983.
12. Hillel, AD and Miller, R: Bulbar amyotrophic lateral sclerosis: Patterns of progression and clinical management. Head Neck 11:51–59, 1989.
13. Hogan, RB, Demarco, DC, Hamilton, JK, et al: Percutaneous endoscopic gastrostomy—to push or pull. A prospective randomized trial. Gastrointest Endosc 32:253–258, 1986.
14. Horner, J and Massey, EW: Managing dysphagia. Special problems in patients with neurologic disease. Postgrad Med 89:203–213, 1991.
15. Howard, L: Parenteral and enteral nutrition therapy. In Isselbacher, KJ, Braunwald, E, Wilson, JD, et al: (eds): Principles of Internal Medicine. McGraw-Hill, New York, 1994, pp 464–472.
16. Hudson, AJ: Outpatient management of amyotrophic lateral sclerosis. Semin Neurol 7:344–351, 1987.
17. Jeejeebhoy, KN: Assessment of nutritional status. In Rombeau, JL and Caldwell, MD (eds): Clinical Nutrition. WB Saunders, Philadelphia, 1990, pp 118–126.
18. Jones, B and Donner, MW: How I do it: Examination of the patient with dysphagia. Dysphagia 4:162–172, 1989.
19. Kasarskis, EJ, Berryman, S, Vanderleest, JG, et al: Nutritional status of patients with amyotrophic lateral sclerosis: Relation to the proximity of death. Am J Clin Nutr 63:130–137, 1996.
20. Logemann, JA: Swallowing physiology and pathophysiology. Otolaryngol Clin North Am 21:613–623, 1988.
21. Mamel, JJ: Percutaneous endoscopic gastrostomy. Am J Gastroenterol 84:703–710, 1988.
22. Mazzini, L, Corra, I, Zaccala, M, et al: Percutaneous endoscopic gastrostomy and enteral nutrition in

amyotrophic lateral sclerosis. J Neurol 242:695–698, 1995.

23. Miller, CL: Immunological assays as measurements of nutritional status. A review. Journal of Parenteral and Enteral Nutrition 2:554–566, 1978.

24. Morgan, DB, Path, MRC, Hill, GL, et al: The assessment of weight loss from a single measurement of body weight. The problems and limitations. Am J Clin Nutr 33:2101–2105, 1980.

25. Nau, KL, Bromberg, MV, Forshew, DA, et al: Individuals with amyotrophic lateral sclerosis are in a caloric balance despite losses in mass. J Neurol Sci 129:47–49, 1995.

26. Park, RHR, Allison, MC, Lang, J, et al: Randomised comparison of percutaneous endoscopic gastrostomy and nasogastric tube feeding in patients with persisting neurological dysphagia. Br Med J 304:1406–1409, 1992.

27. Ponsky, JL and Gauderer, MWL: Percutaneous endoscopic gastrostomy: Indications, limitations, techniques, and results. World J Surg 13:165–170, 1989.

28. Robbins, J: Swallowing in ALS and motor neuron disorders. Neurol Clin 5:213–229, 1987.

29. Rosenfield, D and Barosso, AO: Difficulties with speech and swallowing. In Bradley, WG, Daroff, RB, Fenichel, GM, et al: (eds): Neurology in Clinical Practice. Butterworth-Heinemann, Boston, 1995, pp 155–168.

30. Sasaki, CT and Isaacson, G: Functional anatomy of the larynx. Otolaryngol Clin North Am 21:595–612, 1988.

31. Shulzl, LO: Obese, overweight, desirable, ideal; where to draw the line in 1986? J Am Diet Assoc 86:1702–1704, 1986.

32. Slowie, LA, Paige, MS, and Antel, JP: Nutritional considerations in the management of patients with amyotrophic lateral sclerosis. J Am Diet Assoc 83:44–47, 1983.

33. Sonies, BC and Baum, BJ: Evaluation of swallowing pathophysiology. Otolaryngol Clin North Am 21:637–648, 1988.

34. Wicks, C, Gimson, A, Vlavianos, P, et al: Assessment of the percutaneous endoscopic gastrostomy feeding tube as part of an integrated approach to enteral feeding. Gut 33:613–616, 1992.

CHAPTER 25

PSYCHOLOGICAL MANAGEMENT

The journey from good health to the latter stages of ALS presents a formidable challenge to the patient's spirit and psyche. Although this journey is sometimes solitary, often frightening, and emotionally painful, with honesty and understanding from physicians and friends, the patient can meet its challenges.

This chapter examines psychological management in terms of three stages of change for patients. In the first stage, patients are faced with symptoms but no diagnosis; in the second stage, evaluation leads to diagnosis and explanation of the disease; in the third stage, patients begin to cope with new physical and psychosocial realities and adapt to the ongoing changes and challenges of the disease.

THE EXPERIENCE BEFORE DIAGNOSIS

Before Medical Evaluation

In this early stage, the individual has yet to consult a physician concerning symptoms

and is continuing to live in a normal or nearly normal fashion. For some, twitching in a muscle, cramping in a limb, a mild limp, a minor speech impediment, or slight difficulty swallowing may be physically uncomfortable and psychologically distressing, but concerns about the significance of symptoms are often pushed aside and ignored in the hope they will go away. When symptoms persist or limit daily activities, they usually prompt a physician visit. Physical examination and routine laboratory testing generally follow, and the primary care physician or internist, concerned about the muscle weakness, suggests a neurologic referral.

Meeting the Neurologist— The Diagnostic Process

The first visit with a neurologist may be a time of considerable anxiety for the patient, who is beginning to suspect that the symptoms and signs reflect a neurologic illness. The neurologist's detailed examination and additional blood tests, electromyography (EMG), and neuroimaging (see Chapters 5, 7, and 8) may continue to raise the patient's level of anxiety. There may be two or more visits before the neurologist is prepared to make the diagnosis of ALS. In fact, in the early stages of the disorder or in instances of slow progression, the diagnosis may be suspected or viewed as possible but cannot be made with enough certainty to qualify as probable or definite ALS. We review with our patients the World Federation of Neurology definitions of suspected, possible, probable, and definite ALS (see Chapter 6). Although the diagnosis of possible ALS suggests that an alternative diagnosis is conceivable, we explain that the results of clinical, EMG, neuroimaging, and laboratory examinations make such an eventuality unlikely and that we have not yet clearly identified another explanation for the symptoms.

We also encounter patients from time to time who have seen several physicians, including other neurologists, and yet, in the face of what strikes us as unequivocal clinical and laboratory findings of ALS, have not been given a diagnosis. These patients are extremely frustrated and in despair. We try to comfort them by explaining that the diagnosis of ALS in its early stages is difficult and that we too would have been unable to establish it had we met them at their initial presentation. In fact, in the study of 60 ALS patients,[1a] the mean time to diagnosis was 12.3 months, 27% were initially misdiagnosed, and patients saw an average of 3.7 physicians before the diagnosis of ALS was made.

LEARNING ABOUT THE DIAGNOSIS

In the absence of a family history, patients are generally unfamiliar with ALS and its consequences, so "doctors are charged with a very delicate educational task."[21] However, in most instances, by the time the neurologist is prepared to speak about ALS as definite, probable, possible, or suspected, the patient has an idea of what the problem may be because of discussions with friends and family, his or her own research (which now may include locating information on online bulletin boards), and discussions with the referring physician and neurologist about the meaning of symptoms and signs. It behooves the neurologist to present the diagnosis frankly, with honesty and hope, and only after careful evaluation and testing (see Chapter 18).[2] Rose[20] observes that "a sudden blurting out of the nature of the disease can be shattering and there can be few patients who will face with equanimity being told that they have a progressive disease that may involve breathing muscles." Also, it is preferable that information be provided gradually so that the patient has time to adjust; facts

should not be thrust on the patient until he or she is judged ready for them.[20] Patients find that disclosure is best when they are not overwhelmed with too much information too soon. Written materials may be given to patients and family members to read at their own pace after the initial shock of the diagnosis has lessened. It is also helpful for a nurse to contact patients weekly for a period immediately after diagnosis to provide support and information and to schedule physician appointments if warranted.[2]

At diagnosis, we attempt to provide hope in several ways. First, we and our team of health-care providers clearly state that the patient will not face the disease alone and will never be ignored or abandoned.[2,8a,19] Second, we point out that the conventional wisdom of a rapid course does not necessarily apply to all patients and that slower progression is well documented, with some patients having 5, 10, 15, or more years ahead of them after diagnosis. Third, we find that engaging in short, straightforward lessons about normal nervous system anatomy, the structures that are affected, and, importantly, structures that are spared also fosters hope. Fourth, presenting the current state of knowledge of the pathogenesis of ALS is helpful to some patients. Explaining that one or more control mechanisms that normally maintain motor neuron integrity may have gone awry helps patients understand the rationale of proposed therapies. Participation in clinical trials provides many patients with additional hope. Also, we fully expect that some patients and family members will have doubts that the diagnosis is correct and will want a second opinion, a desire we fully support and facilitate (see Chapter 18).

THE EXPERIENCE AFTER DIAGNOSIS

Studies of Psychological Issues in ALS

Over the last three decades an important literature on the psychological aspects of ALS has developed. It consists of a combination of scientific studies and thoughtful essays by clinicians who have worked closely with patients with ALS. A careful reading of this literature provides insights into the experience of living with ALS and is therefore helpful to professionals devoted to caring for these patients (Table 25–1).

PERSONALITY

In one of the first psychological studies of patients with ALS, 10 patients were evaluated with a series of self-administered psychological tests and psychiatric interviews.[3] Patients with ALS were compared with control subjects with inoperable neoplastic disease. The tests were the Internal-External Control Scale, the Multiple Affect Adjective Check List, and the Minnesota Multiphasic Personality Inventory (MMPI). (The Internal-External Control Scale asks patients to choose between paired statements that either suggest that events are a consequence of their own behavior or that events in an individual's life are beyond their personal control). Patients with ALS showed a significantly higher degree of internality (personal control), not varying with social class, duration of illness, age, sex, or functional impairment than patients with inoperable neoplastic disease. Review of personal histories indicated a high degree of independence and highly competent behavior; generally, these patients had gone to remarkable lengths to continue working. The authors speculated about an association between ALS and an adaptive style that is characterized by hyperindependence, active mastery, and chronic exclusion of an unhappy affect from awareness.

Table 25–1. **SUMMARY OF PSYCHOLOGICAL ISSUES IN ALS**

Study	Major Findings
Brown and Mueller, 1970[3]	• Personality features associated with ALS include high degree of independence, denial of unhappy affect.
Houpt et al, 1977[10] Peters et al, 1978[18]	• No characteristic personality profile emerged from studies of patients with ALS.
Gould, 1980[9]	• Patients with ALS experience three phases in regard to control over their lives as the disease progresses: *Early stage*—External control, with confidence in science and medicine to treat and possibly cure *Intermediate stage*—Traditional medicine is ineffective, need to take personal control *Late stage*—Relinquish control, turn to external control, such as religious faith or existential fatalism
Gould, 1980[9]	• Denial has an important adaptive function: Helps prevent loss of patients' relationships with caregivers. • Denial may mask despair and pessimism. • Patients should be given the opportunity to ventilate to those not directly involved in their care.
Montgomery and Erickson, 1987[15]	• Distress syndrome (anxiety, depression, fatigue, alienation) common among patients with ALS (46%). • Pulmonary dysfunction is a reliable predictor of psychological disturbance.
Armon et al, 1991[1]	• Premorbid psychological or adaptive difficulties are no greater in patients with ALS than controls. • Men with ALS were more likely to have behaved stoically before diagnosis.
McDonald, 1994[13]	• Depression is common in patients with ALS (60%). • Psychological well-being is possible in ALS and may not decline despite progression of the disease.
McDonald et al, 1994[14]	• Psychological status (well-being) correlates with survival time in patients with ALS.

Another psychological study evaluated 40 consecutive patients admitted for evaluation and treatment for ALS who were given psychological tests and had psychiatric interviews.[10] Patients with ALS did not have a high degree of internal control and did not use denial as a defense more often than a group of patients with inoperable neoplastic disease. A third study compared the MMPI profiles of 21 men and 17 women with ALS with the profiles of 50,500 general medical patients. No characteristic personality profile for patients with ALS emerged.[18] The increased defensiveness that had been observed in the earlier study[3] was not confirmed.

A more recent study searched for psychological and adaptation difficulties antedating the diagnosis of ALS by reviewing comprehensive medical records of 45 patients with ALS and 90 control subjects from the same community matched by age, gender, and period of observation.[1] Mild-to-moderate difficulties (e.g., reactive depression, anxiety, tension) were comparable when women with ALS were compared with women in the control group. However, when men with ALS and mild-to-moderate difficulties were compared with controls, contact with a physician was absent or significantly lower for patients, implying a stoicism in men that is not present in women. Others have noted that the personality style of patients with ALS is marked by impressive stoicism, optimism, generosity, and cheer.[15] These traits might be explained in part by partial denial,[9] which allows the patient to redefine reality to exclude more distressing aspects of the disease from awareness to promote psychological coping.

THE RELATIONSHIP BETWEEN INTERNAL CONTROL AND STAGE OF DISEASE

An important finding that came out of the 40-patient study[10] mentioned in the previous section was that the intensity of internal control varied with length of disease: Patients with a length of illness of 1 to 2 years had greater control than those whose length of illness was less than 1 year or greater than 2 years.[10] Based on this observation, Gould[9] proposed three phases of control in the lives of patients with ALS as the disease progressed. Patients with ALS within 1 year of diagnosis (phase I) are more likely to score high for external control, with confidence in medicine, doctors, and hospitals and a conviction that they will get well by following medical instructions. As the first year passes without a cure, the patient enters a second phase in which traditional medicine is viewed as ineffective, and the patient adopts a new perspective "to beat the disease" on his or her own. During this phase, the internal locus of control is strong, as the patient makes intense personal efforts to maintain activity and good nutrition, to exercise and look for new treatments. The second year passes without amelioration of the disease, heralding the third phase when the patient shifts back toward some form of external control, such as religious faith or an existential fatalism.

THE ROLE OF DENIAL

Analysis based on a group of 65 patients with ALS[9] suggested that they maintain a strategy of partial denial throughout their illness. The denial, however, is deemed "healthy" because reality is not actually denied but rather is redefined so that the most distressing aspects of the disease are not a part of ordinary consciousness; in this way, the patient maintains function and hope. Denial might also have an important adaptive function in that patients may consider expression of doubt and discouragement to imply criticism or lack of confidence in their medical care and fear losing their relationship with the treating physician.[9] Because denial may mask despair and pessimism, when it is overridden, major concerns and anxieties may be revealed. The author suggested that patients should be given the opportunity to reflect and ventilate about their condition and express doubt and discouragement with physicians or professionals not directly involved in their care.

PSYCHOLOGICAL DISTRESS AND DEPRESSION

Montgomery and Erickson[15] administered the MMPI to 38 patients with ALS who attended screening evaluations for a clinical trial with thyrotropin-releasing hormone. Of the 38, 18 patients had psychometric evidence of maladjustment. These difficulties appeared more prevalent than previous research had suggested. The average profile for poorly adjusted patients suggested somatic preoccupation plus a distress syndrome that involved anxiety, depression, impaired concentration, fatigue, loss of control, and alienation. However, psychometric determination of depression was not associated with any measure of ALS disease severity, implying that other factors are the primary determinants of depressed mood. Anxiety and general ego disorganization were associated with both upper motor involvement and pulmonary dysfunction, and the latter was thought to be the best single predictor of psychological disturbance. Patients with respiratory compromise had more somatic preoccupation, anxiety, and schizotypic features than patients with normal respiration. Features of hypomania were seen in patients with respiratory dysfunction, which may indicate problems with attention and concentration, as well as restlessness and irritability associated with impaired breathing.

Progression of the physical signs of ALS was associated with increasing problems in multiple psychological domains, including cognitive and memory difficulties, social and emotional alienation, and loss of social and functional control.[15] Massman and colleagues[12a] found that about one-third of their ALS patients displayed notable neuropsychological deficits, especially in the realm of problem solving, attention, visual recognition memory, word generation, and verbal free recall. Neuropsychological deficits were more likely to occur in patients with severe motor deficits and in patients with fewer years of education but, notably, did not correlate with symptoms of depression.

As ALS progresses, respiratory competency is lost, which usually heralds the terminal stages of the disease. At this point, denial and other defenses may fail, and patients may acknowledge and report anxiety and despair. Therefore, patients with ALS seem no less prone to psychological adjustment difficulties than patients with other terminal illnesses, particularly in the latter stages of ALS.[15] The evident stoicism of ALS patients should not blind health-care workers to individual needs; comprehensive management should include repeated psychological evaluations of patients and their families as the disease advances.[15]

PSYCHOSOCIAL-SPIRITUAL ADJUSTMENT

In a comprehensive 18-month study of the psychosocial-spiritual profiles of 144 patients with ALS, depression, hopelessness, perceived stress, anger expression, loneliness, health locus of control, life satisfaction, and sense of purpose in life were evaluated.[13] Scores for each test ranged widely, suggesting variability in psychosocial-spiritual adjustment, but when average scores for these tests were compared to a normal, healthy population, the only differences were that ALS patients had more depression and a more external locus of control. Sixty percent had some level of measurable depression, compared to 16% to 20% in the healthy population.

A variety of factors influenced whether a patient had a sense of well-being or distress. Older patients (over 65 years) had higher levels of depression and hopelessness, perhaps in part because these patients might have been facing end-of-life issues even before the diagnosis of ALS was made, and perhaps because they feared they would burden their families. Mildly ill patients had a higher level of well-being than those more affected, experiencing less depression and perceived stress. Even moderately affected patients who had had ALS for 19 to 60 months felt considerable distress, marked by high levels of depression, hopelessness, perceived stress, and a low sense of purpose in life. McDonald[13] points out that these patients may appear to be coping with their disease but are actually highly distressed, even experiencing psychosocial-spiritual crisis, so that intervention is essential.

Of note, well-being did not necessarily decline as the disease progressed; most patients remained in the same psychosocial-spiritual state throughout the study. Long-term (greater than 5 years) survivors of ALS, representing 31% of the group entering the study, had greater psychosocial-spiritual well-being than those with ALS for a shorter time, even though 21% of this group was severely affected. The 18 (12%) patients who were respirator-dependent did not experience higher levels of depression, loneliness, hopelessness, or perceived stress, and they considered their lives to have purpose and meaning. Rapid decline in neurologic function was associated with the highest levels of psychosocial-spiritual distress, probably because the patients did not have the opportunity "to integrate the loss of one function before another loss was confronted."[13]

For the spouses (79% of 144 patients were married) and the other 10 primary caregivers, as a total group (123 people), the psychosocial-spiritual profile was similar to that of the control spouses except that the spouses of ALS patients had higher depression scores (although much lower than the patients) and a greater loneliness.[13] Some clearly experienced psychosocial-spiritual distress. Eighteen (15%) felt profoundly hopeless and were moderately to severely depressed, 28 (23%) experienced a high degree of loneliness, and 58 (47%) expressed a high degree of stress in their lives. Isolation sometimes generated feelings of resentment and guilt.

PSYCHOLOGICAL WELL-BEING AND SURVIVAL

The role of psychological factors in survival was evaluated in 138 of these patients.[14] Assessment scales measured the degree of hopelessness, depression, loneliness, stress, and expression of anger, as well as sense of purpose in life, locus of control for health (internal vs external), and ways of coping. A psychological status score was derived from these scales, and three groups (high, middle, and low) were identified based on the psychological scores, with the high group representing psychological well-being (34 patients), the middle group a more neutral psychological status (71 patients), and the low group psychological distress (32 patients). Survival status was monitored for 3.5 years. Eleven patients (32%) of the high and 27 (82%) of the low psychological score groups died during the study. When the confounding factors of length of illness, disease severity, and age were controlled for, patients with psychological distress had a greater risk of mortality overall and also a greater risk of dying in any given time period than those with psychological well-being. Median survival time during the study period was also

significantly longer for the high (>1200 days) and middle (609 days) psychological score groups than for the low group (333 days). When the covariates of length of illness, severity of disease, and age were controlled, the relative risk of death per unit time for patients with psychological distress was 2.24 times that for a patient with psychological well-being. The risk of dying associated with psychological distress was greater than the risk associated with increased age and was similar to that of disease severity. Thus, psychological status is an important prognostic factor in ALS that is independent of the length of time since diagnosis, disease severity, and age.[14] (see Chapter 9).

Living with ALS: Promoting Psychological Well-Being

These studies and our own experience in looking after patients with ALS have taught us that despite considerable physical handicaps and innumerable emotional and social challenges, patients with ALS can achieve a good quality of life. Patients who are psychologically well are hopeful and feel that life has purpose.[13] As Smith[21] observed, "they have been able to come to terms with ALS, transcending the ALS experience to find peace in a seemingly arbitrary world." How can we as physicians promote satisfaction with life for our patients and help them to achieve psychological well-being as they live with ALS? As O'Brien and colleagues[17] discuss, part of our task is to help patients realize that they still have potential: "In caring for patients with motor neuron disease, the overall impression is not one of disability and loss, but rather of the immense potential of each individual for growth and creativity in the face of progressive physical deterioration."

Our approach is to try to address seven overlapping areas related to the emotional and social lives of our patients as listed in Table 25–2.

RECOGNIZING AND TREATING DEPRESSION

As we have seen, despair is common in patients with ALS, and clinical depression of varying severity is seen in approximately

Table 25–2. AN APPROACH TO PROMOTING PSYCHOLOGICAL WELL-BEING IN PATIENTS WITH ALS

Recognizing and treating depression

Helping patients recapture purpose in their lives

Fostering a sense of autonomy in the patients

Developing a therapeutic partnership with the patient to restore hope

Overcoming our own sense of professional failure

Facing our own mortality

Supporting the family

60%. We look carefully for indicators of depression and have a low threshold for intervention, recommending counseling or drug treatment, depending on the severity (see Chapter 19).

RECAPTURING PURPOSE IN LIFE

Smith[21] has said that "many patients choose to live with considerable disability not because they are afraid to die but because they have reasons to live." Indeed, the psychological distress caused by severe illness is related more to the disruption of personal relationships than it is to death itself.[24] Thus, in discussion with our patients, we try to ascertain whether they still feel their lives are purposeful. If they do not, we try to help them rediscover the purpose they once had and to again find meaning in their lives. Regaining purpose is also closely tied to rediscovering pleasure in life. Goldblatt points out,[8a] "To move toward developing a successful way of managing progressive illness, the patient does not have to give up pleasure, but it must come from different, often deeper, sources.

Although the course of ALS is one of progressive weakness, we emphasize to patients that cognitive clarity and psychic energy are totally preserved, and that they can compensate for loss of strength and kinetic control by maintaining and even increasing social interaction. We may relate uplifting histories of patients who continued to maintain intellectual vigor and social contacts despite their illness. One of our patients who had traveled extensively before diagnosis is now in a wheelchair and severely weakened by ALS

but continues to be a font of knowledge for family and friends about travel, geography, and local customs; she is consulted frequently for trip planning. A patient we have learned about continues to work as a prize-winning journalist despite severe generalized ALS with bulbar and spinal involvement.[6] Special computer software and a toggle switch have allowed him to continue to use his word processor and do some of his best writing, with only minimal finger movement. One year after the diagnosis of ALS was made, a 41-year-old fitness instructor and college baseball coach had a "storybook season," winning the National Association of Intercollegiate Athletics Independent Conference championship.[23] He noted that his "optimism came back, physically and mentally." He credits his family, his faith, and the support of his team in helping to pull through this period of his life. And, finally, our patients gain inspiration from the life of Sam Filer, eloquently described by David Goldblatt, M.D.[8b] Judge Filer, age 58, who has had ALS for 7 years, is quadripeligic, on a ventilator, and nourished by a feeding gastrostomy. He communicates electronically, working from home and judicial chambers, handling a full case load. The judge views ALS "not as a life-threatening disease but rather as a life-enhancing condition."

FOSTERING AUTONOMY

Cassel[4] has written that "maintaining autonomy for a patient with ALS is critical because patients with this disease have lost many of the characteristics that give them power in the world. It is autonomy that is a key element in living a meaningful life in our culture." This idea is probably true for many patients, especially those with a strong internal locus of control. Autonomy may be somewhat less important for those with an external locus of control, patients who want the health team to direct them, to tell them what course of action should be taken.[13]

We attempt to foster autonomy in patients in various ways, including sharing information, sharing decision making, offering the opportunity to participate in research, and showing respect for the patient's values.[4] As we pointed out previously, describing the nature of the illness helps many patients because knowledge about the disease is "an avenue to power."[4] We find that full, albeit gradual, disclosure of the nature of the disease and its prognosis is helpful in the long run for patient and family. There is truth and wisdom in presenting the disease as manageable if not curable, with the patient moving from being a victim of disease to being a "person-in-charge" who is meaningfully involved in the constant decision making that the course of the disease requires.[12] Thus, the patient must be at the center of decision making for all treatment plans concerning his or her disease. The patient needs to hear what the neurologist thinks is happening so that he or she can realistically confront the situation; no information or only partial disclosure from the neurologist leads to uncertainty and doubt about the true nature of the disease and often to the very opposite of autonomy—helplessness, with its attendant anxiety and despair.[4]

When patients have begun to come to terms with the diagnosis of ALS and have begun to recapture the sense of purpose in their lives, we can help them recognize that unlike a number of other serious illnesses, which present a risk of sudden death at any moment, ALS allows them time to consider various facets of their lives.[4] They have time to deal with the emotional aspects, time to confront mortality and the meaning of life as well as the meaning of death, time to think things over, and time to reconsider grievances and misunderstandings. There is time to make and change decisions about acceptable or desirable forms of medical help. Cassel[4] points out that "medieval Christian philosophy considered that the best death was one that was foreseen, for which a person had ample time to prepare."

ESTABLISHING A PARTNERSHIP TO RESTORE HOPE

Clinicians and patients also have time to develop a therapeutic partnership.[4] The patient has time to work through various reactions he or she experiences and time to develop supportive relationships with physicians, family members, and friends. It is the relationships with the family and friends that are often essential to recapturing the sense of purpose in life. As Smith[21] points out, the neurologist, having established rapport and understanding with the patient and family, has an opportunity to "help the patient make the momentous decision of whether to go on living with ALS or let the disease take its course." However, as mentioned previously, the partnership must be based on honesty and full disclosure, which means that the neurologist must be able to discuss the unpleasant truths concerning prognosis. When the partnership includes information about research efforts and new therapies, it often leads the patient to participate in clinical trials. Participating in a trial enhances both patient and physician morale and the physician's ability to care for patients with ALS.[21] It is critical, however, that the "physician's interest in the patient be linked to the life of the patient rather than the life of the drug trial."[21]

We also agree with Smith[21] that it is helpful to introduce patients to others who have made the choice to live with ALS despite handicaps. These patients and their families speak from a firsthand perspective, and it is difficult for us as treating neurologists to divorce ourselves completely from the physician's point of view concerning how to live with ALS.

During the course of the illness, we repeatedly and clearly convey to the patients that we are interested, that we care and will not abandon them. We inform the patient that no one yet fully understands ALS, that we are uncertain about the cause and pathogenesis but that we are entering a new era of therapies based on evidence from research in the basic sciences. Such sharing of uncertainty about the disease may well enhance patients' trust and promote hope.[4] Although knowledge of ALS is growing rapidly, the large gaps in our understanding behoove us "to never rule out the possibility of a long survival and productive life for ALS patients."[4] A good partnership between physician and patient often raises the level of patient well-being, sometimes simply because the patient knows the physician is available and supportive.[12]

OVERCOMING THE SENSE OF PROFESSIONAL FAILURE

The physician who sees the patient's condition gradually deteriorate and is unable to offer treatment that might have a meaningful impact on the disease course may find establishing a relationship with a dying patient to be difficult and emotionally taxing,[13] because physicians are trained to consider recovery as the major goal of the profession. We need to remind ourselves, however, that "medicine was a healing art long before there were specific effective agents for any illness."[4] It is important for us as caregivers to redefine our concepts of success and failure so they depend less on cure and more on care and attention to the psychological well-being of our patients and their families.[4,7,13] Rabin,[19] a physician with ALS, wrote: "I am often surprised and moved by the acts of kindness and affection that people perform. Fundamentally, what the family and patient needs is the sense that people care. No one else can assume the burden, but knowing you are not forgotten does ease the pain."

ACKNOWLEDGING OUR OWN MORTALITY

As physicians, we must confront our own difficulty in accepting death, our tendency to deal exclusively with technical problems because science offers a sense of control,[4] and our inclination to ignore the emotional aspects of incurable illness.[5] There is a risk that the physician's feelings of impotence and anxiety concerning death will be conveyed to the patient and adversely affect the latter's psychological adjustment.[11] For many of us, therefore, education in psychology and ethics is helpful in dealing with a disease like ALS.[5] Gould[9] points out that obtaining psychiatric support for themselves may help physicians maintain a therapeutic partnership with the patient during the course of the disease.

SUPPORTING THE FAMILY

In most instances, the family has a substantial role in caring for the patient with ALS (see Chapter 18). As Gould[9] discussed, "emotional, financial, and social consequences of ALS to the spouse and children cannot be overstated." Modifications in family life and alterations of the spouse's and children's traditional roles are needed to cope with this prolonged and expensive ill-

ness.[9] The family begins to do the physical caretaking tasks that the patient could previously perform, and they must also shoulder emotional burdens both for themselves and the patient.[8]

Coping becomes even more challenging as the patient's ability to speak becomes progressively more impaired, to the point at which even expressing emotion is difficult. As Finger[8] points out, "the crisis of ALS is a crisis to patient and family that is both pragmatic and emotional." Family members often have to put their lives "on hold" as they devote virtually all their physical and psychic energy to the care of the patient. There is a risk that this virtually full-time involvement will lead to the spouse's isolation and loneliness, and ultimately cause resentment toward the patient.[13] Therefore, we often counsel spouses to find time to take care of their needs, and recommend psychological support when necessary.

In the absence of a definitive treatment and with the progressive loss of motor function, families feel powerless, a feeling that is particularly threatening and defended against with unrealistic guilt.[9] Guilt, in turn, may lead family members to become overly involved and to overextend themselves, which may eventually give rise to anger and resentment. Many families need counseling for these very powerful feelings, which may be displaced on another family member who thus becomes a scapegoat. Gould[9] therefore recommends psychiatric intervention for the family that includes the following:

- Encouraging family members to preserve maximum autonomy for the patient
- Uncovering and exploring family members' feelings of responsibility, guilt, and omniscience
- Assisting in establishing and maintaining appropriate limits
- Facilitating and legitimating ventilation of angry feelings concerning the patient
- Identifying and working through individual conflicts precipitated by the illness
- Supporting the family with knowledge, experience, and empathy

Despite the burdens of the disease, over 30% of patients with ALS note that some aspect of their lives, such as family relationships, had improved during the process of learning to cope with ALS and to accept their own mortality.[13]

One way families can deal with issues related to the illness is through an ALS family support group. Participating in such a group can help families become more confident as caregivers, and feel nurtured and emotionally supported by others who are experiencing similar difficulties, all of which contributes to their ability to function adequately.[8] The major goal of the group is to increase participants' ability to deal with the stress, with the emphasis being on more effective behavior and improved coping skills.

We make every effort not only to inform the patient about the disease but also to inform the spouse. When communication with the spouse is poor, the spouse tends to create personal theories about the disease that ultimately lead to self-blame.[13] They may feel that they did not intervene appropriately to change whatever factor they believed caused the illness. Spouses also must grapple with the change in the relationship from husband and wife to caregiver and patient. They must make every effort to preserve some aspect of the former relationship by sharing activities they have always enjoyed together and finding others to help with physical care.[13]

To conclude, we quote O'Brien and colleagues,[17] who observed that "the majority of patients are cared for at home, a fact that stands as a tribute to the courage and resilience of patients and as a tribute to the dedication and resourcefulness of families and friends."

Comfort at the End of Life

In the latter stages of ALS, when respiratory involvement is pronounced, we have found that the hospice program, with its emphasis on palliative rather than curative care and the philosophy that "dying is a normal process, whether or not resulting from disease," is uniquely suited to assist patients and families with issues surrounding the progressive and eventually fatal nature of ALS.[22] Hospice provides emotional as well as medical support from a team consisting of neurologists, nurses, social workers, clergy, and volunteers (see Chapter 18). The hospice program cares for the family as a whole, not just the patient. Consequently, not only is the patient cared for physically and psychologically, but also the family's fears and anxieties are attended to.[17] The program strives to maintain the patient's dignity and even hope as death approaches. As Nuland[16] has written, "The greatest dignity to be found in death is the dignity of the life that preceded it. Hope resides in the meaning of what our lives have been."

SUMMARY

Our own experience and a review of the literature of the psychosocial-spiritual dimensions of living with ALS and caring for ALS patients suggest that there is no characteristic personality profile in this disease. Clearly, however, when the patient initially learns of the diagnosis, fear and anxiety are quite likely; therefore the diagnosis must be presented with honesty, understanding, and hope. The message to the patient must be clear and unequivocal that the neurologist and medical team are always available for support and treatment. Physicians need to convey strongly that although ALS is not curable, it is manageable and that the patient, if willing, may take center stage in orchestrating his or her care.

Living with the losses engendered by ALS poses innumerable physical and emotional challenges to the patient and family members, so despair is nearly universal, clinical depression is common, and a feeling of overall psychosocial-spiritual distress is prevalent, especially for patients with a rapidly progressive course. Much can be done, however, to ameliorate distress and promote emotional well-being. Such well-being is particularly important, because some evidence indicates that survival in ALS is enhanced by psychological wellness. We vigorously treat depression, and help patients regain a sense of purpose in their lives that may have become blurred or lost after learning of their diagnosis. We strenuously promote autonomy, which for many patients is the cornerstone for restoring purpose and meaning in their lives, and for helping them choose among various treatment options. We strive to develop a therapeutic partnership with the patient that creates trust and hope. We also endeavor to overcome the anxiety of facing our own mortality and to change our perception of our traditional (albeit mythical) role as a powerful healer, for success in caring for ALS patients rests not in cure but in treating symptoms and helping the patients achieve the best psychosocial-spiritual well-being possible.

Last, we support the family and individual family members, especially the spouse; in many instances they are grappling with overwhelming emotional, financial, and social difficulties. Family support groups help to lift the burden of responsibility that family members feel for their loved one and ease the emotional crises that ALS engenders. Toward the end of life, hospice care continues to affirm life by providing medical, emotional, and spiritual comfort for patients and their families.

REFERENCES

1. Armon, C, Kurland, LT, Beard, CM, et al: Psychologic and adaptational difficulties anteceding amyotrophic lateral sclerosis: Rochester, Minnesota, 1925–1987. Neuroepidemiology 10:132–137, 1991.
1a. Belsh JM and Shiffman PL. The amyotrophic lateral sclerosis (ALS) patient perspective on misdiagnosis and its repercussions. J Neurol Sci 139 (suppl.):110–116, 1996.
2. Beisecker, AE, Cobb, AK, and Ziegler, DK: Patients' perspectives of the role of care providers in amyotrophic lateral sclerosis. Arch Neurol 45:553–556, 1988.
3. Brown, WA and Mueller, PS: Psychological function in individuals with amyotrophic lateral sclerosis (ALS). Psychosom Med 32:141–152, 1970.
4. Cassel, C: Patient autonomy as therapy. In Mulder, DW (ed): The Diagnosis and Treatment of Amyotrophic Lateral Sclerosis. Houghton Mifflin, Boston, 1980, pp 325–335.
5. Cesa-Bianchi, M and Ravaccia, F: Psychological prep-aration of the physician for ALS patients. Adv Exp Med Biol 209:311–312, 1987.
6. Cobb, N: Living from word from word. Boston Globe. May 16, 1995, pp 37–42.
7. Ferro, FM, Riefolo, G, Nesci, DA, et al: Psychodynamic aspects in patients with amyotrophic lateral sclerosis (ALS). Adv Exp Med Biol 209:313–316, 1987.
8. Finger, S: The family support group in the treatment of amyotrophic lateral sclerosis. Neurol Clin 5:83–100, 1987.
8a. Goldblatt, D. Caring for patients with amyotrophic lateral sclerosis. In Smith, RA (ed): Handbook of Amyotrophic Lateral Sclerosis. Marcel Dekker, New York, 1992, pp 271–288.
8b. Goldblatt, D. A life-enhancing condition: The honorable Mr. Justice Sam N. Filer. Sem Neurol 13: 375–379, 1993.
9. Gould, BS: Psychiatric aspects. In Mulder, DW (ed): The Diagnosis and Treatment of Amyotrophic Lateral Sclerosis. Houghton Mifflin, Boston, 1980, pp 157–167.
10. Houpt, JL, Gould, BS, and Norris, FH, Jr: Psychological characteristics of patients with amyotrophic lateral sclerosis (ALS). Psychosom Med 39:299–303, 1977.
11. Kelemen, J: Coping with amyotrophic lateral sclerosis. Arch Found Thanatol 9(4):abstract 26, 1981.
12. Kelemen, J and Leach, CF: Amyotrophic lateral sclerosis: The support network. Archives of the Foundation of Thanatology 11:abstract 23, 1984.
12a. Massman, PJ, Sims, J, Cooke, N, et al: Prevalence and correlates of neuropsychological deficits in amyotrophic lateral sclerosis. J Neurol Neurosurg Psychiat 61:450–455, 1996..
13. McDonald, ER: Psychosocial-spiritual overview. In Mitsumoto, H and Norris, FH (eds): Amyotrophic Lateral Sclerosis. A Comprehensive Guide to Management. Demos, New York, 1994, pp 205–227.
14. McDonald, ER, Wiedenfeld, SA, Hillel, A, et al: Survival in amyotrophic lateral sclerosis. The role of psychological factors. Arch Neurol 51:17–23, 1994.
15. Montgomery, GK and Erickson, LM: Neuropsychological perspectives in amyotrophic lateral sclerosis. Neurol Clin 5:61–81, 1987.
16. Nuland, SB: How we die. Reflections on life's final chapter. Vintage Books, New York, 1995.
17. O'Brien, T, Kelly, M, and Saunders, C: Motor neurone disease: A hospice perspective. Br Med J 304:471–472, 1992.
18. Peters, PK, Swenson, WM, and Mulder, DW: Is there a characteristic personality profile in amyotrophic lateral sclerosis? A Minnesota multiphasic personality inventory study. Arch Neurol 35:321–322, 1978.
19. Rabin, D, Rabin, PL, and Rabin, R: Compounding the ordeal of ALS: Isolation from my fellow physicians. N Engl J Med 307:506–509, 1982.
20. Rose, FC: The management of motor neuron disease. Adv Exp Med Biol 209:167–174, 1987.
21. Smith, RA: On behalf of the patient. Adv Exp Med Biol 209:319–322, 1987.
22. Thompson, B: Amyotrophic lateral sclerosis: Integrating care for patients and their families. American Journal of Hospice and Palliative Care 7:27–31, 1991.
23. Wahl, M: Life throws coach a curve. Quest (Muscular Dystrophy Association), 1(1), 12–13, 1994.
24. Weisman, AD: On dying and denying. Behavioral Publications, New York, 1972.

CHAPTER 26

MEDICAL ECONOMICS, LEGALITY, AND MEDICAL ETHICS IN ALS

In the preceding chapters, we discussed symptomatic treatment, clinical trials, physical rehabilitation, nutritional support, communication, respiratory care, and psychological issues. In addition to these mostly medical concerns, physicians caring for patients with ALS must deal with problems of an economic, legal, and ethical nature.[23] For example, the long period of disease and the highly complex care required in ALS bring economic issues to the fore as patients and families look for ways to finance expensive medical costs. At many stages of the disease,

physicians also may face legal and ethical dilemmas, so an understanding of these areas is essential for optimal medical care.

ECONOMIC ISSUES

Medical Expenses

Medical expenses for the diagnosis and care of patients with ALS are costly.[18] For diagnosing ALS, routine tests include electromyography, magnetic resonance imaging, blood chemistry tests, a thyroid function test, and immunofixation electrophoresis. Some patients may need additional sophisticated testing for anti-GM_1 antibodies, a muscle biopsy, or a lumbar puncture; occasionally even a bone marrow biopsy may be required (see Chapter 7). The expense of the diagnostic testing is related to the uncertainty of the diagnosis in the early stages of the disease. The result is repeated medical evaluation as signs become more pronounced until the diagnosis is clear. In the early stages, several tests are ordered that appear unnecessary in retrospect. These include evoked potential testing, electroencephalography, and neuroimaging procedures (see Chapter 7). It is not unusual to see patients with ALS who

448

early in their disease had repeated testing that appears out of character with the eventual diagnosis of ALS. Moreover, when the diagnosis of ALS is established, patients often require a second opinion, which adds to the medical costs.

Drug treatment was limited to symptomatic treatment until January, 1996, when the Food and Drug Administration approved riluzole as the first treatment for ALS. This medication currently costs approximately $700 per month. Many of the possible drug treatments currently being investigated, such as insulin-like growth factor I, are available only in an injectable form. Consequently it is unlikely that these will be any less expensive, because injectable forms are generally more expensive than oral forms. Costs for new drug treatments will have to be covered by patients, insurance companies, or both. In general, Medicare will not cover medication costs. Thus, patients who carry only low-coverage private insurance or those who have only Medicare will face an enormous financial burden. Although some mechanisms, such as the North American Organization of Rare Disorders, assist financially needy patients in obtaining newly approved, expensive medication, expenses for new drugs will certainly increase the overall medical costs of ALS management. Physicians should advise patients to find the least-expensive drug carrier or pharmacy to buy new medications; sometimes financial counselors or ALS nurse coordinators may be helpful in identifying less expensive drug carriers.

In the course of the disease, costly therapeutic interventions, such as enteric feeding or treatment for pneumonia, may become necessary. The medical expenses may be substantially lower when physicians have in-depth knowledge of ALS, because they are able to avoid unnecessary tests and therapies. This is an important reason for managed-care insurance companies to refer patients with ALS to ALS centers, where cost-effective care may be possible.

Table 26–1 lists current price ranges for various types of equipment required in caring for patients with ALS. The single most expensive treatment is long-term ventilator support, as discussed in Chapter 22. The cost of hiring a private nurse or nurse's aide is the single most expensive service.

Financial Resources for Medical Care

Table 26–2 summarizes various sources of financial support for patients and their families. We describe financial resources exclusively in the United States. In other major industrial countries, such as Canada, France, and the United Kingdom, the national or federal health insurance covers most medical expenses for patients with ALS. In Japan, national health insurance, corporate health insurance, or both cover medical expenses. In general, personal assets and support by charitable organizations are an important source for financing some costs in ALS. Every country has its own unique health system, which will not be discussed in this book.

PRIVATE MEDICAL INSURANCE

Private medical insurance provides the primary coverage for most patients with ALS. The level of coverage depends on the individual policy; a detailed discussion of private insurance coverage is beyond the scope of this chapter. It is important, however, to discuss two issues: how to use the insurance coverage and how to deal with the maximum "cap" of the insurance coverage. The cap, or maximum amount the insurance company will pay out over a lifetime, is set by the company and depends on the individual policy. Some policies have no cap, whereas others are low. Recently, we have learned of another cap for patients with ALS, an annual medication cap. The costs of riluzole exceed the annual medication cap for some patients, so that they must use their personal assets or give up taking riluzole. This will create new economic issues for patients with ALS.

Because ALS is a severe chronic disease, costs for treatment and management will consume a large amount of insurance coverage. After the diagnosis of ALS is made, the patient (or policyholder) should meet with a representative of the insurance company and outline how he or she wishes to use the insurance, a process called a *benefit adaptation*. The goal of this process is to conserve the insurance money by making a plan to use the coverage effectively and for a longer period. Most patients may not realize the existence of such a program until their disease progress-

Table 26–1. PRICE LIST OF EQUIPMENT USED WITH ALS PATIENTS

Equipment	Cost (in US dollars) to Purchase (rental/month)
Orthoses and Splints	
Wrist splint	20–35
Soft neck collar	10–20
Modified neck collar	30–80
Ankle-foot orthosis (ready to use)	70–80
Ankle-foot orthosis (custom made)	470–580
Equipment for Mobility	
Cane	5–50
Quad-cane	20–50
Walker	45–400
Rolling walker	200–500
Lift chair	700–2400
Patient lift (Hoyer)	1000–1500
Tub lift	600–700
Transfer bench	80–180
Wheelchair, manual	280–975 (29–78/mo)
Wheelchair, electric	3500–20,000
Electric scooter	2000–3500
Wheelchair ramp	150–2000
Bedroom and Toilet	
Overhead table	75
Hospital bed, manual	1100 (200/mo)
Hospital bed, electric	1600–1900 (300–365/mo)
Grab bars	20–50
Toilet safety rails	65–80
Raised toilet seat	15–90
Portable toilet	70–450
Communication Devices	
Language boards	2–10
Voice amplification	40–250
Text Telephone Yoke (TTY)	200
Speech enhancer	2000–4500
Augmentative system	500–7500
Laptop with software	2500 and up
Nutritional and Expiratory Support	
Enteral pump	4200–5600 (18–35/mo)
BiPAP respirator	1700 (185/mo)
Volume ventilator	11,000 (650/mo)
Pulse oximeter	1750 (95/mo)
Apnea monitor	3200 (330/mo)
Suction machine	520 (65/mo)
In-Exsufflator	2750–3600 (270–330/mo)

Note: This is not an exhaustive list of equipment but rather it is intended to provide an idea of prices of common items. Data were obtained from multiple sources, such as several vendors in Cleveland, Ohio, and recent catalogs. These prices are subject to change and will differ in other parts of the country. Simpler and more basic versions are generally at the low end of the cost ranges, and more elaborate versions are more expensive.

Abbreviations: BiPAP = Bilevel positive airway pressure.

Table 26–2. **POTENTIAL FINANCIAL RESOURCES FOR PAYMENT OF MEDICAL EXPENSES IN ALS**

Major Resources

- Private medical insurance or health maintenance organization insurance
- Personal assets
- Medicaid insurance

Minor Resources

- Medicare insurance
- Disability payments from Social Security
- Medical deductions on income taxes
- Tax liabilities of assets
- Medigap insurance

Other Services

- Equipment bank program run by local voluntary services (ALS Association and Muscular Dystrophy Association)
- Financial support from the Muscular Dystrophy Association for a number of services and equipment, such as wheelchair and augmentative communication devices
- Various volunteer services and government-paid social services

es to the stages that require more financial resources. It is also difficult to make a financial plan when the disease is still in its early stages. Benefit adaptation ensures that the insurance resources are most effectively used. In this way, individual patients become *case-managed benefit recipients* as soon as possible. This plan is particularly helpful when the patient is going to receive costly ventilator care.

HEALTH MAINTENANCE ORGANIZATIONS AND OTHER MANAGED-CARE HEALTH PLANS

These plans focus on preventing illness with a comprehensive system of health services. Benefits may include dental care, prescriptions, vision care, and not having to buy Medigap insurance. Health maintenance organizations (HMOs) or other managed-care health plans save costs by keeping patients in their system and typically restricting the choice of physicians. Thus, it is difficult, if not impossible, to obtain approval by an HMO for referral to an ALS Center.

SOCIAL SECURITY DISABILITY INCOME

Patients who are younger than age 65 but disabled totally and permanently because of disease are eligible for Social Security Disability Income; in the case of ALS, approval is likely to be granted. To obtain approval, the specific motor disabilities and diagnostic tests supporting the diagnosis of ALS must be clearly documented in the application form. A perfunctory description of the patient's condition risks denial of the disability claim. After the date of disability approval, there is a 5-month waiting period before retroactive payments begin. Disability income is relatively small; the size of the payment depends on how much money one has paid into the Social Security system over the years. When the disability continues, the patient may require more medical coverage. There is at least a 2-year waiting period before the patient becomes eligible to apply for Medicare. Such a protracted waiting period for disabled patients may cause serious financial hardship because patients often become unemployed because of functional disability and may be denied private insurance because they have difficulty paying the premium.

MEDICAID INSURANCE

Medicaid is a health-care program for people with low income, cosponsored by the state and the federal government. Benefits include inpatient and outpatient services and nursing home care (skilled and intermediate). Both physicians and state Medicaid review offices determine the level of care needed for each patient. Each state establishes its income and asset eligibility levels for services. For example, in the state of Ohio, a patient's total gross income per month from all resources may not exceed the full cost of nursing home care.[5] Assets may not exceed $1,500 for an individual and $2,250 per couple. The family's house is exempt as long as the spouse or a qualified relative lives in it. The family may keep a motor vehicle under a certain value.

The provisions to protect the spouses of nursing home residents include the following: the spouse may keep from $1,254 to $1,919 of the monthly income and $15,348 or half the couple's combined assets, whichever is greater, up to $76,740. The determination of income and assets can be complicated when the spouse is alive. If the family has substantial assets, it is advisable to seek professional advice from an attorney who specializes in medical expense and elder care law.

When patients require nursing home care, one should know that Medicaid reimbursement to a nursing home is much lower than the rate at which the individual pays privately. Therefore, some nursing homes may limit the number of beds available for those receiving Medicaid, resulting in a shortage of nursing home beds for Medicaid patients.

MEDICARE INSURANCE

Medicare has been the federally funded national health insurance program for the elderly since 1965, and for the disabled since 1973. The program has two components, part A and part B. Part A covers hospital, nursing home, and home health services. Enrollment in Part A is automatic for individuals age 65 or older who receive Social Security benefits. Those with end-stage renal disease or 2 years of total and permanent disability also qualify, even if they are younger than age 65, as discussed previously. Part B extends coverage to physician services, outpatient hospital services, and limited ambulatory care. Part B is voluntary and requires a monthly premium of approximately $30.

Part A hospital insurance covers only 90 days of hospitalization but will be renewed after discharge if the beneficiary is not readmitted for at least 60 days. Otherwise, the coverage requires a substantial coinsurance payment from a private insurer or the patient. In addition, Medicare contains a benefit referred to as "lifetime reserve days," which is coverage for an additional 60 days of hospital care; it requires an additional coinsurance payment, and these lifetime reserve days can be used only once during the beneficiary's life.

Medicare provides coverage for an individual in a skilled nursing facility. The following requirements must be met:
- The skilled nursing facility must be certified by Medicare
- An individual must need daily acute skilled nursing care or rehabilitation services and have the *potential for improvement*
- A minimum 3-day hospitalization must precede the nursing facility admission
- Admission to a nursing home must be approved by the nursing facility's utilization review committee

Patient eligibility is reviewed weekly. When skilled nursing facility admission is approved, Medicare pays all charges for the first 20 days, and for days 21 through 100 the beneficiary is responsible for a $92.00 copayment. The patient's private insurance usually pays 80% of charges not paid by Medicare but may have a deductible or special copayment policy. Beyond 100 days in a nursing home, private insurance, the patient, or both must cover the costs. When the individual becomes terminally ill, however, Medicare will pay up to 210 days of hospice care. The Medicare program will also support home health care, which will encourage the chronically ill to receive as much care as possible outside of the hospital. For a patient to receive home care benefits, physicians must issue a certification of medical necessity for intermittent skilled care, provided by a certified home health agency according to the physician's plan of care. The primary service provided at home is limited to skilled nursing, physical therapy, or speech therapy. Once the primary service is approved, secondary services such as a nurse's aide, occupational therapy, social services, and miscellaneous supplies or durable medical equipment may also be paid.

Although home care is a Medicare benefit,

many patients find it difficult to obtain Medicare support for home care. Not surprisingly, the various regional fiscal intermediaries, such as the Medicare offices and home care services, vary in their interpretation of the medical reviews of the need for this type of care. Although we are not aware of a single case in which a ventilator-dependent patient was denied skilled nursing care or home care, gaining approval for coverage of less dire situations, such as extended visits by a nurse's aide or an expensive piece of adaptive equipment, may require the utmost assertiveness by the beneficiary.[13] Obtaining Medicare approval for home care is particularly difficult for the disabled. For example, patients with ALS who cannot afford to purchase technology to assist in communication depend on Medicare benefits to restore communication capability. Expensive but effective assistive technology has a high potential for denial, but the equipment may be obtained with repeated appeals.[13]

MEDICARE AND "MEDIGAP" INSURANCE

"Medigap" is a widely used insurance term referring to insurance supplementing Medicare. If a service is not covered by Medicare, however, it is usually not covered by Medigap. As with Medicare Part A, there may be only one benefit period. Patients can purchase Medigap insurance policies through any private insurance company. It is illegal to sell a Medigap policy that duplicates other insurance while a private insurance policy is still in effect.[5]

How to Finance Medical Care for ALS

The husband of a patient who has ALS and is ventilator-dependent shared in a pamphlet[32] his experiences and the difficulty he encountered in paying for treatment for his wife, and provided explicit guidance on how to finance the costs of ALS and how to protect one's spouse. Figure 26–1 depicts several routes to finance the costs of ALS. For most patients, the first step is to use private medical insurance until it is exhausted. When private medical insurance covers a limited por-

tion of medical expenses, patients must use private assets to cover the gap. Private insurance can be used for home care or nursing home care, but the coverage can be quite limited. The Social Security Disability Income program should be used also, but the financial support is modest. When private medical insurance is exhausted, the family, the patient, and his or her spouse must pay expenses until they are poor enough to qualify for Medicaid. When the family can no longer pay, the government starts paying part of the costs through Medicaid. At this stage, if the patient is in a nursing home, it absorbs the remaining costs.

For patients who are older than 65 years and carry both private and Medicare insurance, the private insurance will be exhausted first. For example, when the patient is in a nursing home, the private insurance will pay until the cap is reached, and only then will Medicare insurance begin to pay. For patients who are older than 65 and carry only Medicare, coverage may be highly inadequate. If the patient is cared for at home, only a limited time for skilled nursing care is allowed. Personal assets must be used to gain additional coverage. Unfortunately, Medicare does not pay the costs of nursing home care for more than 100 days. At this point, the family has to pay until they reduce their personal assets to a level that qualifies the patient for Medicaid for nursing home care. This process is called a *spend-down* period. If the spend-down is done without careful planning, both the person with ALS and the spouse will be impoverished. By taking careful advantage of the *spousal impoverishment provisions* of Medicaid, the spouse can avoid becoming impoverished.

Lawyers who specialize in elder care law may be needed to help the family prevent impoverishment resulting from medical expenses. When completing the Medicaid application, the crucial step is the assessment of assets, which can be complicated. The interpretation of Medicaid laws and regulations varies from state to state, county to county, and even between Medicaid office case workers. If there is a need to challenge the welfare department's interpretation, lawyers who specialize in such law are indispensable. To negotiate the division of assets between the patient and the spouse, specialized knowl-

A. Patients younger than 65 years with Private Insurance

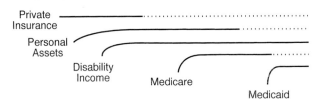

B. Patients older than 65 years with Medicare and Private Insurance

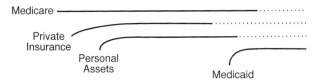

C. Patients older than 65 years with Medicare only

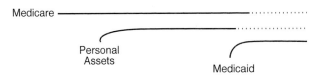

D. Patients of any age with Medicaid and no other insurance or assets

Medicaid ─────────────────────────────

Figure 26–1. Four potential courses for financing ALS treatment using the major resources available in the United States. How to pay medical expenses for a disease like ALS depends on the patient's principal insurance and age. (*A*) If the patient is younger than 65 years old and has private health insurance, the patient and family gradually will have to start using personal assets. The patient will be able to apply for Social Security Disability Income when he or she becomes disabled. After two years' waiting, the patient will be supported by Medicare but will have to "spend down" personal assets, at which point the patient becomes eligible for Medicaid. (*B*) The principal insurance is Medicare, which provides coverage for those over age 65. Again, private insurance is used and personal assets will have to be "spent down" until the patient is eligible for Medicaid. (*C*) Financing is shown for a patient older than 65 with no private insurance. (*D*) Medicaid will cover patients of any age who have no other insurance of any kind and so few assets that they meet the Medicaid asset eligibility criteria.

edge is also required. Furthermore, Medicaid rules are constantly changing. Although hiring a lawyer may be costly, in a chronic disease like ALS, the long-term savings in managing finances may be substantial.

LEGAL ISSUES

Legal issues discussed here pertain to medical practice in the United States. Many other countries, such as Canada and the United Kingdom, practice legal procedures very similar to those of the United States. Full detail is beyond our scope, however.

The advance directive is the most powerful extension of the competent patient's right of self-determination. Physicians have a legal and moral duty to follow relevant and legally authorized advance directives.[3,8] Advance directives are of two principal types: (1) written instructions that express a patient's wishes for treatment in various anticipated clinical situations (the *living will*), and (2) written ap-

pointments designating proxy decision makers whose authority is activated in the event a patient becomes incompetent (*durable power of attorney for health care* or *health-care proxy appointments*).[3] The do-not-resuscitate (DNR) order specifically prohibits cardiopulmonary resuscitation in case of cardiopulmonary arrest. Only competent patients and lawful proxy decision makers for incompetent patients can authorize physicians to write DNR orders.[30]

All 50 states and the District of Colombia have statutory provisions for living wills, health-care proxies, or both. The American Medical Association and American Academy of Neurology support the use of legal advance directives.[3]

There are still significant impediments to the effective use of advance directives, however.[3] Most people would prefer to avoid thinking about and planning for such emotionally upsetting situations.[15] Also, many lack knowledge about advance directives, and the content in an advance directive may be difficult to understand. In one study, less than 40% of the 97 mentally competent patients with a DNR order knew the definition of a living will.[31] The lower the educational level and socioeconomic status of patients, the less frequently they prepare advance directives. Third, until recently, most hospitals have not routinely inquired as to whether patients had prepared advance directives or offered assistance to patients who wished to complete them. Last, the existence of the advance directive may go unknown, or it may not be honored during the hospital admission.[7]

As discussed in Chapter 18, advance directives must be discussed during the early stages of ALS, long before signs of respiratory failure or significant dysphagia develop, but the discussion must occur only after the physicians and patient have had sufficient time to discuss the disease and prognosis, and ideally have established a good relationship.[34] The issues of advance directives should not be discussed in a busy clinic setting.

The Living Will

The written instructional directive, or living will, states the patient's preferences for treatment in certain anticipated circumstances. Commonly, living wills contain language such as "If I am ever terminally ill without reasonable hope for recovery, I wish to be permitted to die naturally without receiving life-sustaining treatment." The precise language of written directives and the regulations regarding their execution and implementation vary from state to state. States have authorized legal forms printed for patients to complete and sign with required cosignatories as witnesses.[3] A living will is not categorically restricted to termination of treatment; it may be designed to indicate someone's wish for maximum medical treatment. In this situation, proper legal documentation is required.

A living will has some disadvantages.[34] The required language is somewhat vague and ambiguous. The extent to which patients understand the meanings and implications of their living wills is a concern.[3] Some directives are quite lengthy and filled with technical details and checklists. Such sophisticated directives can be used successfully only by a minority of highly educated patients. According to Schneiderman and colleagues,[28] patients who make legally executed written directives may respond differently at a later date to questions about their health-care preferences because they interpret the living will language differently. In another study, more than half of participating outpatients could not identify the correct definitions of terms commonly used in the living will.[16]

Another issue arises if the patient's wishes change over time. Periodic updates to written instructional directives help keep the directive up to date. According to Bernat,[3] advance directives are useful in the short term when a patient and physician discuss the details of selected treatment and the meaning of specific treatment choices. For example, the living will of a patient with ALS may become more meaningful after a thorough discussion with their physicians regarding the use of a ventilator rather than a general discussion of life-support measures.

Durable Power of Attorney for Health Care

The written appointment designating proxy decision makers whose authority is activated in the event that a patient becomes incompetent is known variously in different states as "durable power of attorney for health care," "health-care proxy appointments," "health-care agent," "health-care proxy," or "health-care surrogate." The proxy appointment permits a patient, while competent, to authorize another person to make health-care decisions in the event that the patient becomes incompetent in the future. As for the living will, states have authorized legal forms printed for patients to complete and sign with required cosignatories as witnesses. The health-care proxy is specifically restricted to health-care decisions. The "durable" modifier refers to the fact that such appointments are not nullified by subsequent patient incompetence.[3]

Unlike the living will, the health-care proxy appointment permits greater flexibility. The proxy can use his or her discretion to interpret the general wishes of the patient in the context of a specific clinical situation, even a unique and previously unanticipated situation. Conflicts of interest can occur, however, if the proxy's decision is made more in the proxy's own interest than in the interest of the patient. The shortcomings of both the instructional and proxy directives can be minimized if a patient executes both types.[3,9]

Do-Not-Resuscitate Orders

In the 1960s, cardiopulmonary resuscitation (CPR) became a routine procedure for any patient who was dying. However, the futility of CPR was increasingly recognized in patients whose conditions were irreversible. Physicians then were permitted to write DNR orders for such patients at admission or at any time during their hospital stay to prevent futile treatment.

Currently, CPR is performed on patients who suffer cardiopulmonary arrest in the hospital unless a DNR order exists. Physicians can write a DNR order for patients who gave prior advance directives indicating that they wish to die naturally. However, when terminal patients are hospitalized, doctors need to discuss the DNR decision, even if the patient has requested such an order in advance directives, because the patient may have changed his or her mind. Only competent patients and lawful proxy decision makers for incompetent patients can authorize physicians to write the DNR order. Thus, unlike most treatments that require a patient's or proxy's valid consent, CPR requires valid refusal, or it will be performed by default under the doctrine of presumed consent.[30]

The physician should be tactful and compassionate in talking with the patient about these issues. Such discussion is easier when the patient-physician relationship is well-established. The overwhelming majority of patients and proxies will understand the futility of CPR in the case of terminal disease, agree with the DNR decision, and be grateful for the physician's communication and care.[3] If the dying patient or proxy requests CPR despite the physician's best attempts to explain the high likelihood of a poor outcome, ideally the care should be transferred to another physician. If such an arrangement cannot be made, the physician must clearly reiterate the likely consequences, such as

permanent ventilatory support. Although the physician is not morally obligated to order CPR, because ALS is irreversible and fatal, it is best to honor the patient's or proxy's wishes.

ETHICAL ISSUES

ALS is devastating to patients and their families. Treating and managing such a chronic terminal disease raises several difficult ethical issues. Earlier chapters discussed how to present the diagnosis (see Chapters 18 and 25), presymptomatic diagnosis of superoxide dismutase-1–linked familial ALS and genetic counseling (Chapter 10), the use of placebo in clinical trials (Chapter 20), and respiratory and nutritional care (Chapters 22 and 24). In this chapter, we review disclosure of the diagnosis, withholding treatment, end-of-life issues, and palliative care. A recent book, *Ethical Issues in Neurology* by JL Bernat,[3] covers many ethical issues that arise when treating patients with ALS.

Disclosure of the Diagnosis

Disclosure of the diagnosis to patients (and if patients allow, to their families) is the physician's responsibility and in the United States is considered ethical. How to present bad news to patients and families is another matter. Some patients have told us of frightening experiences with neurologists who bluntly pronounced that they have ALS, the prognosis is terminal, nothing can be done, they have only a few years to live, and they should place their business and personal affairs in order. Such an attitude is unacceptable. This behavior not only harms a physician's credibility but also raises the patient's and family's suspicion that the diagnosis may be incorrect. Unfortunately, how to present bad news is seldom taught during medical training, and generally the physician must rely on personal experience, as we have discussed in Chapters 18 and 25. The treating neurologist has an ethical duty to explain the disease and diagnosis compassionately.

In Japan, it has been common to share the diagnosis of ALS with families but not patients. This practice has rapidly changed in recent years, and diagnosing physicians now discuss the diagnosis with the patients more openly (T. Saito, MD, Kitasato University, personal communication, 1996). On the other hand, physicians in France usually consider it better to keep families and patients unaware of the fatal outcome of the disease and therefore withhold the diagnosis. This behavior has grim consequences, the most important of which is that it can prevent provision of the most suitable medical attention and care. It also engenders anxiety in both patients and families.[22]

On rare occasions, we are asked by family members not to disclose the diagnosis to the patient. In such instances, physicians must explain that they have an ethical obligation to the patient to tell the truth. When the diagnosis is concealed, the patient may feel isolated from the family, who becomes anxious in the attempt to hide the truth. Sharing the truth allows the family to mourn the loss, feel and express anger, and ultimately grow together. Our ethical code must center on the patient, and we must not be caught up in a conspiracy of silence, which relatives may feel they prefer because of their own fears and concerns.[26] Prudent physicians take the time needed to resolve such a conflict, helping the family to fully understand the consequences when the diagnosis is not given to the patient.

Withdrawing Treatment

There is a point at which the duty to try to save the patient's life is exhausted. However, this point cannot be readily defined. The decision to limit treatment may depend on a balance between the burdens that the treatment would impose and the benefits that it may produce.[3,9]

The United States Supreme Court in the landmark decision in *Cruzan v. the State of Missouri* (1976) concluded that both competent and incompetent citizens had the constitutional right to refuse any form of medical therapy, including hydration and nutrition.[1a] The American Academy of Neurology Ethics and Humanities Subcommittee also fully agrees that the provision of hydration and nutrition is a form of medical therapy that can be refused by a competent patient.[4] The subcommittee also gives primacy to the autonomy and rights of self-determination of competent patients, and to autonomy's ethical foundation, the doctrine of informed consent. Competent patients ultimately have the right to refuse therapies that physicians recommend for them, even if the refusal will result in death.

A prerequisite for a patient's rational decision to accept or reject life-sustaining therapy is that the physician has conveyed adequate information to the patient. Physicians have an ethical duty to explain compassionately and noncoercively to patients the prognosis and clinical course they may expect with and without life-sustaining treatment. Ethically, physicians have the duty to communicate with absolute clarity with these patients and to ascertain that the patient's decision has been carefully considered and is rational under the circumstances.

End-of-Life Issues

ASSISTED SUICIDE

Although suicide is no longer a criminal offense, assisting or counseling a person to commit suicide is. In struggling with this issue, one must take into account not only the patient's rights and autonomy but also those of the medical profession and the individual physician.

A retired Michigan pathologist, Dr. Jack Kevorkian, has helped patients commit suicide. Kevorkian has been highly successful in bringing this controversial issue to the public's attention but has done so in a way that many people, including physicians, find reprehensible. Although Kevorkian reviewed medical records of patients with terminal illnesses who requested his "help," he was not the physician who cared for them. As a pathologist, his practice was not based on longstanding experience with terminally ill patients. As the number of assisted suicides in which he has participated has increased, public support for him has risen. The public is sending medical professionals a clear message: People are afraid to die in our hospitals, and they do not trust us to let them keep their dignity at the end of life and die in the way they want to.[6]

This phenomenon tells us that physicians may not be paying much attention to the needs of terminally ill patients. Physicians are guided by the Hippocratic oath,[6] "I will neither give a deadly drug to anyone if asked for it, nor will I make a suggestion to this effect. In purity and holiness I will guard my life and my art." Cassel[6] suggests that the Hippocratic oath is much more a statement about a narrow perception of the integrity of the profession than about that patient's need. If we improved the care of patients at the end of life, there would be less demand for assisted suicide. For example, physicians must not fear prescribing medications that make death in terminally ill, suffering patients more comfortable.

In the United States, there was recently an attempt to legalize assisted suicide in Oregon.[21] Ballot Measure 16, "The Oregon Death with Dignity Act," was narrowly approved in the general election in November 1994. Shortly after the election, a lawsuit was filed in federal court, and in August 1995, an Oregon judge ruled that the measure was unconstitutional because it did not give equal protection for terminally ill patients who would not desire assisted suicide. The legal status of this act will remain suspended for some time, possibly until the U.S. Supreme Court decides the fate of assisted suicide in the United States. The Supreme Court review process was scheduled to begin in the spring of 1997.

The Oregon law would have allowed an attending physician to prescribe a lethal dose of medication that is requested by a terminally ill patient for self-administration. The following seven conditions summarize the essential features of the act:[20,21]

1. Competent adult residents of Oregon who are expected to live less than 6 months are eligible.
2. The patient must make two oral requests and one written request during a 15-day period.
3. A second physician must confirm the diagnosis, the patient's decision-making capacity, and the voluntary nature of the request.
4. Referral to a mental health professional is required if the patient's judgment appears to be influenced by depression or some other mental disorder.
5. The physician must ask the patient to disclose the decision to family members, but the patient may refuse to do so.
6. Physicians must report their participation in assisted suicide to the state health division, but they are protected from professional and legal liability.
7. Insurance companies may not withhold death benefits from patients who act in accordance with the law.

Voters' approval of the act has been widely interpreted in Oregon as reflecting a broad rejection of medicine's approach to the care of dying patients more than specifically endorsing assisted suicide. As a consequence, the issues of comprehensive end-of-life care for terminally ill patients are now being seriously addressed in Oregon. Several changes concerning hospice care have already taken place. The campaign enhanced awareness of hospice care among patients, families, and health-care providers; reimbursement for hospice services has improved; and physician reimbursement was increased by reimbursing physicians for phone calls and other oversight activities of hospice patient care.[21]

According to a study by Lee et al.,[20] 46% of 2,761 Oregon physicians who responded to the questionnaire (70% of all eligible physicians) have a favorable attitude toward legalized physician-assisted suicide, but a sizable minority (31%) object on moral grounds to legalization of and participation in assisted suicide. According to this survey, 83% of all physicians surveyed are concerned that financial pressure might be a possible reason for an assisted-suicide request.

EUTHANASIA

Assisted suicide occurs when the physician helps the patient in the act of killing himself or herself, whereas euthanasia is the deliberate and direct action by a physician to end a patient's life at his or her request. Euthanasia, as assisted suicide, is illegal and a criminal offense in the United States. The issue, however, is likely to be debated actively because it is done in the Netherlands[14,19,35] and has been legalized recently in an Australian territory.[27]

The Dutch Model

The Dutch euthanasia guidelines mandate that three criteria be satisfied: (1) the act must be voluntary; (2) the patient must experience unbearable suffering; and (3) the physician must obtain a corroborating consultation.[33] Although euthanasia remains a criminal offense in the Netherlands, it is commonly practiced. The Dutch government decree, which came into effect in early 1994, states that doctors can avoid prosecution in two circumstances: (1) the request to terminate life is made by a patient suffering from a physical or psychiatric disorder, or (2) life is actively terminated without request in a patient suffering from a physical or psychiatric disorder.

The fact that the decree covers both voluntary and nonvoluntary euthanasia and both physical and psychiatric disorders is considered as unequivocal confirmation that the Dutch have clearly progressed down the proverbial slippery slope.[33] According to some critics, there is reason to believe that euthanasia cannot be contained within guidelines or protocols.[17,33,35] According to a study by the Dutch government, almost one-third (1000 of 3300) of the reported euthanasia deaths were cases of active involuntary euthanasia.[33a] The study also found that approximately 4900 (60%) of 8100 deliberate overdoses of morphine were given without patient knowledge or consent because the physician believed the patient had a poor quality of life or because of family distress.[33a] Thus, the idea that voluntary active euthanasia can be practiced within certain guidelines seems to be unsupported.[17] Furthermore, how the physician or family perceives the patient's quality of life can radically differ from the patient's perceptions (see Chapter 22), suggesting a possibility that a physician's decision on end-of-life issues may not rightly reflect the patient's wish.

Recent studies, however, show that the number of acts of euthanasia in the Netherlands has not changed from 1990 to 1995.[33b,33c] Based on these studies, Angell[1] expresses her impression that the Dutch are apparently not on a slippery slope and, as far as we call tell, Dutch physicians continue to practice physician-assisted dying only reluctantly and under compelling circumstances.

The Northern Territory of Australia Model

In 1996, euthanasia was legalized in the Northern Territory of Australia. The essentials are as follows:[27]

1. Patients must be at least 18 years old, of sound mind, suffering from a terminal illness, and "experiencing pain, suffering and/or distress" that is severe and "unacceptable to the patients."

2. A terminal illness is defined as "an injury or degeneration of mental or physical faculties that in reasonable medical judgment will, in the normal course, without the application of extraordinary measures or of treatment unacceptable to the patient, result in the death of the patient."

3. The physician must be satisfied that "any medical treatment reasonably available to the patient is confined to the relief of pain, suffering and/or distress with the object of allowing the patient to die a comfortable death."

4. The physician must believe that the patient has reached his or her decision voluntarily and has considered the possible implications for any family members.

5. The patient must be given information about palliative care by a specialist in that field.

6. The physician is prohibited from assisting in the patient's death if he or she believes that "there are palliative care options reasonably available to the patient to alleviate the patient's pain and suffering to levels acceptable to the patient."

7. A second doctor, independent of the first and with psychiatric credentials, must confirm the diagnosis and prognosis made by the first doctor.

8. The psychiatrist must also confirm that the patient does not have "treatable clinical depression."

9. The patient must wait 7 days before signing a formal certificate of request, the necessary details of which are specified in the act. An additional 48 hours must elapse between the signing of the request and the time the doctor assists in ending the patient's life.

10. The assistance can include prescribing or preparing a lethal substance or providing such a substance directly to the patient for self-administration.
11. Having once decided to take part, the physician is required to provide the assistance personally or remain present while it is given and to remain present until the patient dies.
12. The patient's medical record must contain all necessary documentation described above.

DILEMMAS OF EUTHANASIA

In the past, the debate about euthanasia was generally confined to terminally ill patients in great pain and who personally requested that life be terminated intentionally with a medically administered drug overdose.[33] However, euthanasia has become a superficial and simplistic response to the problem of human suffering and an inappropriate solution to loneliness and poor quality of life.[19] It is not a solution to intractable pain and suffering, problems that can arise very early in the course of an incurable illness.[19]

A number of people have expressed these concerns and also the fear that the most vulnerable patients may feel pressure to request euthanasia. Walton[35] concluded that euthanasia should not be legalized in the United Kingdom, stating that

We concluded that, if legalized, it should be virtually impossible to ensure that all acts of euthanasia were truly voluntary and hence that any liberalization of the law in the UK could not be abused. We also felt that vulnerable people—the elderly, lonely, sick, poor, or distressed—might feel pressure, whether real or imagined, to request early death. Our decision was also influenced by the outstanding achievements of the palliative care movement in the UK.

Scott[29] points out that the request for euthanasia is more often a cry for validation of life, purpose, and meaning than it is a true request to be killed. Some patients may be saying "Let me die," as they have fears that treatment and technological advances will prolong a life with poor quality. Others may mean "I want to die," revealing their own personal anguish and the emotional pain they have suffered. They may also be distressed or fear physical or emotional distress in the future. Caregivers must improve symptom control and allow the patient to express feelings and make some sense of the situation, enabling the patient to gain a sense of purpose.

Some patients may actually be saying "Kill me." This plea again needs to be heard, and it is essential that the desperation and feelings leading to this wish are recognized. Many would feel that active killing is not the answer to this distress but that such requests should be a stimulus to look at how we can improve our care of all patients. With good palliative care, the patient may feel less need to request euthanasia as the distress of the illness is minimized. Whatever our views, patients requesting euthanasia and their families need our time and support, need us to listen and to try to help them make sense of the situation.[26]

Physician-assisted death, including euthanasia and assisted suicide, is one of the most controversial and provocative issues in health care, not just in medical practice but also from legal and ethical standpoints. Angell[1] recently stated:

[A moral distinction between euthanasia and assisted suicide] is important in the United States, where, because of our greater disparities in socioeconomic status and the high cost of medical care, the risk of abuse of euthanasia is undoubtedly greater than it is in the Netherlands. Assisted suicide is considered less liable to abuse. For these reasons, if any form of physician-assisted dying becomes accepted in the United States, it is likely to be assisted suicide, not euthanasia.

The debate will continue.[1,14]

Palliative Care

Palliative care is a program of active compassionate care primarily directed toward improving the quality of life for the dying.[24] At its core is the affirmation of life, even in the face of impending death. Care goals shift from the cure and prolonging of life to the alleviation of psychological and spiritual suffering, the relief of pain and other symptoms, and the enhancement of quality and meaning for the duration of the patient's life.[24–26] Walton[35] states,

While we reject legalized euthanasia, we were wholly supportive of "double effect." We accept that the professional judgment of the health care team can be exercised to enable increasing doses of medication (whether of analgesics or of sedatives, or both) to be given in order to provide relief, even if this shortens life [the "double effect"]. The essential questions are those of motive and intention. If the motive is to relieve pain and distress with no intention to kill, this practice is wholly acceptable, both in medical practice and under the current law.

This view is also the recommendation of the American Academy of Neurology Ethics and Humanities Subcommittee.[4] The subcommittee holds that it is ethically permissible to risk death as long as the physician's primary intent remains to relieve the dying patient of pain, anxiety, and dyspnea, and not purposely to end life. Otherwise, the death is more painful and frightening because of the physician's unwillingness to prescribe adequate doses of medications to make the death more comfortable.

In a response to debate on euthanasia, Twycross[33] clearly delineates the moral and ethical responsibilities of the physician who treats dying patients:

My experiences in 25 years as a hospice doctor have reinforced my belief that when everything is taken into account—physical, psychological, social and spiritual—euthanasia is not the answer. The belief is enhanced by what I see happening in the Netherlands. However, lest it be thought that I have become hardened and indifferent to suffering let me add that, although firmly opposed to euthanasia, I consider that: a doctor who has never been tempted to kill a patient probably has had limited clinical experience or is not able to empathize with those who suffer; and a doctor who leaves a patient to suffer intolerably is morally more reprehensible than the doctor who performs euthanasia.

Preserving life is increasingly meaningless when a terminally ill patient is close to death, and the emphasis on relieving suffering becomes paramount. Even here, however, the doctor is obliged to achieve this objective with minimum risk to the patient's life. Consequently, treatment to relieve pain and suffering that coincidentally might bring the moment of death forward by a few hours or days becomes acceptable (the double effect), but administering a drug such as potassium or curare, with the primary intention of causing death, is not. Neurologists who specialize in the care of patients with ALS are well aware of this practice. The physician must establish a relationship with the patient based on mutual respect and begin the dialogue that embraces end-of-life issues. In the context of a caring physician-patient relationship, discussion of palliative measures or comfort care arises rather naturally, when the patient has chosen not to receive permanent ventilator support. Even for those who use noninvasive positive-pressure ventilation, such discussion is important.

Withdrawal of Ventilator Support

The issue of withdrawing ventilator support has been discussed in Chapter 22. Withdrawing ventilator support and providing palliative care stem from similar considerations.[9–11] A trusting relationship between the physician, patient, and family is an essential prerequisite for both discussions. Physicians must understand the patient's needs, respect his or her wishes, and be willing to withdraw ventilator support if requested. The setting of withdrawal may be in the hospital or at home.[2] Goldblatt and Greenlaw[12] state,

Failure to sustain breathing mechanically or withdrawing artificial support of breathing from a requesting patient who, in the terminal stage of ALS, has become unable to breathe without a mechanical ventilator cannot be called assisted suicide, mercy killing, or either passive or active euthanasia. It is allowing a competent person to die naturally of the incurable illness that afflicts him. The state has no legal interests to be served by intervening in the process, which bears no relationship to issues of malpractice, much less to clinical negligence or homicide. In regard both to starting and to stopping the ventilator, we believe strongly that it is time to lay aside the moral, legal, and ethical conflicts that have needlessly delayed or prevented physicians from complying with the resolute decision that competent patients have made about their own lives. We urge doctors to act in these cases, as in all others, with their best medical judgement.

Inspired by Dr. Goldblatt, we have implemented this philosophy in our practice.[12]

SUMMARY

Diagnostic investigation, newly approved drugs, assistive devices, home equipment, nutritional care, communication devices, and ventilatory support are expensive, as are home care, private nursing, and care in a nursing home. Physicians cannot ignore these issues. For patients and their families, the financing of such expensive medical care poses a formidable challenge. Although the current health-care and insurance systems are rapidly changing, patients and their families must review all potential resources, both major and minor. Possible resources in the United States include private insurance and managed-care payment, and public assistance such as Social Security disability payments, Medicaid, Medicare, and Medigap.

The advance directives are the most powerful extension of the competent patient's right to self-determination. Physicians have a legal duty to follow relevant and legally authorized advance directives. There are still several impediments to the effective use of advance directives. Physicians must make every effort to remove such impediments. The living will is a written instructional directive stating the patient's preferences for future treatment in certain anticipated circumstances. Durable power of attorney for health care is a written appointment directive designating proxy decision makers whose authority is activated in the event that a patient becomes incompetent. In patients whose prognosis is terminal, the futility of cardiopulmonary resuscitation has been increasingly recognized, but only competent patients and lawful proxy decision makers for incompetent patients can authorize physicians to write DNR orders.

Major ethical issues in ALS involve disclosure of the diagnosis and end-of-life concerns. Assisted suicide and euthanasia, which are criminal offenses in the United States, may be superficial and simplistic responses to the problem of human suffering and inappropriate solutions to loneliness and poor quality of life. Furthermore, assisted suicide or euthanasia is likely to expand beyond the boundary of guidelines and protocols. Further debate on physician-assisted death continues.

Palliative care is active, compassionate care primarily directed toward improving the quality of life for dying patients. At its core is the affirmation of life, even in the face of impending death. Treatment to relieve pain and suffering that coincidentally might advance the moment of death by a few hours or days is acceptable (the principle of double effect), but administering a drug with the primary intention of causing death is not. Failure to sustain breathing mechanically, or withdrawing artificial support of breathing from a competent patient in the terminal stage of ALS, who has requested withdrawal, cannot be called assisted suicide, mercy killing, or either passive or active euthanasia. Physicians should use their best medical judgment in such cases.

REFERENCES

1. Angell, M: Euthanasia in the Netherlands—Good news or bad? N Engl J Med 335:1676–1678, 1996.
1a. Annas, GJ: Nancy Cruzan and the right to die. N Engl J Med 323:670–673, 1990.
2. Beal Libby, BT: ALS nursing care management: State of the art. In Mitsumoto, H and Norris, FH, Jr (eds): Amyotrophic Lateral Sclerosis. Demos, New York, 1994, pp 183–197.
3. Bernat, JL: Ethical Issues in Neurology. Butterworth-Heinemann, Newton, 1994.
4. Bernat, JL, Cranford, RE, Kittredge, FI, et al: Competent patients with advanced states of permanent paralysis have the right to forgo life-sustaining therapy. Neurology 43:224–225, 1993.
5. Buckles, L (ed): Senior Living Guide. Guide Publishing, Chagrin Falls, 1996.
6. Cassel, CK: Caring for dying patients: Physicians and assisted suicide. Cleve Clin J Med 62:259–260, 1995.
7. Danis, M, Southerland, LI, Garrett, JM, et al: A prospective study of advance directives for life-sustaining care. N Engl J Med 324:882–888, 1991.
8. Emanuel, LL, Barry, MJ, Stoeckle, JD, et al: Advance directives for medical care—a case for greater use. N Engl J Med 324:889–895, 1991.
9. Glasberg, MR: Amyotrophic lateral sclerosis: Legal and ethical issues. In Mitsumoto, H and Norris, FH, Jr (eds): Amyotrophic Lateral Sclerosis. Demos, New York, 1994, pp 253–265.
10. Goldblatt, D: Decisions about life support in amyotrophic lateral sclerosis. Semin Neurol 4:104–110, 1984.
11. Goldblatt, D: Caring for patients with amyotrophic lateral sclerosis. In Smith RA (ed): Handbook of Amyotrophic Lateral Sclerosis. Marcel-Dekker, New York, 1992, pp 271–288.
12. Goldblatt, D and Greenlaw, J: Starting and stopping the ventilator for patients with amyotrophic lateral sclerosis. Neurol Clin 7:789–806, 1989.

13. Gould, BS: Long-term care: The financial realities. in Mitsumoto, H and Norris, FH, Jr (eds): Amyotrophic Lateral Sclerosis. Demos, New York, 1994, pp 295–300.

14. Helme, T: The euthanasia debate: In reply to Lord Walton. Journal of the Royal Society of Medicine 89:320–323, 1996.

15. Johnston, SC, Pfeifer, MP, and McNutt, R: The discussion about advance directives. Arch Intern Med 155:1025–1030, 1995.

16. Joos, SK, Reuler, JB, Powell, JL, et al: Outpatients' attitudes and understanding regarding living wills. J Gen Intern Med 8:259–263, 1993.

17. Kass, LR: "I will give no deadly drug." Why doctors must not kill. Bulletin of the American College of Surgeons 77:6–17, 1992.

18. Klein, LM and Forshew, DA: The economic impact of ALS. Neurology 47 (Suppl 2): S126–S129, 1996.

19. Latimer, EJ: Euthanasia: A physician's reflections. J Pain Symptom Manage 6:487–491, 1991.

20. Lee, MA, Nelson, HD, Tilden, VP, et al: Legalizing assisted suicide—Views of physicians in Oregon. N Engl J Med 334:310–315, 1996.

21. Lee, MA and Tolle, SW: Oregon's assisted suicide vote: The silver lining. Ann Intern Med 124:267–268, 1996.

22. Meininger, V: Breaking bad news in amyotrophic lateral sclerosis. Palliat Med 7(suppl 2):37–40, 1993.

23. Mitsumoto, H and Norris, FH, Jr (eds): Amyotrophic Lateral Sclerosis. Demos, New York, 1994.

24. O'Brien, T: Palliative care and taboos within motor neurone disease. Palliat Med 7(suppl 2):69–72, 1993.

25. Oliver, D: Bereavement—whose responsibility? Palliat Med 7(suppl 2):73–76, 1993.

26. Oliver, D: Ethical issues in palliative care—An overview. Palliat Med 7:15–20, 1993.

27. Ryan, CJ and Kaye, M: Euthanasia in Australia—the Northern Territory Rights of the Terminally Ill Act. N Engl J Med 334:326–328, 1996.

28. Schneiderman, LJ, Pearlman, RA, Kaplan, RM, et al: Relationship of general advance directive instructions to specific life-sustaining treatment preferences in patients with serious illness. Arch Intern Med 152:2114–2122, 1992.

29. Scott, JF: Lamentation and euthanasia. Humane Medicine: Journal of the Art of Healing 8:116–121, 1992.

30. Senn, JS: Writing "no-CPR" orders: Must resuscitation always be offered? Can Med Assoc J 151:1125–1128, 1994.

31. Stolman, CJ, Gregory, JJ, Dunn, et al: Evaluation of patient, physician, nurse, and family attitudes toward do not resuscitate orders. Arch Intern Med 150:653–658, 1990.

32. Stroud, JS: Financing ALS. [Patient Education Material]. Department of Neurology Cleveland Clinic ALS. Cleveland Clinic Foundation, 1996.

33. Twycross, RG: Euthanasia: Going Dutch? Journal of the Royal Society of Medicine 89:61–63, 1996.

33a. van der Maas, PJ, van Delden, JJM, Pijnenborg, L, and Looman, CWN: Euthanasia and other medical decisions concerning the end of life. Lancet 338: 669–674, 1991.

33b. van der Maas, PJ, van der Wal, G, Haverkate, I, et al: Euthanasia, physician-assisted suicide, and other medical practices involving the end of life in the Netherlands, 1990–1995. N Engl J Med 335: 1699–1705, 1996.

33c. van der Wal, G, van der Maas, PJ, Bosma, JM, et al: Evaluation of the notification procedure for physician-assisted death in the Netherlands. N Engl J Med 335: 1706-1711, 1996.

34. Virmani, J, Schneiderman, LJ, and Kaplan, RM: Relationship of advance directives to physician-patient communication. Arch Intern Med 154:909–913, 1994.

35. Walton, L: Dilemmas of life and death: Part two. Journal of the Royal Society of Medicine 88:372–376, 1995.

INDEX

Note: Page numbers followed by f indicate figures; page numbers followed by t indicate tables.